Chronic Mental Illness and the Changing Scope of Intervention Strategies, Diagnosis, and Treatment

Barre Vijaya Prasad
Dharwad Institute of Mental Health and Neurosciences, India

A volume in the Advances in Psychology, Mental Health, and Behavioral Studies (APMHBS) Book Series

Medical Information Science
REFERENCE
An Imprint of IGI Global

Published in the United States of America by
Medical Information Science Reference (an imprint of IGI Global)
701 E. Chocolate Avenue
Hershey PA, USA 17033
Tel: 717-533-8845
Fax: 717-533-8661
E-mail: cust@igi-global.com
Web site: http://www.igi-global.com

Library of Congress Cataloging-in-Publication Data

Names: Vijaya Prasad, Barre, 1981- editor.
Title: Chronic mental illness and the changing scope of intervention strategies, diagnosis, and treatment / Barre Vijaya Prasad, editor.
Description: Hershey PA : Medical Information Science Reference, [2017] | Includes bibliographical references and index.
Identifiers: LCCN 2016017434| ISBN 9781522505198 (hardcover) | ISBN 9781522505204 (ebook)
Subjects: | MESH: Mental Disorders | Chronic Disease
Classification: LCC RC454.4 | NLM WM 140 | DDC 616.89--dc23 LC record available at https://lccn.loc.gov/2016017434

This book is published in the IGI Global book series Advances in Psychology, Mental Health, and Behavioral Studies (APMHBS) (ISSN: pending; eISSN: pending)

British Cataloguing in Publication Data
A Cataloguing in Publication record for this book is available from the British Library.

Advances in Psychology, Mental Health, and Behavioral Studies (APMHBS) Book Series

Bryan Christiansen
PryMarke, LLC, USA

ISSN: pending
EISSN: pending

Mission

The complexity of the human mind has puzzled researchers and physicians for centuries. While widely studied, the brain still remains largely misunderstood.

The **Advances in Psychology, Mental Health, and Behavioral Studies (APMHBS)** book series presents comprehensive research publications focusing on topics relating to the human psyche, cognition, psychiatric care, mental and developmental disorders, as well as human behavior and interaction. Featuring diverse and innovative research, publications within APMHBS are ideally designed for use by mental health professionals, academicians, researchers, and upper-level students.

Coverage

- Counseling & Therapy
- Psychiatry
- Neurological Disorders
- Developmental Disorders
- Eating Disorders
- Personality Disorders
- Cognition
- Emotional Health
- Human Interaction
- Treatment & Care

IGI Global is currently accepting manuscripts for publication within this series. To submit a proposal for a volume in this series, please contact our Acquisition Editors at Acquisitions@igi-global.com or visit: http://www.igi-global.com/publish/.

The Advances in Psychology, Mental Health, and Behavioral Studies (APMHBS) Book Series (ISSN pending) is published by IGI Global, 701 E. Chocolate Avenue, Hershey, PA 17033-1240, USA, www.igi-global.com. This series is composed of titles available for purchase individually; each title is edited to be contextually exclusive from any other title within the series. For pricing and ordering information please visit http://www.igi-global.com/book-series/advances-psychology-mental-health-behavioral/110200. Postmaster: Send all address changes to above address.

Titles in this Series

For a list of additional titles in this series, please visit: www.igi-global.com

Identifying, Treating, and Preventing Childhood Trauma in Rural Communities
Marion Baker (Center of Hope Arizona, USA) Jacqueline Ford (Center of Hope Arizona, USA & Walden University, USA) Brittany Canfield (Center of Hope Arizona, USA & Fielding Graduate University, USA) and Traci Grabb (Arizona's Children Association, USA & Center of Hope Arizona, USA)
Information Science Reference • copyright 2016 • 306pp • H/C (ISBN: 9781522502289) • US $185.00 (our price)

Handbook of Research on Diagnosing, Treating, and Managing Intellectual Disabilities
Rejani Thudalikunnil Gopalan (Gujarat Forensic Sciences University, India)
Information Science Reference • copyright 2016 • 496pp • H/C (ISBN: 9781522500896) • US $210.00 (our price)

Neuroeconomics and the Decision-Making Process
Bryan Christiansen (PryMarke LLC, USA) and Ewa Lechman (Gdansk University of Technology, Poland)
Business Science Reference • copyright 2016 • 354pp • H/C (ISBN: 9781466699892) • US $195.00 (our price)

Integrating Technology in Positive Psychology Practice
Daniela Villani (Università Cattolica del Sacro Cuore, Italy) Pietro Cipresso (Università Cattolica del Sacro Cuore, Italy & I.R.C.C.S. Istituto Auxologico Italiano, Italy) Andrea Gaggioli (Università Cattolica del Sacro Cuore, Italy & I.R.C.C.S. Istituto Auxologico Italiano, Italy) and Giuseppe Riva (Università Cattolica del Sacro Cuore, Italy & I.R.C.C.S. Istituto Auxologico Italiano, Italy)
Information Science Reference • copyright 2016 • 447pp • H/C (ISBN: 9781466699861) • US $185.00 (our price)

Global Perspectives on Youth Gang Behavior, Violence, and Weapons Use
Simon Harding (Middlesex University, UK) and Marek Palasinski (Liverpool John Moores University, UK)
Information Science Reference • copyright 2016 • 425pp • H/C (ISBN: 9781466699380) • US $185.00 (our price)

Exploring the Collective Unconscious in the Age of Digital Media
Stephen Brock Schafer (Digipen Institute of Technology, USA)
Information Science Reference • copyright 2016 • 316pp • H/C (ISBN: 9781466698918) • US $175.00 (our price)

Psychosocial Studies of the Individual's Changing Perspectives in Alzheimer's Disease
Cordula Dick-Muehlke (University of California, Irvine, USA) Ruobing Li (University of California, Irvine, USA) and Myron Orleans (California State University, Fullerton, USA)
Medical Information Science Reference • copyright 2015 • 434pp • H/C (ISBN: 9781466684782) • US $225.00 (our price)

Editorial Advisory Board

Table of Contents

Detailed Table of Contents

Section 2
Chronic Mental Illness and Comorbidities

Comorbidity refers to presence of one or more additional disorders along with a primary disorder. It affects the prognosis and course of treatment. It is often difficult for clinician to make correct diagnosis in presence of various disorders. The clinical picture of various disorders interferes with treatment process and the outcome. There are some disorders in psychiatry, known as chronic illness. These are schizophrenia, bipolar disorder and obsessive-compulsive disorder. All these three disorder have a major effect on individual's life. Anxiety, depression, substance abuse and panic symptoms are common in schizophrenia; hence the clinical picture changes frequently. While the literature suggests that presence of two or three disorders make treatment worse, hence multidisciplinary treatment need to be used.

There is vast literature available about prevalence and pattern of substance use in patients with Chronic mental illness such as Schizophrenia. Many of these studies have also investigated the issues related to the impact of substance use on the course and prognosis of the mental illness and vice versa. The factors affecting the use and its impact on treatment have also been studied to some extent in the Western countries. Estimates of the prevalence of substance abuse in schizophrenia and major affective disorder vary as a function of settings (e.g., community, hospital-in-patient vs. out-patient), demographic characteristics of the sample and assessment methods, with most prevalence rates ranging between15% to 65%. Patients with Chronic Mental illnesses and Substance use disorders are difficult to treat and many models for their management have been proposed. This chapter will deal with some of these issues.

Section 3
Chronic Mental Illness: Family and Global Burden

The objective of the chapter is to understand the processes involved in care giving for those with a Chronic Mental Illness and to develop an effective intervention incorporating methods and strategies that aims at reducing caregiver stress and burden. OCD is a neurobiological disorder characterized by the presence of symptoms such as obsessions and compulsions. Literature is reviewed on prevalence, intervention and tools that can assess caregiver stress and burden in OCD. Accommodation and Expressed emotion plays key roles in interpersonal relationships that exist in the families of those afflicted with mental illness and may affect the treatment. Psycho education found to be helpful in educating the family about all the relevant aspects of OCD and to determine their role as a caregiver in order to deal with the illness in an effective way. Family intervention beyond the scope of psycho-education programme is required to prepare caregivers to take on the role of care giving more effectively.

In the present study we intend to assess if the expressed emotion perceived by the patients with schizophrenia and bipolar disorder has any effect on their quality of life. Is the burden experienced by the caregivers, has any effect up on their quality of life? To explore these issues, regression was employed to estimate the quantitative effect of the causal variables upon the variable that they influence and the "statistical significance" of the estimated relationships. This study consisted of 120 participants. 30 patients with Schizophrenia Bipolar disorder and two caregiver groups. Administration of tests was done on individual basis. FEICS was administered to assess EE perceived by the patients. WHOQOL (BREF) scale was used to assess quality of life of patients. BAS was given to assess caregiver's burden. For the assessment of data regression analysis was calculated.

Mental disorders are an important cause of long-term disability and dependency. It accounts for over 15% of the disease burden in developed countries, which is more than the disease burden caused by all cancers. Mental illness is a leading cause of suffering, economic loss and social problems. The burden of mental disorders is likely to have been underestimated because of inadequate appreciation of the connectedness between mental illness and other health conditions. Mental disorders increase risk for communicable and non-communicable diseases, and contribute to unintentional and intentional injury, and comorbidity complicates help-seeking, diagnosis, and treatment, and influences prognosis. Consequently, health professionals have trivialized the issue of mental illness. It is essential that researchers and public health professionals work together to resolve the enormous public health crisis presented by mental disorders. In short, we must "mainstream" mental health.

Foreword

As twenty first century is known as a century of stress and anxiety, prevalence of mental disorders is found to be increasing and so is the focus of mental health professionals on their adequate diagnosis and devising successful intervention and treatment strategies. Considering the global data, mental illnesses share more than one tenth of the burden of diseases and their prevalence among the adult population is alarming in the sense that it is fourth among the ten leading causes of disability. Evidences are that around ten percent of the global population is affected by psychological disorders. The cause of concern is that as per the trends, in the coming half decade the prevailing mental and behavioural disorders will come into the category of being classified as chronic and disabling. Although these type of mental illnesses are not out of the sight of the mental health problems, their elimination has not yet become feasible due to various reasons including lacunae in proper diagnostic outcomes and relatively lesser effective treatment and intervention practices.

The efforts of researchers have though been relentless and a dedicated sense of commitment to upkeep human mental health is well evident in the researchers, clinical psychologists, psychiatrists and other mental health problems. However, the reach to the outcomes of their efforts remains quite restricted and such scientific knowledge sharing is relatively scarce. The current edited volume *Chronic Mental Illness and the Changing Scope of Intervention Strategies, Diagnosis, and Treatment* in the book series on 'Advances in Psychology, Mental Health and Behavioural Studies' presents rigorous efforts of the editor Dr. Barre Vijaya Prasad, Associate Professor in bringing together the voluminous current research in the area. The volume addresses under-researched crucial aspects and various correlates of chronic mental illnesses in different populations ranging from childhood through adolescence and adulthood to old age. Having a broad spectrum of coverage at its basis, the volume attempts to uncover and extend to reader wide latitude of scientific knowledge related to chronic mental illnesses.

The very systematic outline of the volume, presented in the form of six logical cohorts beginning with a focus on in-depth conceptual information on the target area and concluding with a synthesis of attention towards advanced treatment strategies, provides the readers and professionals a comprehensive scope of insight into the mental and behavioural disorders with chronic and disabling impacts on human population. The section formation has been very concise and focused clustering of specific issues related to chronic mental illnesses. The editorial competencies are visible in a nice blend of conceptualizations and reconceptualization in light of the changing research scenarios. The conceptual background created in the first section along with an addressal of rehabilitation practices takes a systematic way to proceed smoothly to deliberate upon the issues related to comorbidities existing in relation to the chronic psychological disorders. Issues related to families, caregivers and management practices have also been well documented upon at the relevant places and in the forthcoming sections. Specific focus exists on the current research based intervention strategies for all ages from elderly to down the childhood have been explored, evaluated and synthesized for the optimum use of mental health professionals and researchers so as help improve the quality of life and well of the human race. For reaching this primary objective, the volume's strongest aspect lies in highlighting the newly emerged and emerging advanced treatment strategies to effectively deal with chronic mental illnesses and checking them from causing global disabling effects.

Incorporating 18 specifically dedicated chapters contributed by the eminent scholastic researchers, academicians and practitioners from across the country, the volume is an exemplary academic product which will serve as a path illuminating torch for all kinds of mental health professionals. It will fill a big void and will prove to be a very handy reference to the budding clinical psychology scholars, practicing clinical psychologists, psychiatrists, the scientific acumen of mental health profession. It will also prove to be a beneficial insight provider to the care givers and policy makers to serve the people in need. Most importantly the volumes will guide the emergence of new researches and devising new intervention strategies to cure chronic mental illnesses. I appreciate the enormous efforts of Dr. Barre Vijaya Prasad in bringing in such a comprehensive volume and call the readers to help it reach to the people suffering from mental and behavioural illnesses.

Updesh Kumar
Defence Institute of Psychological Research (DIPR), India

Preface

INTRODUCTION

Mental and behavioural disorders account for 12% of the global burden of disease. The global prevalence of mental and behavioural disorders among the adult population is estimated to be 10% and contributed to four of the ten leading causes of disability. Ten percent of the population across the globe suffers from Mental and behavioural disorders till to date and we have derived many of the intervention strategies to reduce the burden of these illness. In spite of these projected figures for the year 2020, 15% of them will become chronic in nature and disabling, adding to global burden and economic loss and loss of years of functioning. There are multiple factors contributing for chronicity and some of them though identified but ineffective interventions have maintained the illness.

As per standard diagnostic classification systems ICD/DSM, list of Chronic Mental Illnesses (CMI) are (a) Pervasive Developmental Disorders (b) Attention Deficit and Disruptive Behavior Disorders; (c) Feeding & Eating Disorder of Infancy or Early Childhood; (d) Elimination Disorders; (e) Other Disorders of Infancy, Childhood, or Adolescence; (f) Schizophrenia & Other Psychotic Disorders; (g) Mood Disorder; (h) Personality Disorders; or (i) Medication-Induced Movement Disorders. From the list can make out striking contributing factors are the developmental issues. Other than development factors which appear later in the course of illness is not been studied effectively. Early identification of these modifiable factors can reduce the burden of the CMI in the population. There are meager available intervention strategies for the persons who have already acquired disability due to chronicity. Scope of this book tries to look at research which is focused on new research methodologies for identifying and diagnosing the epidemiological factors contributing for CMI in the community. It's also focused on research related to psychopharmacological inventions and interventions for the care of chronic mental illness, disability due to CMI and intervention strategies at mental health institutions, effectiveness of national policies/programmes and its outcome across the countries (South-East Asian, Europe, Australia, USA, Canada, Africa etc.,) in care of CMI, mental health acts across the world in protecting the rights of Persons with CMI.All this issues are analyzed by authors who contribute to this book.

OBJECTIVE OF THE BOOK

Around 18 methodological basis of CMI chapters were included. We asked researchers to submit studies of the changing the scope of intervention strategies, diagnosis and treatment persons with CMI. To look at the epidemiology, factors, prevalence of disability, scope of research in diagnosis/management, and implementation of policy strategies of CMI. Were integrated the findings from the individual studies. We believed that research articles in the collection will make significant contributions to a currently under-researched aspect of CMI, and the collection as a whole were set an agenda at global level to guide ongoing re conceptualizations of the individual's experience and innovative research, practice and care giving in the field of mental health.

Target Audience

The target audiences of this book were composed of professionals and researchers working in the field of mental health including psychiatrists, neurologists, neurosurgeaons, psychologists, social workers, psychiatric nursing, psychosocial rehabilitation therapists, mental health counselors, and general physicians. This book will be useful for undergraduates, graduates and post graduates students in the field of mental health. This book will be a referral book for academic purposes in libraries.This willl also aims at guiding adminstrative and policy matters for the care of persons with CMI. We believed all of these audiences will find helpful materials that reinforce and enhance their work.

ORGANIZATION OF THE BOOK

There are 18 chapters in this book and the chapters are grouped into six main sections. The six sections assist the reader to be guided to a specific area of interest because each section is based on a particular theme. The sections are divided as follows: Section 1 contains chapters that are focused on providing in-depth information on chronic Mental illness and rehabilitation. In this section, CMI and Homelessness, CMI in old age home, dumping patients - concern towards management and psychosocial intervention strategies for patients with schizophrenia are discussed in detail and explored within the contexts of CMI. Section 2 examines the CMI and comorbidities especially treatment issues and were also focused management of substance abuse disorder. In Section 3 CMI: family and global burden were emphasized on understanding and management of caregiver's stress and burden of person with obsessive compulsive disorder. Predictive of expressed emotion, caregiver's burden and quality of life in CMI, it was also highlighted global burden of mental disorders quality of care and unmet needs for treatment of CMI. In Section 4 chapters were depicted mainly CMI: disabilities and legal issues, for example, disabilities in schizophrenia, CMI in prisons global scenario. Another important chapter for this book is majorly Legal Aspects of CMI were elucidated with current legislature amendment. Section 5 explored with CMI: Child and Adolescents were Consisted of Psychosocial intervention strategies Street Children with Substance Abuse, chronic Mental illness and the changing scope of intervention strategies, Diagnosis and treatment in Child and Adolescent Population. In Section 6, were highlighted with CMI: Advanced treatment strategies were explained, suicide in patients with CMI. Cognitive remediation Therapy in Chronic Schizophrenia. Efficacy of art therapy in patients with Paranoid Schizophrenia. Psychotherapeutic interventions in emotional and behavioural problem with adolescent. The description of each chapter is given below:

Although the work is not free from shortcomings, and while many of those were painstakingly amended, some could not because of the practical constraints attached. I am hopeful that they would be taken up by further researchers.

Section 1: Chronic Mental Illness and Rehabilitation

Chapter 1: Chronic Mental Illness and Homelessness

Homeless individuals are the neglected, dispossessed and disenfranchised section of the society and almost one fourth to one third of them have an underlying serious mental illness. Homeless persons with severe mental illnesses are often the most visible but the most difficult to reach and the most difficult to ignore. The prevalence of mental illness amongst homeless is higher than that compared to the general population. Researchers have theorized various stressors related to homelessness as precipitating factors of mental illness. In the chapter entitled "Chronic Mental Illnesses and Homelessness", conceptual issues in definition of homelessness, relationship with mental illness, reasons behind, magnitude of problem, difficulties faced by homeless, barriers in accessing health care and possible interventions were discussed. Authors suggested that integration of health resources, co morbid treatment of substance use, social security benefits, continuum of care approach, inter agency coordination and better service delivery can be possible solutions for the ongoing problem. Commitment by government, private sector, social welfare sector, strong political will and integrated efforts to address the problem of homeless persons with mental illness.

Chapter 2: Chronic Mental Illness in Old Age Homes – An International Perspective

Old age is characterized with reduced physical ability, declining mental ability, the gradual giving up of role playing in socio-economic activities, and a shift in economic status moving from economic independence to economic dependence upon others for support. In the chapter were discusses various aspects morbidities during old age with special mention of dementia, depression, anxiety and substance abuse. Author/s mentioned the need to generate data about mental morbidities in larger studies with culture free tools. There is a global movement towards 'successful' ageing and a model of care for older adults that focus on maximizing health, wellbeing, and social participation in old age. Further they added that there is also a strong need to generate models of care in old age homes so that the old age homes are not just a shelter for care but provide satisfying quality of life in a home like environment.

Chapter 3: Chronic Mental Illness and Dumping Patients – A Concern towards Management

Chronic mental illness brings a lot of suffering, not only the individual who is suffering from chronic mental illness but the families and caretakers also face discrimination, social stigma and pressure from the society. Many families and caretakers face these pressure and stigma with pride and support the person who is suffering from the mental illness. Most families look for the ways and ideas of getting rid from the patient. The best way to get rid from the problem is dumping the patient in the mental institutes. In this chapter "Chronic Mental Illness and Dumping Patients: a Concern towards Management" shares its concern about the conditions of the dumped patients because of their chronic mental illness. The author/s of the chapter discusses about proper vocational training, job perspectives, proper family counselling and other resources can help the patients' families and caretakers to take their responsibility for the chronically ill patients.

Chapter 4: Psychosocial Intervention Strategies in Chronic Mental Illness

Schizophrenia is a chronic, severe, and disabling brain disease. Schizophrenia is found all over the world. The severity of the symptoms and the long-lasting, chronic pattern of schizophrenia often results in disability, and many individuals need ongoing assistance to manage the most basic functions of independent living. The chapter entitled "Psychosocial Intervention Strategies in Chronic Mental Illness" discussed about the psychosocial intervention strategies in chronic mental illness, like individual psychotherapy, cognitive behaviour therapy, cognitive therapy with schizophrenia, behaviour therapy with schizophrenia, group therapy and family interventions were highlighted. In addition to this psychiatric rehabilitation were also discussed with vocational training, social skill training, and community rehabilitation approach. With help of these intervention modalities the utility to prevent frequent hospitalizations and reduces the impact on the individual, family and the economy of the nation as well.

Section 2: Chronic Mental Illness and Comorbidities

Chapter 5: Comorbidity Issues and Treatment in Chronic Mental Illness

Comorbidity refers to presence of one or more additional disorders along with a primary disorder. It affects the prognosis and course of treatment. In the chapter entitled "Comorbidity Issues and Treatment in Chronic Mental Illness " the author discusses about chronic mental illness such as schizophrenia, bipolar disorder and obsessive-compulsive disorder. All these three disorder have a major effect on individual's life. Anxiety, depression, substance abuse and panic symptoms are common in schizophrenia; hence the clinical picture changes frequently. While the literature suggests that presence of two or three disorders make treatment worse, hence multidisciplinary treatment need to be used. This chapter pointed out few important issues which need to handle by the clinicians. The chapter also talks about the changes in treatment approach. A balanced approach need to be adopted by practitioner which would be helpful for patients. A proper assessment to rule out the other disorder is necessary so that required treatment could be started to maintain the follow up. Majority of the comorbid disorders were identified as phobic disorders, posttraumatic stress and major depression.

Chapter 6: Management of Chronic Mental Illnesses and Substance Use Disorders

Substance use disorder is an accepted complication of chronic and severe mental illness and is associated with serious adverse consequences. Recent evidence regarding the general integrated treatment approach is consistent and positive, but much work remains to be done on the organization and financing of integrated programs. This chapter "Management of Chronic Mental Illnesses and Substance Use Disorders" focuses on the development of basic components of integrated treatment case management, close monitoring, substance abuse treatment, family psychoeducation, rehabilitation, housing, and medications. Despite a number of promising treatments, there is still a long way before we know what treatments work for which groups of dual-diagnosis patients. This problem express further need for homogenized diagnostic criteria for dual diagnosis patients in order for clinicians to identify individuals appropriate for integrated treatment to develop an effective modality to treat this complex population with a diverse range of mental disorders.

Section 3: Chronic Mental Illness – Family and Global Burden

Chapter 7: Understanding and Management of Caregivers' Stress and Burden of Person with Obsessive Compulsive Disorder

OCD is a neurobiological disorder characterized by the presence of symptoms such as obsessions and compulsions. Accommodation and Expressed emotion plays key roles in interpersonal relationships that exist in the families of those afflicted with mental illness and may affect the treatment. The next chapter entitled "Understanding and Management of Caregivers' Stress and Burden of Person with Obsessive Compulsive Disorder" aims to understand the processes involved in care giving for those with a Chronic Mental Illness and to develop an effective intervention incorporating methods and strategies that aims at reducing caregiver stress and burden. Psycho education found to be helpful in educating the family about all the relevant aspects of OCD and to determine their role as a caregiver in order to deal with the illness in an effective way. Family intervention beyond the scope of psycho-education programme is required to prepare caregivers to take on the role of care giving more effectively.

Chapter 8: Predictors of Expressed Emotion – Caregiver's Burden and Quality of Life in Chronic Mental Illness

Family caregivers of persons with chronic mental illnesses are a key support system in our country as well as in most of the nonwestern world. Most caregivers feel burdened when caring for relatives with major psychiatric disorders, as these disorders are unpredictable and long-lasting. Not only caregivers but the patients with schizophrenia and bipolar disorder report disturbed quality of life. In the absence of adequate mental health infrastructure, the family caregivers take multiple roles at providing care for persons with mental illnesses. In this chapter entitled "Predictors of Expressed Emotion, Caregiver's Burden and Quality of Life in Chronic Mental Illness", is an empirical study which intends to assess if the expressed emotion perceived by the patients with schizophrenia and bipolar disorder has any effect on their quality of life. Is the burden experienced by the caregivers, has any effect up on their quality of life? To explore these issues, regression was employed to estimate the quantitative effect of the causal variables upon the variable that they influence and the "statistical significance" of the estimated relationships.

Chapter 9: Global Burden of Mental Disorders Quality of Care and Unmet Needs for Treatment of Chronic Mental Illness

Mental disorders are an important cause of long-term disability and dependency. Four of the six leading causes of years lived with disability are due to neuropsychiatric disorders (depression, alcohol-use disorders, schizophrenia and bipolar disorder). Mental illness imposes a huge burden on individuals, families and society. The cost of illness incurred by individuals, employers and governments is enormous. The chapter entitled "Global burden of mental disorders quality of care and unmet needs for treatment of chronic mental illness" aims to critically appraise the way that the burden of disability and premature mortality is apportioned, in WHO's estimates of global burden of disease, between underlying conditions within groups of disorder, and, specifically, to assess whether these estimates account for the full contribution of mental disorder to mortality and disability. The author also reviewed available evidence for interactions between mental disorders and other health conditions. The implications of these links for the future orientation of health policies, health systems, and services were finally discussed.

Section 4: Chronic Mental Illness – Disabilities and Legal Issues

Chapter 10: Disabilities in Schizophrenia – The Psychosocial and Neurocognitive Perspective

This chapter aims to study different aspects of disability in schizophrenia with specific emphasis on neurocognitive and psychosocial functioning. Schizophrenia is characterized by marked disturbances and abnormalities in the domains of thought, perception, speech, emotion and behavior. The varied symptoms across patients and over time, produces disabilities which is quite different from other disabilities. These disabilities associated with chronic mental illness and especially schizophrenia is more difficult to cope up with due to the associated stigma and care burden. The disability in schizophrenia is mostly observed in occupational, social and interpersonal domains and has been closely related with neurocognitive impairment in schizophrenia. The studies have shown similar opinion on predictive value of neurocognitive functions in different psychosocial functions in schizophrenia. Authors have suggested that research is required which focuses in formulating better management plan and reduce the disability.

Chapter 11: Chronic Mental Illness in Prisons – Global Scenario

The psychiatric morbidity among prison inmates is substantially higher than in the general population. Many people with identifiable psychiatric illness do conflict with the law, often by no fault of their own but because of symptoms of their psychiatric illness and end up in jails. The chapter discusses that prisons are detrimental to mental-health, and the standards of psychiatric care are significantly lower than those for the general public. The burden of psychiatric illness in this vulnerable and marginalized population poses a serious challenge. They recommended for remedial measures to be taken identification of magnitude of problem, preventable causes and treatment with proper compliance and follow-up is needed. Certain remedial measures are to be implemented for a better future of prison and community because ultimately these prisoners will be released from prison and become a part of community. Beginning of reforms is the immediate need as a long journey ahead.

Chapter 12: Legal Aspects of Chronic Mental Illness

The mental health is a part of the general health and has a serious concern in the society. A person who suffers mental illness suffers not only for himself but also would bring about suffering for the people who are not only to the family but to the society at large. In the chapter, legal aspects of chronic mental illness, various issues described like disability and mental illness and its differences in terms of legal issues. The author's main focus of the chapter was highlighting various admissions procedures, civil rights of patients, Code of Civil Procedure, private rights, economic rights, criminal law and people with mental disorder. The authors were concluded that the fundamental aim of this legislation is to protect, promote and fulfill the rights of the persons with disability, and protecting the human rights and fundamental rights of people with mental disorders.

Section 5: Chronic Mental Illness – Children and Adolescents

Chapter 13: Psychosocial Intervention Studies for Street Children with Substance Abuse

In this chapter author made an attempt to review the literature and describes various interventions available for street children. The current chapter enlists all the intervention activities carried out for this group. The chapter encourages the discussion under the subthemes of concept of street children, prevalence of street children, reasons for on the street, street life and ways of coping with stress, substance abuse among street children, intervention carried out with street children and substance abuse, suggestions and conclusion. The author discussed psychosocial intervention that are well proven in the general population and effectively tried with street children. It was further suggested that the governments, nongovernmental organizations and other service providers should utilize the psychosocial intervention in their activities to bring change among street children with substance abuse.

Chapter 14: Chronic Mental Illness and the Changing Scope of Intervention Strategies – Diagnosis and Treatment in Child and Adolescent Population

Childhood forms an important phase in the development period of life during which one develops physically, emotionally, socially, intellectually and morally. Chronic and severe mental health problems in children impact the overall development of the child thereby leading to significant and lifelong disability. In this chapter included two important CMI in children mainly Schizophrenia and Bipolar Mood Disorder and discussed the clinical features, course, outcome and treatment strategies. Authors discussed the importance of early interventions. In the clinical dimension, the discussion on the early intervention directed to the first break, with special attention to the period of untreated psychosis, may represent the construction of care instruments and strategies useful in the assistance to the psychopathology of child and adolescents population.

Section 6: Chronic Mental Illness – Advanced Treatment Strategies

Chapter 15: Advanced Intervention Strategies for Suicide in Patients with Chronic Mental Illness

This chapter focuses on various aspect of suicide including neurobiological factors like neurotransmitters, neural circuits, genetic and epigenetic factors, response on pharmacotherapy and newer generation novel treatment strategies and various psychosocial factors. Chronic mental illnesses are common to find in routine clinical practice and suicide is one of the dreaded outcomes. There is rising trend of research on suicide in patient with psychiatric illness in last decade. With such rising trend, it requires specific attention in all domains among public service providers along with specific targeted population of patients suffering from psychiatric illness. A social and public health response to suicide is crucial and should complement a mental health response. Researches stated that twenty-eight countries have established national suicide prevention programs dedicated to suicide research and prevention. However, there is still a need to expand suicide prevention research and anti-suicidal strategies. But due to limited resources especially in under-develop or developing nation, the accessibility to all is still a concern by service providers.

Chapter 16: Cognitive Remediation Therapy in Chronic Schizophrenia

Cognitive impairments are recognized as one of the most ubiquitous features of schizophrenia. Cognitive deficits appear to play a large role in how patients with schizophrenia function in their everyday lives. In the chapter, the role of cognitive deficits in schizophrenia was discussed with special reference to extraordinary difficulty with communication, motivation, self-care, and establishing and maintaining relationships with others. Patients with schizophrenia are often additionally treated with supportive psychotherapy, behavioral management, or social skills training as required. However, the efficacy of these adjunct therapies could be limited in presence of marked cognitive deficits. They further added that remediation programs may be drafted targeting the overall neuropsychological functioning in a comprehensive way. Along with neuropsychological functions, more stress may be put on social and vocational functioning and a combined rehabilitation package should be made in future.

Chapter 17: Efficacy of Art Therapy in Treating Patients with Paranoid Schizophrenia

Paranoid Schizophrenia is a chronic mental illness, which is characterized by the presence of delusion of persecution, suspicious, distrusting, guarded, reserved, tensed, and also sometimes hostile or aggressive. The therapeutic relationship between patient and the professional is integral to the recovery process and the outcome. Good communication on the part of health care professionals is an essential element in developing the strong practitioner-patient relationship necessary in the treatment of schizophrenia. The third chapter entitled describes a case of paranoid schizophrenia in which behavioral therapy, supportive therapy and family therapy along with art therapy is used for such patients. Art therapy proves to be an advance intervention strategy to work with patient as an advanced intervention strategies and treatment. As mentioned by the author the art therapy, even without any formal interpretation during the therapy session communicated a lot of material in the therapy sessions which help the flow of therapy process leading to a successful result. This case reassures the efficacy of art therapy and assures its effectiveness as tool for the management of schizophrenia with medication and family therapy for a complete biopsychosocial intervention.

Chapter 18: Psychotherapeutic Interventions in Emotional and Behavioral Problems with Adolescents

In this chapter the authors discussed the importance of integrated psychotherapeutic approaching improving self-confidence, feeling of security and improving self-esteem, self-respect, confidence and emotional well –being of an adopted adolescent with emotional and behavioral problems. The effectiveness of yoga in improving emotional well- being and anger management was also discussed. The main focus of the chapter was on cognitive behavior techniques adjunct with yoga for stress inoculation and anger management in adolescents.

Barre Vijay Prasad
Dharwad Institute of Mental Health and Neurosciences, India

Acknowledgment

It is important for me to take this opportunity to acknowledge the many people that worked hard to ensure that this special book came to light. I would like to give my heartfelt thanks to each and every one of the authors and reviewers who played vital roles in working to make this book a reality. This book was not only inspired by colleagues, authors and friends; it was also directly improved by their active involvement in its development. I have been most greatly influenced in writing this book by three professional heroes: Sigmund Freud, Carl Rogers and Aron. T. Beck. I am honored to consider Prof. Bahadur Singh Tej, G. Padmaja and Suvashisa Rana as mentors, and I would not have written this book without their inspiring examples of during my academic journey.

I would like to express my gratitude to Srinivas Kosgi for helping me in the process of selection, editing the chapters, in all aspects of design of this book. I would like to express my thanks to Amit Khanna, Pratima Kaushik and Ashwini R.; to the people who dedicated their time to come out of this book; all those who provided support, talked things over, offered comments, remarks and assisted in the editing phase. My special thanks go to Shamsi Akbar who is technically contributed many hours of her attention towards improving this book, as well during the process of proof reading and final submission of the manuscript.

Prior to this, call for chapters was heavily informed by L. Sam S. Manickam who is Indian clinical psychologist yahoo groups' moderator, I thank him for facilitating at digital mail system to spread the words. I sincerely, thank and acknowledge faculty, staff and colleagues from DIMHANS, who have directly or indirectly contributed in synthesis of this book.

Last and foremost, I would like to thank my parents for blessing me throughout my career and writing this book. They have been my inspiration and motivation for continuing to improve my knowledge and move my career forward.

Finally, I would like to thank my publishers IGI to made my dream comes true.

Barre Vijay Prasad
Dharwad Institute of Mental Health and Neurosciences, India

Section 1

Chronic Mental Illness and Rehabilitation

Chapter 1
Chronic Mental Illnesses and Homelessness

Prerna Kukreti
Jamia Hamdard University, India

Prerna Khanna
Pushpanjali Crosslay Hospital, India

Amit Khanna
IHBAS, India

ABSTRACT

Homelessness is a complex socio-economic problem complicated by individual attributes and risk factors. The burning issue of homelessness has been a subject of concern in the modern day world often stretching the existing administrative system to innovate and design models for managing the same. With the changing definitions of homelessness, the estimates have also varied across cultures and countries. Because of the inherent difficulty in studying homelessness, accurate estimates of the number of homeless are lacking. Most studies in the West report that approximately 288 per 10,000 people are homeless. With the accurate data on homelessness lacking, the estimates of mental illness amongst homeless is even more obscure. The prevalence of mental illness amongst homeless is higher than that compared to the general population. Researchers have theorized various stressors related to homelessness as precipitating factors of mental illness. There is dearth of literature on mental illness in homeless population which is representative of the homeless population at a national level.

INTRODUCTION

"Be it sight of dirt covered lady muttering to self-roaming on streets in layers of clothes in summers, or a nude adolescent sitting roadside smiling to self, or an elderly gesticulating to self in rags incarcerated in jail for pelting stones at passersby; these can be few heart rendering, thought provoking scenarios which just give a glimpse of unseen unheard of mentally ill homeless individuals. In some individuals, these scenes invoke sense of fear and apprehension, in some hatred; whereas sympathy and compassion

DOI: 10.4018/978-1-5225-0519-8.ch001

in others but creates turmoil in mind of all." Homeless individuals are the neglected, dispossessed and disenfranchised section of the society and almost one fourth to one third of them have an underlying serious mental illness (Sullivan, Burnam, Koegel, & Hollenberg, 2000; Folsom & Jeste, 2002; Fischer & Breakey, 1991). Homeless persons with severe mental illnesses are often the most visible but the most difficult to reach and the most difficult to ignore.

As compared to general population, prevalence of chronic psychiatric disorders, e.g. substance use disorder, psychosis, depression and personality disorders are higher among homeless persons across the globe (Han et al., 2003; Timms & Balazs, 1997). However, the prevalence of homelessness with mental illness and the strength of association vary across nations (Schutt et al., 2009; Ran et al., 2006; Folsom et al., 2005; Montross et al., 2005). Homeless persons are subjected to poor living standards, physical and sexual assault. But with ongoing daily struggle for basic amenities concerns for mental health care takes a backseat. They are often not even counted in census population and their woes remain unheard of to draw attention of policy makers. But even if seen through the lens of a health economist, studies have shown higher level of psychiatric hospital use (Koege, Sullivan, Burnam, Morton, & Wenzel, 1999; North et al.,1993; Padgett, Struening, & Andrews, 1990) and higher mental health treatment costs (Rosenheck, Frisman, & Gallup,1998) than not homeless patients. So, the problem is an equally big challenge for social scientists, clinicians and policy makers.

In this chapter, conceptual issues in definition of homelessness, relationship with mental illness, reasons behind, magnitude of problem, difficulties faced by homeless, barriers in accessing health care and possible interventions were discussed.

CONCEPT OF HOMELESSNESS

Defining homelessness has long been a topic of debate, but international agreement is elusive and most of the definitions of homelessness in use across the world are not conceptually grounded. Like poverty and unemployment, homelessness is also a relative concept, which "acquires meaning only in relation of the housing conventions of a particular culture" (Chamberlain & Johnson, 1992). Edgar, Doherty and Meert (2003) developed a conceptual model for European Typology of Homelessness and Housing Exclusion (ETHOS), they defined "adequate housing" as per following parameters (Edgar et al., 2003; Edgar et al., 2009):

- **Physical Domain:** Having a decent dwelling (or space) adequate to meet the needs of the person and his/her family,
- **Social Domain:** Being able to maintain privacy and enjoy social relations, and
- **Legal Domain:** Having exclusive possession, security of occupation and legal title.

On basis of these, there can be four headings to classify homelessness or housing exclusion as per European Federation of National Organizations Working with Homeless (FEANTSA) classification proposed in 2007:

- **Roofless:** (e.g. living on streets),
- **Houseless:** (e.g. living in institutional shelters),
- **Insecure:** (e.g. living in refugee camps, under constant threat), and
- **Inadequate accommodation.**

Figure 1. Model for defining a population as homeless, housing excluded, or adequately housed, according to physical, legal, and social domains, and access to adequate housing
(Edgar, 2009)

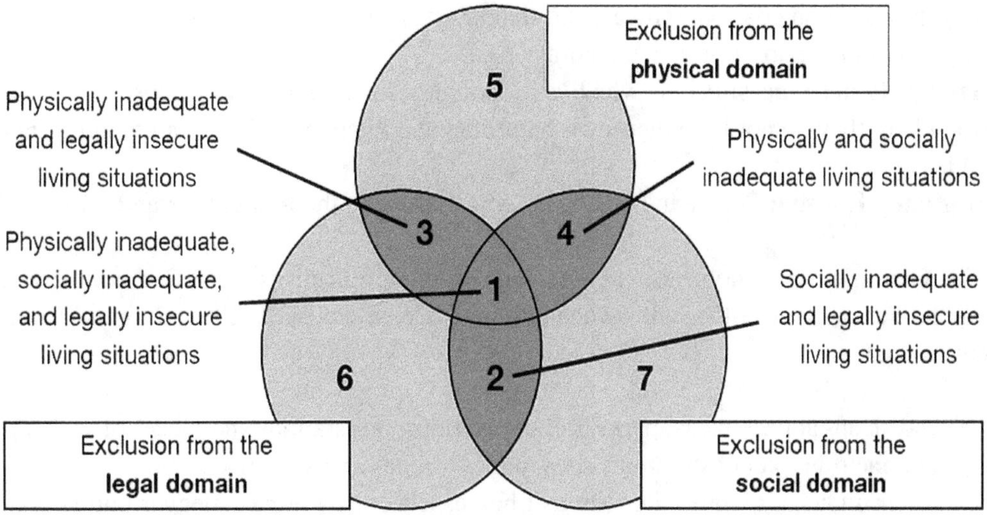

Above things can be conglomerated into two subsets (FEANTSA, 2007):

- **Homelessness:** Roofless and houseless;
- **Housing Exclusion:** Insecure and inadequate.

As per ETHOS and the New Zealand Definition of Homelessness, definition of homelessness includes following (Statistics New Zealand, 2009):

1. Living in a place of habitation (during the reference period) that is below a minimum adequacy standard; and
2. Lacking access to adequate (physical, legal and social domains) housing.

On basis of this, ETHOS suggested following model and situations for homelessness (Statistics New Zealand, 2009; Amore, Baker, & Chapman, 2011):

1. **Homelessness:** Living in a place of habitation that is below a minimum adequacy standard (exclusion from two or more domains) AND lacking access to adequate housing
2. **Housing Exclusion:** Living in a place of habitation that is at or above a minimum adequacy standard but not fully adequate (exclusion from one domain) AND lacking access to adequate housing
3. **Adequate Housing:** Living in a place of habitation that satisfies all three domains

Australian Society on the other hand, defined homelessness as 'not having access to safe, secure and adequate housing'. The Australian Bureau of Statistics (Chamberlain, 1999) identifies following types of homelessness:

- **Primary Homelessness:** People without conventional accommodation such as those who 'sleep out', or use derelict buildings, cars, railway stations for shelter.
- **Secondary Homelessness:** People who frequently move from temporary accommodation such as emergency accommodation, refuges, and temporary shelters. People may use boarding houses or family accommodation just on a temporary basis.
- **Tertiary Homelessness:** People who live in rooming houses or boarding houses, medium or long-term, where they do not have their own bathroom and kitchen facilities and tenure is not secured by a lease.
- **Marginally Housed:** People in housing situations close to the minimum standard.

In India, Census defines 'homeless' as a person not living in 'census houses' or build house, person who do not possess a house, either self-owned or rented (Census of India, 2001; Supreme Court Report, 2001), but instead:

1. Lives and sleeps at pavements, parks, railway stations, bus stations and places of worship, outside shops and factories, at constructions sites, under bridges and so on;
2. Spend their nights at night shelters, transit homes, short stay homes, beggar homes and children homes;
3. Lives in temporary structures without full walls and roof, such as under plastic sheets, or thatch roofs on pavements, parks and other common spaces.

Across several studies, opinions also differ regarding the reference period, frequency and persistence of homelessness to differentiate between short term, long term, chronic and repeated homelessness (Chamberlain & Johnson, 2002). In most nations, measurement of homelessness is limited or non-existent, and the lack of an international, standard definition of homelessness means that there is no credible benchmark for governments to be held to.

Magnitude of the Problem

The homeless population presents special methodological challenges for collecting accurate epidemiological information. Consequently, early estimates of prevalence rates for mental health, substance use, and co-occurring disorders varied greatly by study (Fischer & Breakey, 1991). Across several nations also, prevalence varies considerably. The third national census of homeless school students in Australia (Chamberlain, & MacKenzie, 2008) revealed that 48 to 82 per cent of homeless young people had a diagnosable mental illness and the most common disorders were mood disorders, anxiety disorders, such as post-traumatic stress disorder and substance use disorders. Suicide attempts were present in nearly 28 percent and suicidal ideations were reported by almost one in every 10thhomeless young person. Surprisingly the substance use trends showed a queer trend of declining use in Australian youth in general, but increasing usage in homeless population. Despite the high illness load, help seeking was less in young people experiencing homelessness and to dismay even those who sought help, did not receive adequate response because of their multiple and complex needs, including dual diagnosis and consequently fell between the gaps in service delivery (Chamberlain & MacKenzie, 2008).

Glimpses from United States, another developed country, from other corner of the world showed almost similar trends. According to the United States, Department of Housing and Urban Development's June 2010 Annual Homeless Assessment Report submitted to Congress (Substance Abuse and Mental Health Services Administration or SAMHSA, 2011) 407,966 individuals were homeless in shelters, transitional housing programs or on the streets and of these109,812 individuals were chronically homeless. Predominant homeless clients were single (82%) and males (62%). Of these, 26.2% had chronic severe mental illness and 34.7% had co-occurring substance use problems (SAMHSA, 2011). Another yearlong study conducted in the San Diego, Adult Mental Health Services found 15% as prevalence of homelessness; of these20% of the patients were suffering from schizophrenia, 17% with bipolar disorder and 9% with depression (Folsom et al., 2005) In another cross sectional study, 43% of homeless people in the United States were found to have either a mental health or a substance use problem, and an additional 23% had concurrent mental health and substance use problems (Burt, 2001).

The story from developing nations is also not different. Indian Census of 2001 enumerated 1.94 million as homeless (Census of India, 2001) and 2011 census mentioned 1.7 million as homeless persons that constituted 0.4% of Indian population (Government of India, 2013). Grossly it appeared as good news that there was an overall decline in the houseless population from the last Census though some accounts suggested it to be an under estimation. Between the two census years, not just the numbers changed; rather a new trend emerged of 28% decline of homelessness in rural India with 20% increase in urban homeless people. Nearly a fourth (26%) of the homeless population of urban India was residing in the top five metros of the country (Government of India, 2012-13). Few studies were conducted in different parts of India to assess the prevalence of mental illness in such population. A study reported that of one hundred and forty homeless persons admitted in the department of psychiatry of a north Indian medical university nearly 90.7% had mental illness. Rates of co morbidity were very high, most (55.7%) had more than one psychiatric diagnosis,44.3% had co-morbid substance abuse and 38.6% had co morbid intellectual disability (Tripathi et al., 2013). In another study carried out amongst inpatients of psychiatry centre in Haryana, more than 60% patients met the criteria for at least one psychiatric disorder and at least 30% had serious mental illness (Gupta, Nehra, Kumar, Sharma, & Kumar, 2013).

The high prevalence rates of mental health, substance use, and co-occurring disorders among homeless individuals across the globe highlights the need to screen for both mental health and substance use disorders and to screen routinely for the presence of a second disorder in presence of one disorder in homeless population. A broad range of treatment options should be available to meet the needs of people with co-occurring disorders.

HOMELESSNESS: RELATIONSHIP WITH MENTAL ILLNESS

Relationship of homelessness with mental illness is bidirectional i.e. homelessness leads to deterioration of mental health and in turn mental illness can also lead to homelessness. It forms a vicious cycle from which escape of an individual becomes difficult. It has also been found that more severe the level of homelessness, poorer is the level of mental health (Lester, & Bradley, 2001; Lam, & Rosencheck, 1999). Mental illnesses bring a lot of challenges in the life of people; an extreme end can be turning homeless due to severe untreated illness. Other way, homelessness can also contribute to mental illness. Amongst psychiatric illnesses in homeless mentally ill, as per a north Indian data, psychotic disorders were the most common (65%) followed by substance abuse (44.3%) and bipolar disorder/mania (12.9%) (Tripathi et al., 2013). Other studies have also reported a much higher prevalence of severe mental illnesses in homeless individuals (Folsom, & Jeste, 2002). Substance abuse has also consistently been reported to be associated with vulnerability to homelessness in the United States and other Asian countries (Folsomet al., 2005; Han et al., 2003). Along with younger age and male gender, homelessness has been highly correlated with substance abuse in other studies too (Cuffel, Heithoff, & Lawson, 1993; Lehmanet, Myers, Thompson, & Corty, 1993). Homeless and mentally ill are often diagnosed with many other accompanying disabilities, such as drug addiction, alcoholism, HIV/AIDS, diabetes, and tuberculosis. Mentally ill homeless people tend to be the sickest, the most ragged, and the most difficult people for society to accept. In addition, because rationality itself is compromised by mental illness, they are often the least able to help themselves, either economically or medically, and thus they slide more deeply into danger.

Mentally ill homeless men and women are also vulnerable to attack; they are often victims of violent crime. Some of the crimes against them are examples of the worst behavior imaginable. Many mentally ill homeless also come into contact with the criminal justice system as offenders, get arrested as they engage in such illegal activities as trespassing, petty theft, shoplifting, and prostitution—often crimes of survival under the most desperate of conditions, and sometimes can be direct result of impaired judgment due to mental illness. Given consistent medical and psychosocial treatment along with stable housing, many of them could again function at a high level. But such stability and consistent care are impossible to achieve in background of homelessness. Thus homelessness and mental illness become a vicious circle, one compounding the other in a vortex of suffering for the individual. Unfortunately, without mental health treatment and related support services, it is difficult for mentally ill homeless persons to gain access to, and remain in permanent housing. Often they face stigma associated with their illness and discrimination by potential landlords or neighbors. All of these factors make individuals with serious mental illnesses extremely vulnerable to homelessness and difficult to help once they become homeless (Brown, & Gibbs, 1996).

ASSOCIATION OF HOMELESSNESS AND MENTAL ILLNESS: REASONS BEHIND

Following are the possible reasons behind coexisting mental illness and homelessness.

Administrative and Policy Related Factors

- **Process of Deinstitutionalization Marked the Beginning:** Prior to late 1950s and early 1960s, most persons with mental illness resided in long term state mental asylums not for therapeutic purpose per se, but more as a custodial setting made for protecting society from mentally ill. With the advent of effective treatment by late 1960s (especially psychotropics), the process of deinstitutionalization started to gain momentum. State hospitals were depopulated, criteria for new admissions were made stringent and authority for planning of mental health services shifted from state to local communities. Many mentally ill people were released from institutions without a safety net of assured treatment, supportive services, or appropriate housing lead to chaos. What was thought to be as a transitional step, with sudden implementation without adequate preparedness of community mental health or social welfare resources resulted in increase in homelessness of these patients (Cisneros,1997).

Illness Related Factors

- **Impaired Ability to Take Care of Self Due to Illness:** Severe mental illness disrupts a person's ability to carry out essential aspects of daily life, such as self-care and household management. The most common reason for the patients' becoming homeless and remaining on the street was that patients wandered away from their home due to mental illness that was not treated adequately/timely. This was evident by the fact that most of the patients developed clear symptoms of mental illness before becoming homeless. Data from a few other studies suggest that about one-fifth of the persons had mental illness before becoming homeless (Mental health foundation, London, 2006). Hence, mental illness is an important contributor to homelessness.
- **Disturbed Interpersonal Relationship Due to Illness:** Mental illnesses may also prevent people from forming and maintaining stable relationships or cause people to misinterpret others' guidance and react irrationally. This often results in pushing away caregivers, family and friends who may be the force and social support that keeps the person from becoming homeless. As a result of these factors, people with mental illnesses are much more likely to become homeless than the general population. A study of people with serious mental illnesses by California's public mental health system found that 15% were homeless at least once in a one-year period (Folsom et al., 2005). Patients with schizophrenia or bipolar disorder are particularly vulnerable.
- **Cognitive Deficits:** Increased confusion, memory problems, difficulty planning ahead not related to stress-induced symptom relapse but as part of illness can compound the problem further and can hamper maintaining compliance or link with caregivers or health care system.
- **Untreated Mental Illness:** Serious mental illnesses rapidly deteriorate if effective treatment is not available to the patients. Less than a third of homeless people with mental health problems receive treatment (Bines, 1994). Most patients are mentally ill before leaving their families and only a minority had received treatment. Stigma, misconceptions and lack of accessible and affordable treatment were the common reasons for not initiating proper treatment at outset. A large multi-country survey supported by the World Health Organization (WHO) showed that 35–50% mentally ill in the developed countries and 76–85% patients in less developed countries had received no treatment in the past 12 months (Demyttenaere et al., 2004).
- **Predisposition to Co-Morbid Medical Illnesses:** Mental illness may cause people to neglect taking the necessary precautions against disease and can lead to physical problems such as respiratory infections, skin diseases, or exposure to tuberculosis, sexually transmitted diseases, nutritional deficiencies, HIV or Hepatitis, which can further compound mental illness and reduces ability of client further to take care of self (Tripathi, 2013).
- **Comorbid Substance Abuse:** Some mentally ill people self-medicate using street drugs, which can lead not only to addictions, but also to disease transmission. This combination of mental illness, substance abuse and poor physical health makes it very difficult for people to obtain employment and residential stability (SAMHSA, 2003).

Factors Related to Service Delivery

- **Scarcity of Appropriate Mental Health Resources:** In low and middle income (LAMI) countries, there is a huge scarcity of resources to address the mental health needs of the population (Saraceno & Saxena, 2002). Mental health services still continue to be urban-centered, confined to hospital-based facilities and are fragmented (Thirunavukarasu, 2011).
- **Lag Period in Development in Rehabilitative Facilities:** Even with the advent of time therapeutic facilities developed well, but rehabilitative facilities, especially community outreach services did not catch up well, especially in LAMI countries (Saraceno& Saxena, 2002). Many such persons with homelessness and mental illness are brought to health agencies for acute treatment, improves fairly but the rehabilitation back in community with good follow up care is not ensured; which brings these patients soon in similar state. The coordination between acute treatment and community care and liaison with social welfare agencies needs to be strengthened.

Social Factors

- **Stigma:** The stigma attached to such illness has always been a serious issue. In developing countries, the families approach faith healers or alternative medicine often and earlier in comparison to the proper mental health settings (Trivediand Jilani, 2011). Social isolation, stigma and a perception of being displaced from society make it difficult for this client group to canvas for better services.
- **Lack of Political Will:** The negative social attitudes towards mental health, massive underestimation of the suffering of mentally ill people, lack of political empathy and the lack of mental health leadership increases the challenges in providing appropriate care in LAMI Countries (Saraceno, & Saxena, 2002). The mentally ill because of their affected condition are not only shunned but also receive no support or sympathy of any kind. They often face poor living condition, infection, inaccessibility to basic health services, premature death and so on. Streets have become home to many mentally ill due to lack of social support and care (Anish, 2013). The difficulties of addressing combined substance misuse and mental illness (dual diagnosis) which exists in this group has long been acknowledged but not appropriately dealt with.
- **Problems Faced by Homeless Population with Mental Illness:** Programs for homeless population need to be responsive to a broad range of psychosocial problems that are significantly complicated by the conditions of poverty, homelessness and the presence of co-occurring disorders. These problems may contribute to the onset of homelessness, but they may also result from homelessness. Homeless individuals with co-occurring mental health and substance use disorders face the challenge of living with multiple impairments and disabilities, while also struggling to meet immediate survival needs for food, clothing and shelter. Many of these individuals also experience general medical illnesses, legal problems, histories of trauma, behavioral problems, skill deficits and a lack of connection to meaningful supports (Fischer, 1990). These unstable conditions severely compromise efforts to recover from illnesses and/or addictions. The basic problems of homelessness are the need for personal shelter, warmth and safety; other difficulties include (Rai, 2008).

- **Lack of Basic Amenities:** Lack of personal security and privacy, especially for sleeping, safe-keeping of bedding, clothing and possessions, which may have to be carried at all times, hygiene and sanitary facilities, cleaning and drying of clothes, preparing and storing food, without permanent location or mailing address, hostility and legal powers against urban vagrancy (Supreme Court of India Report, 2001).
- **Poor Self-Care:** The combined effect of psychiatric symptomatology and addiction can influence the person's capacity to attend to self-care needs. In addition, attention to self-care is not a high priority for homeless individuals who must also attend to issues of basic survival.
- **Entanglement with Law Enforcement Agencies:** They get often arrested by police and are often suspected allegiance to and complicity with sex work, drug peddling and the petty crime of the streets. The Indian laws that criminalize the urban homeless include laws against vagrancy (such as the preventive Sections 109 and 151 in the Criminal Procedure Code), begging (such as the Bombay prevention of Begging Act, 1959 and Tamil Nadu Prevention of Begging Act, 1945) and juvenile justice (The Juvenile Justice act, 2006), which provide for arrest, incarceration and custodialization for sleeping or loitering on the streets, for merely having 'no ostensible means of livelihood' or even for simply being a child 'in care of need and protection). In formal studies amongst homeless population, due to stigma, initially very few admit to arrest, but with time it is learnt that in fact many street youths had spent few years in brutalized detention centers and many had run away from these loveless facilities. The livelihoods of many homeless people like street vending and rickshaw pulling are also subject to continuous harassment and extortion by police and municipal authorities. But is still the threat of using these intensely anti-poor legal provisions more than their actual deployment, which holds the homeless populations in cities the throes of habitual fear and submission to public authority (Rai, 2008).
- **Predisposition to Physical Illnesses:** Other negative health consequences experienced by homeless young adults include sexually transmitted infections, poorly controlled chronic mental illness, and lack of immunization for conditions, such as HIV, hepatitis B and (Wright, Campbell, &Tompkins, 2002; Taylor & Goldberg, & Hutchinson, 2000). Homeless young adults also are at increased risk for the development of respiratory disease, thought to be related to exposure to tuberculosis and influenza (Snyder & Eisner, 2004). In addition to the mentioned problems, homeless young adults often experience posttraumatic stress disorder (Crane, 1998), skin disorders, foot problems, and lice (Gill, 2003).
- **Victims to Sexual Assault:** Studies have shown that homeless women with schizophrenia are sexually assaulted at alarming rates, which exposes them to all kinds of deprivation and infections including the HIV virus. A systematic review revealed that homeless adolescents are diagnosed with widely varying rates of mental health disorders and high rates of sexually transmitted infection (King, Feldman, & Waithaka, 2008).

BARRIERS IN ACCESSING HEALTH CARE BY HOMELESS MENTALLY ILL

Barriers experienced by the homeless mentally ill in accessing health care are as follows (Canavanet al., 2012).

Illness Specific Barriers

- **Nature of Severe Mental Illness:** The cyclic or chronic nature of serious mental illnesses can make it difficult for individuals to retain housing and employment when their symptoms recur or worsen. Hence predisposes them for homelessness and in that state further puts them away from caregivers and health care system.

Barriers Specific to Homelessness

- **Lifestyle of Homeless:** One of the important barriers is also difficult and chaotic life circumstances of homeless people itself, including alcohol and substance abuse issues (FEANSTA ETHOS, 2005) and difficulties in maintaining medication compliance (Lam, & Rosencheck, 1999). There is often unwillingness amongst the homeless population to engage with the services (Wright & Tompkins, 2006), often due to a lack of trust in health professionals (Busch-Geertsemaet, Edgar, O'Sullivan, & Pleace, 2010).
- **Lack of Knowledge about Health Benefits and Entitlements:** Most of the homeless are not aware about their entitlement to in the line of healthcare services and hence do not access them (Bianco, & Wells, 2001).
- **Financial Obstacles:** In many countries there may be cost associated to accessing healthcare that makes it inaccessible to homeless people (Bianco, & Wells, 2001) e.g. barriers relating to health insurance are also reported (Patton, 1970), mainly relating to not having insurance or not being registered with a General Practitioner (GP) (Hsieh& Shannon, 2005).
- **Lack of Affordable Housing:** A permanent residence still represents one of the main requirements for registering with the health care systems in a number of European countries which blocks the very first step of physical access (Anderson et al., 2006; FEANTSA, 2006). Homeless people are often reported as having problems registering with health services hence they often access mental health care through accident and emergency services, where it is unlikely to receive appropriate care and treatment (Griffiths, 2002). A stable housing is perhaps the first line of treatment for people with psychiatric disabilities. Yet with limited income, many people with serious mental illnesses are forced to live in overcrowded and often substandard living environments that place them at physical and emotional risk. Due to the ongoing stigma surrounding mental illness, many housing providers, funding societies and neighborhood groups become reluctant to give house to people with disabilities, further marginalizing this section (Bines, 1994).

Health Service System Related Barriers

- **Limitations in Accessing Health Services:** Accessibility not only means physical accessibility, but also services being approachable, appropriate to the need of the concerned group. For homeless mentally ill, limited accessibility is also due to factors such as opening hours, inflexible appointment procedures and location (Griffiths, S., 2002; FEANTSA, 2006).
- **No Continuity of Care:** Lifestyle of homeless persons to be a mobile one, but there is frequently no flexibility in the healthcare system in this regard. A move from one district to another may mean that a homeless person finds himself or herself outside the system again.

- **Difficulty Accessing Drug and Alcohol Services:** Community deaddiction services are insufficient and sometimes have very long waiting times, so are often not utilized extensively (Neale, & Kennedy, 2002)
- **Fragmented Health Care Services:** The homeless people with serious mental illnesses are typically handled by separate agencies due to their complex physical, mental and social needs. Unfortunately these services are fragmented across one hospital or sometimes across different health care and social welfare agencies. Admission and discharge procedures in the health services also appear to be tedious because of absence of liaison between admitting, treating and discharging agency (FEANTSA, 2006).Lack of coordination between mental health, social welfare and homelessness services is a crucial lacunae in this regard (Hsieh, & Shannon, 2005). The burden of coordination often falls on the consumer, but fragmented services are difficult for homeless individuals with serious mental illnesses to negotiate unaided (Wen Hudak, & Hwang, 2007).

Social Barriers

- **Stigma:** Nearly two-thirds of all people with diagnosable disorders do not seek treatment, in part because of the stigma associated with mental illness and the receipt of mental health treatment. Biased societal attitudes make it difficult for people with serious mental illnesses to find housing and jobs, maintain social networks and become accepted in their communities (Trivedi & Jilani, 2011).
- **Discrimination:** Homeless people find it harder to register with a psychiatrist than members of the general public. Requests for a permanent address and other details can constitute a real or a psychological barrier. Also there have been reports of less conducive behavior of therapist and prejudices against homeless people. Homeless people tend to also encounter negative reactions from health professionals when they try to access healthcare services. Trying to deal with administrative personnel in health care system can be particularly difficult (Wen & Hwang, 2007).

STRATEGIES FOR COMMUNITY BASED INTERVENTIONS FOR HOMELESS PERSONS WITH MENTAL ILLNESS

Community-based services for people with serious mental illnesses based on an underlying set of client-centered core values is the answer to complex problems being faced by homeless persons with mental illness. These values include a focus on treatment in the least restrictive setting; access empowerment and responsibility; diversity and flexibility; peer, family, other natural supports and the principles of mental health recovery. The mental health field has developed a well-established set of practices and services to provide community- based care to people with serious mental illnesses. To be effective, the individual service components must be coordinated in a comprehensive, integrated system of care (Dowling, 2006). Such a system includes the following (Cisneros, 1997).

- **Case Management:** It involves coordination of a particular community's care by a case manager with provision of services like access to drop-in center services, temporary housing and rehabilitation services for patients in community itself. Outcome results in greater improvement in psychiatric symptoms and quality of life, compared to usual care. A longitudinal cohort study of clients receiving outreach, case management, and residential treatment found that having more contacts with the program was associated with greater improvements in psychological distress and greater reductions in alcohol and drug problems (Rosenheck, Frisman, & Gallup, 1995).

- **Assertive Community Treatment (ACT):** ACT treatment modality consists of a team of psychiatrists, nurses, and social workers with a low client-to-staff ratio providing comprehensive psychiatric care, medication monitoring, intensive case management and crisis intervention in the community. One of the studies found that ACT was superior to usual care in reducing psychiatric hospitalizations, but not in improving psychiatric symptoms or quality of life (Lehman, Dixon, Kernan, DeForge, & Postrado, 1997). Another study found that ACT was superior to brokered case management in improving certain psychiatric symptoms (Morse, Calsyn, Allen, & Tempelhoff, 1997). An older study found that ACT was superior to drop-in center services or outpatient clinic care in increasing program contacts, but not in improving psychiatric symptoms or substance use (Calsyn, Allen,Tempelhoff, & Smith, 992).

ACCESS TO COMMUNITY CARE AND EFFECTIVE SERVICES AND SUPPORTS (ACCESS):

ACCESS program involves a team similar in constitution to ACT but also with added responsibility of liasioning the health and social welfare services, whose primary goal was to determine if greater integration and coordination among agencies within service systems improved outcomes among mentally ill homeless people receiving ACT. Clients at all sites experienced improvements in mental health and substance use problems. At intervention sites, increased integration among service agencies was achieved but did not affect individual-level health outcomes. (Morse & Tempelhoff, 1997; Rosenheck Lam, &Morrissey, 2002).

- Psychosocial rehabilitation services,
- Community alternatives for crisis care,
- Integrated services for co-occurring substance abuse and serious mental illness,
- Consumer self-help, consumer-operated programmes, consumer advocacy,
- Family self-help and advocacy,
- Housing programmes,
- Income, education, and employment.
- **Health Care Integrated Service Systems:** Interventions providing coordinated treatment and support for homeless adults with mental illness and/or substance abuse usually result in greater improvements in health related outcomes than does usual care.
- **Putting the Pieces Together:** As with so many of society's problems, we do a disservice to this issue by looking for one ultimate solution. Through decades of trial and error, we have come to understand that although there is no one solution to the problem of homelessness, solutions can be crafted as a series of steps that, when taken together, provide real help. Meeting this goal requires a commitment and partnership by government (central, federal, state and local) and the private sector including foundations, philanthropists, researchers, businessmen and women, the media, and the general public to help people with serious mental illnesses achieve full participation in society. They deserve nothing less. Some specific steps that government and private partners can take to make this vision a reality include, but are not limited to, the following (Cisneros,1997):

- Continue research into both effective clinical treatments for serious mental illnesses and successful program design.
- Increase the supply of affordable housing and housing subsidies and replicate successful supported housing programs throughout the country.
- Facilitate entry into treatment and into the full range of services required by people with serious mental illnesses.
- Enhance interagency initiatives to address fragmentation of services, especially around issues of discharge planning.
- Continue to reduce stigma and improve public awareness of effective treatment for serious mental illnesses.
- Create programs and services that are culturally appropriate.

Programs with adequate integration should

- Assertively address mental health, substance abuse and other problems through active outreach and services.
- Closely monitor the need for services.
- Integrate mental health and substance abuse interventions.
- Involve a comprehensive set of services for developing living, interpersonal, vocational and social skills.
- Ensure a stable residential situation with a continuum of housing options that are safe and free of illegal drugs and alcohol.
- Understand that chronic mental health and substance abuse problems need long-term treatment.
- Commit to the belief that improved quality of life is possible for an individual, regardless of the nature and severity of his or her problems.

Components that are basic to Continuum of Care approach which must be in place in order for the continuum to be viable in a community are:

- Outreach and assessment, to identify the needs of individuals or families and to link participants to appropriate facilities and services.
- Emergency shelter, to provide safe alternatives to the streets and referrals to service providers and housing opportunities.
- Transitional housing, with supportive services appropriate to the problems faced by individuals or families not prepared to live on their own. Such services may involve job training, job placement, substance abuse treatment, short-term mental health services, or training in independent living skills.
- Permanent housing, with or without supportive mental health services.

A strong prevention strategy is also a key element of the Continuum of Care. Enabling services to act before mental health problems become severe and intractable has been identified as a crucial component of homelessness prevention (FEANTSA, 2009)

CURRENT SCENARIO AND HOPE FOR FUTURE

The willingness to ignore the existence of homeless mentally ill is common amongst not only policy makers and law enforcing agencies, but among the health-care agencies and public too. Homeless mentally ill have received increasing attention from Non Government Organizations (NGOs) in the last decade. NGOs have developed comprehensive services for the homeless mentally ill in several nations. However, services from NGOs remain available to a very limited region of country and are almost nonexistent in another part of country. Moreover, services provided by NGOs may be difficult to sustain over time and on larger scales (Thara & Patel, 2010). Effective provisions in a national plan are required for care of the homeless and wandering mentally ill individuals whose plight is borne out of a combination of health, socioeconomic and human right issues. Further research regarding the relative effectiveness of different service delivery models would lead to more explicit policy recommendations concerning the role of specific services for homeless people, both compared to generic services but also in relation to a targeted mental health component. Such research would also assist in identifying the most efficient pathways from homeless specific services to the generic services. The integration of both specific and generic services requires high levels of co-ordination, which this study suggests do not currently exist. More comprehensive strategies for the care and treatment of homeless people with mental health problems which address the issues highlighted in this paper are necessary. Targeted policy responses, including a commitment to adequate funding, along with improved structures for coordination and inter-agency working should be developed in order to improve service delivery across globe.

CONCLUSION

Homelessness is a big problem and mental illness makes it worse. Homelessness can lead to and perpetuate mental illness and vice versa. Co morbidities like substance use disorder, other mental illness, and physical illnesses are very high in homeless persons with mental illness. They suffer from physical, sexual assault and get incarcerated often at hands of law enforcement agencies. They face stigma and discrimination not just at the hand of society but also via healthcare agencies. Non availability of appropriate healthcare resources, stigma, discrimination, inadequately developed community resources are significant barriers in health seeking. Integration of health resources, co morbid treatment of substance use, social security benefits, continuum of care approach, inter agency coordination and better service delivery can be possible solutions for the ongoing problem. Commitment by government, private sector, social welfare sector, strong political will and integrated efforts to address the problem of homeless persons with mental illness.

REFERENCES

Amore, K., Baker, M., & Chapman, P. H. (2011). The ETHOS Definition and Classification of Homelessness: An Analysis. *European Journal of Homelessness*, *5*(2), 19–37.

Anderson, I., Baptista, I., Wolf, J., Edgar, B., Benjaminsen, L., & Sapounakis, A. (2006). *The changing role of service provision: barriers of access of health services for homeless people. European Federation of National Organizations Working with Homeless (FEANTSA)*. European Observatory on Homelessness.

Anish, K. R. (2013). An evaluation of psychosocial rehabilitation facilities for homeless mentally ill in India. *Arthraties Journal of Social Sciences, 12*(2), 1–19.

Bianco, C., & Wells, S. M. (Eds.). (2001). *Overcoming Barriers to Community Integration for People with Mental Illnesses. Center for Mental Health Services Substance Abuse and Mental Health Services Administration (SAMHSA)*. U.S. Department of Health and Human Services.

Bines, W. (1994). *The health of single homeless people*. York, UK: Centre for Housing Policy, University of York.

Bombay prevention of begging Act (1959) Complete Act- Bare Act.

Brown, G.K., & Gibbs, J. (1996). *Community Mental Health Centers and Homeless Persons: A report from the office of the Inspector General of HHS*. Washington, DC: U.S. Department of Health and Human Services.

Burt, M. R. (2001). *Helping America's homeless*. Washington, DC: Urban InstitutePress.

Busch-Geertsema, V., Edgar, W., O'Sullivan, E., & Pleace, N. (2010). *Homelessness and Homeless policies in Europe: lessons from research*. In FEANTSA: A report prepared for the European Consensus Conference on Homelessness.

Canavan, R., Barry, M. M., Matanov, A., Barros, H., Gabor, E., Greacen, T., & Priebe, S. et al. (2012). Service provision and barriers to care for homeless people with mental health problems across 14 European capital cities. *BMC Health Services Research, 12*(1), 222. doi:10.1186/1472-6963-12-222 PMID:22838503

Census of India report, homeless population. (2001). Office of registrar general & census commissioner, India.

Chamberlain, C. (1999). *Counting the homeless: Implications for policy development*. Canberra: Australian Bureau of Statistics.

Chamberlain, C., & Johnson, G. (2002). The development of Prevention and early intervention services for homeless youth: Intervening successfully (Position Paper). Melbourne: Australian Urban Housing Research Institute (AUHRI).

Chamberlain, C., & MacKenzie, D. (1992). Understanding Contemporary Homelessness: Issues of Definition and Meaning. *The Australian Journal of Social Issues, 27*(4), 274–297.

Chamberlain, C., & MacKenzie, D. (2008). Youth Homelessness. *Youth Studies*, (27), 17-25.

Cisneros. (1997). Searching for Home: Mentally Ill Homeless People in America. *Cityscape (Washington, D.C.)*, 155–172.

Crane, M. (1998). The associations between mental illness and homelessness among older people: An exploratory study. *Aging & Mental Health, 2*(3), 171–180. doi:10.1080/13607869856641

Cuffel, B. J., Heithoff, K. A., & Lawson, W. (1993). Correlates of patterns of substance abuse among patients with schizophrenia. *Hospital & Community Psychiatry*, *44*, 247–251. PMID:8444435

Current Statistics on the Prevalence and Characteristics of People Experiencing Homelessness in the United States. (2011). SAMHSA.

Demyttenaere, K., Bruffaerts, R., Posada-Villa, J., Gasquet, I., Kovess, V., & Lepine, J. P. (2004). World Health Organization (WHO) World Mental Health Survey Consortium. Prevalence, severity, and unmet need for treatment of mental disorders in the WHO, World Mental Health Surveys. *Journal of the American Medical Association*, *291*, 2581–2590. doi:10.1001/jama.291.21.2581 PMID:15173149

Dowling, S., Manthorpe, J., Cowley, S., King, S., Raymond, V., & Perez, W. (2006). *Person-centred planning in social care: A scoping review*. Joseph Rowntree Foundation, King's College London.

Edgar, B. (2009). *European Review of Statistics on Homelessness*. Brussels: FEANTSA.

Edgar, W., Doherty, J., & Meert, H. (2003). *Second Review of Statistics on Homelessness in Europe*. Brussels: FEANTSA.

FEANTSA. (2006). *The right to health is a human right: ensuring access to health for people who are homeless*. In Feantsa Annual European Report.

FEANTSA & Mental Health Europe. (2009). *Joint statement in homelessness and mental health*. Mental Health Europe. Retrieved September 12, 2014, from http:/www.mhesme.org/assets/files/Common%20 statement%20FEANTSA%20MHE%20.pdf)

FEANTSA European typology on homelessness and housing exclusion (ETHOS) . (2005). Brussels: FEANTSA. Retrieved September 12, 2014, fromhttp://www.feantsa.org/files/ freshstart/Toolkits/ Ethos / Leaflet/EN.pdf

FEANTSA Proposal, . (2007). *A Retrospective Module on Homelessness for Household Surveys*. Brussels: FEANTSA.

Fischer, P. J. (1990). *Alcohol and drug abuse and mental health problems among homeless persons: A review of the literature, 1980-1990*. Rockville, MD: National Institute of Alcohol Abuse and Alcoholism and National Institute of Mental Health.

Fischer, P. J., & Breakey, W. R. (1991). The epidemiology of alcohol, drug and mental disorders among homeless persons. *The American Psychologist*, *46*(11), 1115–1128. doi:10.1037/0003-066X.46.11.1115 PMID:1772149

Folsom, D., & Jeste, D. (2002). Schizophrenia in homeless persons: A systematic review of the literature. *Acta Psychiatrica Scandinavica*, *104*, 1–10. PMID:12059843

Folsom, D. P., Hawthorne, W., Lindamer, L., Gilmer, T., Bailey, A., Golshan, S., & Jeste, D. V. et al. (2005). Prevalence and risk factors for homelessness and utilization of mental health services among 10,340 patients with serious mental illness in a large public mental health system. *The American Journal of Psychiatry*, *162*(2), 370–376. doi:10.1176/appi.ajp.162.2.370 PMID:15677603

Gill, P., & de Wildt, G. (Eds.). (2003). *Housing and Health: The Role of Primary Care*. Oxford, UK: Radcliffe Medical.

Griffiths, S. (2002). *Addressing the health needs of rough sleepers. Homelessness Directorate*. London: Office of the Deputy Prime Minister.

Gupta, R., Nehra, D. K., Kumar, V., Sharma, P., & Kumar, P. (2013). Psychiatric illnesses in homeless (runaway or throwaway) girl inmates: A preliminary study. *Dysphrenia*, *4*(1), 31–35.

Han, O., Lee, H. B., Ahn, J., Park, J., Cho, M., Hong, J., & Kim, C.-Y. et al. (2003). Lifetime and current prevalence of mental disorders among homeless men in Korea. *The Journal of Nervous and Mental Disease*, *191*(4), 272–275. doi:10.1097/01.NMD.0000061151.19363.82 PMID:12695742

Homelessness – Provision of Mental Health and Substance Abuse Services. (2003). *Substance Abuse and Mental Health Services Administration (SAMHSA), Center for Mental Health Services*. Retrieved September12, 2014, from http://mentalhealth.samhsa.gov

Hsieh, H. F., & Shannon, S. E. (2005). Three Approaches to Qualitative Content Analysis. *QHR*, *15*, 1277–1288. PMID:16204405

Justice, J. (Care and protection of children) Amendment Act, 2006 (Act No. 33 of 2006), Ministry of Law and Justice, India.

King, C., Feldman, J., Waithaka, Y., Aban, I., Hu, J., Zhang, S., & Bachmann, L. H. et al. (2008). Sexual risk behaviors and sexually transmitted infection prevalence in an outpatient Psychiatry Clinic. *Sexually Transmitted Diseases*, *35*(10), 877–882. doi:10.1097/OLQ.0b013e31817bbc89 PMID:18607313

Koegel, P., Sullivan, G., Burnam, A., Morton, S. C., & Wenzel, S. (1999). Utilization of mental health and substance abuse services among homeless adults in Los Angeles. *Medical Care*, *37*(3), 306–317. doi:10.1097/00005650-199903000-00010 PMID:10098574

Lam, J., & Rosencheck, R. (1999). Street outreach for homeless persons with serious mental illness: Is it effective? *Medical Care*, *37*(9), 894–907. doi:10.1097/00005650-199909000-00006 PMID:10493468

Lehman, A. F., Dixon, L. B., Kernan, E., DeForge, B. R., & Postrado, L. T. (1997). A randomized trial of assertive community treatment for homeless persons with severe mental illness. *Archives of General Psychiatry*, *54*(11), 1038–1043. doi:10.1001/archpsyc.1997.01830230076011 PMID:9366661

Lehman, A. F., Myers, C. P., Thompson, J. W., & Corty, E. (1993). Implications of mental and substance use disorders: A comparison of single and dual diagnosis patients. *The Journal of Nervous and Mental Disease*, *181*(6), 365–370. doi:10.1097/00005053-199306000-00005 PMID:8388914

Lester, H., & Bradley, C. P. (2001). Barriers to primary healthcare for the homeless: The general practitioner's perspective. *The European Journal of General Practice*, *7*(1), 6–12. doi:10.3109/13814780109048777

Mental health foundation. (2006). Retrieved September12, 2014, fromwww.mentalhealth.org.uk

Ministry of housing & urban poverty alleviation annual report. (2012-13). Government of India.

Montross, L. P., Barrio, C., Yamada, A., Lindamer, L., Golshan, S., & Garcia, P. et al.. (2005). Tri-ethnic variations of co-morbid substance and alcohol use disorders in schizophrenia. *Schizophrenia Research*, *79*, 297–A305. PMID:15978782

Morse, G. A., Calsyn, R. J., Allen, G., Tempelhoff, B., & Smith, R. (1992). Experimental comparison of the effects of three treatment programs for homeless mentally ill people. *Hospital & Community Psychiatry*, *43*, 1005–1010. PMID:1398563

Morse, G. A., Calsyn, R. J., & Klinkenberg, W. D. (1997). An experimental comparison of three types of case management for homeless mentally ill persons. *Psychiatric Services (Washington, D.C.)*, *48*(4), 497–503. doi:10.1176/ps.48.4.497 PMID:9090733

Neale, J., & Kennedy, C. (2002). Good practice towards homeless drug users: Research evidence from Scotland. *Health & Social Care in the Community*, *10*(3), 196–205. doi:10.1046/j.1365-2524.2002.00357.x PMID:12121256

North, C. S., & Smith, E. M. (1993). A systematic study of mental health services utilization by homeless men and women. *Social Psychiatry and Psychiatric Epidemiology*, *28*(2), 77–83. doi:10.1007/BF00802096 PMID:8511667

Padgett, D., Struening, E. L., & Andrews, H. (1990). Factors affecting the use of medical, mental health, alcohol, and drug treatment services by homeless adults. *Medical Care*, *28*(9), 805–821. doi:10.1097/00005650-199009000-00010 PMID:2402175

Patton, M. Q. (1970). *Qualitative Research and Evaluation Methods* (3rd ed.). Thousand Oaks, CA: Sage.

Press note on poverty estimates of 2011-12. (2013). Planning Commission, Government of India.

Rai, A. (2008). Delhi City Report. In H. Mander (Ed.), *Living Rough Surviving City Streets- A study of Homeless Population in Delhi, Chennai, Patna and Madurai (2)*. New Delhi, India: Planning Commission.

Ran, M. S., Chan, C. L. W., Chen, E. Y. H., Xiang, M. Z., Caine, E. D., & Conwell, Y. (2006). Homelessness among patients with schizophrenia in rural China: A 10-year cohort study. *Acta Psychiatrica Scandinavica*, *114*(2), 118–123. doi:10.1111/j.1600-0447.2006.00746.x PMID:16836599

Rosenheck, R., Frisman, L., & Gallup, P. (1995). Effectiveness and cost of specific treatment elements in a program for homeless mentally ill veterans. *Psychiatric Services (Washington, D.C.)*, *46*(11), 1131–1139. doi:10.1176/ps.46.11.1131 PMID:8564501

Rosenheck, R. A., Lam, J., Morrissey, J. P., Calloway, M. O., Stolar, M., & Randolph, F. (2002). Service systems integration and outcomes for mentally ill homeless persons in the ACCESS program: Access to Community Care and Effective Services and Supports. *Psychiatric Services (Washington, D.C.)*, *53*(8), 958–966. doi:10.1176/appi.ps.53.8.958 PMID:12161669

Saraceno, B., & Saxena, S. (2002). A mental health resources in the world: Results from Project Atlas of the WHO. *World Psychiatry; Official Journal of the World Psychiatric Association (WPA)*, *1*, 40–44. PMID:16946821

Schutt, R. K., Hough, R. L., Goldfinger, S. M., Lehman, A. F., Shern, D. L., Valencia, E., & Wood, P. A. (2009). Lessening homelessness among persons with mental illness: A comparison of five randomized treatment trials. *Asian Journal of Psychiatry*, *2*(3), 100–105. doi:10.1016/j.ajp.2009.07.003 PMID:20161434

Snyder, L. D., & Eisner, M. D. (2004). Obstructive Lung Disease among the Urban Homeless. *Chest*, *125*(5), 1719–1725. doi:10.1378/chest.125.5.1719 PMID:15136382

Statistical Standard for Occupied Dwelling Type. (2009b). *Statistics New Zealand*. Wellington: Statistics New Zealand.

Sullivan, G., Burnam, A., Koegel, P., & Hollenberg, J. (2000). Quality of life of homeless persons with mental illness: Results from the course of homelessness study. *Psychiatric Services (Washington, D.C.)*, *51*(9), 1135–1141. doi:10.1176/appi.ps.51.9.1135 PMID:10970916

Tamil Nadu Prevention of Begging Act. (1945). Complete Act- Bare Act.India.

Taylor, A., Goldberg, D., Hutchinson, S., Cameron, S., Gore, S. M., McMenamin, J., & Fox, R. et al. (2000). Prevalence of hepatitis C virus infection among injecting drug users in Glasgow 1990–1996: Are current harm reduction strategies working? *The Journal of Infection*, *40*(2), 176–183. doi:10.1053/jinf.2000.0647 PMID:10841096

Thara, R., & Patel, V. (2010). Role of non-governmental organizations in mental health in India. *Indian Journal of Psychiatry*, *52*(7), S389–S395. doi:10.4103/0019-5545.69276 PMID:21836712

The national report on homelessness for Supreme Court of India. (2001). Supreme Court commissioners WR196/2001

Thirunavukarasu, M. (2011). Closing the treatment gap. *Indian Journal of Psychiatry*, *53*(3), 199–201. doi:10.4103/0019-5545.86803 PMID:22135436

Timms, P., & Balazs, J. (1997). ABC of mental health. Mental health on the margins. *British Medical Journal*, *315*(7107), 536–539. doi:10.1136/bmj.315.7107.536 PMID:9329311

Tripathi, A., Nischal, A., Dalal, P. K., Agarwal, V., Agarwal, M., Trivedi, J. K., & Arya, A. et al. (2013). Sociodemographic and clinical profile of homeless mentally ill inpatients in a north Indian medical university. *Asian Journal of Psychiatry*, *6*(5), 404–409. doi:10.1016/j.ajp.2013.05.002 PMID:24011688

Trivedi, J. K., & Jilani, A. Q. (2011). Pathway of psychiatric care. *Indian Journal of Psychiatry*, *53*(2), 97–98. doi:10.4103/0019-5545.82530 PMID:21772640

Wen, C. K., Hudak, P. L., & Hwang, S. W. (2007). Homeless people's perceptions of welcomeness and unwelcomeness in health-care encounters. *Journal of General Internal Medicine*, *22*(7), 1011–1017. doi:10.1007/s11606-007-0183-7 PMID:17415619

Wright, N. M. J., Campbell, T. L., & Tompkins, C. N. E. (2002). Comparison of conventional and accelerated hepatitis B immunization schedules for homeless drug users. *Communicable Disease and Public Health*, *5*, 324–326. PMID:12564251

Wright, N. M. J., & Tompkins, C. N. E. (2006). How can health services effectively meet the health needs of homeless people? *The British Journal of General Practice*, *56*, 286–293. PMID:16611519

KEY TERMS AND DEFINITIONS

Factors Responsible for Homelessness: There are many factors that contribute to an individual or family becoming homeless: divorce, domestic violence, drug and alcohol related, job loss, lack of affordable housing, lack of child support, low wages, natural disaster/ physical disabilities, post-traumatic stress disorder, poverty, severe depression and tragedy.

Homelessness and Mental Illness: People with serious mental illness are disproportionately affected by homelessness. The consequences of homelessness tend to be more severe when coupled with mental illness. People with mental illnesses remain homeless for longer periods of time and have less contact with family and friends.

Socio-Pathology of Homelessness: The term homeless is given to someone that does not have a suitable and permanent place to spend the night in. This phenomenon is visible in the form of vagrancy, sleeping on the streets, or marginalization. Homelessness occurs as a result of social pathology such as poverty, addiction, meaningless jobs, corruption and prostitution, contractual diseases, migration, natural disasters, political, social upheavals, war, old age and inflation.

Chapter 2
Chronic Mental Illness in Old Age Homes: An International Perspective

Shamsi Akbar
King George Medical University – Lucknow, India

Hitesh Khurana
Pt. B. D. Sharma PGIMS, India

ABSTRACT

Aging is a part of natural developmental process in the life of any living being. For human beings it is not just a biological phenomenon but it has psychological and social implications too. Some of the areas that would be affected include those related to health and health care, family composition, living arrangement, housing and migration. As a result of these socio-demographic evolutions and situations, older adults at times are forced to shift from their own homes to institutions/ Old age homes OAH. Living in OAH evokes a picture of apathy, dependence, and sadness which make the older adults increasingly vulnerable to mental health problems. Further there is also a strong need to develop suitable strategies to implement better mental health programmes and guidelines for the CMI in old age homes.

INTRODUCTION

This is not the end. It is not even the beginning of the end. But it is, perhaps, the end of the beginning. (Winston. S. Churchill)

Aging can generally be described as the process of growing old and is an intricate part of the life cycle. As Shakespeare had put, "Old age is last scene of all that ends this strange eventful history, is second childishness and mere oblivion, sans teeth, sans eyes, sans taste, sans everything." Basically it is a multi-dimensional process and affects almost every aspect of human life. Old age means reduced physical ability, declining mental ability, the gradual giving up of role playing in socio-economic activities, and a shift in economic status moving from economic independence to economic dependence upon others

DOI: 10.4018/978-1-5225-0519-8.ch002

for support. Old age is called "dark" not because the light fails to shine but because people refuse to see it (Gowri, 2003). Aging is a part of natural developmental process in the life of any living being. For human beings it is not just a biological phenomenon but it has psychological and social implications too. With improved economic status and health care facilities, the number of people living beyond age 60 years is rapidly increasing. Various authors define old age starting between 55 to 65 years age in different countries and cultures. However, most of the authors agree upon 65 years and above age as cut off for defining old age (Kinsella & Phillips, 2005). For various welfare issues individuals above age 60 years are considered to be in old age in India (Zachariah, Mathew, & Irudaya, 2000). In developing countries majority of older people still live in rural areas where they are much respected as a wise family member. However, the situation is much changing due to industrialization leading to more migration and disintegration of joint families. With changing economy, social values and support system has also considerably changed. In the traditional societies elderly were highly respected as family members and source of wisdom. But the younger generation now considers elderly people largely unwanted. The elderly people occupy economically lower social status and economically weaker, However, they are less receptive to accept the natural process of growing weaker (Pesic, 2007). Biologically too, old age is characterized by disease disability and dependency. With such vulnerabilities and changing social structure and values, the generation gap is widening and problems of old age are becoming difficult to manage.

Definition of Aging

Although everyone is familiar with aging, defining aging is not a so straight forward. Aging can simply refer to the passage of time and can even have a positive connotation as in "aging wine". For example, Rose (1991) in his seminal book on the evolution of aging defines aging as "a persistent decline in the age-specific fitness components of an organism due to internal physiological degeneration." From my point of view, such a definition of aging is certainly not wrong, but one might say that it is not sufficiently precise.

The aging process is of course a biological reality which has its own dynamic, largely beyond human control. However, it is also subject to the constructions by which each society makes sense of old age. In the developed world, chronological time plays a paramount role. The age of 60 or 65, roughly equivalent to retirement ages in most developed countries is said to be the beginning of old age. In many parts of the developing world, chronological time has little or no importance in the meaning of old age. Other socially constructed meanings of age are more significant such as the roles assigned to older people; in some cases, it is the loss of roles accompanying physical decline which is significant in defining old age. Thus, in contrast to the chronological milestones which mark life stages in the developed world, old age in many developing countries is seen to begin at the point when active contribution is no longer possible" (Gorman, 1999).

Age classification varied between countries and over time, reflecting in many instances the social class differences or functional ability related to the workforce, but more often than not was a reflection of the current political and economic situation. Many times the definition is linked to the retirement age, which in some instances, was lower for women than men. This transition in livelihood became the basis for the definition of old age which occurred between the ages of 45 and 55 years for women and between the ages of 55 and 75 years for men (Thane, 1978). To sum it up, aging is a complex process composed of several features:

1. An exponential increase in mortality with age;
2. Physiological changes that typically lead to a functional decline with age;
3. Increased susceptibility to certain diseases with age.

THEORIES OF AGING

Biological Theories of Aging

Among all the biological theories the genetic theory is the most popular. This theory assumes that the life span of a cell or organism is genetically determined that the genes of an animal contain a "program" that determines its life span, just as eye colour is determined genetically. This theory finds support in the fact that people with parents who have lived long lives are likely to live long themselves. Also, identical twins have life spans more similar in length than do non-twin siblings. The genetic theory of aging centers on telomeres which make the tip of chromosomes. The telomers contain repeated segments of DNA (deoxyribonucleic acid). The number of repeats in a telomere determines the maximum life span of a cell, since each time a cell divides, multiple repeats are lost. Once telomeres have been reduced to a certain size, the cell reaches a crisis point and is prevented from dividing further, consequently, the cell dies (Sadave, Hills, Heller, & Berenbaum, 2011).

Research has shown that telomeres are vulnerable to genetic factors that alter an organism's rate of aging. In humans, variations in a gene known as *TERC* (telomerase RNA [ribonucleic acid] component), which encodes an RNA segment of an enzyme known as telomerase, have been associated with reduced telomere length and an increased rate of biological aging. Telomerase normally functions to prevent the over shortening of telomeres, but in the presence of *TERC* mutations the enzyme's activity is altered. *TERC* also appears to influence the telomere length that individuals possess from the time of birth. Persons who carry *TERC* variations are believed to be several years older biologically compared with no carriers of the same chronological age. This accelerated rate of biological aging is likely also influenced by exposure to environmental factors, such as smoking and obesity, which increase a carrier's susceptibility to the onset of age-related diseases relatively early in adult life. This theory gets support from mutations of genes that affect telomere length. Mutations result in introduction of "errors" in the genetic information coded in the DNA which is translated into synthesis of faulty enzymes. Mutations i.e. the process of alteration in the genetic information in DNA can occur due to various factors that include exposure the radiations, drugs etc. Mutations also occur naturally during cell division. Slight differences induced in the transmission of information from DNA molecules of the chromosomes through RNA molecules (the "messenger" substance) to the proper assembly of the large and complex enzyme molecules could result in a molecule of the enzyme that would not "work" properly. Such alteration in the enzymes makes the individual vulnerable to various metabolic problems and oxidative damage. This is precisely what happens in the instance of mutations in the *TERC* gene. Such mutations disrupt the normal function of the telomerase enzyme. Thus as the cell continues to divide it loses its telomeric repeat sequences. Along with that, besides quantitative reduction in the genetic load, mutations add the errors in information leading to ineffective metabolism making the individual vulnerable to physical ailments (Rogers, 2016).

Psychological Theories

During an individual's life span several changes in behaviour will occur therefore there is no defining psychology of aging theory as everyone's experience will vary. For those who are less fortunate psychological changes in personality and cognition may occur. There is of course the ideal thought that one can continue the journey by living a Ulysses a type lifestyle, this may be harder for those with pathological changes but these individuals may also benefit the most from this approach. I will briefly explain each theory and how it may influence the aging process.

- **Optimization and Compensation (SOC):** Advocated by Baltes and Baltes (1990). This theory suggests that there are psychological gains and losses at every life stage, but that in old age the losses far exceed the gains. Baltes suggests that evolutionary development remains incomplete till the very last stage of life, during which societal supports no longer suffice to compensate for the decline in physiological infrastructure and losses in behavioural functionality (Baltes & Smith, 1999).

Sociological Theories

Sociological theories focus on the changing roles and relationships that accompany aging. These theories discuss how these changing roles, relationships, and status impact the older individual's ability to adapt. In this chapter briefly discussed the following sociological theories: disengagement, activity, and continuity.

- **Disengagement Theory:** The theory was formulated by Cumming and Henry in 1961 in the book Growing Old, and it was the first theory of aging that social scientists developed. The disengagement theory of aging states that "aging is an inevitable, mutual withdrawal or disengagement, resulting in decreased interaction between the aging person and others in the social system he belongs to". The theory claims that it is natural and acceptable for older adults to withdraw from society. Thus, this theory has historical significance in gerontology. Since then, it has faced strong criticism since the theory was proposed as innate, universal, and unidirectional (Vern & Norella, 2009).

The disengagement theory is one of three major psychosocial theories which describe how people develop in old age (Priscilla, 2005). The other two major psychosocial theories are the activity theory and the continuity theory, and the disengagement theory comes to odds with both.

- **Activity Theory:** Developed by Havighurst and associates in 1953, asserts that remaining active and engaged with society is pivotal to satisfaction in old age. This mentality is diametrically opposed to the Disengagement Theory. Successful aging equals active aging. Activity can be physical or intellectual in nature, but mainly refers to maintaining active roles in society. To maintain a positive self-image, the older person must develop new interests, hobbies, roles, and relationships to replace those that are diminished or lost in late life. This theory proposes that an older person should continue a middle-aged lifestyle, denying the limitations of old age as long as possible. Likewise, society should avoid the injustice of ageism by applying the same norms to old age as it does to middle age. Society should not demand declining involvement of its aging members (Joe, 2015).

- **Continuity Theory of Aging:** George, (1968) and Robert (1971) are most closely associated with the continuity theory (Boundless, 2015).The Continuity Theory of aging relates that personality, values, morals, preferences, role activity, and basic patterns of behavior are consistent throughout the life span, regardless of the life changes one encounters. This theory builds upon and modifies the activity theory. Unlike the other two sociological theories, the continuity theory offers the backdrop of life perspective to describe normal aging. The latter part of life is simply a continuation of the earlier part of life, a component of the entire life cycle (Boundless, 2015).

Within the sociological theories of aging, variables of ethnicity, gender, lifestyle, and socioeconomic status are only minimally considered, if taken into account at all. None of the three theories can be supported with evidence-based data (Joe, 2015).

Cognitive Theories

Cognitive theories of aging attempt to explain the nature of age-related differences in cognition. In the past 20 years, several dominant frameworks have emerged: reduced processing resources, general slowing, inhibition deficits, and transmission deficits.

1. **Reduced Processing Resources:** People have a limited pool of processing resources from which they can draw when performing cognitive tasks and the amount of available resources decreases as we get older. Therefore, age related declines in cognitive performance are expected whenever a cognitive task requires more of these resources, e.g., more complex tasks (Salthouse, 1991).
2. **General Slowing:** Theory of general slowing, suggests that a major factor contributing to age-related differences in cognitive functioning is a reduction in older adults' processing speed, or the speed of executing cognitive operations. This age-related slowing occurs in the central nervous system and therefore affects all tasks regardless of complexity. Although most researchers accept the idea that speed of processing slows with age, there is considerable debate over whether this slowing is the cause of all age differences (Salthouse, 1991).
3. **Inhibition Deficits:** Third cognitive theory of aging proposes that older adults have a deficit in their inhibitory processes: Aging impairs the ability to inhibit or suppress irrelevant information that becomes activated in the course of cognitive processing. Inhibitory processes serve two functions: to prevent irrelevant information from entering working memory and to delete information that is no longer relevant to the task at hand. When inhibitory processes are impaired, people will get more interference from irrelevant information because of their inability to suppress it (Kensinger, 2004).
4. **Transmission Deficits:** Older adults often have difficulties retrieving the appropriate name for a person, place, or thing. These word-finding problems can be manifest in various ways: excessive use of pronouns (due to difficulty generating the proper nouns), decreased accuracy and increased reaction time when asked to name items, and increased tip of the tongue experiences. The tip-of-the-tongue state occurs when a person has access to a word's meaning, but not the phonological features of the word. The word seems just out of reach. Older adults tend to have more tip-of-the-tongue experiences than young adults, particularly for proper names, and the accuracy of the phonological information available during a tip-of-the-tongue state (e.g., the first letter of the word, the number of syllables) tends to be more accurate for young adults than for older adults (Grady & Craik, 2000).

AGING PROCESS AND CHRONIC MENTAL ILLNESS

The aging process, old age people are more vulnerable to suffer with many chronic diseases and chronic disease are not generally prevented by vaccines or cured by medication, nor do they just disappear. To a large degree, the major chronic disease killers – heart disease, cancer, stroke, and diabetes are an extension of what people do, or not do, as they go about their daily lives. Eighty-eight percent of those over 65 years of age have at least one chronic health condition. Health damaging behaviours, particularly tobacco use, lack of physical activity, and poor eating habits, are major contributors to the nation's leading chronic diseases. Sometimes these chronic diseases may lead to severe mental health problems. Older adults experience many challenges and adjustments. Good mental health enables a person to face these changes and deal with them. This does not mean that an older person never experiences any problems or disease, but that symptoms are treated and controlled, and do not interfere with leading a rewarding life. Unfortunately, many older people still believe the myth that mental health problems result from personal failure or weakness. This stigma means that they may not want to admit that a problem or symptom exists, and do not seek help. Mental illness is a health term used for a group of mental conditions that cause severe disturbances in thinking, behavior, feeling and relating, often resulting in a substantially diminished capacity to cope with the ordinary demands of life and distress. Mental illness can affect persons of any age and social strata and can occur in any family.

In addition, many people mistake the symptoms of depression, anxiety and other mental health problems for the aging process itself. Unfortunately, many people think that confused thinking, irritability, depressed mood, and loss of energy are just signs that someone is getting older rather than signs that someone needs help. The truth is that normal aging involves changes, but most changes are gradual. The aging process does not cause sudden personality changes, loss of intellect, or confusion.

The following factors can interact with each other and lead to or escalate mental health problems, such as: dementia, anxiety, depression, alcoholic beverages, and prescription medications - some may cause depression or anxiety, over-the-counter drugs - some may interact with prescriptions, stress of change and loss and physical illness.

COMMON CHRONIC MENTAL DISORDERS IN OLDER ADULTS

Dementia

Dementia is a syndrome involving deterioration in memory, thinking, behaviour and the ability to perform everyday activities such as dressing, eating, personal hygiene and toilet activities (WHO, 2010). It generally affects older people, although it is not a normal part of aging. A report by WHO and the Alzheimer Disease Association International (ADI) in 2012 suggest a crude estimated prevalence of 4.7% among people 60 years and over. This indicates that 35.6 million people are living with dementia (WHO, 2012). The total number of people with dementia is projected to almost double every 20 years. That is, to 65.7 million by 2030 and up to 115.4 million by 2050 (WHO, 2012). Much of this increase is attributable to the rising numbers of people with dementia living in low- and middle-income countries. There are significant social and economic implications in terms of direct medical costs, direct social costs and the costs of informal care. The total cost as a proportion of GDP varied from 0.24% in low-income countries to 1.24% in high-income countries (WHO, 2012). Though no cure is available, much can be done for people with dementia and their caregivers. A range of pharmacological and several non-pharmacological interventions are available and can be delivered by even non-specialized health providers (WHO, 2010; Seitz et al., 2012).

Depression

Depression in old age is an emerging public health problem leading to morbidity and disability worldwide (Rajkumar, 2009). According to World Health Organization, Depression is a common mental disorder, characterized by sadness, loss of interest or pleasure, feelings of guilt or low self-worth, disturbed sleep or appetite, feelings of tiredness and poor concentration. The WHO estimated that the overall prevalence rate of depressive disorders among the elderly generally varies between 10 and 20%, depending on the cultural situations (Rangaswamy, 2001; Singh & Misra, 2009). Although India is the second-most populated country in the world, in terms of elderly population of 60 years and above, elderly depression is not yet perceived as a public health problem in India (Rangaswamy, 2001; Singh & Misra, 2009). Many people experience depression in old age, either as a result of living alone or due to lack of close family ties and reduced connections with their culture of origin, which results in an inability to actively participate in the community activities (Maulik & Dasgupta, 2012). Social and cultural shift has also encroached the rural India which for centuries has boasted of a joint family system with high respect for its elderly members (Grimier, 2012). Depression in elderly lowers the productivity and increases health care financial burden to the family members (Nandi, Banerjee, Mukherjee, Nandi, & Nandi, 1997). Finding out prevalence of depression among older adults living in old age home and community provides the information about the impetus we should give on mental health care. Effective psychological and pharmacological treatments exist; however, great care needs to be taken when prescribing antidepressants to this age group. Health care providers should prescribe reduced initial doses of antidepressants and finish with lower final doses (WHO, 2010). If severe, depression may lead to suicide. Comorbidity with alcohol use disorders increases the likelihood (Blow, Brockmann., & Barry, 2004).

Anxiety

Anxiety disorders occur in about 4% to 10% of community samples of older adults, and anxiety symptoms that do not meet criteria for a disorder affect 15% to 20%. (Cohen, Magai, Yaffee., & Walcott-Brown, 2006). Generalized anxiety disorder (GAD), characterized by persistent worry and associated physical symptoms lasting 6 months or longer, is the most common of the pervasive anxiety disorders in later life. Its community prevalence (in all age groups) is estimated to be 4% to 7% and 3% to 11% in older patients in the primary care setting (Wittchen, Kessler., & Beesdo, 2002). These figures may be significant underestimates, given that many older adults deny psychological problems and emphasize somatic complaints (Lenze, Karp, & Mulsant, 2005). Increased rates of anxiety are typical for older adults with a medical illness, as is higher prevalence among the homebound, nursing home residents, and patients with chronic illness (Lenze, Karp., & Mulsant, 2005; Junginger, Phelan, Cherry., & Levy, 1993). Anxiety symptoms are reported in as many as 40% of older patients with disabilities or chronic medical conditions, and poor health outcomes are associated with anxiety, including decreased levels of physical activity, poorer perception of health, memory difficulties, and increased dependence (Brenes, Guralnik., & Williamson, 2005). Increased rates of coronary artery disease and mortality are also associated with anxiety (Brenes, Ritchevsky. & Mehta, 2007).

Anxiety is also pervasive in older adults with dementia. Symptoms of anxiety occur in 8% to 71% of patients with dementia, and 5% to 21% have a DSM anxiety disorder (Seignourel, Kunik. & Snow, 2008). These wide ranges in population estimates result to some degree from differences in population characteristics and measurement strategy, and from lack of clarity about appropriate diagnostic criteria (Starkstein, Jorge, Petracca, & Robinson, 2007). Older adults can present with anxiety or worries about physical health (illness, changes in vision or hearing), cognitive difficulties, finances, and changes in life status (widowhood, care-giving responsibilities, retirement). Clinicians need to be aware that older adults may deny psychological symptoms of anxiety (fear, worry) but endorse similar emotions with different words (worries, concerns). As noted above, older adults also tend to emphasize somatic rather than psychological symptoms of anxiety (Lenze, Karp & Mulsant, 2005)

Other Mental Disorders

Alcohol abuse and misuse is the major substance abuse problem among older adults. "In the United States, it is estimated that 2.5 million older adults have problems related to alcohol, and 21 percent of hospitalized adults over age 60 have a diagnosis of alcoholism with related hospital costs as high as $60 billion per year" (Schonfeld & Dupree, 1995, p. 1819). In 1990, those over the age of 65 comprised 13 percent of the U.S. population; by the year 2030, older adults will account for 21 percent of the population (U.S. Bureau of the Census, 2009). This projected population explosion has serious implications for both the number of alcohol-related problems likely to occur among older adults and the subsequent costs involved in responding to them.

Though substance abuse problems are thought of as young people's problems, they should not be neglected in older adults. Substance abuse problems among the elderly are often overlooked or misdiagnosed. In Europe, the number of older adults with such problems will double from 2001 to 2020 (European Monitoring Centre for Drugs and Drug Addiction [EMCDDA], 2008). According to IHME (2010) data, the absolute Disability Adjusted Life Years (DALYs) for alcohol disorders for people over 60 is about 1.5 million years. This constitutes about 0.3% of total DALYs for this age group (IHME, 2010). The corresponding figures for other substance use disorders are 338.000 years and 0.1%. Availability of maintenance treatments and better health care has contributed to an increased number of older adults who survive early onset drug use. Stressful life events such as retirement, marital breakdown or bereavement, social isolation, financial problems, mental disorders and some chronic physical conditions are main contributing factors to substance abuse. Physiological changes associated with aging and increased use of other medicines, especially sedatives, may make drinking in lower doses more harmful for older adults through inducing more liver damage and causing more accidents and injuries (European Monitoring Centre for Drugs and Drug Addiction [EMCDDA], 2008). Prescribing for older adults is common. Some prescribed medicines such as benzodiazepines and opioids have a potential for abuse or dependence and this may occur within or outside a medical context. Treatment of substance use disorders in older adults is at least as effective as in younger adults. Treatment of health conditions due to substance use, especially management of withdrawal states or substance-induced psychoses, should be delivered in a supportive and, if necessary, medical environment, with proper consideration given to interactions between psychoactive substances and prescribed medicines as well as to other health complications. Although there is little research on the abuse of other illicit substances (e.g., heroin, cocaine, marijuana) by older adults, therapists and health care personnel are seeing older adults who present with symptoms of illicit drug abuse.

AGING TRENDS IN THE WORLD

As cited by Pesic (2007) almost all developed countries will experience aging of their populations. Peterson described this demographic change as a "gray dawn". In the developed world, every sixth person is over 65 years of age. In the next 30 years it will be every fourth person. Up to 2030, the proportion of those over 65 will be 33% in Australia, or 50% in Germany. The number of "very old" i.e. those over 85, is increasing more rapidly than the number of "old"– those below 85. In the next 50 years, the number of people over 85 years of age will increase by six times. All countries in the world have experienced marked increase in proportion of people living beyond 60 years' age. This trend started earlier in developed countries. The World Assembly on Aging in Vienna in 1982 highlighted that aging cannot be recognized as a phenomenon of the west alone. It was evident from the demographic changes taking place that the aging process was occurring at an unprecedented rate in most developing countries (Sen, 1994). In recent years, the number of people aged 65 or over has risen by 2 per cent a year and the fastest-growing age group is people over 80(Commission for Architecture and the Built Environment, 2009). In UK, 11 per cent of those aged 65 or over are often or always lonely 48 per cent of those aged 65 or over say the television is their main company 12 per cent of those aged 65 or over say they are trapped in their own home. The number of people aged 75 and over living alone will increase by over 40 per cent in the next 20 years (One Vioce, 2009).

India, with 1.27 billion people is the second most populous country in the world. We have a population growth rate at 1.58%, With this growth rate the extrapolated population of India by the end of 2030 is predicted to be more than 1.53 billion people by the end of 2030. The share of India's population aged 60 and older is projected to climb from 8 percent in 2010 to 19 percent in 2050, according to the United Nations Population Division (UN, 2011) with improving economy and health care facilities the absolute figures as well as proportion of elderly population in the country are on rise. Demographers have presumed that by the year 2050 more than 40%of people would only be elders in India (Ramesh & Sridhara, 2013). They are largely rural based (Bhushan & Sachdeva, 2002). The enormous growth in the proportion of older adults in the country, change in family structure and other contemporary changes in the psycho-social matrix and values often compel the elderly to live alone or to shift from their own homes to institutions/ old age homes [OAH]. Many epidemiological studies have been conducted in India to estimate the psychiatric morbidity in general population but only a few have taken specifically the elderly population into consideration (Dotty et al., 1992).

HEALTH STATUS OF ELDERLY LIVING IN THE OLD AGE HOMES

Studies in the West have demonstrated advancing age along with higher cognitive and functional impairment as predictors of entry to various supported long-term care facilities.(Greene, & Ondrich,1990; Branch, Wetle, & Scherr, 1988) Considering the need to find out the present situation of the inhabitants of OAH multiple stressful factors like loss of physical vigor, occupation, and death of spouse, feeling of loneliness, dissatisfaction in life and changes in living arrangements would lead to disturbance in the psychic equilibrium, producing mal-adaptive patterns of adjustment including physical and mental disorders, especially depression (Agarwal & Jhingan, 2002; Ghosh, 2006).Many studies have revealed that depression in elderly is associated with widowed state or staying alone (Nandi, Banerjee., & Mukherjee, 1997).

Depression is a common problem of OAH inmate in the west. About 13-15% inmates in European OAH report depressive symptoms (Ames, 1990; Martha et al., 2002) besides this a number of studies worldwide have estimated the prevalence of depression in non-demented elderly to be around 40% (Mann, Graham., & Ashby, 1984; Mann, Schneider, Mozley., 2000). Chalise (2014) using geriatric depression scale found depression to be prevalent in 57.8% of the inmates of OAH in Nepal. A statistically significant correlation was found between feelings of depression and age, sex, previous family type, ethnicity, feeling of loneliness and instrumental activities of daily living. Regression analysis shows that being women, feeling of loneliness and higher the dependency in IADL were predictors of depression among elderly inmates. As cited by (Jané-Llopis, & Gabilondo, 2008) there is no clarity as to whether the prevalence of depression or anxiety increases or decreases with age, these conditions have been found to be high in later life. Depression affects 10-15% of persons over age 65 years but the numbers might be even higher if the whole spectrum of depressive syndromes, including sub clinical depression and depressive symptoms, is considered. Yet this condition is often under-diagnosed and this is particularly true of residents in care homes. Further, co-morbid depression in older people also increases the frequency and cost of professional help and the risk of premature placement into chronic care homes.

The many studies reporting mental health problems were not designed to screen for problems. Rani, Palani and Sathiyasekaran (2012) found 96.7% of elders in OAH suffering from one or other health problems. However, they report only 20.5% of inmates having neurological and mental health problems. The mental health problems reported by them include neurosis (3.3%), senile dementia (3.3%), personality & character disorder (0.5%). Insomnia as separate health problem was found in 19.5% of inmates with higher prevalence among females. It is remarkable that no tool to screen for mental health problems or any diagnostic criteria were used in studies focusing on multiple morbidities.

STRATEGIES TO IMPROVE MENTAL HEALTH PROBLEMS IN OLD AGE HOMES

Rapid socioeconomic changes are forcing the young people to leave their homes and take economically more productive role, leaving frail elderly at home. Institutionalization of elderly has its own problems and still not adequately accepted by all. However, at times there is no better alternative than OAH for the elderly. We need to change the attitude of younger population towards those living in OAH. Elderly living in OAH feel that younger generation lacks respect for them, and perceives them as burden. It might lead to overall efficiency, sociability, degree of involvement in work and hobbies (Dubey, Bhasin, Gupta., & Sharma, 2011).

Elderly are more likely to get institutionalized due to mental and nervous system related problems as these lead to inability to take care at home (Rani et al., 2012). The authors in this study also found health care facilities existing in both governments managed and private OAH. They chose nursing homes randomly. However as pointed out by Gupta et al. (2014), the health facilities are better in paid OAH ensuring the inmates a statistically better quality of life. Ironically only few of those in need of OAH placement can afford to pay Underestimating the mental health issue can impede the management of physical health issues also as mental and physical health problems can also interact in older people making their overall assessment and management more difficult (Jane-Llopis & Gabilondo, 2008). Hence a multidimensional approach focusing at predisposing factors and disability reduction needs to be utilized. Some of these measures can be as follows.

Providing Better Medical Facilities

The international colloquium on the oldest old (2009) observed that those aged 80 years and above have more morbidities and disabilities. Therefore, the current structure of OAH is inadequate. Old age institution with good health care and counselling facilities is the requirement for this age group. Old age health problems present differently from the similar problems of the adults. The response to moderate stresses may also be exaggerated requiring special precautions and care. The data above suggests that more than most of the inmates would have mental health problems and nearly all would have physical health problems (Tiwari et al., 2012). Notwithstanding this fact, most of the OAH have only primary level health care facilities which may also be inadequate. The OAH should be developed in the vicinity of some multispecialty hospital ensuring periodic regular visits by the specialist free of cost or at affordable price. Psychiatrist should be an essential member of the team for geriatric health care. The hospitals should also reserve some minimum number of beds for the elderly persons in case of emergencies.

The Psychosocial Interventions

Social participation is an important component of healthy aging. It involves social contact and engagement in meaningful activities. Socially active older adults have improved quality of life, health, and wellbeing, and are less likely to be depressed or isolated (Perrin & May, 2001). Psychosocial interventions such as cognitive, behavioural, music and supportive interventions can facilitate more active aging and rehabilitation in older adults. The importance of social participation in older adults would be beneficial of three major health problems: dementia, depression, anxiety and substance abuse considered in both home and old age home environments.

Recognizing Elderly as a Vulnerable Group

Elderly age as mentioned above is associated with vulnerabilities. Additionally, the environment of OAH itself is also stressful. The elderly people are predisposed to develop disability for a variety of reasons including mental morbidity. The vulnerabilities and needs of this group should always be considered while formulating any social welfare policy. Additionally, the environment of OAH itself is also stressful. Therefore, as far as possible, migration of elderly to OAH should be prevented or delayed. Ancient Indian scriptures glorify services to elders. "One who always serves and respects elderly is blessed with four things: Long Life, Wisdom, Fame and Power" Manusmriti. Many ancient societies including Indian and Chinese, observed gerontocracy wherein the power is held by a family's oldest members (Mahajan & Ray, 2013). However in recent times the older people prefer shifting to OAH for a variety of reasons which comprise neglected and living alone (36.9%); physical insecurity (16.5%); neglect after decreased income contribution (10.7%); lower medical care expenses and living costs in old-age homes as compared to living alone independently (9.7%); physical and verbal abuse and insults by daughter-in-law and son (8.7%); neglect by family due to high treatment costs and care (6.8%); poverty (5.8%); peaceful and spiritual life (1.9%); drug addict or abusive son (1%); schizophrenic son (1%) and belongings lost in the recent floods (1%).The main reason being the unwillingness of the family to care for aged (Kumar, Bansal., & Bansal, 2008).

A National Policy on older persons in India was announced in January 1999 which identified a number of areas of intervention-financial security, healthcare and nutrition, shelter, education, welfare, protection of life and property for the wellbeing of older persons. The Integrated Program for older people and maintenance of parents and senior citizen act (2007) of India motivates the younger generation for taking care of elderly. Parents are also legally protected against maltreatment by younger generation. Parents cannot be evicted from a house without legal intervention if they have been staying there from before. There are three enactments in India that prevent children from abusing their parents. Under section 125 of the CrPC, a magistrate can order a child to maintain his old parents under the maintenance of parents and senior citizen act (2007). The Hindu Adoptions and Maintenance Act say an aged parent can demand maintenance from children in the same way that a wife can demand it from her husband. The Protection of Women from Domestic Violence Act' 2005 too provides parents with the right to seek relief from any kind of abuse.

Family and Community Support

Many individuals decide to move to the OAH because they feel ignored or not respected by the by the younger generation. Many also feel economically deprived and exploited. At policy level in India the maintenance of parents and senior citizen act (2007) provide guidelines for children to take care of their elderly family members. There should be mutual participation of the younger's and elderly persons in the family and community affairs. For the similar reasons, the OAH should not be just considered as a sheltered place for physical care. The community should be sensitized to visit OAH frequently. A model should be developed for OAH and orphan homes to be in close proximity of each other where the elderly can get a involved in caring for lonely children and the children can get the care and affection from the elderly supplementing the each other's requirements.

Empowering the Old

Not all elderly are disabled, nor a disabled elderly is completely disabled. Many elderly persons openly express their desire to work, make their livelihood and contribute to the community. The OAH management team should involve the inmates who are physically fit for community activates. The old age pension should be permissible to them which should be utilized for their welfare only. Across the world for several decades, number of women joined the workforce is increasing. More married couples earned double incomes during their working years and saved more money for their retirement. In US, private employers and governments began offering better retirement programs. By 1990, senior citizens reported earning 36 percent more income on average than they did in 1980; that was five times the rate of increase for people under age 35 (U.S. Census Bureau, 2009). Government of India discontinued pension to government employees 2006 onwards and offered cumulative provident fund scheme in lieu of that. This decision also leaves the elderly open to financial exploitation of elderly.

However Indian government introduced National Policy on Senior Citizens in 2011 with the policy objectives: The foundation of the new policy, known as the "National Policy for Senior Citizens 2011" is based on several factors. These include the demographic explosion among the elderly, the changing economy and social milieu, advancement in medical research, science and technology and high levels of destitution among the elderly rural poor (51 million elderly live below the poverty line). A higher proportion of elderly women than men experience loneliness and are dependent on children. Social deprivations and exclusion, privatization of health services and changing pattern of morbidity affect the elderly. All those of 60 years and above are senior citizens. This policy addresses issues concerning senior citizens living in urban and rural areas, special needs of the oldest old and older women.

Health care, research, creation of awareness and training facilities to geriatric caregivers have also been enumerated under this policy. The main objective of this policy is to make older people fully independent citizens.

This policy has resulted in the launch of new schemes such as:

1. Strengthening of primary health care system to enable it to meet the health care needs of older persons.
2. Training and orientation to medical and paramedical personnel in health care of the elderly.
3. Promotion of the concept of healthy aging.
4. Assistance to societies for production and distribution of material on geriatric care.
5. Provision of separate queues and reservation of beds for elderly patients in hospitals.
6. Extended coverage under the Antyodaya Scheme with emphasis on provision of food at subsidized rates for the benefit of older persons especially the destitute and marginalized sections.

The Integrated Programme for Older Persons is a scheme that provides financial assistance up to 90 per cent of the project cost to non-governmental organizations or NGOs as on March 31, 2007. This money is used to establish and maintain old age homes, day care centres, mobile Medicare units and to provide non-institutional services to older persons. The scheme also works towards other needs of older persons such as reinforcing and strengthening the family, generation of awareness on related issues and facilitating productive aging.

Another programme of the government is the Scheme of Assistance to Panchayati Raj Institutions voluntary organisations and self-help groups for the construction of old age homes and multi service centres for older persons This scheme provides a onetime construction grant. Central Government Health Scheme provides pensioners of central government offices the facility to obtain medicines for chronic ailments up to three months at a stretch. The National Mental Health Programme [NMHP] focuses on the needs of senior citizens who are affected with Alzheimer's and other dementias, Parkinson's disease, depression and psycho geriatric disorders (Policies & Schemes, 2015).

Care of the Care Givers

Caring for elderly people can be very exhausting experience, which may give rise to severe emotional problems and burn out among the non-formal care givers. The OAH should periodically address the problems and needs of the care givers so as to sufficiently empower them to work for the elderly. Training sessions should be held to ensure their competency in the latest developments. There should be adequate shift duty arrangements and time outs in their routine. However, the knowledge of psychiatric problems at the institutional level requires to be tackled with utmost care. Multidisciplinary approach with mental health profession as an important element in the intervention of the psychopathological problem is the need of the hour. Institutionalization/OAH is here to stay in our society. We need to improvise the needs, merits and an interventional perspective beyond psychopathology. The issue is not just prevention of a problem, but also promotion of general health and mental health is an essential aspect of care of the aged. Hence, perspective on quality of life, subjective well-being and emotional support are key concerns for the elderly in the modern era, irrespective of scientific advances in medical care (Parkar, 2015).

FUTURE RESEARCH DIRECTION

To facilitate a transition into old age with dignity and wellbeing, research is crucial to determine which bio-psychosocial interventions are useful and provide best value for money. This will include an assessment of the comparative effects of interventions to develop methodologies, and improve implementation and effectiveness. Not only is the development of existing psychosocial interventions crucial but it is also vital to take advantage of technological advances in designing new interventions in terms of new model old age homes.

CONCLUSION

This is no controversies to the fact that old age is a special vulnerable group of the community, which is rapidly increasing its proportion in the population. With rapid economic and industrial advancements this group is rapidly getting segregated from the rest of community and left to self for its care. Such socioeconomic change is forcing members of this vulnerable group to seek shelter in OAH for physical mental and emotional reasons. Consequently, OAH are becoming the place for most disabled elderly people of the community. In comparison with community the OAH inmates have higher prevalence of chronic mental illness. The prevalence figures reported for these morbidities are different in different studies. However, dementia, depression, anxiety and substance abuse are the most prevalent morbidities in most of the studies. There is a need to generate data about mental morbidities in larger studies with culture free tools. There is a global movement towards 'successful' aging and a model of care for older adults that focus on maximizing health, wellbeing, and social participation in old age. As with old age care, there has been a shift towards a more psychosocial model of care for older adults, emphasizing the potential for adaptation, rehabilitation and positive change. Further there is also a strong need to generate models of care in OAH so that the OAH are not just a shelter for care but provide satisfying quality of life in a home like environment.

REFERENCES

Agarwal, N., & Jhingan, H. P. (2002). Life events and depression in elderly. *Indian Journal of Psychiatry*, *44*, 34–40. PMID:21206879

Ames, D. (1990). Depression among elderly residents of local authority residential homes.It's nature and efficacy of intervention. *The British Journal of Psychiatry*, *156*(5), 667–675. doi:10.1192/bjp.156.5.667 PMID:2095943

Baltes, P. B., & Baltes, M. M. (Eds.). (1990). *Successful Aging: Perspectives from the Behavioural Sciences*. New York: Cambridge University Press. doi:10.1017/CBO9780511665684

Baltes, P. B., & Smith, J. (1999). Multilevel and systemic analyses of old age: theoretical and empirical evidence for a fourth age. In Handbook of Theories of Aging. Springer.

Bhushan, V., & Sachdeva, D. R. (2002). *An Introduction to Sociology* (34th ed.). Allahabad, India: Kitab Mahal.

Blow, F. C., Brockmann, L. M., & Barry, K. L. (2004). Role of alcohol in late-life suicide. *Alcoholism, Clinical and Experimental Research, 28*(5Suppl), 48S–56S. doi:10.1111/j.1530-0277.2004.tb03603.x PMID:15166636

Boundless. (2015). Continuity Theory. *Boundless Sociology*. Retrieved 20 Dec. 2015 from https://www.boundless.com/sociology/textbooks/boundless-sociology-textbook/aging-18/the-functionalist-perspective-on-aging-128/continuity-theory-723-3593/

Branch, L. G., Wetle, T. T., Scherr, P. A., Cook, N. R., Evans, D. A., Hebert, L. E., & Taylor, J. O. et al. (1988). A prospective study of incident comprehensive medical home care use among the elderly. *American Journal of Public Health, 78*(3), 255–259. doi:10.2105/AJPH.78.3.255 PMID:3124639

Brenes, G. A., Guralnik, J. M., Williamson, J. D., Fried, L. P., Simpson, C., Simonsick, E. M., & Penninx, B. W. J. H. (2005). The influence of anxiety on the progression of disability. *Journal of the American Geriatrics Society, 53*(1), 34–39. doi:10.1111/j.1532-5415.2005.53007.x PMID:15667373

Brenes, G. A., Kritchevsky, S. B., & Mehta, K. M. (2007). Scared to death: Results from the Health, Aging, and Body Composition study. *The American Journal of Geriatric Psychiatry, 15*, 262–265. PMID:17322138

Chalise, H. N. (2014). *Depression among elderly living in Briddashram (OAH). Advances in Aging Research*. AAR.

Cohen, C. I., Magai, C., Yaffee, R., & Walcott-Brown, L. (2006). The prevalence of anxiety and associated factors in a multiracial sample of older adults. *Psychiatric Services (Washington, D.C.), 57*(12), 1719–1725. doi:10.1176/ps.2006.57.12.1719 PMID:17158485

Commission for Architecture and the Built Environment .(2009). Independent living by design CABE London

Dubey, A., Bhasin, S., Gupta, N., & Sharma, N. (2011). A Study of elderly livingin old age home and with infamily set-up in Jammu. *Studies on Home and Community Science, 5*(2), 93–98.

European Monitoring Centre for Drugs and Drug Addiction (EMCDDA). (2008). *Substance use among older adults: a neglected problem.* Available at http://www.emcdda.europa.eu/html.cfm/ index50563EN.html

Ghosh, A. B. (2006). Psychiatry in India: Need to focus on geriatric Psychiatry. *Indian Journal of Psychiatry, 48*(1), 4–9. doi:10.4103/0019-5545.31612 PMID:20703408

Gorman, M. (1999). Development and the rights of older people. In J. Randel et al. (Eds.), *The aging and development report: poverty, independence and the world's older people* (pp. 3–21). London: Earthscan Publications Ltd.

Gowri, G. B. (2003). Attitudes towards old age and aging as shown by humor. *The Gerontologist, 17*(2), 220–226.

Grady, C. L., & Craik, F. I. M. (2000). Changes in memory processing with age. *Current Opinion in Neurobiology, 10*(2), 224–231. doi:10.1016/S0959-4388(00)00073-8 PMID:10753795

Greene, V. L., & Ondrich, J. I. (1990). Risk factors for nursing home admissions and exits: A discrete-time hazard function approach. *Journal of Gerontology Social Science*, *45*(6), 275–276. PMID:2229951

Grimier, H. (2012). Are elderly people living in old age home, less depressed than those of community? Findings from a comparative study. *Journal of Chitwan Medical College*, *1*(2), 2–8.

Gupta, A., Mohan, U., Tiwari, S. C., Singh, S. K., Manar, M. K., & Singh, V. K. (2014). Home away from Home: Quality of Life, Assessment of Facilities and Reason for Settlement in OAH of Lucknow, India. *Indian Journal of Community Health*, *26*(2), 165–169.

Gupta & Sharma. (1992). The oldest old and the use of institutional long term care from an international perspective. New York: Oxford University Press.

IHME. (2010). *Global Burden of Disease Study: Data Downloads*. Retrieved from http://ghdx.healthmetricsandevaluation.org/global-burden-diseasestudy-2010-gbd-2010-data-downloads

Jané-Llopis, E., & Gabilondo, A. (Eds.). (2008). Mental Health in Older People. Consensus Paper. Luxembourg: European Communities.

Joe, V. (2015). *Theories of Aging (Part 3) - Sociological Theories*. Retrieved 20 Dec. 2015 from http://allnurses-breakroom.com/geriatrics-aging-elderly/theories-of-aging-412760.html

Junginger, J., Phelan, E., Cherry, K., & Levy, J. (1993). Prevalence of psychopathology in elderly persons in nursing homes and in the community. *Hospital & Community Psychiatry*, *44*, 381–383. PMID:8462948

Kensinger, E. A. (2004). *Remembering emotional information: Effects of aging and Alzheimer's disease. In Progress in Alzheimer's Disease Research*. Nova.

Kinsella & Phillips. (2005). Global Aging: The Challenge of Success. Population Bulletin, 60(1).

Kumar, M., Bansal, R. K., & Bansal, M. (2008). Need to Support Old-age Home Residents. *Indian Journal of Community Medicine*, *33*(2), 131. doi:10.4103/0970-0218.40887 PMID:19967043

Lenze, E. J., Karp, J. F., & Mulsant, B. H. (2005). Somatic symptoms in late-life anxiety: Treatment issues. *Journal of Geriatric Psychiatry and Neurology*, *18*(2), 89–96. doi:10.1177/0891988705276251 PMID:15911937

Mahajan, A., & Ray. (2013). *Hindu scriptures*. Retrieved from www.hindubooks.org/scriptures/manusmriti/ch2/ch2_121_130.html

Mann, A. H., Graham, N., & Ashby, D. (1984). Psychiatric illness in residential homes for the elderly: A survey in one London borough. *Age and Aging*, *13*(5), 257–265. doi:10.1093/ageing/13.5.257 PMID:6496236

Mann, A. H., Schneider, J., Mozley, C. G., Levin, E., Blizard, R., Netten, A., & Todd, C. et al. (2000). Depression and the response of residential homes to physical health needs. *International Journal of Geriatric Psychiatry*, *15*(12), 1105–1012. doi:10.1002/1099-1166(200012)15:12<1105::AID-GPS252>3.0.CO;2-W PMID:11180466

Martha, L., Gail, J., Patrick, J., Ellen, L., Barnett, S., & Denis, J. (2002). Major depression in elderly home health care patients. *The American Journal of Psychiatry*, *159*(8), 1367–1374. doi:10.1176/appi.ajp.159.8.1367 PMID:12153830

Maulik, S., & Dasgupta, A. (2012). Depression and Determinents in rural elderly of west Bengal-a cross sectional study. *International Journal Biological Medicine Research*, *3*(1), 1299–1302.

Nandi, P. S., Banerjee, G., & Mukherjee, S. P. (1997). A study of psychiatric morbidity of elderly population of a rural community in West Bengal. *Indian Journal of Psychiatry*, *39*, 122–129. PMID:21584058

Parkar, S. R. (2015). Elderly mental health: Needs. *Mens Sana Monographs*, *13*(1), 91–99. doi:10.4103/0973-1229.153311 PMID:25838727

Perrin, T., & May, H. (2001). *Wellbeing in dementia: An occupational approach for therapists and carers*. Edinburgh, UK: Churchill Livingstone.

Pesic, L. (2007). Social and health problems of the elderly. *ActaMedica Medianae*, *46*, 45–48.

Policies & Schemes. (2016). Retrieved January 18, 2016, from, Phttp://www.archive.india.gov.in/citizen/senior_citizen/senior_citizen.php?id=12

Priscilla, E. (2005). *Gerontological nursing and healthy aging*. Elsevier Health Sciences.

Rajkumar, A. P., Thangadurai, P., Senthilkumar, P., Gayathri, K., Prince, M., & Jacob, K. S. (2009). Nature, Prevalance and Factors Associated with Depression among the Elderly in Rural South Indian Community. *International Psychogeriatrics*, *21*(2), 372–378. doi:10.1017/S1041610209008527 PMID:19243657

Ramesh, K.G., & Sridhara, m.v. (2013). *Health Status of Elderly Living in the Old Age Homes: An Overview JMSD*. Academic Press.

Rangaswamy, S. M. (2001). Geneva, Switzerland: The World Health Organization; World Health Report on Mental Health: New understanding New Hope. *Indian Journal of Psychiatry*, *43*(1), 1–4. PMID:21407829

Rani, M., Palani, G., & Sathiyasekaran, B. W. C. (2012). Morbidity profile of elders in OAH in Chennai. *National Journal of Community Medicine*, *3*(3), 458–464.

Rose, M. R. (1991). *Evolutionary Biology of Aging*. New York: Oxford University Press.

Sadava, D., Hillis, D., Heller, C., & Berenbaum, M. (2011). *Life: The science of biology* (9th ed.). Sunderland, MA: Sinauer Associates Inc.

Salthouse, T. A. (1991). The processing-speed theory of adult age differences in cognition. *Psychological Review*, *103*(3), 403–428. doi:10.1037/0033-295X.103.3.403 PMID:8759042

Schonfeld, I., & Dupree, I. W. (1995). Treatment approaches for older problem drinkers. *The International Journal of the Addictions*, *30*(13-14), 1819–1842. doi:10.3109/10826089509071057 PMID:8751320

Seignourel, P. J., Kunik, M. E., & Snow, L. (2008). Anxiety in dementia: A critical review. *Clinical Psychology Review*, 7. PMID:18555569

Seitz, D. P., Brisbin, S., Herrmann, N., Rapoport, M. J., Wilson, K., Gill, S. S., & Conn, D. et al. (2012). Efficacy and feasibility of nonpharmacological interventions for neuropsychiatric symptoms of dementia in long term care: A systematic review. *Journal of American Medical Directorate Association, 13*(6), 503–506. doi:10.1016/j.jamda.2011.12.059 PMID:22342481

Sen, K. (1994). *Aging: Debates on Demographic Transition and Social Policy*. London: Zed Books Ltd.

Singh, A., & Misra, N. (2009). A study on Loneliness, Depression and Sociability. *Industrial Psychiatry Journal, 18*(1), 51–52. doi:10.4103/0972-6748.57861 PMID:21234164

Starkstein, S. E., Jorge, R., Petracca, G., & Robinson, R. G. (2007). The construct of generalized anxiety disorder in Alzheimer disease. *The American Journal of Geriatric Psychiatry, 15*(1), 42–49. doi:10.1097/01.JGP.0000229664.11306.b9 PMID:17194814

Thane, P. (1978). The muddled history of retiring at 60 and 65. *New Society, 45*(826), 234–236.

Tiwari, S. C. (2012). Geriatric Psychiatric Morbidity in Rural Northern India: Implications for the Future. *International Psychogeriatrics, 12*(1), 35–48. doi:10.1017/S1041610200006189 PMID:10798452

United Nations Population Division (UN). (2011). *World Population Prospects: The 2010 Revision*. Accessed at http://esa.un.org/unpd/wpp/index.htm

U.S. Census Bureau. (2009). *Webinar on 2008 Income, Poverty, and Health Insurance Estimates from the Current Population Survey*. Retrieved February 13, 2012 (http://www.census.gov/newsroom/releases/archives/news_conferences/2009-09-10_remarks_johnson.html)

Vern, L. B., & Norella, P. (2009). *Handbook of theories of aging*. Springer Publishing Company.

Voice, O. (2009). *Shaping our aging society*. Help the Aged and Age Concern.

WHO. (2010). *mhGAP-IG*. Retrieved from http://whqlibdoc.who.int/publications/2010/9789241548069_eng.pdf

WHO. (2012). *Dementia: a public health priority*. World Health Organization, Alzheimer's disease International. Retrieved from http://apps.who.int/iris/bitstream/10665/75263/1/9789241564458_eng.pdf

Wittchen, H. U., Kessler, R. C., & Beesdo, K. (2002). Generalized anxiety and depression in primary care: Prevalence, recognition, and management. *The Journal of Clinical Psychiatry, 63*(8), 24–34. PMID:12044105

Zachariah, e. t. k. c., Mathew, s., & Irudaya, r. (2000). *Socio-Economic and Demographic Consequenes of Migration in Kerala*. Academic Press.

KEY TERMS AND DEFINITIONS

Aging: A multi-dimensional process and affects almost every aspect of human life.

Anxiety: Anxiety refers to pervasive anxiety which is not restricted to specific external situations and is not associated with the consistent and extensive avoidance behaviour which characterizes phobia.

Dementia: Dementia is a syndrome involving deterioration in memory, thinking, behaviour and the ability to perform everyday activities such as dressing, eating, personal hygiene and toilet activities.

Depression: Depression refers to a range of mental conditions characterized by persistent low mood, absence of positive affect (loss of interest and enjoyment in ordinary things and experiences), and a range of associated emotional, cognitive, physical and behavioural symptoms.

Old Age Home (OAH): A modern day shelter for aged individual. Who may spend their late life willingly or forcefully in that place.

Substance Use Disorder (SUD): Also known as drug use disorder, SUD is a condition in which the use of one or more substances leads to a clinically significant impairment or distress.

Chapter 3
Chronic Mental Illness and Dumping Patients:
A Concern towards Management

Jyoti Mishra Pandey
RINPAS, India

Preeti Mishra
Sri Mahant Indiresh Medical College, India

Shobit Garg
Sri Mahant Indiresh Medical College and Hospital, India

Bholeshwar Parshad Mshra
DMC Ludhiana, India

ABSTRACT

Patients with mental illness don't take care of themselves, are dependent not only for medicine intake but also for their day to day requirements including their personal hygiene. All these issues and many more put a heavy psychological burden on the families. When they become overburdened with these responsibilities and problems they find it easy to dump patients in the mental institutes. There are very few mental health institutes in India but the number of patients with chronic mental illness is very high. The common problems are poor social environment, hostile family environment, unaffordable prices of medicines Few efforts like proper psycho-education, frequent phonic follow-ups from the professionals, proper guidance, family therapy, supportive psychotherapy etc. can be done. The government should also take some steps to manage the chronically ill patients like following strict rules to avoid dumping patients in the mental health institutes. Proper vocational training and job perspective should be planned for these populations so that they can be less dependent on their families.

The mentally ill people frighten and embarrass us...and so we marginalize the people who most need our acceptance. What mental health needs is more love, more affection and more unashamed conversation. (Anonymous)

Any kind of illness whether medical or psychological puts a lot of stress not only on the patient but also on people living with them like their families and care takers. Situation becomes all the more different and difficult when it comes to any psychiatric illness. The attitude and behaviour changes not only of

DOI: 10.4018/978-1-5225-0519-8.ch003

the families and caretakers of the patient but also of the society towards them. It is known that a human is a social animal and without society it is difficult to survive. Therefore, any deviation from the social norms and standard is either changed or excluded from the society. Mental illness is one of those major social stigmas which have excluded many families of the persons who are suffering from mental illness from the society. Not only the social stigma but other social issues like economical condition, disturbed family environment, and chronicity of illness are the major issues which give rise to a very serious situation called "dumping". Dumping patients in the mental institutes has become a very serious issue of our society. It has become a very easy way out for those families and caretakers who take these chronically ill mental patients as burden and because of this the institutions are becoming overloaded with dumped patients. Who is at fault for these dumping; the family or the society? The question is why this is happening? Why families or care takers are running away from their responsibilities? What problems are the caretakers facing with the chronically ill mental patients? Is it avoidable? What step or change is required to stop these patients dumping? The focus of the current topic would be to understand the seriousness of dumping and those factors that are leading to this dumping and what can be done to avoid this situation.

INTRODUCTION

Mental health is psychological well-being of a person. There is no fixed definition of mental illness. As defined by WHO, "health is state of complete physical, mental and social well-being and not merely the absence of disease or infirmity" (WHO, 2006). At its Sixty-fifth session, held in May 2012, the World Health Assembly adopted a resolution calling on WHO to develop, in consultation with Member States, a comprehensive action plan that actively addresses not only the need for early identification and appropriate care for persons with mental disorders, but also assesses vulnerabilities and risks as a basis for developing the mental health plan (WHO, 2012). Chronicity of mental illness is very prolonged and severe in nature. It involves severe psychotic disorders like schizophrenia, mood disorders like mania and depression and other behavioural disorders etc. Prevalence of mental disorders as per World Health Report, 2001 is around 10% and it is predicted that burden of disorders is likely to increase by 15% by 2020 (Indian Council of Medical Research [ICMR], 2005). A study showed that about one in four United States [U.S.] adults (26.2%) age 18 and older, in any given year, has a mental disorder (e.g., mood disorder, anxiety disorder, impulse control disorder, or substance abuse disorder) (Kessler, Chiu, Demler., & Walters, 2005), meaning that mental disorders are common and can affect anyone. Many adults with common chronic medical conditions such as arthritis, cancer, diabetes, heart disease experience concurrent depression and anxiety—further complicating self-management of these disorders and adversely affecting quality of life (Chapman, Perry., & Strine, 2005; El-Gabalawy, Cox, Clara., & Mackenzie, 2010; IOM, 2012). In another study it was seen that the police officers frequently encounter people with mental illness—approximately 5 percent of U.S. residents have a serious mental illness, and 10 to 15 percent of jailed people have severe mental illness (Lamb, Weinberger., & Gross, 2004). The Lincoln (Nebraska) Police Department found that it handled over 1,500 mental health investigation cases in 2002, and that it spent more time on these cases than on injury traffic accidents, burglaries, or felony assaults (Lincoln Police Department, 2004). The New York City Police Department responds to about 150,000 "emotionally disturbed persons" calls per year (Waldman, 2004).

It is a common notion that chronically ill mental patients cannot live a normal life and they do not have emotional aspect and are unable to use their thinking ability in their daily life. Chronicity of any illness does not mean that his or her reasoning or thinking capacity becomes zero. When it comes to mental illness, except for few disorders, the patients have and can use their intelligence and thinking process and a very important aspect is that they have and they can show emotional ability or feelings. They also feel humiliated when they are discriminated by the society. The pain becomes intolerable when they are not accepted even by their own family members. Some families find these mentally ill patients especially older patients useless and a burden to the family. If a visit is given to the mental hospitals, it will be shocking to know that some patients are dumped to the mental hospitals before independence. Few of them when they were dumped to the hospital they were just in their teens but now they are in their 70s and 80s. Some of them have died in the mental hospitals but nobody has turned up from their families. The condition of women, whether mentally healthy or unhealthy, is very dreadful in Indian society. A mentally healthy woman faces various social and family expectations and pressure in their entire life. One can imagine the plight of mentally ill women which is even worse. A report by NDTV India (2014) gave a very startling revelation. They interviewed 52 women and girls who had been institutionalized because for their mental disabilities in two years, as well as their families, staff members and doctors at the institutions where the patients were treated in four Indian states. They reported 31 cases of electroconvulsive therapy administered "without consent," though in many cases familial consent replaces patient consent. It was also reported that 38 cases of physical abuse, with many patients reporting that they were beaten with sticks. The group's researchers witnessed this in three institutions where patients were beaten if they did not walk fast. Researchers also found four cases of sexual abuse reported in residential institutions. Sadly, many cases of sexual exploitations and ill treatment of mentally ill woman remain unreported and even if it is reported the police does not listen to them as they say that how can they take the complains of those who are mentally unhealthy. Surprisingly, majority of such abuse takes place at home by some of their relatives than in the institutions and they remain unnoticed and unreported. The families of mentally ill female try to dump the patients in the institution because they think that nobody will marry her and she will be a burden for them for life long.

Women and girls with intellectual disabilities or mental illness in India are subject to forced institutionalization, most of the times in overcrowded and unsanitary conditions, verbal and physical abuse, and medication without consent. Nobody from their family members is even bothered to come and see them. The cases that are managed well in the institutions their problem increases when they are discharged and come back to social life. Their family do not accept them or take it as a burden that nobody will marry her and will waste money on their medicines. Unemployment and dependency on family members, social rejection, pressure and stigma puts a lot of pressure on the mental condition of the women and that often worsens the condition and leads to frequent relapses. Sadly, they live with the illness in the society and at the end they die with the illness unattended and unwanted.

A very common problem that family and caretakers face is non-compliance of the patient towards medicine and frequent relapses, making the illness more chronic and serious. A very common mistake usually done by the patients and family members is that when thc patient is maintaining well after taking medicine, they stop the medicine immediately that often leads to relapse. Another issue is that the patients and families don't come for follow up that makes the condition of the illness even poorer. The reasons for this could be many but the commonest reason could be the financial constraints or the distance of mental institutes from their residence. When it comes to medical illness, the cases are handled very carefully but when it comes to mental illness instead of dealing with carefully the additional pressure has been attached to them like stigma, social isolation and marginalisation. How would it be if a person were treated as a second-class patient just because of the type of illness that he had? The attitudes and beliefs about mental illness are shaped by personal knowledge about mental illness, knowing and interacting with someone living with mental illness, cultural stereotypes about mental illness, media stories, and familiarity with institutional practices and past restrictions (Corrigan, Markowitz., & Watson, 2004; Wahl, 2003).

Chronic mental illness is a serious concern in our society. It makes the patient dependent and less functional in their day to day activities. Patients' chronic mental illness puts a heavy burden on the families and care takers. Patients with mental illness are perceived as a disturbance in the family, they don't take care of themselves, are dependent not only for medicine intake but also for their day to day requirements including even their personal hygiene. All these issues and many more put a heavy psychological burden on the families. When they become overburdened with these responsibilities and problems they find it easy to dump patients in the mental institutes. If these problems are not handled properly then this can be a very serious issue and the mental institutes in India will be overloaded with dumped patients. There are very few mental health institutes in India but the number of patients with chronic mental illness is very high.

INDIAN SCENARIO

India is a place where psychiatric illness is seen as a contagious disease. Social stigma and discrimination put a lot of pressure on the patients. According to various community based surveys, prevalence of mental disorders in India is 6-7% for common mental disorders and 1-2% for severe mental disorders. In India the rate of psychiatric disorders in children aged between 4 to 16 years is about 12% and nearly one-third of the population is less than 14 years of age. With such a magnitude of mental disorders it becomes necessary to promote mental health services for the well being of general population, in addition to provide treatment for mental illnesses. Treatment gap for severe mental disorders is approximately 50% and in case of Common Mental Disorders it is over 90% (Ministry of Health and Family Welfare [MHFW], 2013). The condition of mental patients in India is very distressing. Even in the institutions the treatment of mentally ill patients is not satisfactory. A report by Sharma (2013) stated that in India mentally ill population are often locked away in understaffed institutions where they are deprived of even basic human rights. Others are picked up by quacks who torture them in the name of religious healing, or they dump them in the jungle. She has reported that in a Mental Hospital in a metro city of India, about 30 male patients in tattered clothes struggle in a dormitory. The foul smell from the bathrooms nearby is nauseating. On the next floor, two female patients lie unattended on the corridor outside a female dormitory. At another Mental Hospital, about 400 patients share 250 beds. Patients at a severe stage of mental illness are locked up in small overcrowded cubicles. To kill body lice patients are stripped and sprayed with insecticides which are used for killing pests. The funds that come to the hospital for food, clothing and medicines are taken away by the officials. Most mental hospitals are in a deplorable condition. According to the National Human Rights Commission (NHRC, 2015), there are only 43 government mental hospitals in India, of which hardly half a dozen are in a liveable condition. The NHRC was asked to report on the condition of mental hospitals in the 1990s. They brought out the first report in 1999; the condition of most mental hospitals was shocking. Even after two decades, it remains the same. It shows poor attitude towards the mental health care in the country. The fact is the NHRC's reports in

1999 and 2011 look almost similar. Most hospitals lacked, and still lack, even clean water and hygiene. At least 100 million people suffer from mental illness in India. About 10 million need hospitalization. There are only 4,000 psychiatrists in the country and 70 percent of them practice in private hospitals in urban areas. There is a severe shortage of paramedics. In 2008, according to an NHRC report, one single psychiatrist was found operating the 331-bed hospital in Varanasi. There are physicians and even gynaecologists who are in charge of mental hospitals. These doctors don't understand the intricacies of a psychiatric illnesses and the comprehensive care the patients require.

In Indian scenario as far as mental illness is concerned, the faith healers come before a psychiatrist (Bathla, Chandan, Bathla, & Kaloiya, 2015). The faith healers are making money without any knowledge and education because of the prevalent superstitions in Indian culture. The way the faith healers in India deal with the mentally ill patients is very horrifying. The patients are beaten up severely, they are asked to inhale smoke of burnt chilli and they are chained, sometimes even for life time. In 2001, a fire in a coastal village of Tamil Nadu charred to death 26 mental patients, who could not escape the fire as they were chained (Sharma, 2013). It is also very shocking to know that the female mental patients are often sexually abused by the faith healers and sadly because of the mental illness they cannot complain. When the families and caretakers don't see any improvement, the best way they find is dumping them in either the institutions or would let them wonder aimlessly in the society.

FACTORS AFFECTING DUMPING PATIENTS

It is said that for any problem there is a particular cause or factor that are responsible for the occurrence of the problem or the illness and at the same time no single factor contributes to any illness especially mental illness. When we talk about chronic mental illness multiple factors plays its role, such as the environment, the society and the family.

Social Factors

Environment plays a very important role in shaping one's behaviour and personality. Society is a very important institution when we talk about environmental factor. In terms of chronic mental illness, society plays a very vital role. As per the social definition, those who do not fall in the socially defined norms and conditions are either punished or leftover by the society. The society marginalizes those who are different from them. They are not allowed to attend social functions. Other members create distance from their family members. They don't marry in that family where a mentally ill patient live. In a study it was reported that when stigma leads to social exclusion or discrimination (experienced stigma), it results in unequal access to resources that all people need to function well: educational opportunities, employment, a supportive community, including friends and family, and access to quality health care (Link & Phelan, 2001; Corrigan, Markowitz., & Watson, 2004). Therefore, many families because of the social stigma and pressure either leave the patient to wonder in the society or dump the patient in the mental institution. These individuals even if they have recovered or become asymptomatic they still face social ignorance and can't live their life as normal as others in the society are living. When they come out or discharged from the hospital, they are not accepted by them. They don't get jobs and also face humiliation by the society. Therefore, because of these individual factors a significant pressure comes on the person suffering from chronic mental illness and on their families and caretakers. This leads to emotional and psychological break down of the person and the family member and end result comes up with either throwing the mentally ill person out of the house, or are being dumped either in the mental institutes or in the jails or prison. It is also seen that many patients who are admitted in the mental institutes themselves do not want to go back to their homes because of the humiliation, social pressure and social stigma. A study has shown that being unemployed, living at or below the poverty line, being socially isolated, and living with other social disadvantages can further deflate self-esteem, compounding mental illness symptoms, and add to the burden of stigma (Sartorius, 2005) and it was also found in a study that an increased risk of death at younger ages for people with mental illness (Colton & Manderscheid, 2006).

Society is a place which reflects all the positive and negative aspects of life. Positively, the society grows when a person grows but negatively, it also stops a person who wants to grow. It stops a person who is deviant from the social norms and standards. Chronic mental illness is a situation where a person who is suffering from the illness is negatively accepted by the society. After coming from the mental health institutions, the society does not give a warm welcome to the patient. There are many questions that the society arises for themselves, for the families and for the individual who is suffering from chronic mental illness. The society thinks whether he or she is safe for the other people living in the society? Is he or she become normal? What example will they set for other normal people? Do they deserve a second chance to live in the society? What if they break the expectations of the society? Are the other members of the family safe under a single roof? What other children and young generation will learn after seeing his or her abnormal behaviour? How the financial issues like money for the medicine, regular follow up will be managed? On the other hand, the individual who is suffering from chronic mental illness thinks that will I be accepted by the family members and the society?

So, society has a very significant role to play when it comes to chronic mental illness. Even if a mentally ill patient is roaming or wandering around the street, very few will come in front to take them to the hospital or will report to the police. In a study it was reported that attitudes toward mental illness can also influence how policymakers allocate public resources to mental health services, pose challenges for staff retention in mental health settings, result in poorer quality of medical care administered to people with mental illness, and create fundraising challenges for organizations who serve people with mental illness and their families (Kadri & Sartorius, 2005; Pescosolido et al., 2010; Stuart, 2005).

Individual Factors

A person's life starts even before birth that is pre-natal phase, even there the environmental factor can severely affect a growing foetus. These are genetic factors, maternal infections like rubella leading to microcephaly, maternal stress, and intake of teratogenic drugs during pregnancy. After this pre-natal phase, the neonatal and childhood phase comes where various other factors like medical issues or psychological issues can affect a person significantly. These issues are any infection or illness, non- congenial and hostile family environment and many more. The adolescent phase comes with major storming physical and psychological changes. Positive changes would lead to positive mental health and negative changes would lead to negative mental health like mental illness. During the adolescent phase a very major concern is intake of drugs or substance abuse. The peer pressure makes an individual more vulnerable to indulge in various other activities which can make an adolescent's mental health poorer, such as, getting bullied or being terrorized by others, substance abuse and very importantly unsafe sex and HIV/AIDS. The next phase after adolescent is adulthood, where various psychological and environment pressure takes place. The family pressure and burden, over expectation by others, relationship problems, financial issues, any medical problem, hostile family environment and marital issues are those factors that influence a person significantly. Apart from these issues a very common issue is isolation in adulthood, for example, divorce, separation or death of a spouse and a very limited group or friend circle. These factors can either cause mental illness or can be a co-morbid condition of any medical illness like Diabetes, cancer or HIV/AIDS etc. with these medical illnesses depression is a very common mental co morbidity. The next phase comes with old age, where a significant change takes place, for example, cognitive decline and dementia, Parkinson's disease. Older adults are also particularly at high risk of social isolation, retirement, unsteady income, and also become more susceptible to chronic disease which may deprive them of their mobility, independence and cognitive skills. These often gives rise various psychiatric illness. So, the individual risk factors which forms a cycle and start from *prenatal -to-neonatal -to- childhood -to- adolescent -to- adulthood -to- old age.* This cycle can get triggered at any stage of life cycle and can psychologically hamper a person significantly.

The other individual factor is secure and supportive environment, and a healthy childhood behind them. An adolescent personality is also a very confounding factor. His or her self-esteem, emotional control or vulnerability, way of dealing with the challenging situation, healthy coping mechanism, attribution style, parental care, healthy family environment, healthy peer group, social intelligence and many more factors can make an individual's emotional and psychological condition healthier. However, non-congenial and hostile family environment makes the mental health poor. A child with parents who has a mental illness or substance use disorder is placed at a high risk of experiencing family discord and psychiatric problems. The other confounding factors are persistent beating, severe bullying, parental loss or abuse - can cause a level of trauma that has many a times an ineradicable effect over the rest of the person's life. Other environmental conditions like poor housing or living conditions, lack of opportunities for productive learning and social interaction, may increase their exposure to disease and infections and illnesses.

The genetic and environment plays a significant role in mental health, both can make the environment healthier or it can make the environment even more badly. Similarly, if the genetic risk is high but the environment condition is very healthy then the chance of getting any psychiatric illness reduces. In contrast, if the genetic risk is nil but the environment risk factor is very high and worse than the chance of getting mental illness is very high. Fortunately, the environmental condition can be controlled by an individual. So, mental illness can be controlled or reduced by controlling or by making the environment healthy.

To summarize, the individual factors leading to dumping patients in the institutions are;

1. The *humiliation and discrimination* from the society and family increases the chance of dumping patients in the institutions.
2. Many a time patients feel *safer in institution* then in the home and society.
3. The chronic mental patients get *basic needs of life* in the institution which they know that they will not get from the family and from the society.
4. *Fear of isolation* and difficulty to restart their life in the society forces them to live in the institutions.
5. *Difficulty in fulfilling expectations* of the families and society

Family Factors

The home is a place where a person comes back from all the loads and responsibility of the external world and the family members at the home are those who motivate a person to go out, work and secure the future of the family members. Family member ties a very emotional knot with each other. Miserably if the family environment becomes disturbed then that emotional bond becomes emotional burden on the family members when a person is diagnosed with some mental illness. As the symptom of mental illness is different from the symptoms of medical illness the family members face various difficulties while dealing with the mentally ill patients. Very common issues are financial burden, over emotional expression, hostile environment, overloaded responsibility and many more. These factors are the major and common cause of dumping patients in the mental institute. It was reported by Lewis (2014) that there are 10 times more mentally ill Americans in prisons and jails than in state psychiatric hospitals. Adding to that those individuals' condition often deteriorate while they are imprisoned. In 2012, there were an estimated 356,268 inmates with severe mental illnesses in U.S. prisons and jails. There were only 35,000 mentally ill individuals in state psychiatric hospitals. Some mentally ill prisoners refuse treatment because they are unaware of their illness, which worsens their symptoms. Treatment for mental illness is a right affirmed by the U.S. Supreme Court (Lewis, 2014). Perhaps, the reason could be that if the family member admits the patient to the mental institute then they have to take the economical responsibility of admission and for medicine of the patient but if they will be in prison then the responsibility would be of police and administration and not of the family members. The patient because of the illness is unable to say anything and on the other hand the family members would not come to the prison to take them out. This is a very easy way out of the family members and caretakers to avoid responsibility. They also think that as they are good for nothing, so by taking them home will add more to the problem and from their behaviour the children and the young members of the family will also learn hostile behaviour. As the mentally ill person often show a very high emotional expression, their psychotic symptoms like suspiciousness and aggressive behaviour creates a very hostile environment in the family. They demand more attention and care for all their needs and requirement and thus because of these issues family members and caretakers try to avoid and shrink the responsibility of the patient and that give rise to dumping the chronically ill mental patients to the institutes.

To summarize, there are some key factors that affect chronic mental illness and increasing chances to dump chronically ill mental patients' in the mental institute:

- *Dependency* on the families and caretakers is a significant factor of dumping patients in the mental institutes.
- *Lifelong intake of medicine* of the patients and related financial issues and burden is another major cause of dumping patients in the mental institutes.
- *Psychotic behaviour* creating chaos, difficulty, disturbing the mental piece of the family members and creating unhealthy environment in the family is another factor giving rise to dumping patients in the mental institutes.
- *Disturbing the privacy* of the families and caretakers is another factor of dumping patients in the mental institutes.
- *Unemployment* of the patients making the condition worse and increasing the chances of dumping patients in the mental institutes.

- *Social stigma and pressure* on the family members and caretakers for having mental patients at home creates shame in families also leads to dumping the patients in mental institutes.

Unemployment

Unemployment is a huge problem with vast repercussions, where even a mentally fit and healthy person is regarded as worthless in a society. India is a place where because of the over population, a large chunk of population is unemployed and dependent on others. In such a scenario providing job perspectives to the chronically ill mental patients can be a very difficult goal to achieve. On the other hand, leaving this population unemployed can create burden on mentally ill patients' families, caretakers and society. An individual who is not working and at the same time because of symptoms of his mental health creates chaos or unhealthy environment in the family, their dependency on the family members for their daily requirement puts a lot of financial burden on the family members. As the psychiatric medicines are costly and in many cases the patient requires lifelong medication, the family members do not take care of the patients properly and do not give medicine regularly. This often leads to relapse of the patients. The family members and caretakers often do not go for the patients' follow up sessions because of the fees and travelling charges. These financial burden and dependency of the patients mainly the unemployment of the patients plays significant role in dumping them in the institutions.

MISUSE OF SERVICE BY FAMILY

Institutions and the hospitals are the place where patients' either come by themselves or brought by the family members or caretakers for the treatment and to live a healthy life. The doctors and the mental health workers take treating patients as worshiping God. However, the situation becomes reverse when families and care takers misuses the advantages and the facilities of the given hospital or the institute. They leave or dump the patient to the hospital and for this they give false information to the doctors so that they cannot trace the address and ask or force them to take their patients back at home. It is very distressing that because of the chronicity of the illness families or care takers are running away from their responsibilities. The best way for the family to get rid of their problems is to just dump the patient in the mental institute. This is a very common pattern of dumping patients. The mental health institutions are overloaded with the dumped patients.

The institutions' capacities are very less in numbers in comparison to the population suffering from mental illness. The institutions are also having less quality and quantity of manpower. The institutions because of the overburdened patients and less staff members for their care have inadequate facilities. These overcrowded facilities are often unmonitored. As per the NDTV (2014) report a government-run institution in New Delhi operating at nearly three times its capacity. At Pune Mental Hospital, there were just 25 working toilets for more than 1,850 patients. Shockingly, even the institutions are taking money by the families and caretakers of the mentally ill person for keeping them in the institutions, no matter whether they have resources or not. It was reported by an Indian Journalist Sharma (2013) that the mentally ill patients are getting dumped in jungles also, especially in the forest reserves of south India. Families, mostly from the north, pay lorry drivers to 'drop' these hapless victims, including children and women, in the forest ranges. Social activists in reserves such as Wayanad and Bandipur say drivers rape the female victims before dumping them at the mercy of nature. In some countries, people with severe mental disorders are inappropriately locked up in prisons simply because of the lack of mental health services. People with substance abuse disorders or people who, at least in part due to a mental disorder, have committed minor offences are often sent to prison rather than treated for their disorder. These disorders therefore continue to go unnoticed, undiagnosed and untreated (WHO, 2007)

ROLE OF VARIOUS DOMAINS

Role of Government

Chronic mental illness is not only a family or a society's issue but the government should be equally concerned about them. The government has various schemes and plans for the chronically ill mental patients on the basis of their functional disability because of the prolonged mental illness. Various facilities and concessions are given to them by the government on the basis of their functional ability. However, the main problem is majority of the population is unaware about the facilities available for them. The large piece of mental health professionals does not even bother to give proper information and counselling to the families of mentally ill patients. The government should plan various other programs for mentally ill patients so that the problem that they and their families are facing can be controlled. Like, plan to provide good job opportunities when they come out from institution after treatment. The government should also plan strict action and a law for those who are dumping them and creating discrimination for them. Other issues like the mental illness treatment are very expensive because of its chronicity and prolonged intake of medicine. Insurance companies cover medical illness but avoid covering for mental illnesses.

Many of the mentally ill patients instead of going for the treatment, they are send to the prisons. The reason is the unawareness among general public regarding mental illness and it is an associated with co morbidity. Their aggressive behaviour, hostile and abusive nature, some anti-social traits are considered a crime and are send to prisons and the vicious cycle of dumping. Prisons are the wrong and worst place for many people in need of mental health treatment, since the criminal justice system emphasizes on punishment rather than treatment and care. This results in worsening of the clinical condition of the mental patients and they start deteriorating. Laws can be introduced which allows for the shifting of prisoners who have been wrongly detained to psychiatric facilities at all stages of trial (arrest, prosecution and imprisonment). For prisoners who are mentally ill who have been charged with minor offences, the introduction of ways and means to divert them towards mental health services before they reach prison will ensure that they receive the treatment they need and also help in reducing the prison population. The imprisonment of people with mental illness due to deficiency of public mental health services should be strictly prohibited by law. Mental health legislation can be a powerful measure to protect the rights of people with a mental illness, including prisoners. Mental health laws are outdated and fail to address the mental health needs of the prison population. The development of legal provisions that deal with mental health needs of mentally ill person include: the right to quality treatment and care, to maintain confidentiality, to protection from discrimination and violence, and to protection from torture and other cruel, inhuman and humiliating treatment (WHO, 2007).

Role of Institutions

The institutions are overloaded with the patients who are dumped by their families and caretakers. The families are fudging from their responsibility and taking an easy way out to either throw the patient out of their house or let them roam around or dump the patients in either in the hospital or in the institution. Many a times even in the hospitals and institutions the mental patients are not treated well or completely. Some hospitals have been accused of not even stabilizing patients before sending or discharging them as they do not take the patients as their own responsibility. They are often discharged without any documentations and proper pre- discharge counselling sessions.

If we see these problems, it is essential to think that where is the system lacking in dealing with such situations? First, the institutions whether private or government require more doctors, more psychologists, more social workers and better infrastructure for them because the mentally ill patients are very high in numbers but the resources to deal with it is very less. Secondly, there are few cautions that every institute should take from their side to avoid dumping patients like admitting patients for a very limited period of time, various formalities and detailed information of the relatives and care takers of the patients should be taken. After the patient shows improvement, the relatives and care takers are being informed about the patient discharge through proper channel. However, despite of all the precautions, dumping of patients in the mental hospitals are increasing day by day. Even if they are not dumped in the hospitals we can see them wandering around in the society.

Mental health promotion program can be done with the aim to reduce the risk factors that contribute to poor mental health and enhance the protective factors, which contribute to good mental health. With this effort a serious problem of dumping patients in the institutions can be avoided. The mental health professionals should work together as a team to avoid this situation. The promotion of mental health also produces many other benefits like health, social, and economic benefits. Interventions to promote good mental health include: strengthening parenting skills in early childhood; preventing or reducing bullying in schools, social awareness campaign, reducing stigma and discrimination and many supportive interventions. The absence of protective factors in the presence of risk factors can result in behaviours associated with poor mental health, such as increased crime, low educational attainment, problematic substance use, depression and suicide, all of which have broader social and economic consequences. Both risk and protective factors can exist at the individual, community, and structural levels, as well as in different settings and situations (NeLMH, 2004). For example, some of the protective factors at the individual level for the entire population include self-esteem, a sense of coherence, personal coping skills, social support, sense of mastery or control, ability to form and sustain satisfying relationships, resilience, sense of belonging, and optimism. (MHPU, 2003; Moodie & Jenkins, 2005). These are also indicators of good mental health. Risk behaviours, social and economic problems, and rates and severity of physical and mental illness can be reduced by strengthening protective factors for good mental health (NeLMH, 2004). So, the role of the institution should not be limited to dealing with mental illness but also to the promotion of mental health. Promotion of mental health and awareness among society and its members regarding mental illness can help to reduce stigma and can increase the acceptance of patients among society.

Role of Society

The society is a family where all the members live together. As it is well known that man is a social animal and living against society and its' norms will be difficult for any member of the society including those members also who are not mentally healthy. Social stigma and mental illness has become a part of a mentally ill person's life and because of this their life has become more complicated. This is also a major obstacle in their treatment and recovery. Social isolation, unemployment, poor economic conditions, poor housing are the additional factors worsening the condition of the chronically ill mental patients. However, it is said that many of the mental health problems of the individuals can be recovered if proper care and support is given to them and mainly the acceptance from the family and society. The situation has been made difficult not only by the society but also by their families, caretakers, friends and workplace. Therefore, the people suffering from chronic mental illness faces problems in finding work, maintain a healthy and positive relationships, are not included in any social gathering or in main stream society and they do not live a respectful life in the society. The focal reason of their suffering is many a time these social stereotyped views and behaviour. Majority of the social members think that the chronic mental ill patients are dangerous and violent to others but in reality the mentally ill people themselves are more prone to these violence and attacks.

Apart from society and its stigma and discrimination, the condition of the mentally ill person is exacerbated by the role of the media. The media plays as a role model for the society but media has presented a very cruel and bad picture of mentally ill person. There is a wrong belief in the society that these individuals cannot live a normal and healthy life. So, leaving mentally ill person free in the society can be dangerous and harmful for other mentally healthy person. A study by Centers for Disease Control and Prevention [CDC], (2010), found that most adults (>80%) in the states surveyed agreed that mental illness treatment is effective, but substantially fewer adults (35%–67%) agreed that people are caring and sympathetic to people with mental illness. In general, adults with mental illness symptoms, including those receiving treatment for a mental health problem were less likely to agree that people are caring and sympathetic to people with mental illness. This attitude and perception of the society for chronically ill mental patients give rise to dumping patients in the mental institutes.

The families and caretakers of the mentally ill person often try to hide the fact from others that they have mentally ill person in their home. Therefore, because of the social pressure, stigma and shame, they don't visit the services for the treatment. A study in United States reported that only about 20% of adults with a diagnosable mental disorder (Wang et al., 2005) or with a self-reported mental health condition (Hennessy, Green-Hennessy, & Marshall, 2012) saw a mental health provider. Embarrassment associated with accessing mental health services is one of the many barriers that cause people to hide their symptoms and to prevent them from getting necessary treatment for their mental illness symptoms (U.S. Department of Health and Human Services, 1999; 2001; Greene-Shortridge, Britt., & Castro, 2007; Nadeem et al., 2007). Stigma poses a barrier for public health primary prevention efforts designed to minimize the onset of mental illness, as well as with secondary prevention efforts aimed at promoting early treatment to prevent worsening of symptoms over time (Weiss, Ramakrishna, & Somma, 2006).

As the society plays a role of the senior member of the family, their acceptance and rejection puts a lot of pressure on the family members and on the mentally ill patient. If the society is receptive and gives a warm welcome to the chronically ill patients after they return from the health institution, it becomes very easy for them to start a new life and this decreases the chance of relapse also. So, as the society accepts a person when he or she recovers from any medical illness, they should also accept the mentally ill person in the same way. There should not be any discrimination on the basis of medical or psychological illness. There should be strict action against those who are creating obstacle for the mentally ill individual. If society takes this essential step in promoting mental health and supporting person with chronic mental illness, then a very serious problem of dumping patients in the institutions can be avoided.

The Role of Family

A person's innate as well as learned ability to deal with thoughts and feelings helps them to manage their daily life issues and circumstances by using all aspects of intelligence; cognitive intelligence, emotional intelligence and social intelligence. This includes the capacity to deal with the social world around by contribution in social activities, taking responsibilities or respecting the views of others. The chances of success increases if with this effort, the effort of family members of the mentally ill patients included by taking the responsibility to provide help to them to readjust in the society, help them to develop healthy and supportive relationships. They should involve in community and other group activity engagements and access to economic resources like work, education, housing and money.

The common problems that family members are facing are poor social environment, hostile family environment, economical issues, unaffordable prices of medicines, dependency and many more. The chronicity of the illness itself is a big concern. It requires lifelong medicine, proper self and emotional care, frequent hospital visits for follow ups. Families who have poor financial background have difficulty to follow proper management chart. We should also understand that the chronicity of the medical illness is different from the mental illness. In the medical illness the patients are able to use their cognition and intelligence which is lacking in mental patients. The patients with medical illness can understand their illness and are more functional and less dependent on their families or care takers. In contrast, the mentally ill patients require frequent care and guidance for their medicine. There is a huge difference in the family environmental conditions of the chronicity of medically and mentally ill patients. Providing awareness about the chronic mental illness among family members helps them to understand the emotional and psychological turmoil of the patients mainly in depression. If family members are with the patients then there no social discrimination and stigma can affect the harmony of the family and this would also decrease the chances of dumping patients in the institutions.

SUGGESTIONS

Chronic mental illness is certainly a very serious and distressing condition. The reason is not merely the illness itself but the stigma and marginalization associated with it is more traumatizing. The individual, the family, the society and the nation, all have a vital responsibility towards mentally ill population and this should not be the duty of the families and caretakers alone. By taking few preventive steps we can stop many unacceptable behaviour of the society towards mentally ill people. Acceptance, respect and independent life are the few requirements that a chronically ill mental patient expect from the family and society. There are few suggestions for those persons or the society who are dealing with this population, so that something better could be done for our mentally ill population. These suggestions are;

1. There should be proper guidelines and protocols for the management of chronically ill mental patients. Apart from the role of medicine, the role of clinical psychologist and psychiatric social workers are very important. Few efforts like proper psycho-education, frequent phonic follow-ups from the professionals, proper guidance, family therapy, supportive psychotherapy, the post discharge counselling and management etc can be done.
2. A very common reason for dumping patients is burden on the family and caretakers. Providing appropriate job perspective, vocational training, affordable medicine cost from the government and private organizations can give hope to the patients as well as to their family members. There is ample number of works in the schools, private and government companies and the hospitals which the mentally ill patients are capable to do either independently or with some supervision.
3. The management should not be limited to the institution but also involve proper community based management plans to the module. The reason is that the targeted management plan is limited to the institution and also the management is often symptom based. So, when they get discharged from the institution or the hospital they often relapse when they face the community life because they are unable to fulfil and adjust to the demands of the family and the society.
4. It is very important to verify the details and the identity of the patients and also of their guardian before admitting the patient to the hospital. The identity proof and the address proof should be in a visual form, for example ration card (photo with the family) or voter ID or adhaar card.
5. A very important step that can avoid patient dumping is that before admitting the patient, the consulting doctor should take one guardian of the patient with them for at least one to two days. During that period someone should either visit the given address or reassure the address from authentic resources or police verification can be done.
6. Even if the preventive step fails, the institute should always be ready with the second step. Suppose the patient is dumped in the hospital, the management plan would be to make them more functional and independent on the community level. For example proper vocational training should be planed specially targeting the patient's ability and interest and also the society when they will live their life after discharge. With this training they can survive in the community without becoming a burden.
7. The private companies should also take some step for their better future and secure few positions especially for those who have some chronic mental illness but maintain well or those who recovered but dumped by their families and caretakers.
8. There should be a group of patients who are dumped by their families, so that they can interact with each other and feel that there are others who are like them. A self help group for chronic mental patients is that voluntary association of people who share a common desire to overcome mental illness or otherwise increase their level of cognitive or emotional wellbeing.
9. The family and the society should get awareness that these illnesses are like any other medical illness and can happen to anybody at any particular time. If a family member is diagnosed with some medical illness, the other members get all the treatments done and help the affected person to recover soon but this situation gets reverse when the person is diagnosed with some mental illness like depression, mania or schizophrenia. The difference between the two diagnoses is the medically ill patient is able to use his cognition but the mentally ill patient is less unable to do so. Other than this, both require similar attention, affection, respect and care.
10. Making a group these families would help them to share their feeling and emotions with each other. With this they will not feel that they are alone in facing this problem. This would also help them to share the strategies to handle the affected person at home in a much better way.

11. Internet is a source which can unite the entire person in the world on a single platform. The mentally ill person lives all around the world, so establishing contact with their families becomes a very difficult task. In that case, with the help of internet the families and affected person can make contact with each other and they can share their thoughts and feeling with each other even without meeting.
12. A home visit program to families of chronically ill mental patients can also be helpful for reducing social stigma and dumping patients. This will help them to have a better understanding of their emotional response. They should be given practical intervention and strategies to minimize the negative aspect and information regarding when and how to seek help for a mental disorder.
13. In view of the fact that the range of risks to mental health is wide, responses and management would become more difficult and multi-layered. Broad strategies include: prevention of the mental illness to occur, promotion of positive interactions; social protection, promotion of the rights, opportunities and care of individuals with mental disorders.
14. Special management plan to support women mental health and to reduce the ill treatment of the society towards them.

CONCLUSION

Chronic mental illness is a very serious issue. Not only the individual who is suffering from chronic mental illness but the families and caretakers also face discrimination, social stigma and pressure from the society. Many families and caretakers face these pressure and stigma with pride and support the person who is suffering from the mental illness. However, there are other families and caretakers who take these pressure and stigma as a shame. They try to avoid telling others that their one family member is suffering from chronic mental illness. They make a very miserable life of the chronically ill mental patient. They look for the ways and ideas of getting rid from the patient. The best way to get rid from the problem is dumping the patient in the mental institutes. As a result, the institutions are overloaded with dumped patients. Dumping them would not give solution to the problem. On the other hand, it will add more problems to the nation. Everyone including the individual himself, the families and caretakers and the society should take their own responsibility towards the chronically ill mental patient. The main concern would be towards the conditions of the dumped patients because of their chronic mental illness. Why families and care takers are shrinking their responsibility towards these patients and dumping them in the mental institutes. What step we can take on the community level and what resources we can provide to them to avoid dumping patients to the mental hospitals. Proper vocational training, job perspectives, proper family counselling and other resources can help the patients' families and caretakers to take their responsibility for the chronically ill patients. As we all know that it is very easy to say but difficult to follow but nothing is impossible. If everyone takes their own responsibility, we can easily avoid dumping patients in the mental institutes. There is still a long way to go.

There are few take home messages for everyone to follow:

1. Every problem comes with a solution. The only effort is to look for that solution instead of avoiding and shifting the responsibility on others.
2. Mental illness is not a contagious disease. So, do not discriminate them.
3. Treat the mentally ill patients as a human being and give them a warm welcome in the society.

4. Help them to stand again in the society.
5. Help them to live their life independently.
6. Respect their basic rights.
7. Spread the awareness of mental health and illness among all the members of the society.

REFERENCES

Bathla, M., Chandan, S., Bathla, J., & Kaloiya, G. S. (2015). Faith healers in morden psychiatric practice: Result of a four year study. *Delhi Psychiatric Journal*, 18(10).

Centers for Disease Control and Prevention. (2010). Attitudes toward Mental Illness-35 States, District of Columbia, and Puerto Rico, 2007. *Morbidity and Mortality Weekly Report*, *59*(20), 619–625. Available from http://www.cdc.gov/mmwr/preview/mmwrhtml/mm5920a3.htm

Chapman, D. P., Perry, G. S., & Strine, T. W. (2005). The vital link between chronic disease and depressive disorders. *Preventing Chronic Disease*, *2*(1). Available from http://www.cdc.gov/pcd/issues/2005/jan/04_0066.htm PMID:15670467

Colton, C. W., & Manderscheid, R. W. (2006). Congruencies in increased mortality rates, years of potential life lost, and causes of death among public mental health clients in eight states. *Preventing Chronic Disease*, *3*(2). Available from http://www.cdc.gov/pcd/issues/2006/apr/05_0180.htm PMID:16539783

Corrigan, P. W., Markowitz, F. E., & Watson, A. C. (2004). Structural levels of mental illness: Stigma and discrimination. *Schizophrenia Bulletin*, *20*(3), 481–491. doi:10.1093/oxfordjournals.schbul.a007096 PMID:15631241

El-Gabalawy, R., Cox, B., Clara, I., & Mackenzie, C. (2010). Assessing the validity of social anxiety disorder subtypes using a nationally representative sample. *Journal of Anxiety Disorders*, *24*(2), 244–249. doi:10.1016/j.janxdis.2009.11.003 PMID:19963338

Greene-Shortridge, T. M., Britt, T. W., & Castro, C. A. (2007). The stigma of mental health problems in the military. *Military Medicine*, *172*(2), 157–161. doi:10.7205/MILMED.172.2.157 PMID:17357770

Hennessy, K. D., Green-Hennessy, S., & Marshall, C. (2012). Datapoints: Receipt of reported mental health specialty care in the 2010 Health Styles Survey. *Psychiatric Services (Washington, D.C.)*, *63*(4), 306. doi:10.1176/appi.ps.20120p306 PMID:22476296

Indian Council of Medical Research. (2005). *Mental health research in India*. Author.

Institute of Medicine (IOM). (2012). *Living well with chronic illness: A call for public health action*. Washington, DC: The National Academies Press.

Kadri, N., & Sartorius, N. (2005). The global fight against the stigma of schizophrenia. *PLoS Medicine*, *2*(7), 597–599. doi:10.1371/journal.pmed.0020136 PMID:16033301

Kessler, R. C., Chiu, W. T., Demler, O., & Walters, E. E. (2005). Prevalence, severity, and comorbidity of 12-month DSM-IV disorders in the National Comorbidity Survey Replication. *Archives of General Psychiatry*, *62*(6), 617–627. doi:10.1001/archpsyc.62.6.617 PMID:15939839

Lamb, H., Weinberger, L., & Gross, B. (2004). Mentally Ill Persons in the Criminal Justice System: Some Perspectives. *The Psychiatric Quarterly*, *75*(2), 107–126. doi:10.1023/B:PSAQ.0000019753.63627.2c PMID:15168834

Lewis, R. (2014). *US prisons home to 10 times as many mentally ill as in state hospitals: New report slams lack of treatment for seriously ill inmates as 'inhumane,' calls for reforms*. Extracted from http://america.aljazeera.com/articles/2014/4/8/mental-illness-prison.html

Lincoln Police Department. (2004). Emergency Protective Custody Issues for the Police. Mimeo.

Link, B. G., & Phelan, J. C. (2001). Conceptualizing stigma. *Annual Review of Sociology*, *27*(1), 363–385. doi:10.1146/annurev.soc.27.1.363

Mental Health Promotion Unit (MHPU) of the Public Health Agency of Canada. (2003). *Mental Health Promotion: Frequently Asked Questions*. Retrieved February 22, 2007 from http://www.phac-aspc.gc.ca/mh- sm/mhp-psm/faq_e.html

Ministry of Health and Family Welfare (2013). *Annual report 2012-13*. Author.

Moodie, R. & Jenkins, R. (2005). I'm from the government and you want me to invest in mental health promotion. Well why should I? *Promotion and Education: The evidence of mental health promotion effectiveness: Strategies for action,* 37-41.

Nadeem, E., Lange, J. M., Edge, D., Fongwa, M., Belin, T., & Miranda, J. (2007). Does stigma keep poor young immigrant and U.S. born black and Latina women from seeking mental health care? *Psychiatric Services (Washington, D.C.)*, *58*(12), 1547–1554. doi:10.1176/ps.2007.58.12.1547 PMID:18048555

National electronic Library for Mental Health (NeLMH). (2004). *Defining mental health promotion: risk and protective factors.* Retrieved March 27, 2007 from http://www.nelmh.net/page_view.asp?c=22&did=2358&fc=004002

National Human Rights Commission. NHRC, (2015). Extracted from http://nhrc.nic.in/disparchive.asp?fno=13716

NDTV. (2014). *Harsh conditions found in Indian mental health facilities for women*. Extracted from http://www.ndtv.com/india-news/harsh-conditions-found-in-indian-mental-health-facilities-for-women-708087

Pescosolido, B. A., Martin, J. K., Long, J. S., Medina, T. R., Phelan, J. C., & Link, B. G. (2010). A disease like any other? A decade of change in public reactions to schizophrenia, depression, and alcohol dependence. *The American Journal of Psychiatry*, *16*(11), 1321–1330. doi:10.1176/appi.ajp.2010.09121743 PMID:20843872

Sartorius, N. (2005). Stigma and discrimination because of schizophrenia: A summary of the WPA Global Programme Against Stigma and Discrimination because of Schizophrenia. *World Psychiatry; Official Journal of the World Psychiatric Association (WPA)*, *4*(1), 11–15.

Sharma, G. (2013). *Mentally ill suffer a horrible fate in India*. Extracted from http://www.dw.com/en/mentally-ill-suffer-a-horrible-fate-in-india/a-17007499

Stuart, H. (2005). Why stigma matters and why it should be beaten. *World Psychiatry; Official Journal of the World Psychiatric Association (WPA)*, *4*(1), 4–5.

U.S. Department of Health and Human Services. (1999). *Mental health: A report of the Surgeon General*. Rockville, MD: U.S. Department of Health and Human Services, Substance Abuse and Mental Health Services Administration, Center for Mental Health Services, National Institutes of Health, National Institute of Mental Health.

U.S. Department of Health and Human Services. (2001). *Mental health: Culture, race, and ethnicity—A supplement to mental health: A report of the Surgeon General*. Rockville, MD: Author.

Wahl, O. F. (2003). News media portrayal of mental illness. *The American Behavioral Scientist*, *46*(12), 1594–1600. doi:10.1177/0002764203254615

Waldman, A. (2004). Police struggle with approach to the mentally ill: recent killings have led to calls for better tracking and treatment of the mentally ill and more training for officers. *The Christian Science Monitor.* Accessible at www.csmonitor. com/2004/0317/p11s02-usju.htm

Wang, P. S., Lane, M., Olfson, M., Pincus, H. A., Wells, K. B., & Kessler, R. C. (2005). Twelve-month use of mental health services in the United States: Results from the National Comorbidity Survey Replication. *Archives of General Psychiatry*, *62*(6), 629–640. doi:10.1001/archpsyc.62.6.629 PMID:15939840

Weiss, M. G., Ramakrishna, J., & Somma, D. (2006). Health-related stigma: Rethinking concepts and interventions. *Psychology Health and Medicine*, *11*(3), 277–287. doi:10.1080/13548500600595053 PMID:17130065

WHO. (2006). *Constitution of the World Health Organization*. WHO.

WHO. (2007). *Mental health in prisons*. Retrieved from http://www.who.int/mental_health/policy/services/en/index.html

WHO. (2012). *Risks to mental health: An overview of vulnerabilities and risk factors*. Retrieved from www.who.int/about/copyright

KEY TERMS AND DEFINITIONS

Chronic: An illness lasting for longer period of time.

Community: People living in the same place sharing similar characteristics and ideas.

Dumping: Disowning / leaving chronic mentally ill people by family members in hospitals/institutes in order to avoid any responsibility of taking care of them.

Health: A state of complete physical, mental, social and spiritual well-being and not merely an absence of disease or infirmity (WHO).

Hospital: A place for providing medical care and treatment to patients.

Institution: An organization devoted to the service of mankind, particularly mentally ill patients.

Prison: A place for legal confinement of people for punishment.

Social: An activity of meeting and developing relationships with other members of society.

Chapter 4
Psychosocial Intervention Strategies for Patients with Schizophrenia:
In Chronic Mental Illness

Ashwini R.
Dharwad Institute of Mental Health and Neurosciences, India

Barre Vijay Prasad
Dharwad Institute of Mental Health and Neurosciences, India

Srinivas Kosgi
Dharwad Institute of Mental Health and Neurosciences, India

ABSTRACT

Throughout recorded history, the disorder we now known as schizophrenia has been a source of bewilderment. Schizophrenia is a chronic, severe, and disabling brain disease. Schizophrenia is found all over the world. The severity of the symptoms and the long-lasting, chronic pattern of schizophrenia often results in disability, and many individuals need on going assistance to manage the most basic functions of independent living. Schizophrenia most often includes hallucinations and/or delusions, which reflect distortions in the perception and interpretation of reality. In this chapter the authors were discussed psychosocial interventions like, individual psychotherapy, cognitive behaviour therapy, cognitive therapy with schizophrenia, behaviour therapy with schizophrenia, group therapy and family interventions were highlighted. In addition to this psychiatric rehabilitation were also discussed with vocational training, social skill training, and community rehabilitation approach. Further common causes of repeated hospitalization and implementation measures were described.

DOI: 10.4018/978-1-5225-0519-8.ch004

INTRODUCTION

Throughout recorded history, the disorder we now know as schizophrenia has been a source of bewilderment. Schizophrenia is a chronic, severe, and disabling brain disease. Schizophrenia is found all over the world. The severity of the symptoms and the long-lasting, chronic pattern of schizophrenia often results in disability, and many individuals need ongoing assistance to manage the most basic functions of independent living. Those suffering from the illness once were thought to be possessed by demons and were feared, tormented, exiled or locked up forever. Schizophrenia most often includes hallucinations and/or delusions, which reflect distortions in the perception and interpretation of reality. The resulting behaviours may seem bizarre to the casual observer, even though they may be consistent with the schizophrenic's abnormal perceptions and beliefs. The kinds of symptoms that are utilized to make a diagnosis of schizophrenia differ between affected people and may change from one year to the next within the same person as the disease progresses. Different subtypes of schizophrenia are defined according to the most significant and predominant characteristics present in each person at each point in time. The result is that one person may be diagnosed with different subtypes over the course of his illness.

Schizophrenia is a mental disorder characterized by a breakdown of thought processes and by poor emotional responsiveness (Oxford University Press, 2010). Common symptoms include auditory hallucinations, paranoid or bizarre delusions, or disorganized speech and thinking, and it is accompanied by significant social or occupational dysfunction. The onset of symptoms typically occurs in young adulthood, with a global lifetime prevalence of about 0.3–0.7% (Van, Kapur, & Lancet, 2009). Diagnosis is based on observed behaviour and the patient's reported experiences. It is approximately 1 percent of the population develops schizophrenia during their lifetime – more than 2 million Americans suffer from the illness in a given year. Although schizophrenia affects men and women with equal frequency, the disorder often appears earlier in men, usually in the late teens or early twenties, than in women, who are generally affected in the twenties to early thirties. People with schizophrenia often suffer terrifying symptoms such as hearing internal voices not heard by others, or believing that other people are reading their minds, controlling their thoughts, or plotting to harm them. These symptoms may leave them fearful and withdrawn. Their speech and behaviour can be so disorganized that they may be incomprehensible or frightening to others. Available treatments can relieve many symptoms, but most people with schizophrenia continue to suffer some symptoms throughout their lives; it has been estimated that no more than one in five individuals recovers completely (Van, & Lancet, 2009). The disorder is thought mainly to affect cognition, but it also usually contributes to chronic problems with behaviour and emotion. People with schizophrenia are likely to have additional (comorbid) conditions, including major depression and anxiety disorders; the lifetime occurrence of substance use disorder is almost 50% (Carson & Saunders, 2000). Social problems, such as long-term unemployment, poverty, and homelessness are common. The average life expectancy of people with the disorder is 12 to 15 years less than those without, the result of increased physical health problems and a higher suicide rate (about 5%).

WORLD SCENARIO

National and international health statistics do not reflect the enormous toll of misery from mental disorders because these conditions are not the immediate cause of death. Few studies have mapped the specific economic costs of mental illness. The cost comparisons made in the USA showed (Greenberg, Stiglin,

Finkelstain, & Berndt, 1993) that the cost burden from depression is about the same as that from heart disease. The Disability-Adjusted Life Year (DALY) measure combines burden from premature mortality with that from living with disability, and provides a more comprehensive assessment of burden of illness. The global burden of disease for neuropsychiatric disorders, as measured by the loss of DALYs, was estimated (World Bank, 1993) to be 6.8% worldwide in 1990. Psychiatric disorders account for 5 of 10 leading causes of disability as measured by years lived with a disability. The overall DALYs burden for neuropsychiatric disorders is projected (Murray & Lopez, 1996) to increase to 15% by the year 2020 and this increase is proportionately larger than for cardiovascular disease. The number of persons with major mental illnesses will increase substantially in the decades to come, for two reasons. First, the number of people living in the age groups of risk for certain illnesses are increasing because of changes in demographics. Thus the number of persons with schizophrenia will increase substantially because of increase in the population between 15 and 45 years of age the world over. No current data provide a clear model of preventable social or biological factors that account for the onset of schizophrenia. Although research has provided little evidence for understanding the social origins of schizophrenia, it does provide strong support for the hypothesis that social and cultural factors affect the course and prognosis of schizophrenia. In a two year follow up study (World Health Organization, 1979) in eight countries of people diagnosed as suffering from schizophrenia, it was found that the outcome varied enormously. Patients in low income countries did far better than those in North America and Europe. For example, two years after the first treated episode of schizophrenia, 50% patients were reported to have recovered in India and 58% in Nigeria, whereas only 8% were reported as recovered in Denmark. Similar findings were reported at 5 years follow up in this eight country study. The differences in prognosis are attributed to a myriad of environmental and other psychosocial factors interacting with the individual and illness. Research has advanced the understanding of the disorder and made major contributions to the treatment of schizophrenia. Treatments are both of a biological nature (*eg* medication) as well as psychosocial (*eg* psycho education of the family and rehabilitation). The helplessness of the past has been replaced by considerable hope since conditions that once were treated in closed institutions are being treated through interventions at home, in community services, and general hospitals. Early treatment is essential for better recovery. In India for a population of nearly one billion people, there are an estimated four million people with schizophrenia, with different degrees of impact on some 25 million family members. India has a national mental health programme, which was formulated in 1982 and adopted as the mental health policy. A decade back 10th Five- Year Plan of India for the Years 2002–2007 emphasized some strategies for the National Mental Health Programme as saying "…..and to shift the focus from the present custodial model to a community-based approach with extension of basic mental health care through outreach facilities."

SYMPTOMOTALOGY

A person diagnosed with schizophrenia may experience hallucinations (most reported are hearing voices), delusions (often bizarre or persecutory in nature), and disorganized thinking and speech. The latter may range from loss of train of thought, to sentences only loosely connected in meaning, to incoherence known as word salad in severe cases. Social withdrawal, sloppiness of dress and hygiene, and loss of motivation and judgment are all common in schizophrenia (Wiley, 2003). There is often an observable pattern of emotional difficulty, for example lack of responsiveness (Brunet & Decety, 2006) Impairment in social cognition is associated with schizophrenia, (Wiley, 2003) as are symptoms of paranoia; social isolation commonly occurs (Ungvari, Caraft, & Gerevich, 2010). Difficulties in working and long-term memory, attention, executive functioning, and speed of processing also commonly occur (Van, Kapur & Lancet, 2009). In one uncommon subtype, the person may be largely mute, remain motionless in bizarre postures, or exhibit purposeless agitation, all signs of catatonia (Addington, Cadenhead, & Cannon, 2007).

Late adolescence and early adulthood are peak periods for the onset of schizophrenia, (Van & Lancet, 2009) critical years in a young adult's social and vocational development (Cullen, Kumra, & Regan, 2008). In 40% of men and 23% of women diagnosed with schizophrenia, the condition manifested itself before the age of 19 (Amminger, Leicester & Yung, 2006). To minimize the developmental disruption associated with schizophrenia, much work has recently been done to identify and treat the prodromal (pre-onset) phase of the illness, which has been detected up to 30 months before the onset of symptoms (Addington, Cadenhead, & Cannon, 2007). Those who go on to develop schizophrenia may experience transient or self-limiting psychotic symptoms and the non-specific symptoms of social withdrawal, irritability, dysphoria, (Coyle, 2006) and clumsiness during the prodromal phase.

POSITIVE AND NEGATIVE SYMPTOMS

Schizophrenia is often described in terms of positive and negative (or deficit) symptoms (Kneisl & Trigoboff, 2009). Positive symptoms are those that most individuals do not normally experience but are present in people with schizophrenia. They can include delusions, disordered thoughts and speech, and tactile, auditory, visual, olfactory and gustatory hallucinations, typically regarded as manifestations of psychosis (American Psychiatric Association, 2000). Hallucinations are also typically related to the content of the delusional theme (Velligan & Alphs, 2008). Positive symptoms generally respond well to medication (Velligon & Alphs, 2008).

Negative symptoms are deficits of normal emotional responses or of other thought processes, and respond less well to medication (Wiley, 2003). They commonly include flat or blunted affect and emotion, poverty of speech (alogia), inability to experience pleasure (anhedonia), lack of desire to form relationships (asociality), and lack of motivation (avolition). Research suggests that negative symptoms contribute more to poor quality of life, functional disability, and the burden on others than do positive symptoms (Smith, Weston & Lieberman, 2010). People with prominent negative symptoms often have a history of poor adjustment before the onset of illness, and response to medication is often limited (Wiley, 2003; Drake & Lewis, 2005).

TYPES OF SCHIZOPHRENIA

The kinds of symptoms that are utilized to make a diagnosis of schizophrenia differ between affected people and may change from one year to the next within the same person as the disease progresses. Different subtypes of schizophrenia are defined according to the most significant and predominant characteristics present in each person at each point in time. The result is that one person may be diagnosed with different subtypes over the course of his illness.

Paranoid Subtype

Paranoid schizophrenia is the most common subtype. People diagnosed with the paranoid subtype may not appear odd or unusual and may not readily discuss the symptoms of their illness. Typically, the hallucinations and delusions revolve around some characteristic theme, and this theme often remains fairly consistent over time. A person's temperaments and general behaviours often are related to the content of the disturbance of thought. For example, people who believe that they are being persecuted unjustly may be easily angered and become hostile. Often, paranoid schizophrenics will come to the attention of mental health professionals only when there has been some major stress in their life that has caused an increase in their symptoms. At that point, sufferers may recognize the need for outside help or act in a fashion to bring attention themselves. Since there may be no observable features, the evaluation requires sufferers to be somewhat open to discussing their thoughts. If there is a significant degree of suspiciousness or paranoia present, people may be very reluctant to discuss these issues with a stranger. There is a broad spectrum to the nature and severity of symptoms that may be present at any one time. When symptoms are in a phase of exacerbation or worsening, there may be some disorganization of the thought processes. At this time, people may have more trouble than usual remembering recent events, speaking coherently or generally behaving in an organized, rational manner. While these features are more characteristic of other subtypes, they can be present to differing degrees in people with the paranoid subtype, depending upon the current state of their illness. Supportive friends or family members often may be needed at such times to help the symptomatic person get professional help (Bengston, 2013).

Disorganized Subtype

As the name implies, this subtype's predominant feature is disorganization of the thought processes. As a rule, hallucinations and delusions are less pronounced, although there may be some evidence of these symptoms. These people may have significant impairments in their ability to maintain the activities of daily living. Even the more routine tasks, such as dressing, bathing or brushing teeth, can be significantly impaired or lost. Often, there is impairment in the emotional processes of the individual. For example, these people may appear emotionally unstable, or their emotions may not seem appropriate to the context of the situation. They may fail to show ordinary emotional responses in situations that evoke such responses in healthy people. Mental health professionals refer to this particular symptom as blunted or flat affect. Additionally, these people may have an inappropriately jocular or giddy appearance, as in the case of a patient who chuckles inappropriately through a funeral service or other solemn occasion. People diagnosed with this subtype also may have significant impairment in their ability to communicate effectively. At times, their speech can become virtually incomprehensible, due to disorganized thinking. In such cases, speech is characterized by problems with the utilization and ordering of words in conversational sentences, rather than with difficulties of enunciation or articulation. In the past, the term hebephrenic has been used to describe this subtype (Bengston, 2013).

Catatonic Subtype

The predominant clinical features seen in the catatonic subtype involve disturbances in movement. Affected people may exhibit a dramatic reduction in activity, to the point that voluntary movement stops, as in catatonic stupor. Alternatively, activity can dramatically increase, a state known as catatonic excitement. Other disturbances of movement can be present with this subtype. Actions that appear relatively purposeless but are repetitively performed, also known as stereotypic behaviour, may occur, often to the exclusion of involvement in any productive activity. Patients may exhibit an immobility or resistance to any attempt to change how they appear. They may maintain a pose in which someone places them, sometimes for extended periods of time. This symptom sometimes is referred to as waxy flexibility. Some patients show considerable physical strength in resistance to repositioning attempts, even though they appear to be uncomfortable to most people. Affected people may voluntarily assume unusual body positions, or manifest unusual facial contortions or limb movements. This set of symptoms sometimes is confused with another disorder called tardive dyskinesia, which mimics some of these same, odd behaviours. Other symptoms associated with the catatonic subtype include an almost parrot-like repeating of what another person is saying (echolalia) or mimicking the movements of another person (echopraxia). Echolalia and echopraxia also are seen in Tourette's syndrome (Bengston, 2013).

Undifferentiated Subtype

The undifferentiated subtype is diagnosed when people have symptoms of schizophrenia that are not sufficiently formed or specific enough to permit classification of the illness into one of the other subtypes. The symptoms of any one person can fluctuate at different points in time, resulting in uncertainty as to the correct subtype classification. Other people will exhibit symptoms that are remarkably stable over time but still may not fit one of the typical subtype pictures. In either instance, diagnosis of the undifferentiated subtype may best describe the mixed clinical syndrome (Bengston, 2013).

Residual Subtype

This subtype is diagnosed when the patient no longer displays prominent symptoms. In such cases, the schizophrenic symptoms generally have lessened in severity. Hallucinations, delusions or idiosyncratic behaviours may still be present, but their manifestations are significantly diminished in comparison to the acute phase of the illness. Just as the symptoms of schizophrenia are diverse, so are its ramifications. Different kinds of impairment affect each patient's life to varying degrees. Some people require custodial care in state institutions, while others are gainfully employed and can maintain an active family life. However, the majority of patients are at neither of these extremes. Most will have a waxing and waning course marked with some hospitalizations and some assistance from outside support sources. People having a higher level of functioning before the start of their illness typically have a better outcome. In general, better outcomes are associated with brief episodes of symptoms worsening followed by a return to normal functioning. Women have a better prognosis for higher functioning than men, as do patients with no apparent structural abnormalities of the brain. In contrast, a poorer prognosis is indicated by a gradual or insidious onset, beginning in childhood or adolescence; structural brain abnormalities, as seen on imaging studies; and failure to return to prior levels of functioning after acute episodes (Bengston, 2013).

As a result of their illness, people with a diagnosis of schizophrenia have difficulty maintaining many of the essential life roles and resources that most others take for granted. These essential life roles and resources include satisfactory, stable, independent housing and relationships, particularly, close interpersonal relationships with friends and relatives. This loss of life roles and resources seriously impacts on the mental health of people with schizophrenia (American Psychiatric Association, 1994). Hence, psychosocial intervention strategies are very crucial along with pharmacological intervention for chronic mental illness patients.

Expressed Emotion

Expressed emotion is a huge factor during the recovery process of those diagnosed with psychological illnesses. The three attitudes pertaining to expressed emotion are known as hostile, critical, and emotional over-involvement. These attitudes of the relatives determine the direction of the illness after treatment. The relatives influence the outcome of the disorder through negative comments and nonverbal actions. These particular interactions between family members that are dealing with a patient with a psychological disorder are stressful on the recovering patient. The stress from the family for the patient to recover and end certain behaviours causes the person a relapse in their illness. They do not know what else to do during this sensitive time of recovery because of the criticism and pity from others. This negativity from loved ones does not help the family member to improve the state of their health (Vaughn & Leff, 1976). Expressed emotion is a measure of how well relatives of a psychological patient express their attitude towards them while they are not present (Hooley & Hoffman, 1999). In order to measure this expressed emotion, the family is interviewed to carefully watch their expressions and comments while answering questions. This interview is known as the Camberwell Family Interview. The family is taped so that the right type of expressed emotion is carefully concluded by someone that has training in coding the attitude being expressed. The tape is watched closely, particularly to see how critical the remarks are towards the recovery process and anything having to do with the disorder of the patient. There are two outcomes of the opinion of the relative: high expressed emotion or low expressed emotion. This is determined by the amount of critical comments made by the relative. High Expressed emotion is when the relative makes six or more critical comments during the interview. Low expressed emotion is considered to be less than six critical (Hooley & Hiller, 2000). Those who have high expressed emotion tend to be more negative than the ones who are low. The interview helps to find out if the environment that the patient will live in after rehabilitation might contribute to a relapse.

Expressed Emotions and Factors

- **Hostility:** Hostility is a negative attitude directed at the patient because the family feels that the disorder is controllable and that the patient is choosing not to get better. Problems in the family are often blamed on the patient and the patient has trouble problem solving in the family. The family believes that the cause of many of the family's problems is the patient's mental illness, whether they are or not.
- **Emotional Over-Involvement:** It is termed emotional over-involvement when the family members blame themselves for the mental illness. These family members feel that any negative occurrence is their fault and not the disorders. The family member shows a lot of concern for the patient and the disorder. This is the opposite of a hostile attitude and a show that the family member is open minded about the illness, but still has the same negative effect on the patient. The pity from the relative causes too much stress and the patient relapses to cope with the pity.
- **Critical Comments:** Critical attitudes are combinations of hostile and emotional over-involvement. It shows openness that the disorder is not entirely in the patients control but there is still negative criticism. Critical parents influence the patient's siblings to be the same way. Family members with high expressed emotion are hostile, very critical and not tolerant of the patient. They feel like they are helping by having this attitude. They not only criticize behaviours relating to the disorder but also other behaviours that are unique to the personality of the patient. High expressed emotion is more likely to cause a relapse than low expressed emotion.

PSYCHOSOCAL INTERVENTIONS

In the recent years there are lot of studies which support combination of drug treatment and psychosocial interventions for better compliance to medication, recovery process and outcome with improvement in quality of life and less relapse rate (McGorry, Yung, & Phillips, 2002). A number of psychosocial intervention strategies have been developed in the recent years. These interventions in a broader sense can be classified into:

1. Individual approach,
2. Cognitive,
3. Behaviour,
4. Group approach,
5. Family approach,
6. Community approach including rehabilitation.

Individual Psychotherapy

Individual psychotherapy involves regularly scheduled talks between the patient and a mental health professional such as a psychiatrist, psychologist, psychiatric social worker, or nurse. The sessions may focus on current or past problems, experiences, thoughts, feelings, or relationships. By sharing experiences with a trained empathic person – talking about their world with someone outside it – individuals with schizophrenia may gradually come to understand more about themselves and their problems. They can also learn to sort out the real from the unreal and distorted. Mental health professionals often do not suggest psychotherapy for individuals with schizophrenia, thinking that it is not effective. That is probably true of the insight-oriented psychotherapies that are non-directive, and rely on the client to spontaneously identify problems and discuss them. However, recent studies indicate that supportive, reality-oriented, individual psychotherapy, and cognitive-behavioural approaches that teach coping and problem-solving skills, can be beneficial for outpatients with schizophrenia. However, psychotherapy is not a substitute for antipsychotic medication, and it is most helpful once drug treatment first has relieved a patient's psychotic symptoms.

Cognitive-Behavioural Psychotherapy

Cognitive psychotherapy, often incorporating behavioural therapy techniques, has been found to be more effective than other types of psychotherapy in treating several specific types of psychological problems, including depression and panic attacks. Sometimes this treatment approach is called cognitive-behavioural psychotherapy because of the ease with which the two approaches combine to effectively treat a variety of psychological problems. This combination of treatment techniques is also effective in the treatment of schizophrenia. The basic premise of cognitive therapy is that beliefs, expectations, and cognitive assessments of self, the world, and the nature of personal problems in the world affect how we perceive ourselves and others, how we approach problems, and ultimately how successful we are in coping in the world and in achieving our goals. Schizophrenia results in distorted perceptions of the world, including self, and disordered or disorganized thinking. It seems reasonable that a cognitive treatment approach would be helpful in treating schizophrenia, assuming that medication is also employed to alleviate psychotic thought processes which would interfere with any psychotherapeutic interventions. The study by Freeman, Dunn, Startup, Pugh, Cordwell, and Mander (2015) published in The Lancet Psychiatry, examined 150 NHS patients who had been diagnosed with schizophrenia or a similar mental illness. The participants all had severe paranoia despite having been medicated (schizophrenia patients are typically prescribed antipsychotic drugs, which don't cure the illness but can reduce symptoms). They took part in six sessions of cognitive behavioral therapy targeting worry and the researchers found that this greatly lessened the intensity of persecution fears, in addition to increasing the patients' levels of happiness.

Cognitive Therapy with Schizophrenia

The misinterpretation of events in the world is common in schizophrenia. Using cognitive therapy with schizophrenia requires the psychologist to accept that the cognitive distortions and disorganized thinking of schizophrenia are produced, at least in part, by a biological problem that will not cease simply because the "correct" interpretation of reality is explained to the client. Cognitive therapy can only be successful if the psychologist accepts the client's perception of reality, and determines how to use this "misperception" to assist the client in correctly managing life problems. The goal is to help the client use information from the world (other people, perceptions of events, etc.) to make adaptive coping decisions. The treatment goal, for the cognitive therapist, is not to "cure" schizophrenia, but to improve the client's ability to manage life problems, to function independently, and to be free of extreme distress and other psychological symptoms.

Behaviours Therapy with Schizophrenia

Behaviour therapy assumes that certain skills increase our ability to function in the world, and to solve problems as they arise. Many psychosocial skills develop as a consequence of our experiences in the world. We "learn from our mistakes" and from our successes in managing different types of problems. Since people have different life experiences, some people learn skills well, and others do not learn as many skills. Another individual difference is our ability to learn from our experiences. In order to learn from experience, we must correctly analyze what was effective and what was not effective in solving a problem. We can also "learn" ineffective or maladaptive responses to problems, especially if those responses lead to immediate reduction of pain or embarrassment, despite having no effect on the long term solution to the problem. The learning of maladaptive responses top problems is often the result of cognitive distortions or making mistakes in assessing cause and effect. That is why cognitive therapy and behavioural therapy are often combined. Individuals with schizophrenia often make incorrect assessments of cause and effect. Also, they often do not learn as well from experience because of their disordered and disorganized thinking. Behaviour therapy teaches them the social skills they never learned, and helps them understand when to apply those skills to problems in the world. *Examples of Behavioural Skills Training*: stress management training, assertiveness training, communication skills training, and problem solving skills.

Group Therapy

In group therapy approaches the focus is on the group as a whole. Every member gets a chance to participate and share his experiences. Group therapies have their benefits as well as limitations. One of the important benefits include it save time and group setup itself acts as therapeutic. One of the difficult tasks is to develop that relatedness in schizophrenia patients which is important part of group therapy. Group approach usually uses different principles and techniques of individual approach in group set up with some modification as the focus is not the individual but group as a whole. There are different types of group as well as different kinds of group therapy. The different types of groups include homogenous or heterogeneous, small or large, closed or open etc. Group therapy approach have adopted mostly for use in psychoeducation, self-help group, social skills training, occupational and recreational therapy. The consensus of clinicians, with support from empirical studies, is that group therapy is most effective during the post treatment and outpatient phase of schizophrenia (May, 1976). A review of the literature dealing with the empirical research of group psychotherapy by Burlingame, Fuhriman, and Johnson (2001) argued that group psychotherapy is effective in schizophrenia and other psychiatric disorders. Social skill training is one of the structured forms of group therapy in schizophrenia with good results. Here the goal is to teach the patient how to behave in different social situation. Behaviourally based instruction, modeling, corrective feedback and contingent social reinforcement aimed to improve social competence. It is characterized by highly interactive, structured, systematic, educational and incremental approach to skills acquisition. Initially the patient is taught simple skills like greeting, making a request and listening to others to highly complex skills like being assertive, coping and negotiating in different situations. Group format enable the patient to learn through vicarious learning by observing his peers (Bellack, Mueser, Gingerich, & Agresta, 2004; Heinssen, Liberman, & Kopelowicz, 2000).

Family Interventions

Family interventions involves family members and relatives involved or living with patient. One such intervention includes family therapy which originated from the research on schizophrenic families. These researchers highlight the role of family in development and maintenance of schizophrenia. It refers to any intervention focusing on the family as whole rather than the individuals. Family is itself seen as patient the presenting members being viewed as a sign of family psychopathology. There are different schools of family therapy with different intervention strategy but goals have common agenda of strengthening family bonding, share burden, problem solving, improve interpersonal skills of the patient and family communication (Anderson, Reiss & Hogarty, 1986; Falloon, Boyd, & McGill, 1984). Work of Leff and Vaughen (1985) proved that high risk of relapse rate in families with high expressed emotions like hostility, criticality, and over-involvement. Falloon, et al. (1984) highlights the importance of family participation and commitment for long term which leads to better outcome. Studies have reported that patients who received family therapy had significantly fewer relapse rate on two year following a hospitalization than who received routine care (Falloon, Boyd, & McGill, 1985; Goldstein, 1985; Leff, 1985). In family interventions, a mental health professional provides support and understanding of the illness for the affected individual and family members. They work together on planning treatment, provide mutual support and understanding of the disease. Family intervention gives the family insight into the symptoms that warn of an impending acute episode so that medication may be adjusted with the aim of averting a relapse. Family interventions also help the family to cope with a chronically mentally ill member as well as reduce the burden faced by the families.

Although there is not a unique approach for family interventions, evidence-based family therapies usually include psychoeducation, stress reduction, emotional processing, cognitive reappraisal, and structured problem solving. Intervention consists of a combination of psychotherapeutic strategies for working with the relatives of people who suffer from psychosis, and it aims to develop a collaborative relationship between the family and the treatment team in order to help patients make progress toward recovery (Mueser, Deavers, Penn, & Cassisi, 2013). Interventions are always delivered by mental health professionals but can differ in theoretical orientation, modality, or length. More than 50 controlled trials have been conducted to test the efficacy of these kinds of interventions ((Mueser, Deavers, & Cassisi, 2013; National Institute for Clinical Excellence, 2009). Principal findings have proven that family therapy has a positive impact on the patient's recovery, with a significant reduction in readmission and relapses, as well as an improvement in their social functioning (Pharoah, Mari, Rathbone & Wong, 2010).

Psychiatric Rehabilitation

Psychiatric rehabilitation (also known as psychosocial rehabilitation and biopsychosocial rehabilitation) is the process of assisting people to acquire and to use, the internal and external skills, supports, and resources necessary to be successful and satisfied living, learning, and working in the environment(s) of their choice. At its most basic level, psychiatric rehabilitation seeks to help people to determine and prioritize their goals, to identify paths for achieving these goals, and to develop the needed skills and supports to achieve these goals (Anthony, Cohen, & Farkas, 1991). Derived from concepts from physical rehabilitation, psychiatric rehabilitation focuses on the disability or impairment resulting from an individual's psychiatric disorder which affects the person's ability to fulfil role expectations. The goal of psychiatric rehabilitation is to help individuals to function "despite" their disability to compensate for or to eliminate deficits in functioning, interpersonal barriers, and environmental barriers created by the disability, and to restore ability for independent living, socialization, and effective life management. Perceived deficits frequently fall into several categories: daily living skills, social interactions, accommodations, vocational productivity, and problem solving (cognitive processes).

Psychiatric rehabilitation services offer 1) skill development, and 2) environmental resource development, in order to help individuals capitalize on their personal strengths, to develop effective coping strategies, and to develop supportive environments so that they may function as independently as possible. Service and support activities are designed to be integrated with the real activities one engages in daily. Rehabilitation services may be offered in a facility setting or "off-site" in the community-at-large or in an individual's home (Hughes, 1994). Rehabilitation services may be offered parallel to, independently of, or integrated with psychopharmacology and other forms of psychiatric treatment.

- **Vocational Training:** Vocational activities may include sheltered work experiences, placement into volunteer jobs, or transitional employment placement to learn work skills. Participants may be taught how to complete a job application form, what they do and do not have to tell employers about their illness, and how to develop a resume. Job interviewing skills are often taught, as individuals with schizophrenia frequently are deficient in the social skills needed to make a good impression in an interview.

- **Social Skill Training:** Basic training in communication skills and interpersonal social skills is often needed because the perceptual impairments and disordered thinking of schizophrenia often interferes with the "natural" learning of these skills through interpersonal interactions and feedback.
- **Community Rehabilitation Approach:** In community rehabilitation approach usually the focus is to put patient back to community which is only possible when individual and family issues have been resolved through different approaches discussed earlier. Community approach goal is to rehabilitate the patient back to his community which is only possible when symptoms have subsided and patient is able to carry out his work to some extent. The de-institutionalization of care for mentally ill gained momentum in fifth decade and peaked at 70's resulted in massive shift in caring the patient in community (Donald, 1963). The services emphasize continued provisions of psychiatric treatment to prevent re-hospitalizations but also the curability of stable and severe housing and systematic efforts reintegrate the patient in to the community. Individual suffering from schizophrenia can develop skill deficits in two forms. Firstly individual after onset of the illness does not use skills, thereby causing the atrophy of the skills. Second due to the early onset of illness the patient might not have learned the skills necessary for living. So they require training to be successful in society. This training is provided in different setups. Some of them are discussed below. Vocational Rehabilitation is probably one of the most well developed psychosocial interventions given in its well established role in psychiatric rehabilitation. Vocational rehabilitation is done taking into consideration both the real and potential abilities as well as limitations of the patients using different questionnaires and observation. It aims at training or re-training patients on a given task to perform at their optimal capacity. Teaching them necessary skills to be competitive in terms of functioning and holding a job. Models of vocational rehabilitation training include job club, Boston university model, supported employment model etc. Social Support Network is process of providing emotional support to people with schizophrenia through social support network as the trend towards de-hospitalization has been growing in psychiatry. Gradually they develop skills and confidence through different activities. Participation in different group and community meeting enhances sense of responsibility and accountability in discharging the work assigned to them. Role-play, role modeling and guided instructions with corrected feedback are used. Group session to express their concerns and feeling help them to learn appropriate and acceptable ways of expressing emotions; Quarter way homes is a facility specifically for patients who have been placed successfully in job market or are functional enough to undergo training outside center. The focus is on helping the patients to make decisions, take accountability for his actions and to gradually learn to cope with work situation.

THE INDIAN SCENARIO

India's contribution in the field of schizophrenia is not limited to medical research only. It has decisively acted in a number of social issues related to the human rights of the mentally ill. High court and Supreme court has taken number of actions in improving the mental hospitals in Ranchi, Thiruvaanthapuram, Gwalior etc. In 1993 the Supreme Court of Indian gave a historic judgment that it is unconstitutional to keep a non-criminal mentally ill person in prison (Wig & Srinivasa Murthy, 1994). By an act of the parliament, mental illness is now included as one of the medical disabilities for the purpose of disability benefits by the government. Many schizophrenic patients and their families are likely to benefit by this legislation in coming years. One area where the Indian contributions are most impressive is the community care of schizophrenic patients. It was realized that in compare with the number of psychiatric patients, the institutional facilities were less, so during 1950s Dr. Vidya Sagar showed the way by involving families in the care of the patients. The rise of NGO's human rights groups is an important social phenomena of the last two decades which is likely to greatly influence the treatment and rehabilitation of schizophrenic patients. In spite of all suitable psychiatric services, still some other problems are also existed.

Common Causes of Repeated Hospitalization

Schizophrenia is a chronic and disabling illness, with the majority of patients experiencing multiple relapses during the course of the illness (Robinson et al., 1999). Relapse, characterised by acute psychotic exacerbation, may have serious implications. For example, there is a risk of patients harming themselves or others, of jeopardising personal relationships, education or employment status (Kane, 2007) and of further stigmatisation of the illness. Additionally, relapse may carry a biological risk. It has been proposed that active psychosis reflects a period of disease progression insofar as patients may not return to their previous level of function and treatment refractoriness may emerge (Wyatt, 1997; Lieberman et al., 1996). Multiple factors contribute to increasing the risk of relapse. In a systematic review and meta-analysis of longitudinal studies it was found that non-adherence with medication, persistent substance use, carers' criticism and poorer premorbid adjustment significantly increased the risk for relapse in first-episode psychosis (Alvarez-Jimenez, 2012). In a prospective, 5 yr follow-up of first-episode psychosis patients it was found that the most common risk factor by far was antipsychotic medication discontinuation (Robinson et al, 1999). In clinical settings disengagement from treatment is common, even and perhaps particularly, in the early stages of illness (Coldham, Addington, & Addington, 2002; Miller, Bodenheimer & Crittenden, 2011). In recognition of the associated risks, improving medication adherence and relapse prevention have been emphasised as key components of the management of schizophrenia (Kane, 2007). However, there remain many unanswered questions regarding the nature of relapse making further study of this component of the illness imperative. During recent studies of relapse in schizophrenia, Emsley, Oosthuizen, Koen, Niehaus, and Martinez (2013) were conducted and struck by several observations:

1. Relapse rates are very high after treatment discontinuation, even after a single episode of psychosis.
2. A longer treatment period prior to discontinuation does not reduce the risk of relapse.
3. Many patients relapse very soon after treatment discontinuation.
4. The transition from remission to relapse may be abrupt, with few early warning signs.
5. Once illness recurrence occurs symptom severity rapidly returns to levels similar to the initial psychotic episode.
6. While most patients respond promptly to re-introduction of antipsychotic treatment after relapse, the response time is variable and frank treatment failure may emerge in a subset of patients.

IMPLEMENTATION

Research is gradually leading to new and safer medications and unraveling the complex causes of the disease. Scientists are using many approaches from the study of molecular genetics to the study of populations to learn about schizophrenia. Methods of imaging the brain's structure and function hold the promise of new insights into the disorder. Ensuring that a person with schizophrenia continues to get treatment after hospitalization is also important. A patient may discontinue medications or stop going for follow-up treatment, often leading to a return of psychotic symptoms. Encouraging the patient to continue treatment and assisting him or her in the treatment process can positively influence recovery. Without treatment, some people with schizophrenia become so psychotic and disorganized that they cannot care for their basic needs, such as food, clothing, and shelter. All too often, people with severe mental illnesses such as schizophrenia end up on the streets or in jails, where they rarely receive the kinds of treatment they need.

It may also be useful for those who know the person with schizophrenia well to keep a record of what types of symptoms have appeared, what medications (including dosage) have been taken, and what effects various treatments have had. By knowing what symptoms have been present before, family members may know better what to look for in the future. Families may even be able to identify some "early warning signs" of potential relapses, such as increased withdrawal or changes in sleep patterns, even better and earlier than the patients themselves. Thus, return of psychosis may be detected early and treatment may prevent a full-blown relapse. Also, by knowing which medications have helped and which have caused troublesome side effects in the past, the family can help those treating the patient to find the best treatment more quickly.

In addition to involvement in seeking help, family, friends, and peer groups can provide support and encourage the person with schizophrenia to regain his or her abilities. It is important that goals be attainable, since a patient who feels pressured and/or repeatedly criticized by others will probably experience stress that may lead to a worsening of symptoms. Like anyone else, people with schizophrenia need to know when they are doing things right. A positive approach may be helpful and perhaps more effective in the long run than criticism. This advice applies to everyone who interacts with the person.

CONCLUSION

As mental health professionals dealing with the psychosocial intervention strategies and this knowledge can be effectively utilized to augment the gains of intervention and prevent frequent hospitalizations that can have a telling impact on the individual, family and the economy of the nation as well.

REFERENCES

Addington, J., Cadenhead, K. S., Cannon, T. D., Cornblatt, B., McGlashan, T. H., Perkins, D. O., & Heinssen, R. et al. (2007). North American prodrome longitudinal study: A collaborative multisite approach to prodromal schizophrenia research. *Schizophrenia Bulletin*, *33*(3), 665–672. doi:10.1093/schbul/sbl075 PMID:17255119

Alvarez-Jimenez, M., Priede, A., Hetrick, S. E., Bendall, S., Killackey, E., Parker, A. G., & Gleeson, J. F. et al. (2012). Risk factors for relapse following treatment for first episode psychosis: A systematic review and meta-analysis of longitudinal studies. *Schizophrenia Research*, *139*(1-3), 116–128. doi:10.1016/j.schres.2012.05.007 PMID:22658527

American Psychiatric Association. (1994). *Diagnostic and statistical manual of mental disorders* (4th ed.). Washington, DC: Author.

American Psychiatric Association. (2000). *Task Force on DSM-IV: Diagnostic and statistical manual of mental disorders*. Author.

Amminger, G. P., Leicester, S., Yung, A. R., Phillips, L. J., Berger, G. E., Francey, S. M., & McGorry, P. D. et al. (2006). Early onset of symptoms predicts conversion to non-affective psychosis in ultra-high risk individuals. *Schizophrenia Research, 84*(1), 67–76. doi:10.1016/j.schres.2006.02.018 PMID:16677803

Anderson, C. M., Reiss, D. J., & Hogarty, G. E. (1986). *Schizophrenia in the Family: A Practitioner's Guide to Psychoeducation and Management*. New York: Guilford Press.

Anthony, W., Cohen, M., & Farkas, M. (1991). *Psychiatric Rehabilitation*. Boston, MA: Boston University, Centre for Psychiatric Rehabilitation.

Bellack, A. S., Mueser, K. T., Gingerich, S., & Agresta, J. (2004). *Social skills training for schizophrenia: A step-by-step guide* (2nd ed.). New York: Guilford Press.

Bengston, M. (2013). Types of Schizophrenia. *Psych Central*. Retrieved on February 4, 2016, from http://psychcentral.com/lib/types-of-schizophrenia

Brunet, G. E., & Decety, J. (2006). Social brain dysfunctions in schizophrenia: A review of neuroimaging studies. *Psychiatry Research, 148*(2-3), 75–92. doi:10.1016/j.pscychresns.2006.05.001 PMID:17088049

Burlingame, G. M., Fuhriman, A., & Johnson, J. E. (2001). Cohesion in group psychotherapy. *Psychotherapy (Chicago, Ill.), 38*(4), 373–379. doi:10.1037/0033-3204.38.4.373

Carson, V. B., & Saunders, W. B. (2000). *Mental health nursing: the nurse-patient journey*. Schizophrenia.

Coldham, E.L., Addington, J., & Addington, D. (2002). *Medication adherence of individuals with a first episode of psychosis*. Academic Press.

Coyle, J. (2006). The Neurochemistry of Schizophrenia. In *Basic Neurochemistry: Molecular, Cellular and Medical Aspects* (7th ed.; p. 876). Burlington, MA: Elsevier Academic Press.

Cullen, K. R., Kumra. S., & Regan, J. (2008). Atypical Antipsychotics for Treatment of Schizophrenia Spectrum Disorders. *Psychiatric Times, 25*(3).

Donald, B. (1963). *Skid Row in American Cities*. Chicago: Community and Family Studies Centre, University of Chicago.

Drake, R. J., & Lewis, S. W. (2005). Early detection of schizophrenia. *Current Opinion in Psychiatry, 144*, 718–726. PMID:16639167

Falloon, I. R., Boyd, J. L., & McGill, C. W. (1984). *Family Care of Schizophrenia*. New York: Guilford Press.

Falloon, I. R. H., Boyd, J. L., & McGill, C. W. (1985). Family management in the prevention of morbidity of schizophrenia: I. Clinical outcome of a two-year longitudinal study. *Archives of General Psychiatry, 42*(9), 887–896. doi:10.1001/archpsyc.1985.01790320059008 PMID:2864032

Freeman, D., Dunn, G., Startup, H., Pugh, K., Cordwell, J., Mander, H., & Kingdon, D. et al. (2015). Effects of cognitive behavior therapy for worry on persecutory delusions in patients with psychosis (WIT): A parallel, single-blind, randomized controlled trial with a mediation analysis. *The Lancet Psychiatry*, *2*(4), 305–313. doi:10.1016/S2215-0366(15)00039-5 PMID:26360083

Goldstein, M. (1985). Family factors that antedate the onset of schizophrenia and related disorders: The results of a fifteen year prospective longitudinal study. *Acta Psychiatrica Scandinavica*, *71*(319), 7–18. doi:10.1111/j.1600-0447.1985.tb08520.x PMID:3863461

Greenberg, P., Stiglin, L., Finkelstain, S., & Berndt, E. (1993). Depression: A neglected major illness. *The Journal of Clinical Psychiatry*, *54*, 419.

Heinssen, R. K., Liberman, R. P., & Kopelowicz, A. (2000). Psychosocial skills training for schizophrenia: Lessons from the laboratory. *Schizophrenia Bulletin*, *26*, 21–46.

Hooley, J. M., & Hiller, J. B. (2000). Personality and expressed emotion. *Journal of Abnormal Psychology*, *109*(1), 40–44. doi:10.1037/0021-843X.109.1.40 PMID:10740934

Hughes, R. (1994). In IAPSRS Publications Committee (1994). An Introduction to Psychiatric Rehabilitation. Columbia, MD: IAPSRS individuals with a first episode of psychosis. *Acta Psychiatrica Scandinavica*, *106*, 286–290.

Kane, J. M. (2007). Treatment strategies to prevent relapse and encourage remission. *The Journal of Clinical Psychiatry*, *68*(14), 27–30. PMID:18284275

Kneisl, C., & Trigoboff, E. (2009). Contemporary Psychiatric- Mental Health Nursing (2nd ed.), London.

Leff, J. P., & Vaughn, C. (1985). *Expressed emotion in families*. New York: Guildford Press.

Lieberman, J. A., Alvir, J. M., Koreen, A., Geisler, S., Chakos, M., & Sheitman, B. (1996). Psychobiologic correlates of treatment response in schizophrenia. *Neuropsychopharmacology*, *14*(3), 13S–21S. doi:10.1016/0893-133X(95)00200-W PMID:8866739

McGorry, P. D., Yung, A. F., Phillips, L. J., Yuen, H. P., Francey, S., Cosgrave, E. M., & Jackson, H. et al. (2002). Randomized controlled trial of interventions designed to reduce the risk of progression to first-episode psychosis in a clinical sample with subthreshold symptoms. *Archives of General Psychiatry*, *59*(10), 921–928. doi:10.1001/archpsyc.59.10.921 PMID:12365879

Miller, B. J., Bodenheimer, C., & Crittenden, K. (2011). Second-Generation Antipsychotic discontinuation in first episode psychosis: An updated review. *Cliincal Psychopharmacological Neuroscience*, *9*(2), 45–53. doi:10.9758/cpn.2011.9.2.45 PMID:23429653

Mueser, K. T., Deavers, F., Penn, D. L., & Cassisi, J. (2013). Psychosocial treatments for schizophrenia. *Annual Review of Clinical Psychology*, *9*(1), 465–497. doi:10.1146/annurev-clinpsy-050212-185620 PMID:23330939

Murray, C. J. L., & Lopez, A. D. (1996). *The Global Burden of Diseases: A Comprehensive Assessment of Mortality and Disability from Diseases, Injuries and Risk Factors in 1990 and Projected to 2020.* Boston: Harvard School of Public Health, World Health Organization and World Bank.

National Institute for Clinical Excellence. (2009). *Schizophrenia (update) Clinical Guidelines CG82*. NICE. Available from: http://www.guidance.nice.org.uk/CG82

Oxford University Press. (2010). "Schizophrenia" Concise Medical Dictionary. Oxford Reference Online.

Pharoah, F., Mari, J., Rathbone, J., & Wong, W. (2010). Family intervention for schizophrenia.[*Cochrane Database of Systematic Reviews*, (12): CD000088. PMID:21154340

Philip, R. (1976). When, what, and why? psychopharmacotherapy and other treatments in schizophrenia. *Comprehensive Psychiatry*, *17*(6), 683–693. doi:10.1016/0010-440X(76)90016-X PMID:186230

Robinson, D., Woerner, M. G., Alvir, J. M., Bilder, R., Goldman, R., Geisler, S., & Lieberman, J. A. et al. (1999). Predictors of relapse following response from a first episode of schizophrenia or schizoaffective disorder. *Archives of General Psychiatry*, *56*(3), 241–247. doi:10.1001/archpsyc.56.3.241 PMID:10078501

Smith, T., Weston, C., & Lieberman, J. (2010). Schizophrenia (maintenance treatment). *American Family Physician*, *75*(12), 1821–1829. PMID:20704164

Ungvari, G. S., Caroff, S. N., & Gerevich, J. (2010). The catatonia conundrum: Evidence of psychomotor phenomena as a symptom dimension in psychotic disorders. *Schizophrenia Bulletin*, *36*(2), 231–238. doi:10.1093/schbul/sbp105 PMID:19776208

Van, O. J., & Kapur, S. (2009). Schizophrenia. *Lancet*, *374*(9690), 635–645. doi:10.1016/S0140-6736(09)60995-8 PMID:19700006

Vaughn, C., & Leff, P. (1976). The influence of family and social factors on the course of psychiatric illness. A comparison of schizophrenia and depressed neurotic patients. *The British Journal of Psychiatry*, *129*(2), 125–137. doi:10.1192/bjp.129.2.125 PMID:963348

Velligan, D. I., & Alphs, L. D. (2008). Negative Symptoms in Schizophrenia: The Importance of Identification and Treatment. *Psychiatric Times*, *25*(3), 1–6. PMID:19590742

Wig, N. N., & Murthy, S. (1994). From Mental Illness to Mental Health. *Health for the Millions*, 2–4.

Wiley, B. (2003). Schizophrenia. Author.

World Bank. (1993). *World Development Report. Investing in Health*. New York: Oxford University Press.

World Health Organization. (1979). Schizophrenia: An International Follow-up Study. WHO.

Wyatt, R. J. (1997). Research in schizophrenia and the discontinuation of antipsychotic medications. *Schizophrenia Bulletin*, *23*(1), 3–9. doi:10.1093/schbul/23.1.3 PMID:9050108

KEY TERMS AND DEFINITIONS

Cognitive Behaviour Therapy: A form of psychotherapy. It was originally designed to treat depression, but is now used for a number of mental disorders. It works to solve current problems and change unhelpful thinking and *behavior*.

Expressed Emotions: The critical, hostile, and *emotionally* over-involved attitude that relatives have toward a family member with a disorder. The *expressed emotion* can be high or low, which is decided by a taped interview known as the Camberwell Family Interview.

Family Intervention: Family intervention includes family members in therapeutic sessions with the goal of improving all family members' mental health and understanding of the disorder. This type of intervention aims to enhance the capacity of both patients and their families for problem solving and illness management. Family interventions have a focus on providing information about the disorder, and emphasizing instructions for medication and treatment adherence. Therapeutic sessions can also involve cognitive behavioural interventions to improve problem solving and communication skills and to reduce familial expressed emotion.

Group Therapy: Group psychotherapy or group therapy is a form of psychotherapy in which one or more therapists treat a small group of clients together as a group.

Individual Therapy: Also known as psychotherapy, talk therapy, or counseling—is a collaborative process between therapist and client that aims to facilitate change and improve quality of life.

Intervention Strategies: Intervention strategy is a systematic plan of action consciously adapted in an attempt to address and reduce the causes of any illness.

Schizophrenia: A long-term mental disorder of a type involving a breakdown in the relation between thought, emotion, and behaviour, leading to faulty perception, inappropriate actions and feelings, withdrawal from reality and personal relationships into fantasy and delusion, and a sense of mental fragmentation.

Section 2

Chronic Mental Illness and Comorbidities

Chapter 5
Comorbidity Issues and Treatment in Chronic Mental Illness

Deepika Srivastav
Institute of Human Behaviour and Allied Sciences, India

Tej Bahadur Singh
Central University of South Bihar (CUSB), India

ABSTRACT

Comorbidity refers to presence of one or more additional disorders along with a primary disorder. It affects the prognosis and course of treatment. It is often difficult for clinician to make correct diagnosis in presence of various disorders. The clinical picture of various disorders interferes with treatment process and the outcome. There are some disorders in psychiatry, known as chronic illness. These are schizophrenia, bipolar disorder and obsessive-compulsive disorder. All these three disorder have a major effect on individual's life. Anxiety, depression, substance abuse and panic symptoms are common in schizophrenia; hence the clinical picture changes frequently. While the literature suggests that presence of two or three disorders make treatment worse, hence multidisciplinary treatment need to be used.

INTRODUCTION

Comorbidity is generally defined as the presence of one or more additional disorders along with a primary disorder. It was first introduced by Feinstein in 1970; to denote some cases in which some additional symptoms occurred during the course of a particular illness. Psychiatric comorbidity is defined as "the co-occurrence of two psychiatric disorders in presence of other illness in the same person" (First, 2005). The nature of symptom is overlapping and do not necessarily imply that one is caused by the other (Feinstein, 1970). It also affects the prognosis and course of treatment. Anxiety, depression, and substance abuse are mostly common illness, that make symptoms worse. The clinical picture of various disorders occasionally changes in subsequent visits. It is found that the symptoms of panic disorders, psychosis, chronic depression and personality disorders are more common with paranoid schizophrenia

DOI: 10.4018/978-1-5225-0519-8.ch005

(Bayle, 2001). There is high risk of developing psychotic symptoms in presence of affective illness as well. Bipolar disorder is highly prevalent and heterogeneous that incorporates psychiatric and medical comorbidities (Bhagwagar, 2007). Earlier the prevalence was less than other psychiatric disorder and the symptoms were characterized by episode of depression and euphoric excitement. It was easy for clinicians to diagnose and treat. Presently, the scenario is completely different. Obsessive Compulsive Disorder is one of the most debilitating disorders that disturb sufferer's entire life. DSM 5 separated OCD from anxiety disorder in the view of the nature of symptomatology and higher prevalence. As all these three illnesses disturb individual a lot and required long term treatment, hence been considered as chronic mental illness. Chapter includes detailed discussion of schizophrenia, bipolar disorder and obsessive compulsive disorder.

SCHIZOPHRENIA

Schizophrenia is a cluster of disorders that alters an individual's thoughts, perception, affect and behaviour. The concept of schizophrenia was formulated by the work of Benedict-Auguste Morel and Karl Kahlbaum in the mid-nineteenth century (Shorter, 1997). The term 'Demence Precoce' was coined by Auguste Morel to define a disorder characterized by cognitive impairments and progressive deterioration observed in young people. The detailed description of schizophrenia was highlighted by Emil Kraepelin. He suggested that the illness begins at an early age ('praecox') and have a relatively chronic course that is characterized by cognitive and social impairment ('dementia'). In 1857 he proposed that the pathognomic symptom of schizophrenia is fragmenting of the thinking. Hedivided symptoms into two groups i.e., fundamental and secondary group. Kurt Schneider proposed first rank symptoms that are characterized by loss of autonomy, such as thought insertion or delusions of being controlled by outside forces (Fish, 1967).

Incidence and Prevalence

Schizophrenia is a relatively common illness and most common form of psychotic disorder. In epidemiological studies, the mean incidence of schizophrenia is reported. It is a disorder with low incidence but a relatively high prevalence, and costs are reflected by its chronicity in many patients (Knapp, Mangalore, & Simon, 2004). The diagnosis is limited to core criteria and corrected for age, is 0.11 per 1000 (range 0.07-0.17 per 1000) (Jablensky, 1992). The mean age of onset is about 5 years greater in women although a lower female rate in adolescence with a second smaller peak after the menopause. The lifetime prevalence is between 0.4 and 1.4% (Cannon & Jones, 1996). Recent studies showed variation in incidence and prevalence rate. The annual incidence is 0.16-1.00 per 1000 population; which is comparatively lower than previous studies (Jablensky et al., 2011), see the changes diagnostic criteria in Table 1.

Diagnostic Criteria

Table 1. Changes in diagnostic criteria from DSM-IV in DSM-V

DSM-IV: Diagnostic Criteria	DSM-V: Diagnostic Criteria
Criterion A: Characteristic symptoms. Two (or more) of the following, each present for a significant portion off time during a 1-month period (or less if successfully treated): • Delusion • Hallucinations • Disorganized speech • Grossly disorganized or catatonic behaviour • Negative Symptoms (i.e., affective flattening, alogia or avolition. **Note:** Only one criterion A symptoms is required if delusions are bizarreor hallucinations consist of a voice keeping up a running commentary on the person's behaviour or thoughts, or two or more voices conversing with each other.	**Criterion A:** Characteristic symptoms: (Minor change). Two (or more) of the following each present for a significant portion of time during a 1-month period (or less if successfully treated). At least one of these should have: • Delusion • Hallucination • Disorganized speech • Grossly disorganized or catatonic behaviour • Negative symptoms (i.e., diminished emotional expression or avolition).
Criterion B: Social/occupational dysfunction (No changes)	
Criterion C: Duration of 6 months (No Changes)	
Criterion D: Schizoaffective and mood disorder exclusion (No changes)	
Criterion E: Substance/general mood condition exclusion (No changes)	
Criterion F: Relationship to global developmental delay or autism spectrum disorder: If there is a history of autism spectrum disorder, the additional diagnosis of schizophrenia is made only if prominent delusions or hallucinations are also present for at least 1 month (or less if successfully treated).	**Criterion F:** Relationship to global Developmental Delay or Autism spectrum disorder (minor changes). If there is a history of autism spectrum disorder or a communication disorder of childhood onset, the additional diagnosis of schizophrenia is made only if prominent delusions or hallucinations, in addition to the other required symptoms of schizophrenia, are also present for at least 1 month (or less if successfully treated).

American Psychiatric Association (2000, 2013)

ETIOLOGY

Neurobiological Theories

Functional excess of dopaminergic activity is related to the development of schizophrenia so it is called Dopamine hypothesis of schizophrenia. It suggests the excess of dopamine in the brain is responsible for schizophrenia. Norepinephrine, a neurotransmitter in peripheral nervous system is widely distributed in the brain. It is related most with hypothalamus, thalamus, cerebellum and limbic system. Increased norepinephrine activity plays an important role in schizophrenia. Several studies reported low level of serotonin concentration in blood of schizophrenia patients (Howes & Kapoor, 2009).

Psychological Theories

There are various psychological theories have explained the causes of schizophrenia, these are as follows:

- **Psychodynamic Theories:** Studies have suggested following two theories (i) Descriptive-Homeostatic: These theories focused on here and stay closet. These theories explain the causation and understand how the disease works as a homeostatic system. (ii) Etiological-Facilitative: These theories explain the broader view of schizophrenia over the course of lifetime. These theories are comprehensive as it explains how OCD is generated and maintained in life. For ex. Klein, (1946) theorized that fixation in early infancy developmental stage is related with paranoid-schizoid phase and also correlated with genesis of schizophrenia.

- **Psychoanalytical Theories** *:* Sigmund Freud in 1904 postulated that psychological conflict between drive i.e., wishful impulses, antithetical wishes and conscience generate defenses against the wishful impulses. Deficiency or deficit model explains in cases of schizophrenia that libidinal energy is invested in the patient's fantasized objects. It is also suggested that the hostility inherent in any form of intense ambivalence toward an object could be projected into feelings of being persecuted by that object (McGlashan, 2009).

Psychiatric Co-Morbidities

- **Substance Abuse and Alcoholism:** Studies suggest an association between schizophrenia and alcoholism. The comorbidity of schizophrenia and alcoholism are at the risk with criminality on a larger scale. Schizophrenic patients have been found violent offenders compared with subjects with schizophrenia who did not abuse alcohol. Literature suggests that for the prevention of the crimes committed by people with schizophrenia, a clinician should also watch for comorbid alcohol abuse (Rasanen, Tiilhonen., & Isohanni, 1998). Rates of comorbidity with substance-related disorders are high in schizophrenia. Over half of individuals of this disorder have tobacco-use disorder and smoke cigarettes regularly (American Psychiatric Association [APA], 2013)
- **Panic Disorder:** Studies reported 45% prevalence of panic attacks in patients with schizophrenia. With paranoid schizophrenia, the symptoms of panic attacks are common (Labbate & Young., & Arana, 1999). Further these panic symptoms are associated with increased suicidal ideation and increased vulnerability to comorbid substance use (Goodwin & McGrath, 2006).
- **Depression:** In recent years attention has been given to depressive mood disorder associated with schizophrenia (Planansky & Johnston, 1978).The recognizable symptoms during schizophrenia are characterized as sadness; feeling of emptiness, impairment of interpersonal relations, suicidal ideas, striking passivity and neurasthenic complaints (McGlashan & Carpenter, 1976).One hospital based clinical study suggests that out of 529 patients; 34% patients were found to have depressive symptoms. These Patients were followed up for 6 to 48 months; among them 10% subjects develop depressive symptoms, 3% developed schizoaffective disorders (Raju, 1986).
- **Personality Disorder:** Patients with personality disorder have an increased risk of mortality through suicide, homicide and accidents. Schizotypal personality disorder is considered to be an attenuated manifestation of schizophrenia (Saran, 2010).
- **Anxiety, OCD and Panic Disorder:** Comorbidity with anxiety disorders is increasingly recognized in schizophrenia. OCD and panic disorders are elevated in individuals with schizophrenia compared with the general population. Schizotypal or paranoid personality disorder may sometimes precede the onset of schizophrenia (Balye, Krebs, Epelbaum, Levy., & Hardy, 2001).

TREATMENT

Earlier until the 1950s, the treatment of schizophrenia generally took place in large asylums where people remained confined for much of their lives. Various community programmes have been launched by government regarding the treatment of schizophrenia.

Pharmacological Treatment

The efficacy of this treatment is well-established for the treatment of acute psychotic episodes and relapse prevention overtime. Clozapinereduces primary and negative symptoms. It decreases relapses along with suicidal behaviour and improves stability in the community. It is also helpful in reducing preexisting tardive dyskinesia. Risperidonereduces the psychotic symptoms. Olanzapineimproves cognitive functions and also works on positive and negative symptoms. Quetiapine, Ziprasidone, Aripiprazole, and Ziprasidone all medicines are effective on positive and negative symptoms. The randomized control trial revealed that antipsychotic agents are associated with 20% improvement in symptoms (Lindenmayer, Khan, Iskander, Abad., & Parker, 2007).

Psychosocial Interventions

- **Psychoeducation:** Psychoeducation can be targeted on the patient to improve outcomes, enhance compliance, and increase knowledge, including on early relapse recognition, thereby contributing to a better sense of well-being. Illness needs to explain to patients as it reinforces patient's comprehension level. Studies revealed that psychoeducation helps in reducing relapse and readmission (Pekkala & Merinder, 2002).
- **Cognitive Behaviour Therapy:** The desired end-point in treating schizophrenia is not only the symptoms reduction whereas the improvement of global functioning via amelioration of cognitive deficits i.e., impaired vigilance, attention, planning and decision–making; needs to applied in adjunctive management (Hayes & McGrath, 2000). Techniques of cognitive behaviour therapy are helpful in dealing with symptoms of panic disorder, anxiety, delusions, auditory hallucinations and negative symptoms. Socratic questioning, identifying and challenging thoughts, exposure of fearful stimulus, vivo, vitro exposure are beneficial in symptoms reduction (Kaplan, 2010).
- **Insight-Oriented Therapy:** Literature suggested the efficacy of insight-oriented psychotherapy in schizophrenia for adaptive functioning. This therapy helps in increasing insight and awareness about symptoms and treatment (Rathod, Kingdom, Smith., & Turkington, 2005).
- **Family Intervention:** In schizophrenia, the criticism and hostility from a close relative (expressed emotion) is the main cause of relapse prevention. Families are the key elements of support for most patients, hence the main task of therapist is to help family members in a positive and constructive ways Psychosocial interventions aimed at developing an alliance with focus on reducing emotional distress, boundary setting and instillation of realistic expectations of patients and services. Thus the aim is to maintain patients in contact with services, and also to reduce frequency and duration of admission, improve outcomes, especially social functioning and quality of life (Leff et al., 1990).

- **Group Therapy:** The group therapy sessions generally take place in clinics, hospitals or in private offices. The goals of group therapy are to emphasis insight, behavioural change, skills development, social support, maintenance and participation in recreational activities. Patients have an opportunity to express their feelings in group and can improve faster (Maurice, 1970).
- **Social Skill Training:** Social skills training are defined as required interpersonal behaviour to attain instrumental goals necessary for community survival, independence and to establish, maintain, and deepen supportive and socially rewarding relationship. Affective, cognitive, verbal and behavioural domains of functioning are most of the time impairs a person's potential for enjoying and sustaining interpersonal relationships. Social skill training is based on a structured learning-oriented approach that aimed to acquisition of skills relevant to the individual and related with his/her environment. It also includes video-modelling, role-play, and other specific homework to solve problem-solving skills (Robertson, Connaughton., & Nicol, 1998). Vocational training is also an important part of social training, however is not dependent on social skill training. Studies reported that specialist vocational training remains scarce component of long-term illness management in most services (Crowther, Marshall, Bond., & Huxley, 2001).
- **Psychosocial Rehabilitation:** Psychosocial rehabilitation emerged during the late 1940s when former patients began to meet together in a social club in New York City to satisfy their needs for acceptance and emotional support. During rehabilitation, patients create their own social support network and the members of psychosocial club design some activities that build experiences of mutual ownership and needs (Chandrasekhar, Prashanth, Kasthuri & Madhusudan, 2010).

BIPOLAR DISORDER

Bipolar disorder affects one's mood very badly. There is little difference in mood and affect which are related with bipolar disorder. Mood is a pervasive and sustained feeling experienced internally that influences a person's behaviour and perception of the world. The external expression of mood is called affect. The symptoms are characterized by unusual shifts in mood, energy, activity levels etc. These symptoms fluctuate from time to time. The person suffering with bipolar disorder can live productive life, if treated properly (Rao, 2010).

Incidence and Prevalence

The domains of bipolar disorder are reflected by depressive episodes with mania or hypomania. One of five women and one of ten men are affected by depression at some time in their life. One percent of the general population is account for bipolar disorder whereas 5 percent of the population and up to 50 percent of population (of bipolar disorder) account for depression. Bipolar II subtype (depression plus hypomania rather than mania) is detected frequently in clinical population. Approximately 15 percent of depressive patients are disabled and commit suicide. Young and elder population are high in committing suicide, despite the availability of effective treatment. Life time prevalence rate of bipolar I disorder, bipolar II (see the Table 2 for diagnostic criteria for Bipolar Disorder*)* and major depressive disorder respectively is 0-2.4%, 0.3-4.8% and 5-17%. Manic episodes are common in men whereas bipolar I disorder is almost equal in occurrences among both men and women (Rihmer & Angst, 2005).

Table 2. Diagnostic criteria for Bipolar Disorder

DSM4	DSM5
Bipolar disorder	Bipolar Disorder 1: It is necessary to meet the provided criteria for manic episodes. This episode may have been preceded by and may be followed by hypomanic or major depressive episodes.
Criteria for manic episode (Minor Changes). A distinct period of abnormality and persistently elevated, expansive, or irritable mood, lasting at least 1 week or any duration if hospitalization is necessary	Criteria for manic episode: **A**. A distinct period of abnormally and persistently elevated, expansive, or irritable mood and abnormally and persistently increased goal-directed activity or energy, lasting at least 1 week and present most of the day, nearly every day or any duration if hospitalization is necessary.
Criteria B: (No changes)	**B.** During the period of mood disturbance and increased energy or activity, three or more of the following symptoms four if the mood is only irritable are present to significant degree and represent a noticeable change from usual behaviour. 1. Inflated self-esteem or grandiosity. 2.Decreased need for sleep e.g., feels rested after only 3 hours of sleep 3. More talkative than usual or pressure to keep talking. 4. Flight of ideas or subjective experience that thoughts are racing. 5. Distractibility i.e., attention too easily drawn to unimportant or irrelevant external stimuli. As reported or observed. 6. Increase in goal-directed activity either socially, at work or school, or sexually or psychomotor agitation (i.e., purposeless non-goal directed activity). 7. Excessive involvement in activities that have a high potential for painful consequences
Criteria C: The symptoms do not meet criteria for a mixed episode	**C.** The mood disturbance is sufficiently severe to cause marked impairment in social or occupational functioning or to necessitate hospitalization to prevent harm to self or others, or there are psychotic features.
Criteria D: (No changes)	**Criteria D:** The episode is not attributable to the physiological effects of a substance e.g., a drug of abuse, a medication, other treatment or to another medical condition.
Note: Manic like episodes that are clearly caused by somatic antidepressant treatment (e.g., medication, ECT, Light therapy) should not count towards a diagnosis of bipolar 1 disorder.	**Note: a** full manic episode that emerges during antidepressant treatment (e.g., medication, electroconvulsive therapy) but persists at a fully syndromal level beyond the physiological effect of that treatment is sufficient evidence for a manic episode and therefore, a bipolar 1 diagnosis.
	Note: criteria A-D constitute a manic episode. At least one lifetime manic episode is required for the diagnosis of bipolar 1 disorder.
	A. criteria have been met for at least onemanic episode (criteria A-D under "Manic episodes" above). **B.** The occurrence of the manic and major depressive episode is not better explained by schizoaffective disorder, schizophrenia, schizophrenic form disorder, delusional disorder, or other specified or unspecified schizophrenia spectrum and other psychotic disorder.

American Psychiatric Association (2000, 2013)

ETIOLOGY

- **Psychodynamic Theories:** Several etiological factors are mentioned under psychodynamic theories, such as:
    - **Anger turned Inward:** Sigmund Freud mentioned in his paper "mourning and melancholia" that due to real or imagined object loss, the individual's anger turned towards self. An actual object loss is present in external reality in cases of grief. Whereas in cases of depression, the lost object is emotional rather than real. Depressed patients experience profound self-depreciation and deficit self-esteem.
    - **Introjection:** Has an important place in psychodynamic field. The patients internalize the lost object so that it becomes an internal presence. Through introjection, the ego gives up a valued and loved object, later, Freud noted. Departed love object is perceived by depressed person as having abandoned them, hence feeling of hatred and anger are intermingled with feeling of love (Strachey, 1914).

Freud's theory extended by Abraham, (1911) gave 'The classical view of depression' which includes 4 key points:

1. During oral phase of 12 to 18 month, disturbances in infant-mother relationship.
2. -Loss of real or imaginal object.
3. Use of introjection to deal with the distress connected with the object loss.
4. Anger with mixture of love and hate is directed inward at the self.

Feelings related with loss objects are related with a mixture of love and hate, anger is directed towards self. Edith Jacobson (1971) suggested that depression is a result of weak and helpless ego wherein the superego is supreme and control ego. According to Jacobson the negative aspects of the object is experienced by self and cruel superego that keeps all the qualities as depressed person identified with ambivalently regarded lost love objects. Individual is captured in a fusion of the bad self with the bad object as the boundary between self and object disappeared. Arieti (1959) studied severely ill patients those were unresponsive for treatment. On the basis of his observation, he proposed a term "dominant other" i.e., the person for whom depressed patients live. The dominant other is generally the spouse or a parent but sometimes a principle, an organization and an ideal serves similar psychodynamic functions. He refereed this structure as "the dominant ideology or the dominant goal". Lewin (1950) referred purified pleasure ego for the ego of hypomanic patients. Unpleasant perceptions, affects and distressing psychic realities related with self-punishments are unaccepted by using the denial defense mechanism. Klein (1948) suggested hypomania as defensive reaction to depression. This includes omnipotence, denial, idealization and contempt. Bibring, (1953) proposed that manic elation is a reaction secondary to serve depression. Narcissistic aspirations to be loved, worthy, superior, and virtually flawless is fulfilled by mania unconsciously.

Psychiatric Comorbidity

Earlier bipolar disorder was relatively rare psychiatric illness, characterized by episodes of euphoric excitement and depressive retardation. This was easy to diagnose and as well as to treat. Gradually the complexity of disorder increased and it has become very difficult to handle. Some Indian studies reported 50% of the patients with comorbid substance abuse. Highest prevalence of cannabis used disorder was 26.7% whereas the commonest comorbid drug was alcohol with 23.8% at abuse level (Kumar & Raju, 1998).

- **Substance Dependence:** Among alcohol-abusing and alcohol-dependent patients, prevalence rates for psychiatric comorbidity of between 57% and 84% have been reported (Lejoyeux & Marinescu, 2006). Approximately 37% of bipolar II disorders have a substance use disorder. Mood disorders with alcohol dependence occur frequently. In various studies individuals with substance-use disorder were found to meet the criteria for major depression. Alcoholics with independent major depression were found to be more likely to attempt suicide than those with substance-induced depression.
- **Mental Retardation, Pervasive Developmental Disorder:** Children with mental retardation found to have psychiatric comorbidity. In cases of mild level of mental retardation mood disorder is very common. 57% of cases have been found to have psychiatric comorbidity in cases of mental retardation (Khess, Dutta, Chakrabarty, Bhattacharya, das., & Kothari, 1988). Children with pervasive developmental disorders were observed to have attention deficit hyperactivity disorder, anxiety disorder and bipolar affective disorder (Girimaji, Biju, Srinath., &Seshadri, 2005).
- **Eating Disorder:** This is very common disorder that occurred in cases of bipolar mood disorder. In presence of this disorder, the clinician needs to be aware regarding the challenges for treatment (Sengupta, 1992). 14% of individuals have at least one lifetime eating disorder in bipolar II disorder. The common eating disorder in bipolar disorder is Binge-eating disorder than bulimia nervosa and anorexia nervosa (DSM V, 2013).
- **Anxiety Disorder:** Anxiety disorder is most common associated disorder with bipolar I and especially bipolar II. Approximately 75% of individuals with bipolar disorder have an anxiety disorder. Children and adolescents have higher rate of comorbid anxiety disorder. Anxiety disorder has a strong correlation with mood. The fluctuations in mood affected by anxiety, hence further effect the treatment (DSM V, 2013).

TREATMENT

Pharmaco-Therapeutic Treatment

Long-term treatment of bipolar disorder covers medications and psychotherapeutic approach. Selective-serotonin reuptake inhibitors are helpful in mood regulation as these reduce mania and also work on depression. Valproate, lithium, olanzapine and lamotrigine reduce the occurrence of mania. During mania lithium, valproic acid and carbamazepine improve overall psychomotor activity, grandiosity, irritability and insomnia. To control the cycle of depression and mania, generally clinicians add bupropion, inositol and choline as well. When the disease increased, antipsychotic drugs are helpful but these have a less primary role in the long-term management of bipolar disorder

Psychotherapies

- **Cognitive Behavior Therapy:** Cognitive behaviour therapy is valuable in helping patients to accept their illness and the need for continuous treatment. Randomized study revealed that psychoeducation, a part of psychotherapy helps in reducing the rates of manic illness in bipolar patients over 18 months by 30 percent. Initial sessions include the education of identifying early sign of depression. The overall aim of cognitive behaviour therapy across disorder is described as (1) To help patient in gaining greater awareness regarding their functional relationship between their thinking, emotional and behavioural difficulties along with proper education about their conditions. (2) To learn and master more adaptive ways of coping with their problems (Perry, Tarrier, Morriss, McCarthy., & Limb, 1999).

In majority of the cases, bipolar disorder patient switch from one episode to another. During depressive episode individual have selective recall of mood-congruent negative memories and are more likely to minimize the significance of a positive event. Patient might tend to personalize and overgeneralize-or think more globally –about the impact of a negative life event. When these individual switch into mania and hypomania, the change in mood states would be associated with underestimation of risk, overestimation of opportunities and/or probabilities for success, and a mood-dependent impairment in the ability to perceive the impact that one's behaviour has on others. During manic episodes the ability to perceive risk is impaired. Overestimation of opportunity, underestimation of risk and probability for success are associated with changes in mood states. Patients don't realize the impact of their behaviour on others. Thus the information processing errors maintain the pathological mood disturbances. Therapist needs to identify surface thoughts, ideas and mental images associated with mood state, referred as 'automatic thoughts' and the "deeper" thoughts referred as dysfunctional belief or schema (Beck, 1976). In this view there are some techniques that are used to treat mood disorder, which are explained in Table 3.

Table 3. Combined cognitive behaviour therapy for Bipolar I and Bipolar II disorder

Behavioural Techniques	Explanations	Cognitive Techniques	Explanations
Behaviour and mood recording	To help people get moving and as a practical means to help people get moving and a platform that help individual to identify the relationship between dysfunctional pattern of thinking and symptoms.	Downward arrow	This technique is used to identify the usual way of a problem situation and unpleasant emotions experienced by patients within a particular situation.
Monitoring activity	Self-monitoring helps therapist and patient to test the thoughts and their activities.	• Distraction techniques • Sensory awareness • Mental exercises • Pleasant memories and Fantasies	This method teach patient to get away from the disturbing thoughts.
Graded task assignment	This method is the practice of maximizing the chances of success by breaking tasks down into small, manageable steps.	Daily Record of Dysfunctional thoughts	A record of negative and dysfunctional thoughts help patient to work on it.

- **Interpersonal Therapy:** Interpersonal therapy (IPT) was developed by Gerald Klerman and Myrna Weismann (1969). The theoretical basis of IPT includes the work of Adolf Meyer and Harry Stack Sullivan. It deals with relationship issues along with the adaptation of environmental changes. This approach involves three interacting components: symptom formation, social and interpersonal experiences and enduring personality pattern. Interpersonal therapy has two goals:
    - To reduce depressive symptoms and improve self-esteem,
    - To help patients in developing more effective strategies for dealing with social and interpersonal relations. This approach recognizes the importance for early developmental experience and also emphasizes interpersonal relationships in the current life situation (Markowitz & Weissman, 2010).

Behavioural Strategies and Techniques for Depression

- **Maintain Records:** Recording positive and negative mood and activities, is essential part of behavioural therapies. Patients monitor immediate and long-term consequences of particular behaviour.
- **Activity Schedule:** Daily record helps therapist to encourage their participation in activities that are related with pleasure.
- **Manage Unpleasant Events:** Feelings are triggered by various situations and interactions. These feelings could be identified by daily record. Patients learn to substitute positive thoughts and prepare to tackle unpleasant situation.
- **Develop New Self-Reinforcement Patterns:** Goal-directed activities are rewarded by increasing it and by learning to reward for themselves.
- **Enhancing Social Skills:** Assertiveness training, modeling, role play, feedback and rehearsal helps in addressing the deficits in social skills.
- **Cognitive Skills Training:** To decrease negative thinking and to increase positive thinking cognitive skills is required. To monitor their thinking and to discriminate between positive and negative thoughts, necessary and unnecessary thoughts and constructive and deconstructive thoughts, specific techniques that include thought-stopping, disputing irrational thoughts and correcting errors in attribution regarding causes of successes and failures.
- **Time Management:** To plan and prepare necessary participation in pleasant events is an important part of therapy. An effort is made to work out appropriate balance between activities that patients have to do and they feel to do (Fennel, 1998).
- **Interpersonal and Social Rhythm Therapy:** This therapy is an adaptation of interpersonal therapy for depression. Poor interpersonal functioning, disruption into sleep/wake cycles are associated with bipolar disorder. Therapy has two objectives:
    - Resolution of key interpersonal problems related to grief, role disputes, interpersonal conflicts or interpersonal deficits.
    - Stabilize social rhythms (day routine, regularity of sleep, exercise and socialization). Therapy helps in gaining insight about bi-directional relationship between moods and interpersonal events. It reduces the frequency of episodic recurrence of disorder.

Interpersonal Problem Areas in Interpersonal and Social Rhythm Therapy

- **Phase 1:**
    - **Grief:** Unresolved grief also referred as "complicated Bereavement". Therapist address unresolved feelings around death of an important person in patient's life
    - **Role Transitions:** Social role transitions include life cycle transitions and social transition
        - Adolescence, childbirth, menopause, decline of physical activity all are part of life cycle transition. Role Transition II includes;
        - Grief at loss of old role i.e., job loss, retirement and moving.
        - Poor adaptation to new Role i.e., promotion at work or in school, parenting
        - Rejection of new Role i.e., unemployment, homemaking, parenting and leaving home.
    - **Interpersonal Deficits:** Patients have a history of impoverished relationship.
        - Grief for the "lost healthy self".

Therapist should help patient in focusing on her true objective along with exploring patient's sadness and frustration. To teach patient to maintain social rhythm stability. (Frank, 2005)

- **Intermediate Phase:**
    - To stabilize social rhythms and identify the most unstable rhythms and set goals for change, set reasonable expectations for change, search for triggers to rhythm disruption.
    - Balance needs to maintain
    - Planned routine needs to adapted and be prepared for unexpected routine.
    - Sleep pattern should be the primary focus of social rhythm matrices biology of sleep should be explained to patient.

Strategies in IPT

1. To select problem areas.
2. Work on grief and role transition see in Table 4.

OBSESSIVE-COMPULSIVE DISORDER

Obsessive-compulsive disorder is characterized by recurrent obsessional thoughts and compulsive acts. There are some thoughts, ideas, images and impulses which enter into individual's mind again and again in a stereotyped form are known as obsessional thoughts. These are very distressing as these are violent, obscene or perceived as senseless. These thoughts are involuntary however recognized as individual's own thoughts. Compulsive acts are stereotyped behaviour which is done repeatedly. These acts are not enjoyable and not related with any useful task yet individual find himself bound to do it.

Incidence and Prevalence

Males are affected more by OCD in childhood period whereas females are more affected during adulthood. The disorder has a prevalence rate of 1.2% on 12 month with a similar prevalence internationally

Table 4. Strategies in IPT in grief and role transition

Problem Areas	Goals	Strategies
Grief	• To facilitate mourning process • To help patient to manage the loss by re-establishing interest and develop new relationships	Review depressive symptoms Psychoeducate patient about the associated symptoms and death of a loved one • Take a description from patient about the events just prior to, during and after the death. Accompany him for the death scene and rituals. • Reconstruct patient's relationship with deceased (listen to stories, ask patient to bring pictures etc) • To encourage patient to have contact and make friends and also to indulge in other interested activities.
Interpersonal disputes	• To identify dispute • Choose a plan of action • To bring a satisfactory resolution by modifying expectations or problematic communication	• To review depressive symptoms • Explain patient about the relationship between onset to the covert or overt dispute and the symptoms • To establish the stage of dispute
Role transitions	• Mourn the loss of the old role • To look at the positive aspect of the new role • To gain mastery of a new role by developing necessary new skills.	• To review depressive symptoms • Assess the difficulty in coping with new life situation • Provide an understanding about positive and negative aspects of old and new roles. • Explore the opportunities in new role and mourn the loss of the old role. • To facilitate movements into new role
Interpersonal deficits	• To reduce patient's social isolation • To encourage patients to form new relationship.	• To review symptoms • To relate symptoms to isolation • To understand the positive and negative aspect of the relationship. • To assess the past and present relationship. • Help patients in gaining an insight about the patterns in relationship • Use of role-play and feedback.

(Frank, 2005).

(1.1% -1.8%). 25% of cases experience OCD by age of 14 years. The mean age at onset is 19.5 years. After age 35 the onset is rare, however occur. Mostly the onset of symptoms is gradual but sometimes it could be acute as well. Prevalence rate in children and adolescents is 2.7%. Earlier onset is occurred in males rather than females (Soomro, 2012).

ETIOLOGY

Pierre Janet worked on OCD and proposed a theoretical model. His work was published in two volume named as 'obsessions and psychasthenia. According to Janet, (1903) the central disturbance lay in a pathological shrinking of mental energy that resulted in a disintegration of the normal organization of mental functions which further led to the failure of the highest of those functions will and attention, which enabled individual to control their thoughts and action, to perceive themselves and their environment realistically, and to perform actions appropriate to that correctly perceived reality. When these higher mental functions were impaired (emotions, motoric correlates), they are out of control. Without regard for reality, lower functions made their appearance in a chaos of mental anarchy. They operated with energy that was normally and naturally theirs and with an additional quantum of energy derived from the higher functions.

Psychoanalytic perspective explains the role of defense mechanism that determines the form and quality of obsessive-compulsive symptoms. These are Isolation, undoing and reaction-formation. *Isolation* is a defense mechanism that protects an individual from anxiety-provoking affects and impulses. In isolation, the affect and the impulse of which it is a derivative, are separated from the ideational component and pushed out of consciousness. If isolation is completely successful, the impulse and associated affect are totally repressed. Undoingdefense mechanism helps in reducing anxiety. It is a compulsive act that is performed in an attempt to prevent or undo the consequences that the patient irrationally anticipates from a frightening obsessional thought or impulse. *Reaction formation* manifest pattern of behaviour and consciously experience attitudes that are exactly the opposite of the underlying impulses. Often, these patterns appear to an observer to be highly exaggerated and, at times, quite inappropriate. This defense mechanism is responsible for many of the personality traits characterized by control that make up the obsessive-compulsive character (Steketee & Lam, 1993).

- **Psychogenic Factors:** Patients with OCD are occupied with aggression or dirt which is related with symptoms and the associated cause lie behind it. The disturbances in normal growth and development of Anal-sadistic phase are related with psychogenesis of obsessive-compulsive disorder. The impulses associated with the anal-sadistic phase are modified in the oedipal and succeeding stages of development. The disturbed developmental process includes unmodified anal-sadistic impulses remains as a component of the individual's psychological makeup. Fixation at particular points under some circumstances gives rise to the difficulties (Geller et al., 2001).
- **Regression:** In OCD, patients begin with a conflict over the oedipal genital impulse. The impulse aroused by an environmental stimulus. Rather than repressing and converting that impulse, a difference maneuver is employed to avoid the associated anxiety with genital impulse. The genital impulses are abandoned and regressed to the earlier anal-sadistic phase of psychosexual development. The distortions that occurred during childhood development are responsible to return to earlier stage due to remained fixation point. Regressive movement of psychic energy reinforced anal-sadistic impulses from the earlier phase of development, hence new anxieties and new conflicts are aroused in behaviour by the pressure of reactivated anal and aggressive impulses. An alteration in the quality of the energy is caused by regression with which the psychic apparatus deal and in the nature of the defenses controlling that energy.
- **Learning Theories:** Learning theory proposed a view of anxiety as a conditioned or learned response to specific stimuli or sets of stimuli and so has developed behavioural accounts of the acquisition and maintenance of anxiety disorders. Mowrer 1969, theory holds that neutral stimuli become associated with fear or anxiety through a process of respondent conditioning by becoming paired with events that are by nature noxious or anxiety producing. Thus, in OCD, previously neutral objects and thoughts become conditioned stimuli capable of provoking anxiety or discomfort. The stage of symptom development is complete when avoidance or escape behaviours are established to reduce the discomfort attached to the obsession thoughts and maintained by anxiety reduction.

Psychiatric Comorbidity

- **Obsessive Compulsive Disorder and Mood Disorder:** Since the nineteenth century, the association between OCD and depression is acknowledged. Literature suggests that one-third of patients with OCD have concurrent major depressive disorder at the time of clinical evaluation and 10times more prevalent in OCD cases (Denys, Tenney, vanMegen, de Geus, & Westenberg, 2004). Additionally, 60-80% of OCDcases experienced a depressive episode in their life. The comorbidity of bipolar disorder in OCD influence symptoms and make disorder complicated (D'Ambrosioetal, Albert, Bogetto., & Maina, 2010).15-35% expected overlap between OCD and BPD has been found by studies consistently. The evidence of a higher-than-expected overlap between OCD and BPAD is highlighted through the epidemiological catchment area study in adult cases. It revealed that 23% of cases with BPAD also met criteria for OCD (Robins & Price, 1991). Other published studies from 1997 to 2004 concluded that the rate of lifetime comorbid BD is up to 21.5% in clinical and epidemiological samples of patients with OCD along with the presence of cyclothymic traits and/or some lifetime hypomanic symptoms (Hantouche et al., 2003).
- **Personality Disorder and OCD:** It has been reported that schizotypal personality disorder is related with the severity of obsessive-compulsive disorder. Cognitive, perceptual and disorganized factors of schizotypal personality are related with OCD(Yamamoto et al., 2012).In a sample of 54 subjects, it was found the higher comorbidity of depression and OCD in axis 1 disorder (Kalra et al., 2008). The profile of schizo-obsessive patients had higher rates of paranoid symptoms, personality disorders and disability (Rajkumar, Reddy., & Kandavelal, 2008).
- **OCD and Psychosis:** Literature review suggests the growing evidences of patient with comorbid OCD and schizophrenia (Hwang & Hollander, 1993). The clinical picture of such cases are little different. Studies suggest that onset of OCD co-occurred with the onset of schizophrenia in 47-76% of the cases (Poyurovsky, Faragian, Shabeta., & Kosov, 2008). Case studies revealed that obsessive doubts, suicidal thoughts contaminated obsessions and compulsions are common in OCD with psychosis (Ganesan et al., 2001).
- **OCD and Other Anxiety Disorders:** Data suggest life time comorbidity between OCD and other anxiety disorder has been identified as follows: 22% for specific phobia, 18% for social phobia, 12% for panic disorder and 30% for generalized anxiety disorder (Pigott, Heureux, Dubbert, Bernstein., & Murphy, 1994). Generalized anxiety disorder makes treatment worse by affecting the clinical symptoms. In adults, this comorbidity is high. There is a lifetime history of GAD with OCD in over 30% of adults (Andrews, Morris-Yates, Holt, &Henderson., 1990). Indian studies suggest 17% major depression, 6% dysthymia and 7% any anxiety disorder among 218 OCD subjects (Bhattacharya, Prasanna, Khanna, JanardhanRedy., & Sheshadri, 2005). The clinical symptoms of post-traumatic disorder and OCD are almost similar in nature. The symptoms are characterized with repeated intrusive thoughts, including avoidant behaviour that interferes with daily functioning, compulsions to reduce the anxiety. OCD and PTSD are associated with classical conditioning to an anxiety-provoking stimulus; this connection between stimulus and anxiety lead reinforcement by behaviour that reduce anxiety. However, the content of the obsessions is different from the intrusive symptoms of PTSD. Case series revealed the difference between general obsessive thoughts and PTSD. Fear of contamination, disgust of dirt and doubt are common in OCD whereas in PTSD the fears are more common (Zohar, Fostick ., & Juyen-wetzler, 2009).

- **OCD and Neurological Diseases:** Evidences suggest that Individual with neurological illnesses have anxiety disorder frequently. Panic disorder, generalized anxiety disorder, social phobia and OCD are common anxiety disorder (Davies, Gabbert., & Riggs, 2001). Most of the time these disorders are untreated as they are unrecognized and attributed to be a normal response of a neurological illness. These disorders should be treated as they can affect the morbidity and mortality in patients with neurological illness.10-22% of Patients with temporal lobe epilepsy (TLE) show a high rate of contaminated obsessions and compulsions, ordering and symmetrical obsessions (Kaplan, 2010).

Patients with basal ganglia dysfunctions, such as Tourette's syndrome, Huntington's disease, and Sydenham's chorea have been associated with an acute onset of OCD (Ogai, Iyo, Mori, &Takei, 2005, Miguel, Rauch, & Jenike,1997). One-third to one-half of children experience comorbid OCD throughout their lifetime. The clinical symptoms are characterized with repeated, symmetry, counting ordering and arranging obsessions and compulsions in presence of tic disorder (March et al., 2007). The comorbidity of OCD has been found in Parkinson's disease. The reason of this comorbidity is highlighted in terms of pathophysiology of OCD in PD along with common correlation of basal ganglia (Harbishettar, Kumar, Janardhan Reddy., & Thennarasu, 2005).

- **Obsessive-Compulsive Disorder and Attention Deficit Hyperactivity Disorder:** Attention deficit hyperactivity disorder is a common childhood-onset neurodevelopmental disorder that occurs in 5% of the population that co-occurs with OCD (Faraone, Sergeant, Gillberg., & Biederman, 2003). Both of the conditions are present symptoms of inattention, attentive symptoms. ADHD and OCD are comorbid with TS (De Geus, Denys, Sitskoorn., & Westenberg, 2007) with prevalence of 0.5-1% (Stewart et al., 2009). Prevalence of ADHD rate varies widely from 0 to 51% among OCD patients. Although the differences exist in the nature of clinical population (Geller et al., 2001; Jaisoorya, Janardhan, Reddy., & Srinath, 2003). Childhood onset OCD have higher rate of ADHD than in general ADHD population sample. The clinical symptoms show the presence of hoarding obsessions/behaviour. Few case studies revealed total 41.9% of participants with ADHD have been found with hoarding behaviours compared to 29.2% of participants without ADHD (Sheppard et al. 2010). 18-40% OCD cases have been found the co-occurrence of hoarding obsessions with comorbid ADHD (Frost, Krause., & Steketee, 1996).

TREATMENT

Pharmacotherapy

Evidences suggested that Tricyclic antidepressant clomipramine is effective for the treatment of OCD. Clomipramine is an effective antiobsessional rather than anti-depressant. Desipramine (Norpeamin), nortriptyline (pamelor), amitriptyline (Elavil), clorgyline and imipramine (Tofranil) are effective in the treatment of OCD. Serotonin reuptake blocking agemts like: Nontricyclic, fluoxetine, clomipramine are effective to control obsessions.

Psychological Intervention

Psychotherapy has been very effective treatment to treat various disorders, although it is very difficult and take time (long term treatment). Patient generally drop out during the treatment and seek help when their symptoms get worse. Thus these are the challenges for clinicians to handle. Literature suggested that patients with major depression along with coexisting axis I, II or III conditions that called, "compound depression". There are other factors also exist like: female gender, family history, severity of illness, early or late age of onset and chronicity of illness. Patients with comorbid anxiety respond poorly to treatment: they tend to have incomplete remission of symptoms and slower response to medication; hence the assessment should include screening for anxiety symptoms and disorders. There is significant overlap between OCD and depression that are often missed by clinician. Noncompliance issues have been associated with eating disorders as well as antidepressant therapies along with cognitive behavior therapy has been found very effective.

Cognitive Behaviour therapy

- **Aversive Procedure:** To eliminate obsessional thoughts aversive therapy is good. The occurrence of a noxious event or punishment immediately follows a behaviour that decreases the likelihood of that behaviour again.
- **Systematic Desensitization:** Systematic-Desensitization is an anxiety-reduction procedure. During systematic-desensitization patients are exposed to a graded hierarchy of anxiety-provoking stimuli in imagination or in vivo that maintain a state of calm through deep muscle relaxation or a variety of other methods applied to induce a countering relaxation.
- **Exposure Response Prevention:** To combat obsessions and compulsion, prolonged exposure and response prevention is used. Obsessional cues are exposed and carefully prevented from engaging in compulsive behaviour. Thus, an attempt is to reduce the anxiety-provoking valence of the obsessions while simultaneously blocking the reinforcement of anxiety reduction that accompanies the carrying out of compulsive behaviours. The combination treatment approach repeatedly exposes patients for prolonged periods to events or thoughts that provoke anxiety while strictly preventing ritualistic behaviours (Salkovskis & Krik 1988).

Insight Psychotherapy

The important components of therapy are; the prominence of situational precipitating events, the capacity to relate to the physician, evidence of good relationships with others, stable work parents, the capacity to tolerate anxiety and depression, the ability to express emotion, intelligence, the ability to be introspective, flexibility in thinking and behaviour and motivation for change (Rathod, 2005).

DISCUSSION

The above description shows the comorbid conditions in schizophrenia, bipolar disorder and obsessive compulsive disorder. As studies clearly show some common comorbid disorders i.e., anxiety, depression and eating disorder. Substance abuse, personality disorder and depression are more common in schizophrenia. Antipsychotic medications are effective in treatment of these disorders. Evidences suggested group therapy, cognitive behaviour therapy and family therapy, insight oriented psychotherapies are helpful in symptoms reduction. Since the publication of DSM 5, the diagnostic criterions have been changed. Obsessive-compulsive disorder has been separated from the cluster of anxiety disorder. Mood disorders are more common in OCD that interfere the process of treatment. There is a need to assess comorbid conditions thoroughly as it affects the process of treatment and a main cause of relapse. Selective serotonin reuptake inhibitor (SSRI) helps in dealing with mood disorder. Increased recognition of psychotherapy is an important aspect of many psychiatric and medical conditions that should be used widely (Sriram, 1990).

CONCLUSION

While the literature suggests that presence of two or three disorders make treatment worse, hence multidisciplinary treatment need to be used which would be helpful. This chapter pointed out few important issues which need to handle by the clinicians. The chapter also talks about the changes in treatment approach. A balanced approach need to be adopted by practitioner which would be helpful for patients. A proper assessment to rule out the other disorder is necessary so that required treatment could be started to maintain the follow up. Majority of the comorbid disorders were identified as phobic disorders, posttraumatic stress and major depression. Life time disorders included antisocial personality disorder (40%), phobia (34%), posttraumatic stress (27%) and major depression (23%), anxiety disorder (76%) with histories of affective disorders (Halikas, 1994).

REFERENCES

Abraham, K. (1911). Notes on the psychoanalytic investigation and treatment of manic-depressive insanity and allied conditions. In *Selected papers on psychoanalysis.* Hogarth Press and the Institute of Psychoanalysis.

American Psychiatric Association. (2013). Diagnostic and Statistical Manual of mental Disorders (5th ed.). Washington, DC: American Psychiatric Association.

Andrews, G., Stewart, G., Morris-Yates, A., Holt, P., & Henderson, S. (1990). Evidence for a general neurotic syndrome. *The British Journal of Psychiatry*, *157*(1), 6–12. doi:10.1192/bjp.157.1.6 PMID:2397364

Arieti, S. (1959). Manic-Depressive Psychosis. American Handbook of Psychiatry, (1), 419-454.

Balye, F.J., Krebs, M.O., Epelbaum, C., Levy, D., & Hardy, P. (2001). Clinical Features of panic attacks in schizophrenia. *European Psychiatry: The Journal of the Association of European Psychiatrist*, (6), 349-353.

Beck, A. T. (1976). Cognitive therapy and the emotional disorders. International University Press.

Bhagwagar, Z. (2007). Bipolar disorder and its comorbidities. *Medscape Psychiatry.* Retrieved from http://www.medscape.org/viewarticle/558733

Bhattacharyya, S., Prasanna, C. L. N., Khanna, S., Janardhan Reddy, Y. C., & Sheshadri, S. (2005). A family Genetic study of clinical subtypes of obsessive-compulsive disorder. *Psychiatric Genetics*, *15*(3), 175–180. doi:10.1097/00041444-200509000-00007 PMID:16094251

Bibring, E. (1953). The Mechanism of Depression. In P. Greenacre (Eds.), Affective disorders. New York: The University Press.

Cannon, M., & Jones, P. (1996). Schizophrenia. *Journal of Neurology, Neurosurgery and Psychiatry,* (60), 604-613.

Chandrashekar, H., Prashanth, N.R., Kasthuri, P., & Madhusudan, S. (2010). Psychiatric Rehabilitation. *Indian Journal of Psychiatry, 52*(1), 278-280.

Crowther, R., Marshall, M., Bond, G., & Huxley, P. (2001). Vocational Rehabilitation for people with severe mental illness. *Cochrane Database of Systematic Reviews*, *2*, CD00380. doi:10.1002/14651858.CD003080 PMID:11406069

D'ambrosio, V., Albert, U., Bogetto, F., & Maina, G. (2010). Obsessive-compulsive disorder and cyclothymic temperament: An exploration of clinical features. *Journal of Affective Disorders*, *127*(1-3), 295–299. doi:10.1016/j.jad.2010.06.007 PMID:20591494

Davies, R. D., Gabbert, S. L., & Riggs, P. D. (2001). Anxiety disorders in neurologic illness. *Current Treatment Options in Neurology*, *3*(3), 333–346. doi:10.1007/s11940-001-0038-1 PMID:11389804

De geus, F., Denys, D. A., Sitskoorn, M.M., & Westenberg, H.G. (2007). Attention and cognition in patients with obsessive-compulsive disorder. *Psychiatry and Clinical Neuroscience, 61*(1), 45-53.

Denys, D., Tenney, N., vanMegen, H. J., de Geus, F., & Westenberg, H. G. (2004). Axis I and II comorbidity in a large sample of patients with obsessive-compulsive disorder. *Journal of Affective Disorders*, *80*(2-3), 155–162. doi:10.1016/S0165-0327(03)00056-9 PMID:15207928

Diagnostic and Statistical Manual of Mental Disorders. (1994). Washington, DC: American psychiatric association.

Faraone, S. V., Sergeant, J., Gillberg, C., & Biederman, J. (2003). The worldwide prevalence of ADHD: Is it an American condition? *World Psychiatry; Official Journal of the World Psychiatric Association (WPA)*, *2*, 104–113. PMID:16946911

Feinstein, A.R. (1970). The pre-therapeutic classification of co-morbidity in chronic disease. *Journal of Chronic Disease,* (23), 455-468.

Fennell, M. J. V. (1998). Depression. In Cognitive behaviour therapy for psychiatric problems a practical guide. Oxford University Press.

First, M. B. (2005). Mutually Exclusive versus co-occurring Diagnostic Categories: The challenge of diagnostic comorbidity. *Psychopathology*, *38*(4), 206–210. doi:10.1159/000086093 PMID:16145276

Fish, F. (1967). Clinical psychopathology: Sign and symptoms in psychiatry. Bristol, UK: John Wright & Sons.

Frank, E. (2005). *Treating Bipolar Disorder: A clinician's guide to Interpersonal and social rhythm therapy*. New York: Guilford.

Frost, R. O., Krause, M. S., & Steketee, G. (1996). The hoarding and obsessive-compulsive symptoms. *Behavior Modification*, *20*(1), 116–132. doi:10.1177/01454455960201006 PMID:8561769

Ganesan, V., Kumar, R., & Khanna, S. (2001). Obsessive compulsive disorder and psychosis. *Canadian Journal of Psychiatry*, (46): 750–754. PMID:11692979

Geller, D. A., Biederman, J., Faraone, S., Agranat, A., Cradock, K., Hagermoser, L., & Coffey, B. J. et al. (2001). Developmental aspects of obsessive-compulsive disorder: Findings in children, adolescents and adults. *The Journal of Nervous and Mental Disease*, *189*(7), 471–477. doi:10.1097/00005053-200107000-00009 PMID:11504325

Girimaji, S.R., Biju, S.T., Srinath, S., & Seshadri, S.P. (2005). Co-morbid psychiatric disorders in pervasive developmental disorders. *Journal of Indian Association for Child and Adolescent Mental Health, 1*(2), 7.

Goodwin, R. D., & Roy Byrne, P. (2006). Panic and suicidal ideation and suicidal attempts: Results from the National Comorbidity Survey. *Depression and Anxiety*, *23*(3), 124–132. doi:10.1002/da.20151 PMID:16502406

Halikas, A. J., Crosby, D. R., Pearson, L. V., Nugent, M. S., & Carlson, A. G. (1994). Psychiatric co-morbidity in treatment-seeking cocaine abusers. *The American Journal on Addictions*, *3*(1), 25–35. doi:10.1111/j.1521-0391.1994.tb00223.x

Hantouche, E. G., Angst, J., Demonfaucon, C., Perugi, G., Lancrenon, S., & Akiskal, H. S. (2003). Cyclothymic OCD:a distinct form? *Journal of Affective Disorders*, *75*(1), 1–10. doi:10.1016/S0165-0327(02)00461-5 PMID:12781344

Harbishettar, V., Kumar, P., Janardhan Reddy, Y. C., & Thennarasu, K. (2005). Is there a relationship between Parkinson's disease and obsessive-compulsive disorder? *Parkinsonism & Related Disorders*, *11*(11), 85–88. doi:10.1016/j.parkreldis.2004.07.006 PMID:15734665

Hayes, R., & McGrath, J. (2000). *Cognitive rehabilitation for people with schizophrenia and related conditions (Cochrane Review).* Oxford, UK: Update Software.

Howes, O. D., & Kapur, S. (2009). The dopamine hypothesis of schizophrenia:version III- the final common pathway. *Schizophrenia Bulletin*, *3*(3), 549–562. doi:10.1093/schbul/sbp006 PMID:19325164

Hwang, M.Y., & Hollander, E. (1993). Schizo-obsessive disorders. *Psychiatric Annals, 23*(7), 396-401.

Jablensky, A. (2011). *People living with psychotic illness 2010, Australian national survey*. Retrieved from https://www.health.gov.au/internet/main/publishing.nsf/.../psych10.pdf

Jablensky, A., Sartorious, N., Ernberg, G., Anker, M., Korten, A., Cooper, J. E., ...Bertelsen, A. (1992). Schizophrenia: Manifestations, incidence and course in different cultures: A world Health Organization ten-country study. Cambridge, UK: Cambridge University Press.

Jaisoorya, T. S., Janardhan Reddy, Y. C., & Srinath, S. (2003). Is Juvenile obsessive-compulsive disorder a developmental subtype of the disorder. Findings from an Indian study? *European Child & Adolescent Psychiatry*, *12*(12), 290–297. doi:10.1007/s00787-003-0342-2 PMID:14689261

Janet, P. (1903). Les obsessions et la psychasthenie (vol. 2). Felix Alcan.

Kaplan, P. W. (2010). Epilepsy and Obsessive-compulsive disorder. *Dialogues in Clinical Neuroscience*, (12), 241–248. PMID:20623928

Khess, C.R., Dutta, I., Chakrabarty, I., & Bhattacharya, P., Das, J., & Kothari, S. (1998). Comorbidity in children with mental retardation. *Indian Journal of Psychiatry*, (40), 289–294. PMID:21494486

Knapp, M., Mangalore, R., & Simon, J., (2004). The Global Costs of Schizophrenia. *Schizophrenia Bulletin,* (30), 279-293.

Kumar, S.P.N. (1998). Impact of substance abuse comorbidity on psychopathology and pattern of remission in mania. *Indian Journal of Psychiatry, 40*(4), 357-363.

Labbate, L. A., Young, P. C., & Arana, G. W. (1999). Panic disorder in schizophrenia. *Canadian Journal of Psychiatry*, (44), 488–490. PMID:10389611

Leff, J., Berkowitz, R., Shavit, N., Strachan, A., Glass, I., & Vaughn, C. (1990). A trial of family therapy versus a relatives' group for schizophrenia.Two year follow-up.Comparative study journal article. *The British Journal of Psychiatry*, *157*(4), 571–577. doi:10.1192/bjp.157.4.571 PMID:2131140

Lejoyeux, M., & Marinescu, M. (2006). Alcohol dependence and abuse and psychiatric disorders. *La Revue du Praticien, 56*(10), 1081-1085. Retrieved from http://www.ncbi.nlm.nih.gov/pubmed/16836203.oyeux

Lewin, B. D. (1950). *The Psychoanalysis of elation*. New York: W.W.Norton.

Lindenmayer, J. P., Khan, A., Iskander, A., Abad, M. T., & Parker, B. (2007). A randomized controlled trial of olanzapine versus haloperidol in the treatment of primary negative symptoms and neurocognitive deficits in schizophrenia. *The Journal of Clinical Psychiatry*, *68*(3), 368–379. doi:10.4088/JCP.v68n0303 PMID:17388705

March, J. S., Franklin, M. E., Leonard, H., Garcia, A., Moore, P., Freeman, J., & Foa, E. (2007). Tics moderate treatment outcome with sertraline but not cognitive-behaviour therapy in pediatric obsessive-compulsive disorder. *Biological Psychiatry*, *61*(3), 344–347. doi:10.1016/j.biopsych.2006.09.035 PMID:17241830

Markowitz, J. C., & Weissman, M. M. (2010). Interpersonal Psychotherapy: Past, Present and Future. *Clinical Psychology & Psychotherapy*, *19*(2), 99–105. doi:10.1002/cpp.1774 PMID:22331561

Maurice, J. K. (1970). group therapy in schizophrenia. *The International Journal of Social Psychiatry*, *16*(4), 266–274. doi:10.1177/002076407001600402

McGlashan, T. H. (2009). Psychosis as a disorder of reduced cathectic capacity: Freud's analysis of the schreber case Revisited. *Schizophrenia Bulletin*, *35*(3), 476–481. doi:10.1093/schbul/sbp019 PMID:19357240

Mcglashan, T.H., & Carpenter, W.T. (1976). Post psychotic depression in schizophrenia. *Archives of General Psychiatry,* (33), 231-239.

Miguel, E. C., Rauch, S. L., & Jenike, M. A. (1997). Obsessive Compulsive Disorder. *The Psychiatric Clinics of North America, 20*(4), 863–883. doi:10.1016/S0193-953X(05)70349-X PMID:9443354

Mowrer, O. H. (1969). Psychoneurotic defenses (including deception) as punishment avoidance strategies. In Punishment and aversive behavior. New York: Crofts-Crofts.

Ogai, M., Iyo, M., Mori, N., & Takei, N. (2005). A right orbitofrontal region and OCD symptoms: A case report. *Acta Psychiatric Scandiavica,* (111), 74-7610.

Pekkala, E. T., & Merinder, L. B. (2002). *Psychoeducation for schizophrenia (Cochrane Review).* Oxford, UK: Update Software.

Perry, A., Tarrier, N., Morriss, R., McCarthy, E., & Limb, K. (1999). Randomized controlled trial of efficacy of teaching patients with bipolar disorder to identify early symptoms of relapse and obtain treatment. *British Medical Journal, 318*(7177), 149–153. doi:10.1136/bmj.318.7177.149 PMID:9888904

Pigott, T. A., L' Heureux, F., Dubbert, B., Bernstein, S., & Murphy, D. L. (1994). Obsessive-compulsive disorder: Comorbid conditions. *The Journal of Clinical Psychiatry*, (55): 15–27. PMID:7961529

Planansky, K., & Johnston, R. (1978). Depressive syndrome in schizophrenia. *Acta Psychiatrica Scandinavica, 57*(3), 207–218. doi:10.1111/j.1600-0447.1978.tb06887.x PMID:645411

Poyurovsky, M., Faragian, S., Shabeta, A., & Kosov, A. (2008). Comparision of clinical characteristics, co-morbidity and pharmacotherapy in adolescents with and without obsessive-compulsive disorder. *Psychiatry Residence, 159*, 133–139. doi:10.1016/j.psychres.2007.06.010

Rajkumar, R. P., Reddy, Y. C. J., & Kandavel, T. (2008). Clinical profile of "schizo-obsessive" disorder; a comparative study. *Comprehensive Psychiatry, 49*(3), 262–268. doi:10.1016/j.comppsych.2007.09.006 PMID:18396185

Rao, P.G. (2010). An overview of Indian research in bipolar mood disorder. *Indian Journal of Psychiatry, 52*(1), 173-177.

Rasanen, P., Tiilhonen, J., & Isohanni, M. (1998). Schizophrenia, Alcohol abuse and violent behaviour: A 26 year follow-up study of an unselected birth cohort. *Schizophrenia Bulletin, 24*(3), 437–441. doi:10.1093/oxfordjournals.schbul.a033338 PMID:9718635

Rathod, S., Kingdom, D., Smith, P., & Turkington, D. (2005). Insight into schizophrenia: the effects of cognitive behavioural therapy on the components of insight and association with sociodemographics-data on a previously published randomized controlled trial. *Schizophrenia Research, 74*(2-3), 211-219.

Rihmer, Z., & Angst, J. (2005). Mood disorders: Epidemiology. In Kaplan & Sadock (Eds.), Comprehensive Textbook of Psychiatry (8th ed.; pp. 1646-1651). William & Wilkins.

Robertson, L., Connaughton, J., & Nicol, M. (1998). Life skills programmes for chronic mental illnesses. *Cochrane Database of Systematic Reviews*. doi:1.1002/14651858.CD000381

Robins, L., & Prince, R. K. (1991). Adult disorders predicted by childhood conduct problems: Results from the NIMH epidemiologic catchment area project. *Psychiatry*, *54*, 116–132. PMID:1852846

Salkovskis, P. M., & Kirk, J. (1988). Obsessional disorders: cognitive behaviour therapy for psychiatric problems A practical guide. Oxford University Press.

Saran, P. (2010). an overview of Indian Research in Personality Disorders. *Indian Journal of Psychiatry*, *52*(1), 250–254. doi:10.4103/0019-5545.69241 PMID:21180410

Sengupta, S. N., Das, P., Kamble, M. V., & Saxena, S. (1992). Dysmorphophobia with bipolar affective disorder: A case report. *Indian Journal of Psychiatry*, (34): 57–68. PMID:21776101

Sheppard, B. A., Chavira, D., Azzam, A., Grados, M. A., Umana, P., Garrido, H., & Mathews, C. A. (2010). ADHD prevalence and association with hoarding behaviour in childhood-onset OCD. *Depression and Anxiety*, *27*(7), 667–674. doi:10.1002/da.20691 PMID:20583294

Shorter, E. (1997). A History of Psychiatry from the era of the Asylum to the age of Prozac. New York: Wiley.

Soomro, G. M. (2012). Obsessive Compulsive disorder. *British Medical Journals. Clinical Evidence*, *1*(18), 1–25.

Sriram, G. T. (1990). Psychotherapy in developing countries: A public Health perspective. *Indian Journal of Psychiatry*, (2), 138–144. PMID:21927442

Stektee, G., & Lam, J. (1993). Obsessive Compulsive Disorder. In Handbook of effective psychotherapy, (pp. 253-278). Springer US.

Stewart, S. E., Illmann, C., Geller, D. A., Leckman, J. F., King, R., & Pauls, D. L. (2009). A controlled family study of attention-deficit/hyperactivity disorder and Tourette's disorder. *Journal of the American Academy of Child and Adolescent Psychiatry*, *45*(11), 1354–1362. doi:10.1097/01.chi.0000251211.36868.fe PMID:17075358

Strachey, J. (1914). Mourning and melancholia, the standard edition of the complete psychological works of Sigmund Freud. London: Hogarth Press.

Yamamoto, H., Tsuchida, H., Nakamae, T., Seiji, N., Sakai, Y., Fujimori, A., & Narumoto, J. (2012). Relationship between severity of obsessive-compulsive symptoms and schizotypy in obsessive-compulsive symptoms and schizotypy in obsessive-compulsive disorder. *Neuropsychiatric Disease and Treatment*, *8*, 579–583. doi:10.2147/NDT.S38450 PMID:23248572

Zohar, J., Fostick, L., & Juyen-Wetzler, E. (2009). Obsessive compulsive disorder. In New Oxford Textbook of Psychiatry (2nd ed.; pp. 765-773). New York: Oxford University Press.

KEY TERMS AND DEFINITIONS

Comorbidity: When two disorders or illness occur in the same person, simultaneously or sequentially.

Cognitive Behavior Therapy: A 'talking therapy' that helps to manage the problems by changing the way of an individual's thinking and behavior. It is commonly used to treat depression and anxiety.

Depression: A state of low mood in a person that affects his or her thoughts, feelings and behavior.

Etiology: Used to find out the causes and the origins of the diseases.

Interpersonal Therapy: A therapy to regain control mood of a depressed person. It is a short term period treatment and very structured.

Insight Psychotherapy: A type of therapy that occurs between the client and the therapist through a conversation. It is a counselling service for the client which makes him to overcome with his or her problems regarding feelings, unhealthy thoughts and behavior.

Mania: Excessive excitement and craze for a particular thing. It is an extreme interest towards a particular thing.

Obsessive Compulsive Disorder: A mental disorder in humans and they feel the need to check the things again and again and repeat it.

Pharmacological Treatment: A treatment that studies the disease and the drugs related to that particular disease. It also studies the uses, preparation and effects of the drugs on the particular disease.

Schizophrenia: A mental health condition characterized by false ideas, hallucinations, and delusion.

Chapter 6

Management of Chronic Mental Illnesses and Substance Use Disorders

Pallavi Sinha
Institute of Human Behaviour and Allied Sciences (IHBAS), India

Amit Garg
Institute of Human Behaviour and Allied Sciences (IHBAS), India

Prerna Khanna
Pushpanjali Crosslay Hospital, India

Amit Khanna
Institute of Human Behaviour and Allied Sciences (IHBAS), India

ABSTRACT

There is vast literature available about prevalence and pattern of substance use in patients with Chronic mental illness such as Schizophrenia. Many of these studies have also investigated the issues related to the impact of substance use on the course and prognosis of the mental illness and vice versa. The factors affecting the use and its impact on treatment have also been studied to some extent in the Western countries. Estimates of the prevalence of substance abuse in schizophrenia and major affective disorder vary as a function of settings (e.g., community, hospital-in-patient vs. out-patient), demographic characteristics of the sample and assessment methods, with most prevalence rates ranging between15% to 65%. Patients with Chronic Mental illnesses and Substance use disorders are difficult to treat and many models for their management have been proposed. This chapter will deal with some of these issues.

INTRODUCTION

During the period following deinstitutionalization in 1950's, psychiatrists started focusing on patients with chronic mental disorders who left institutions and were in the process of getting rehabilitated in the community. By the late 1980s, mental health professionals began to attend to this new younger population of persons with severe mental illness leading to the emergence of the concept of co-occurring disorders or dual diagnosis (Ridgely et al., 1987). As a consequence of deinstitutionalization along with other risk factors like poverty, poor education, poor social skills, lack of vocational skills and opportunities,

DOI: 10.4018/978-1-5225-0519-8.ch006

and residence in drug-infested neighborhoods, such patients experienced a high rate of regular exposure to psychoactive substances and of social pressures to use them. Exposure of these patients with severe mental illness to the drug culture in the community led to the development of another entity of patients having co-morbid substance abuse with psychiatric disorders. Such individuals were discussed under the rubric of dual diagnosis but were also called mentally ill chemical abusers or substance-abusing mentally ill persons (Drake & Wallach, 2000).

There is no single form of dual diagnosis. There are numerous types of psychiatric illness along with different patterns of alcohol or drug abuse. Most of these patients would fall within the following four categories:

1. Those who are severely disabled by comorbid mental health and substance use disorders and will require a coordinated and integrated approach by both mental health and drug and alcohol services,
2. Those who are severely disabled by mental health disorders and adversely affected by problematic substance use disorders
3. Those who are disabled by substance use disorders and adversely affected by mental health problems
4. Those who are mildly disabled by mental health disorders and substance use disorders and who will be treated primarily by a general practitioner but may also require access to either mental health or substance abuse services at various times (Burnam & Watkins, 2006; Drake et al., 2001; Todd et al., 2004).

It is therefore necessary to be clear that dual diagnosis is not a diagnosis in itself. Instead it simply implies that a person has both psychiatric and substance use issues. Among dual-diagnosis patients, substance-use disorders range from single drug abuse to a cocktails of substances, whereas mental health problems can include a wide array of disorders, from those defined as "high-prevalence and low- impact therapeutic", such as anxiety and depression, to those defined as "low prevalence, high-impact therapeutic", such as psychosis and major mood disorders (Canaway & Merkes, 2010). Although the "low impact" group is the most represented among dual-diagnosis patients, the "high impact" group, even if smaller, requires more intensive and expensive treatment programs.

Despite being perceived as a difficult to manage group, and perhaps untreatable, those with dual diagnosis are a disadvantaged and vulnerable group. Accumulating evidence suggests that co-occurring substance abuse leads to relapse and hospitalization, disruptive behavior and violence, familial problems, homelessness, decreased functional status, HIV infection, and medication noncompliance (Drake, Mercer-McFadden, Mueser, McHugo, & Bond, 1998). Substance abuse along with medication non-compliance has been found to be predictors of violent behaviour in patients with mental illness (Torrey, 1994). Homelessness is a major issue for patients with dual diagnosis. Mentally ill persons with substance abuse tend to congregate in urban areas where availability of drugs are higher but housing options are few. The McKinney Research Demonstration Programs for homeless mentally ill adults showed that alcohol or other drug abuse was the reason that patients were unable to find or retain housing and not because of their mental illness per se (Making a Difference, 1995). Studies have also shown that problems related to substance use tend to persist over the long term amongst patients with severe mental illness (Kozaric-Kovacic, Folnegovic-Smalc, Folnegovic, & Maruic, 1995; Morse, Calsyn, Allen, Tempelhoff., & Smith, 1992). The economic burden of dual diagnosis has also become evident. Research has shown that the treatment cost of patients with dual diagnosis is higher than treatment costs for patients with single disorders because they are high users of the expensive hospital and emergency services (Dickey & Azeni, 1996).

EPIDEMIOLOGY

The occurrence of dual diagnosis is quite common. However, the estimates of current and lifetime substance abuse prevalence in Chronic Mental illnesses such as Schizophrenia and Major Affective Disorders vary as a function of setting where the samples are taken, the diagnostic criteria and the variable assessment protocols used.

The largest prevalence study was the Epidemiologic Catchment Area (ECA) study (Regier et al., 1990) which involved over 20,000 structured interviews. The ECA study revealed that 37% of people with alcohol disorders and 53% with other drug disorders had co-morbid psychiatric conditions. Kessler et al. (1997) found that persons affected by alcohol or illegal drug dependence presented a mental disorder 4.1 times and 4.9 times more frequently, respectively, than other non–alcohol-dependent people. Amongst persons seeking treatment for alcohol-related disorder, over 40% had a comorbid mood disorder and 33% had an anxiety disorder while amongst treatment seekers with drug-related disorder, over 60% had a comorbid mood disorder and over 42% had an anxiety disorder (Grant et al., 2004). Substance use disorders have also been strongly associated with externalizing rather than internalizing mental disorders (Kessler et al., 2003; Kessler et al., 2001). In accordance with the above findings, the anxiety-mood disorder most significantly associated with substance use disorder is bipolar depression. A number of community epidemiologic surveys have consistently suggested that mental disorders typically start at an earlier age than substance use disorders (Kessler et al., 2003; Sareen, Chartier, Kjernisted., & Stein, 2001).

Personality disorders are considered to be the most important predictors of treatment outcome in persons with substance abuse. Borderline personality disorder is associated with elevated lifetime rates of substance abuse as well as higher-than-expected rates of charges for various drug-related crimes and criminal behavior (Sansone, Watts, & Wiederman, 2014). The National Epidemiologic Survey on Alcohol and Related Conditions highlighted that individuals with drug use disorder were 2.2 times more likely to present a comorbid personality disorder (Conway, Compton, Stinson, & Grant, 2006). Multiple studies have found that individuals with dual diagnosis have high rates of family history for substance use and/or psychiatric diseases, which can effect the severity and consequences of dual diagnosis (Mroziewicz & Tyndale, 2010; Wilson, Bennett, & Bellack, 2013). Other researchers suggested that the vulnerability to substance abuse increases among individuals with mental illness who were subjected to childhood abuse (Maniglio, 2009; Wilson, 2010) and that this relationship resulted in a range of negative outcomes like earlier onset and longer duration of substance abuse, poor physical health, and more interpersonal problems (Schafer & Fisher, 2011; Sideli, Mule, La Barbera, & Murray, 2012).

The relationship between mental disorders and substance use has been deliberated upon regarding which of the two diseases could most influence the onset of the other. In adolescents and young adults with first psychotic episode, co-occurring substance use was reported in 74% of all cases and was associated with limited response to treatment, decreased medication adherence and worsened illness course (Goerke & Kumra, 2013). Studies have consistently shown that psychosis and the onset of substance use are often linked: one-third of patients experienced their first psychotic episode before the age of 19 years, and adolescence represents the peak time period for use and experimentation with alcohol, cannabis, and other illicit substances, the capability of which to induce psychotic symptoms have been well established. Amongst the myriad of psychoactive substances, cannabis may represent a significant risk factor for the development of psychotic illness in vulnerable individuals (Arias et al., 2013; Morgan & Curran, 2008; Zammit, Allebeck, Andreasson, Lundberg., & Lewis, 2002).

The comorbidity of mood and substance use disorders is also common with a lifetime prevalence rate of all bipolar disorders and substance use disorders at 47.3% and, in particular, for bipolar I and substance use disorders at 60.3%. Comorbid substance use disorder is common in major depression, with lifetime rates of 40.3% for alcohol use and 17.2% for all other associated substance use disorders (Gros, Milanak, Brady, & Back, 2013; Heffner et al., 2013; Maremmani et al., 2013)

Over the years the researches that have been conducted in India, like in the west, clearly reflect that psychiatric illness and drug abuse co-existed more frequently than by chance only. In one prospective study (Desai & Gupta,1999) involving 72 patients, 46% of alcohol abusers had a co-morbid psychiatric disorder, 16.6% had psychosis, 23.6% had a depressive disorder and 48.6% had depressive signs and symptoms. In another study (Ray, 1989) of 147 patients of alcohol abuse, 40% had a psychiatric disorder, 29.2% had co-morbid psychosis, 8.8% had a depressive disorder and 45% had depressive symptoms. Gangadhar et al. (2007) reported a studyon 207 schizophrenia patients. None had a history of using illicit substance in their lifetime. The lifetime co-morbid prevalence of alcohol dependence/harmful use was 17.2%. It was 31.4% among males and 2.1% among females. Sokhlet and Sharma (1998) in another study found high rates of depression and antisocial personality disorder (ASPD) in patients with opioid dependence.

COMMON PSYCHIATRIC CO-MORBIDITIES

The commonest substance of abuse in patients with chronic mental illnesses, in most studies across different demographic and geographical locations is nicotine, alcohol followed by cannabis, with the use of stimulants, psychedelics and intravenous drug use being low but rising.

Nicotine

Nicotine being a licit drug easily available and socially acceptable to certain extent is seen to be widely used by patients with mental illness. Schizophrenia is associated across nations with a higher rate of tobacco smoking as compared to the general population and also other mental illnesses after correction for confounding factors like antipsychotic medications, institutionalization or other drug use (LLerena, la Rubia, Penas-Lledo, Diaz., & de Leon, 2003; McCreadie & Scottish Comorbidity Study Group, 2002). Smoking tobacco has been studied in the context of schizophrenia where it has been hypothesized to be used as self- medication. Though numerous animal studies support this hypothesis however clinical studies present a contradictory picture (Hughes, 2000). The self medication hypothesis proposes that smoking reduces the side-effects of antipsychotics and that nicotine improves the negative, cognitive and/or depressive symptoms of schizophrenia (Taiminen et al., 1998). Evidence from animal studies have suggested that smoking results in nicotine to cause dopamine release in the mesolimbic and mesocortical system which may transiently compensate for the hypodopaminergic state seen in schizophrenia (Drew, Derbez., & Werling, 2000). In-vivo human studies state that nicotine induced enzymatic induction of antipsychotics results in decreased blood levels of the antipsychotic thereby decreasing the antipsychotic induced side-effects (Salokangas et al., 2000). These proposed mechanisms have been the basis for the self-medication hypothesis of schizophrenia. However, despite the animal studies, clinical data is limited in support of nicotine and reduction of negative symptoms of schizophrenia while the data for nicotine improving the sensory gating abnormalities and smooth pursuit eye movements in schizophrenia or cognitive abnormalities induced by anti- psychotics are somewhat stronger (Dalack, Healy, & Meador-

Woodruff, 1998). In a naturalistic study by Aguilar, Gurpegui, Diaz and de Leon, (2005), the beneficial effects of nicotine was proposed to be restricted to mildly dependent smokers, especially those patients who were on low dose typical anti-psychotics with higher sensitivity towards extra pyramidal side-effects.

Alcohol

The issue of co-morbidity is a major focus of research in alcohol use disorders. Both epidemiological and clinic based studies have demonstrated comorbidity in alcohol use disorders. Studies have shown that an epidemiological relationship between anxiety, depression and alcohol use. The Epidemiological Catchment Area study showed that alcohol dependence, anxiety disorders and affective disorders coexist commonly with alcohol use disorders (Regier et al., 1990). This coexistence was also found in the National Comorbidity Survey by Kessler et al. (1997). Which showed that more than 25% of individuals diagnosed with alcohol dependence met the criteria of a depressive episode in the previous year. It stands that anxiety disorders and depressive disorders in subjects with alcohol dependence are the direct consequences of ethanol on the central nervous system. Suicidality has also been studied in persons with alcohol dependence and studies reveal that the risk of suicide among addicts is higher than in the general population (Wilcox, Conner, & Caine, 2004). According to some researchers, risk of suicide in alcohol-dependent subjects is even higher than in patients with depression varying from 7% to 18% (Inskip, Harris, & Barraclough, 1998). In regard to Bipolar disorder, co-morbid diagnosis in alcohol dependent persons stands at 1.9% (Kessler et al., 1996). Research evidence also suggests that having an additional psychiatric diagnosis has implications for the prognosis and treatment of alcohol dependence and the associated psychopathology (Mueller et al., 1994).

Cannabis

Cannabis use once considered to be relatively harmless is now proposed to play a role in triggering, causing and maintaining a wide array of psychiatric disorders. With the discovery of the endocannabinoid system, psychiatric research has now focused on the role of cannabis in schizophrenia, bipolar disorder and depression. Cannabis use is common in patients with bipolar disorders though not much is known about its role as a risk factor for development of bipolar disorder. Studies investigating young bipolar disorder patients showed that rates of cannabis use disorders equal or exceed those of alcohol abuse or alcohol dependence (Strakowski et al., 2005). A seminal study by Strakowski et al. (2007) a significant effect of previous cannabis abuse in first-episode mania on the course of the disease was seen. They proposed an association of alcohol use with depressive episodes and that of cannabis use with manic episodes. In a study by Henquet, Krabbendam, de Graaf, Have, and van Os (2006) showed that cannabis use at baseline significantly increased the risk for manic symptoms during follow-up.

The current scientific evidence for an increased higher risk for major depressive disorder in people using cannabis is less convincing. However, some weak evidence has emerged for a relationship between cannabis use with major depressive disorder and anxiety disorders (Agosti, Nunes, & Levin, 2002). The evidence from longitudinal studies is mixed, although most have reported that regular cannabis use is predicted to increase the risk of depression and/or anxiety in later life (Patton et al., 2002). Similarly, in a longitudinal study by van van Laar, van Dorsselaer, Monshouwer, and de Graaf (2007), cannabis use predicted a modest increase in the risk of a first major depression and a somewhat greater increase in the risk of a first bipolar disorder in the adult population. However, none of the studies could conclusively comment on upon causality between cannabis use and mood disorders. It may also be that the apparent association between cannabis use and depression may actually reflect the association between cannabis use and bipolar disorder, as bipolar disorder is frequently misdiagnosed as major depressive disorder in the initial years.

In contrast to the mixed evidence for association between cannabis use and major depression and bipolar disorder, cannabis has been more conclusively associated with schizophrenia. Two clinical links have been proposed between cannabis use and schizophrenia. Firstly, it has been proposed to significantly increase the risk of development of schizophrenia. Longitudinal studies from Sweden, the Netherlands, New Zealand, and Israel (Andreasson, Allebeck, Engström, & Rydberg, 1987; Arseneault et al., 2002; van Os et al., 2002; Zammit et al., 2002) report that cannabis use during childhood and adolescence doubles the risk of later appearance of psychosis or schizophrenia. These epidemiological studies have used different epidemiological strategies that suggest an overall increased risk of development of schizophrenia with frequent cannabis use. These studies suggest that cannabis has a causal role in the development of psychosis and that heavy cannabis use in early adolescence is strongly associated with the development of later psychotic illness. Furthermore, in schizophrenia, the abuse of cannabis seems to trigger psychotic symptoms and may worsen the outcome of the disease (Gregg, Barrowclough, & Haddock, 2007). Genetic studies have suggested that a functional polymorphism in the catechol-O-methyltransferase (COMT) gene—an enzyme involved in the breakdown of dopamine in the synapse may be associated with schizophrenia. Individuals carrying this COMT polymorphism have been observed to be at least five times more likely to exhibit psychotic symptoms and to develop schizophreniform disorder if they used cannabis frequently (Caspi et al., 2005). The second clinical link in between cannabis and schizophrenia is that schizophrenia patients are more likely than healthy individuals to abuse cannabis (Kovasznay et al., 1997). In contrast to nicotine, there is no substantial evidence that cannabis abuse serves as a kind of self-medication for patients with schizophrenia, although greater support has been found in self-report studies thatpatients see substance use as means to alleviate dysphoria (Gregg & Haddock, 2007).

Research on the neurobiology of drug abuse and schizophrenia indicates that the mesolimbic dopamine system is involved in both cannabis abuse and schizophrenia (Chambers, Krystal, & Self, 2001). Dysregulation in the cortical, temporal, limbic and meso-accumbens a circuit has been implicated in both schizophrenia and in substance abuse disorders (Andreasen, 1999; Wenger, Moldrich, & Furst, 2003). It is plausible that this developmental neuropathology in the hippocampal and prefrontal cortical pathways contributes to vulnerability to both schizophrenia and cannabis use, via dysfunctional interactions with the nucleus accumbens. The endocannabinoid system has also been studied in its role in development of schizophrenia. The density of the CB1 cannabinoid receptors has been found to be increased in the anterior cingulate cortexand the dorsolateral prefrontal cortex in schizophrenia patients (Dean, Sundram, Bradbury, Scarr, & Copolov, 2001). These findings were independent of cannabis use. Genetic studies on the central CB1 cannabinoid receptor have reported an association between polymorphisms of the CNR1 gene and schizophrenia (Leroy et al., 2001). The levels of the endogenous cannabinoid anandamide have also been found to be elevated in the bloodand cerebrospinal fluidof patients with schizophrenia, independent of cannabis use (Giuffrida et al., 2004). All of these findings point to possible functional impairment in the endogenous cannabinoid system in schizophrenia patients.

OPIOIDS

Opioid dependence like other substance use disorders has also been proposed to have high rates of psychiatric co-morbidity. Depression has been found to be common among illicit opioid users (Wild et al., 2005), with heavy opioid use being associated with more severe depression. These rates of depression decrease once people enter treatment for opioid dependence, in particular maintenance pharmacotherapies. In contrast to depression, the prevalence of comorbid psychosis and opioid use is generally low (Gregg et al., 2007). However, comorbid psychosis and opioid use is associated with increased mortality and high levels of dysfunction (Sorensen, Jepsen, Haastrup, & Juel, 2005). In a meta-analysis done on the psychiatric co-morbidity in opioid dependent persons, 78% had at least one co-morbid psychiatric disorder at least once in their lifetime. Personality disorders had a high prevalence (42%) followed by mood disorders (31%) and anxiety disorders (8%) (Frei & Rehm, 2002). Opioid dependent persons with personality disorders have noted to have more severe substance dependence, multiple drug abuse, high risk behaviors like intravenous drug use, high involvement in criminal activities and high suicidality (Havens & Strathdee, 2005).

Etiology

The etiology of dual diagnosis seems to be many and diverse and rather co-morbidity specific. Four models have been hypothesized to depict the relationship between substance use disorders and psychiatric disorders. These are:

1. **Direct Causality Models:** These models depict how a primary disorder leads to secondary disorders. There are two direct causal models:
    a. Secondary mental disorders i.e. primary substance use disorders causing secondary mental disorders.
    b. Secondary substance use disorders i.e. Primary mental disorders leading to substance use disorders.
2. **Indirect Causal Models:** Extend the direct causal models by the concept that a primary disorder may develop a risk factor that provokes a secondary disorder to set in.
3. **Common Factor Models:** Claim that both disorders may share etiological conditions such as genetic predisposition or exposure to environmental factors (Parental substance use disorders or family violence.
4. **Bidirectional Causal Models:** Frequently depict vicious cycles in which two disorders interact (see the Table 1).

From the neurobiological aspect, the key role in the development of addiction is the central nervous system's reward pathway via the dopaminergic mesocorticolimbic circuit. The vulnerability to addiction development is frequently associated with genetic factors and personality traits. Recent studies have highlighted that both alcohol-dependent and opiate-dependent patients have common genetic variants in dopamine D2 receptors and serotonin-transporter–linked promoter region associated with higher frequency to novelty-seeking personality traits. Impulsivity, one of the most extensively studied personality trait represents a predictor of future problems with substance use, due to its biologically-based link to addictive core processes.

Table 1. Evidence based causal models for co-morbid mental disorders and substance use disorders

Comorbidity with Substance Use Disorder	Characteristics of Causal Model
Anxiety disorders (excluding PTSD)	Complex bidirectional vicious cycle models that integrate hypothesis on anxiety reduction, self-medication, anxiety induction. Integrated causal models with direct and bidirectional pathways act as explanation for development and maintenance of comorbidity.
Post-Traumatic Stress Disorder PTSD	Bidirectional causal model. Self-medication used to alleviate symptoms of PTSD and this substance use disorder leads to deterioration in symptoms of PTSD
Depression	Complex model with direct and indirect causal pathways with hypothesis on substance induced depression, secondary depression and secondary substance use disorders.
Schizophrenia	Common factor model with evidence suggesting that ASPD accounts for the excesses in rates of comorbid substance use disorder in patients with severe mental disorders. Alternatively, a secondary substance use models based on the supersensitivity model, i.e. an increased sensitivity to the effects of substances amongst individual with vulnerability for schizophrenia.
Antisocial personality disorder	Direct causal model with common factors such as conduct disorder, behavioural disinhibition and antisocial behavior.
Borderline personality disorder	Bidirectional causal model with impulsivity and emotional dysregulation provoking the development of substance use disorder which in turn maintaining or deteriorate impulsivity and emotional instability.

(Stohler & Rossler, 2005)

Studies in basic sciences indicate that psychomotor responses to addictive drugs are involuntarily enhanced in animal models of psychiatric illness that involve differential forms of temporal-limbic circuit dysfunction, consistent with augmented progression of neuroplastic changes implicated in addictive disease. Animal studies have confirmed the unitary nature of the neuro-circuits that regulate both major psychiatric syndromes and enhanced addiction vulnerability. A vital implication of this integrated neurocircuit theory is that many genetic and environmental risk factors for mental illness, SUDs, or dual diagnosis disorders could be identical.

DUAL DIAGNOSIS TYPOLOGY

Dual diagnosis typology was developed so as to classify patients into clinically meaningful sub-groups to which treatments approaches could be matched.

1. **Reis Typology (Reis, Sloan, & Miller, 1997):** This is based on the severity of psychiatric disorders compared to substance use disorders.
    a. **Type I:** High-severity psychiatric - high - severity- substance.
    b. **Type II:** High-severity psychiatric - low - severity- substance.
    c. **Type III:** Low-severity psychiatric-high -severity- substance.
    d. **Type IV:** Low-severity psychiatric - low - severity- substance.

High psychiatric severity would include severe mental illness having considerable psychosocial impairment while low psychiatric severity would include common mental disorders. High severity substance would include patients with substance dependence while low severity substance would include substance users with quantifiable but marginal psychosocial impairment.

2. **Zimberg Typology (1999) :** This typology is based on the relative prominence of the two types of disorders.
   a. **Type I:** Primary psychiatric disorder, with substance use only when psychiatrically symptomatic (self-medication).
   b. **Type II:** Primary substance use disorder with substance-induced psychiatric symptoms.
   c. **Type III:** Psychiatric and substance use disorders both of long duration that are co-occurring or present at different times.

The type III category is considered to be the true representatives of the dual diagnosis disorder.

MANAGEMENT

The management of patients with dual diagnosis is riddled with challenges. These range from issues pertaining to the patient, to those associated with the illness and physician related factors. The presence of psychotic symptoms both positive and negative can interfere in treatment process. In comparison to those with substance abuse only, people with dual diagnosis have less motivation to change, are harder to engage, drop out of long-term programs more easily, make slow progress and have a narrow repertoire of coping skills and a low tolerance for stressors. Issues of housing, social support and income, pose additional difficulties in the treatment of patients with dual diagnosis. The distinction between mental health providers and substance abuse therapists can further complicate the management with each group not being equipped to deal with both psychiatric and substance use problems simultaneously. These factors pose significant challenges in managing the dual diagnosis patient. The two fundamental problems that may be faced by patients with dual diagnosis are that their substance use disorders were not addressed in the treatment process and if they did receive treatment, it was not tailored to the needs of a person with co-morbid psychiatric disorder. Table 2 enumerates the substance use related risks that need to be assessed by the clinician in dual diagnosis patients to develop an effective management plan.

MODELS OF MANAGEMENT

With the recognition of dual disorders as a distinct entity requiring specialized care, a number of models were developed for the treatment of such patients.

1. **Sequential Model:** The sequential or serial model follows that the patient is treated for one condition followed by the other. Different clinicians provide the treatment for psychiatric and substance use disorders. The disadvantage with this model is that the differing needs of the patients are not met with. Separate treating teams could provide differing and contradictory information to the patient. More importantly, this model became a common clinical justification for exclusion from either the treatment modalities.
2. **Parallel Model:** The parallel model provides treatment for both the psychiatric and substance use disorders at the same time by different clinical teams working in isolation with each other. The parallel model was the starting point towards integration of management of psychiatric and substance use disorders. However, this service failed to address the cross-service planning and participation needed in managing patients with dual diagnosis.

Table 2. Substance use-associated risks should be assessed in six domains (American Society of Addiction Medicine)

Domain I – Risks associated with pattern of substance use, presence of dependence, intoxication and withdrawal	• The drug(s) used amounts, route and site of administration. • Effects of intoxication e.g. accidents, • Effects of withdrawal e.g. withdrawal seizures • Re-instatement of problematic use after a period of abstinence.
Domain II –Biomedical problems	• Hypertension, hyperthermia, stroke, hepatitis. • Other injecting related risks e.g. thrombosis • Sexual health and sexually transmitted diseases. • Amnesia and cognitive impairment
Domain III –Impact on psychiatric symptoms and type of risk behaviour	• Pathological jealousy • Anti-social personality disorder • Borderline personality disorder.
Domain IV- Degree of motivation for change of substance use	• Assessment / structured non –judgemental feedback alone can be very effective in promoting change. • Matching services to clients pace of change and desired goal are more effective than trying to "force" change.
Domain V – Recovery potential	• Length and severity of addiction including previous periods of abstinence / attempts to change. • Previous response to treatment • Personal strengths and resources • Family, community and other ecological resources.
Domain VI – Potential for relapse or continued use	• Lack of structure, routine, housing, employment. • Ongoing stressors or life events (including active psychiatric illness). • Presence of external triggers/cues e.g. paraphernalia at home.

3. **Integrated Model:** By the late 1980s, the problems plaguing the sequential and parallel model became evident and this gave rise to the development of the integrated model. Integrated treatment targets both conditions simultaneously but through either the coordinated interaction between service providers or their working together as one team within an inclusive setting (Drake, Mueser, Brunette, & McHugo, 2004). It involves a flexible combination of treatments from the mental health and addiction fields that are combined to cater to the needs of people with dual diagnoses. This includes detoxification, medication management, cognitive behavioral therapy, motivational interviewing and other psychosocial interventions. Integration is often accomplished through the use of multidisciplinary teams who share the responsibility for treatment and cross-training. Pharmacotherapy aims at controlling psychiatric symptoms, withdrawal along with a focus on potential medications of abuse. Numerous models for providing integrated treatment have evolved. Although the models vary, they have several common service features, beyond the basic commitment to integration of services. First, they are mostly developed as outpatient services. Second, awareness of SUD is insinuated into all aspects of the existing mental health program. Third, they address the difficulty that dual diagnosis patients have in linking with services and maintaining treatment adherence by providing continuous outreach and close monitoring techniques. Fourth, integrated programs recognize that recovery tends to occur over months or years in the community (Drake, Mueser, Clark, & Wallach, 1996). Fifth, most dual-diagnosis programs recognize that the majority of psychiatric patients have little readiness for abstinence-oriented SUD treatments (Mercer-McFadden, Drake, & Brown, 1997). Rather than just treat the highly motivated patients, these programs incorporate motivational interventions aimed at patients with low motivation to maintain abstinence. Therapy progresses slowly, in accordance with the cognitive deficits, positive

and negative symptoms, vulnerability to confrontation, and the greater need for support. The goal of dual diagnosis intervention is recovery from not only the chronic mental illness but also the substance use disorder. In this context, "recovery" means that the individual with a dual diagnosis learns to manage both illnesses so that he or she can pursue meaningful life goals (Minkoff, 1989).

COMPONENTS OF INTEGRATED TREATMENT MODELS

Suggested by Drake et al. (2001)

1. **Staged Intervention:** Effective programs incorporate the concept of stages of treatment (McHugo, Drake, Burton, & Ackerson, 1995; Osher & Kofoed, 1989). It includes forming a trusting relationship (engagement), helping the engaged client develop the motivation to become involved in recovery-oriented interventions (persuasion), helping the motivated client acquire skills and supports for controlling illnesses and pursuing goals and helping the client in stable remission develop and use strategies for maintaining recovery (relapse prevention).
2. **Assertive Outreach:** Assertive community treatment (ACT) is described as a structured health care service approach to working with dual-diagnosis clients—in particular, by adapting a conventional model of case management to the needs of this client cohort (Mueser, 2005). The case-manager responsibilities are to develop a working alliance with clients and to link them into relevant other services. By keeping contact and providing ongoing assessment, case managers are central to client engagement, treatment, and retention.
3. **Motivational Interventions:** Most dual diagnosis clients have little readiness for abstinence-oriented treatment at the onset (Ziedonis & Trudeau, 1997). Effective programs therefore incorporate motivational interventions that are designed to help clients become ready for more definitive interventions aimed at illness self-management (Carey, 1996). Motivational interventions involve helping the individual identify his or her own goals and to recognize, through a systematic examination of the individual's ambivalence and that not managing one's illnesses interferes with attaining those goals (Miller & Rollnick, 1991). Along with the use of MI at the outset of treatment, many teams use cognitive-behavioral therapy [CBT] (Baker et al., 2006). CBT deals with following issues that individuals with dual diagnoses must address: recognizing escalating symptoms and other warning signs; coping with cravings; coming up with healthy alternative activities; normalizing substance-use lapses; developing plans for lapse or relapse; and cognitive restructuring to counteract positive beliefs about substance use.
4. **Counselling:** Once clients are motivated to manage their own illnesses, they need to develop skills and supports to control symptoms and to pursue an abstinent lifestyle. Effective programs provide some form of counseling, either individual or group, that promotes cognitive and behavioral skills at this stage.
5. **Social Support:** Intervention Integrated treatment programs also need to strengthen the immediate social environment of patients to help them modify their behavior. These activities include family interventions or social networking (Drake & Wallach, 2000). Housing and employment are key issues. Programs need to be oriented towards improving social and vocational skills of the index patients.

Table 3. The Integrated Dual Diagnosis Treatment (IDDT) model

Regardless of their specific structure or orientation, integrated dual diagnosis programs reflect the following principles:
• Co-occurring disorders are expected and welcomed. • Treatment is based on an attitude of hope and empathy, with a commitment to maintaining continuity of care throughout the recovery process. • Each diagnosis should be treated as a primary diagnosis, with equally intensive care. • Treatment plans must be individualized according to the patient's diagnosis, level of functionality, and other factors. • Clinicians receive equal training in substance abuse treatment and mental health. • Clients are treated according to their readiness to change. Therapists accept that patients with mental illness may be slower to accept the need for rehab, and they adjust the treatment plan accordingly. • Therapy is collaborative, with client and therapist working together throughout the treatment process. • Therapists adopt a motivational attitude, encouraging their clients through compassionate listening. • Clients receive substance abuse education and counseling along with psychotherapy. • Aftercare programs and intensive case management are provided to ensure continuity of care and prevent relapse.

6. **Long Term Perspective:** Effective programs recognize that recovery tends to occur over months or years in the community. People with severe mental illness and substance abuse do not usually develop stability and functional improvements quickly, even in intensive treatment programs, unless they enter treatment at an advanced stage (Drake et al., 1998). Instead, they tend to improve over months and years in conjunction with a consistent dual diagnosis program. Effective programs therefore take a long-term, community-based perspective that includes rehabilitation activities to prevent relapses and to enhance gains.
7. **Comprehensiveness:** Learning to lead a symptom-free, abstinent lifestyle that is satisfying and sustainable often requires transforming many aspects of one's life for example, habits, stress management, friends, activities, and housing. Inpatient hospitalization, assessment, crisis intervention, medication management, money management, laboratory screening, housing, and vocational rehabilitation incorporate special features that are tailored specifically for dual diagnosis patients.
8. **Cultural Sensitivity and Competence:** Cultural sensitivity and competence is critical to engaging clients in dual diagnosis services (Mercer-McFadden, 1997). Persons from varying backgrounds can be engaged in dual diagnosis services if the services were tailored to their particular racial, cultural, and other group characteristics.

Though the integrated treatment modalities for dual diagnosis was ushered in with encouraging research, a review of different treatment modalities suggested that the evidence for efficacy of integrated treatment programs over treatment as usual was low (Tiet & Mausbach, 2007). This could however be due to the paucity of data and the heterogeneity of team-dependent integrated treatments.

PHARMACOLOGICAL APPROACHES

1. **Pharmacotherapy for SUD and Depression:** There are a substantial number of studies examining treatments for depression or alcohol-related disorders separately. These studies revealed that Selective Serotonin Reuptake Inhibitors (SSRIs) and atypical antidepressants showed mixed results for both depression and alcohol-related outcomes. The review by Quyen, Tiet, and Mausbach (2007) found that the existing efficacious treatments for reducing psychiatric symptoms (e.g., TCA for depressive symptoms) also tend to work in dual-diagnosis patients. However, the benefits of tri-

cyclic antidepressants must be weighed against their decidedly higher side-effect profiles. Murthy and Chand, (2012) proposed that the combination of naltrexone and sertraline was found to be effective in patients with depressive disorder and alcohol dependence. Torrens, Fonseca, Mateu, and Farre (2005) reviewed five studies of the effectiveness of antidepressants among patients with comorbid cocaine dependence and depression and reported that antidepressants are somewhat effective for reducing depressive symptoms but not effective for reducing cocaine use. Treatment for comorbid opioid dependence and depression has focused on studies that included patients on methadone maintenance. Seven reviewed studies found that treatment with antidepressants was not effective for treatment of depression among depressed patients with opioid dependence Torrens et al. (2005). Therefore, while primary treatments such as methadone, buprenorphine and residential treatment have been associated with improvements in depression, studies do not consistently support the effectiveness of antidepressants for reducing depression or opioid use.

2. **Pharmacotherapy for SUD and Schizophrenia:** For patients with schizophrenia or psychotic symptoms, antipsychotic medications are the mainstay of pharmacological treatment. Typical antipsychotic medications probably do not decrease SUD behaviors and, according to some researchers, it may actually precipitate or worsen SUD (Voruganti, Heslegrave, & Awad, 1997). Second generation antipsychotics are more effective for treatment of schizophrenia and comorbid substance abuse and current literature suggests clozapine, olanzapine and risperidone are among the best (Kelly, Daley, & Douaihy, 2012). Clozapine appears to be the most effective of the antipsychotics for reducing alcohol, cocaine and cannabis abuse among patients with schizophrenia. Clozapine's effect in these patients may be related to its ability to decrease the brain reward circuit dysfunction (Kelly et al., 2012). Petrakis et al. (2004) conducted a double-blind randomized clinical trial on the efficacy of naltrexone on 31 patients with a DSM-IV diagnosis of either schizophrenia or schizoaffective disorder and co-occurring alcohol abuse or dependence. The results indicated that those receiving naltrexone reported significantly fewer heavy drinking days, and alcohol cravings compared with those in the placebo condition
3. **Pharmacotherapy for SUD and Bipolar Disorder:** Pharmacotherapy of comorbid SUD and bipolar disorder typically involves use of mood stabilizers or atypical antipsychotics and antidepressants for the mood disorder and concomitant use of a medication specifically for the SUD, e.g., naltrexone for alcohol use disorder. Levin and Hennessy, 2004 reviewed treatments for bipolar disorder and SUD and noted that use of add-on medications such as anticonvulsants to lithium have primarily shown some effectiveness in reducing cravings but not actual substance use. In contrast to the Levin and Hennessy (2004) review, lithium has been found to be effective against relapse among patients with bipolar disorder and alcohol dependence (Maremmani et al., 2013) and lithium+valproate has been found to reduce drinking among bipolar patients (Salloum et al., 2005).
4. **Pharmacotherapy for SUD and Anxiety Disorders:** Many symptoms of withdrawal from substances can be mistaken for anxiety and that detoxification from substances, often result in the clearing of what appear to be anxiety-related symptoms. Tricyclic antidepressants have received the most empirical support for treatment of anxiety disorders, but their high side effect profiles and toxicity precludes their use as a first-line treatment (Brady & Verduin, 2005). The SSRIs or SNRIs are generally considered first-line treatments along with tricyclics. Cornelius and colleagues (Cornelius, Bukstein, Salloum, & Clark, 2003) reviewed the literature and report that buspirone has been found to be effective for alcohol dependent patients with comorbid anxiety. Due to the high risk for addiction, the use of benzodiazepines is not recommended for substance-abusing popula-

tions (Fatseas, Denis, Lavie, & Auriacombe, 2010). Related to this is the important consideration of using medications that are not likely to contribute to potentially toxic interactions with drugs and alcohol (Brady & Verduin, 2005).

5. **Pharmacotherapy for SUD and PTSD:** It appears that the substance-related co-morbidities of PTSD patients may be with harder drugs such as amphetamines and opioids, rather than with alcohol and cannabis (Mills, Teesson, Ross, & Peters, 2006). One caveat to this is that alcohol use disorders are quite high among combat veterans with PTSD (Jacobsen, Southwick, & Kosten, 2001). SSRI antidepressant medications and topiramate may be effective pharmacologic treatments for the PTSD but there is little evidence that SSRIs are effective against alcohol dependence (Brady & Verduin, 2005).

CONCLUSION

Co-morbid substance use disorder is an accepted complication of chronic and severe mental illness and is associated with serious adverse consequences. Recent evidence regarding the general integrated treatment approach is consistent and positive, but much work remains to be done on the organization and financing of integrated programs. Furthermore, the basic components of integrated treatment case management close monitoring, substance abuse treatment, family psychoeducation, rehabilitation, housing, and medications are still being developed and refined. Despite a number of promising treatments, there is still a long way before we know what treatments work for which groups of dual-diagnosis patients. This problem express further need for homogenized diagnostic criteria for dual diagnosis patients in order for clinicians to identify individuals appropriate for integrated treatment and also to develop an effective modality to treat this complex population with a diverse range of mental disorders.

REFERENCES

Agosti, V., Nunes, E., & Levin, F. (2002). Rates of psychiatric comorbidity among U.S. residents with lifetime cannabis dependence. *The American Journal of Drug and Alcohol Abuse*, *28*(4), 643–652. doi:10.1081/ADA-120015873 PMID:12492261

Aguilar, M. C., Gurpegui, M., Diaz, F. J., & de Leon, J. (2005). Nicotine dependence and symptoms in schizophrenia: Naturalistic study of complex interactions. *The British Journal of Psychiatry*, *186*(3), 215–221. doi:10.1192/bjp.186.3.215 PMID:15738502

Andreasen, N. C. (1999). A unitary model of schizophrenia: Bleuler's "fragmented phrene" as schizencephaly. *Archives of General Psychiatry*, *56*(9), 781–787. doi:10.1001/archpsyc.56.9.781 PMID:12884883

Andréasson, S., Allebeck, P., Engström, A., & Rydberg, U. (1987). Cannabis and schizophrenia. A longitudinal study of Swedish conscripts. *Lancet*, *2*(8574), 1483–1486. doi:10.1016/S0140-6736(87)92620-1 PMID:2892048

Arias, F., Szerman, N., Vega, P., Mesias, B., Basurte, I., Morant, C., & Babin, F. (2013). Abuse or dependence on cannabis and other psychiatric disorders. Madrid study on dual pathology prevalence. *Actas Españolas de Psiquiatría*, *41*(2), 122–129. PMID:23592072

Arseneault, L., Cannon, M., Poulton, R., Murray, R., Caspi, A., & Moffitt, T. E. (2002). Cannabis use in adolescence and risk for adult psychosis: Longitudinal prospective study. *BMJ (Clinical Research Ed.)*, *325*(7374), 1212–1213. doi:10.1136/bmj.325.7374.1212 PMID:12446537

Baker, A., Bucci, S., Lewin, T. J., Kay-Lambkin, F., Constable, P. M., & Carr, V. J. (2006). Cognitive-behavioural therapy for substance use disorders in people with psychotic disorders: Randomised controlled trial. *The British Journal of Psychiatry*, *188*(5), 439–448. doi:10.1192/bjp.188.5.439 PMID:16648530

Brady, K. T., & Verduin, M. L. (2005). Pharmacotherapy of comorbid mood, anxiety, and substance use disorders. *Substance Use & Misuse*, *40*(13-14), 2021–2041, 2043–2048. doi:10.1080/10826080500294924 PMID:16282091

Burnam, M. A., & Watkins, K. E. (2006). Substance abuse with mental disorders: Specialized public systems and integrated care. *Health Affairs (Project Hope)*, *25*(3), 648–658. doi:10.1377/hlthaff.25.3.648 PMID:16684728

Canaway, R., & Merkes, M. (2010). Barriers to comorbidity service delivery: the complexities of dual diagnosis and the need to agree on terminology and conceptual frameworks. *Australian Health Review: A Publication of the Australian Hospital Association, 34*(3), 262–268.

Carey, K. B. (1996). Substance use reduction in the context of outpatient psychiatric treatment: A collaborative, motivational, harm reduction approach. *Community Mental Health Journal*, *32*(3), 291–306, discussion 307–310. doi:10.1007/BF02249430 PMID:8790970

Caspi, A., Moffitt, T. E., Cannon, M., McClay, J., Murray, R., Harrington, H., & Craig, I. W. (2005). Moderation of the effect of adolescent-onset cannabis use on adult psychosis by a functional polymorphism in the catechol-O-methyltransferase gene: Longitudinal evidence of a gene X environment interaction. *Biological Psychiatry*, *57*(10), 1117–1127. doi:10.1016/j.biopsych.2005.01.026 PMID:15866551

Chambers, R. A., Krystal, J. H., & Self, D. W. (2001). A neurobiological basis for substance abuse comorbidity in schizophrenia. *Biological Psychiatry*, *50*(2), 71–83. doi:10.1016/S0006-3223(01)01134-9 PMID:11526998

Conway, K. P., Compton, W., Stinson, F. S., & Grant, B. F. (2006). Lifetime comorbidity of DSM-IV mood and anxiety disorders and specific drug use disorders: Results from the National Epidemiologic Survey on Alcohol and Related Conditions. *The Journal of Clinical Psychiatry*, *67*(2), 247–257. doi:10.4088/JCP.v67n0211 PMID:16566620

Cornelius, J. R., Bukstein, O., Salloum, I., & Clark, D. (2003). Alcohol and psychiatric comorbidity. Recent Developments in Alcoholism: An Official Publication of the American Medical Society on Alcoholism, the Research Society on Alcoholism, and the National Council on Alcoholism, 16, 361–374.

Dalack, G. W., Healy, D. J., & Meador-Woodruff, J. H. (1998). Nicotine dependence in schizophrenia: Clinical phenomena and laboratory findings. *The American Journal of Psychiatry*, *155*(11), 1490–1501. doi:10.1176/ajp.155.11.1490 PMID:9812108

Dean, B., Sundram, S., Bradbury, R., Scarr, E., & Copolov, D. (2001). Studies on [3H]CP-55940 binding in the human central nervous system: Regional specific changes in density of cannabinoid-1 receptors associated with schizophrenia and cannabis use. *Neuroscience*, *103*(1), 9–15. doi:10.1016/S0306-4522(00)00552-2 PMID:11311783

Desai, N. G., & Gupta, D. K. (1999). Substance use disorders. In *Textbook of post graduate Psychiatry* (2nd ed., pp. 76–89). New Delhi: Jaypee Publishers.

Dickey, B., & Azeni, H. (1996). Persons with dual diagnoses of substance abuse and major mental illness: Their excess costs of psychiatric care. *American Journal of Public Health*, *86*(7), 973–977. doi:10.2105/AJPH.86.7.973 PMID:8669521

Drake, R. E., Goldman, H. H., Leff, H. S., Lehman, A. F., Dixon, L., Mueser, K. T., & Torrey, W. C. (2001). Implementing evidence-based practices in routine mental health service settings. *Psychiatric Services (Washington, D.C.)*, *52*(2), 179–182. doi:10.1176/appi.ps.52.2.179 PMID:11157115

Drake, R. E., Mercer-McFadden, C., Mueser, K. T., McHugo, G. J., & Bond, G. R. (1998). Review of integrated mental health and substance abuse treatment for patients with dual disorders. *Schizophrenia Bulletin*, *24*(4), 589–608. doi:10.1093/oxfordjournals.schbul.a033351 PMID:9853791

Drake, R. E., Mueser, K. T., Brunette, M. F., & McHugo, G. J. (2004). A review of treatments for people with severe mental illnesses and co-occurring substance use disorders. *Psychiatric Rehabilitation Journal*, *27*(4), 360–374. doi:10.2975/27.2004.360.374 PMID:15222148

Drake, R. E., Mueser, K. T., Clark, R. E., & Wallach, M. A. (1996). The course, treatment, and outcome of substance disorder in persons with severe mental illness. *The American Journal of Orthopsychiatry*, *66*(1), 42–51. doi:10.1037/h0080153 PMID:8720640

Drake, R. E., & Wallach, M. A. (2000). Dual diagnosis: 15 years of progress. *Psychiatric Services (Washington, D.C.)*, *51*(9), 1126–1129. doi:10.1176/appi.ps.51.9.1126 PMID:10970914

Drew, A. E., Derbez, A. E., & Werling, L. L. (2000). Nicotinic receptor-mediated regulation of dopamine transporter activity in rat prefrontal cortex. *Synapse (New York, N.Y.)*, *38*(1), 10–16. doi:10.1002/1098-2396(200010)38:1<10::AID-SYN2>3.0.CO;2-T PMID:10941136

Fatséas, M., Denis, C., Lavie, E., & Auriacombe, M. (2010). Relationship between anxiety disorders and opiate dependence--a systematic review of the literature: Implications for diagnosis and treatment. *Journal of Substance Abuse Treatment*, *38*(3), 220–230. doi:10.1016/j.jsat.2009.12.003 PMID:20116963

Frei, A., & Rehm, J. (2002). The prevalence of psychiatric co-morbidity among opioid addicts. *Psychiatrische Praxis*, *29*(5), 258–262. doi:10.1055/s-2002-32713 PMID:12101492

Gangadhar, B. N., Thirthali, J., Venkatesh, B. K., Naveen, M. N., & Arunchala, U. (2007). Co-morbid substance use disorder in Schizophrenia: Results from a community survey. *Indian Journal of Psychiatry*, *49*, S30.

Giuffrida, A., Leweke, F. M., Gerth, C. W., Schreiber, D., Koethe, D., Faulhaber, J., & Piomelli, D. (2004). Cerebrospinal anandamide levels are elevated in acute schizophrenia and are inversely correlated with psychotic symptoms. *Neuropsychopharmacology: Official Publication of the American College of Neuropsychopharmacology*, *29*(11), 2108–2114. doi:10.1038/sj.npp.1300558 PMID:15354183

Goerke, D., & Kumra, S. (2013). Substance abuse and psychosis. *Child and Adolescent Psychiatric Clinics of North America*, *22*(4), 643–654. doi:10.1016/j.chc.2013.06.001 PMID:24012078

Grant, B. F., Stinson, F. S., Dawson, D. A., Chou, S. P., Dufour, M. C., Compton, W., & Kaplan, K. (2004). Prevalence and co-occurrence of substance use disorders and independent mood and anxiety disorders: Results from the National Epidemiologic Survey on Alcohol and Related Conditions. *Archives of General Psychiatry*, *61*(8), 807–816. doi:10.1001/archpsyc.61.8.807 PMID:15289279

Gregg, L., Barrowclough, C., & Haddock, G. (2007). Reasons for increased substance use in psychosis. *Clinical Psychology Review*, *27*(4), 494–510. doi:10.1016/j.cpr.2006.09.004 PMID:17240501

Gros, D. F., Milanak, M. E., Brady, K. T., & Back, S. E. (2013). Frequency and severity of comorbid mood and anxiety disorders in prescription opioid dependence. *The American Journal on Addictions / American Academy of Psychiatrists in Alcoholism and Addictions, 22*(3), 261–265.

Havens, J. R., & Strathdee, S. A. (2005). Antisocial Personality Disorder and Opioid Treatment Outcomes: A Review. *Addictive Disorders & Their Treatment*, *4*(3), 85–97. doi:10.1097/01.adt.0000155725.14375.6e

Heffner, J. L., Anthenelli, R. M., Adler, C. M., Strakowski, S. M., Beavers, J., & DelBello, M. P. (2013). Prevalence and correlates of heavy smoking and nicotine dependence in adolescents with bipolar and cannabis use disorders. *Psychiatry Research*, *210*(3), 857–862. doi:10.1016/j.psychres.2013.04.010 PMID:23684537

Henquet, C., Krabbendam, L., de Graaf, R., ten Have, M., & van Os, J. (2006). Cannabis use and expression of mania in the general population. *Journal of Affective Disorders*, *95*(1-3), 103–110. doi:10.1016/j.jad.2006.05.002 PMID:16793142

Hughes, J. F. (2000). Evidence for and against the self-medication hypothesis for smoking. *Journal of Neuropsychopharmacology*, *3*, S58–S59.

Inskip, H. M., Harris, E. C., & Barraclough, B. (1998). Lifetime risk of suicide for affective disorder, alcoholism and schizophrenia. *The British Journal of Psychiatry*, *172*(1), 35–37. doi:10.1192/bjp.172.1.35 PMID:9534829

Jacobsen, L. K., Southwick, S. M., & Kosten, T. R. (2001). Substance use disorders in patients with posttraumatic stress disorder: A review of the literature. *The American Journal of Psychiatry*, *158*(8), 1184–1190. doi:10.1176/appi.ajp.158.8.1184 PMID:11481147

Kelly, T. M., Daley, D. C., & Douaihy, A. B. (2012). Treatment of substance abusing patients with comorbid psychiatric disorders. *Addictive Behaviors*, *37*(1), 11–24. doi:10.1016/j.addbeh.2011.09.010 PMID:21981788

Kessler, R. C., Aguilar-Gaxiola, S., Andrade, L., Bijl, R., Borges, G., & Caraveo-Anduaga, J. J. et al.. (2001). Mental-substance comorbidities in the ICPE surveys. *Psychiatria Fennica*, *32*, 62–80.

Kessler, R. C., Barker, P. R., Colpe, L. J., Epstein, J. F., Gfroerer, J. C., Hiripi, E., & Zaslavsky, A. M. et al. (2003). Screening for serious mental illness in the general population. *Archives of General Psychiatry*, *60*(2), 184–189. doi:10.1001/archpsyc.60.2.184 PMID:12578436

Kessler, R. C., Crum, R. M., Warner, L. A., Nelson, C. B., Schulenberg, J., & Anthony, J. C. (1997). Lifetime co-occurrence of DSM-III-R alcohol abuse and dependence with other psychiatric disorders in the National Comorbidity Survey. *Archives of General Psychiatry*, *54*(4), 313–321. doi:10.1001/archpsyc.1997.01830160031005 PMID:9107147

Kessler, R. C., Nelson, C. B., McGonagle, K. A., Liu, J., Swartz, M., & Blazer, D. G. (1996). Comorbidity of DSM-III-R major depressive disorder in the general population: Results from the US National Comorbidity Survey. *The British Journal of Psychiatry. Supplement*, (30): 17–30. PMID:8864145

Kovasznay, B., Fleischer, J., Tanenberg-Karant, M., Jandorf, L., Miller, A. D., & Bromet, E. (1997). Substance use disorder and the early course of illness in schizophrenia and affective psychosis. *Schizophrenia Bulletin*, *23*(2), 195–201. doi:10.1093/schbul/23.2.195 PMID:9165630

Kozaric-Kovacic, D., Folnegovic-Smalc, V., Folnegovic, Z., & Maruic, A. (1995). Influence of alcoholism on the prognosis of schizophrenic patients. *Journal of Studies on Alcohol*, *56*(6), 622–627. doi:10.15288/jsa.1995.56.622 PMID:8558893

Leroy, S., Griffon, N., Bourdel, M. C., Olie, J. P., Poirier, M. F., & Krebs, M. O. (2001). Schizophrenia and the cannabinoid receptor type 1 (CB1): Association study using a single-base polymorphism in coding exon 1. *American Journal of Medical Genetics*, *105*(8), 749–752. doi:10.1002/ajmg.10038 PMID:11803524

Levin, F. R., & Hennessy, G. (2004). Bipolar disorder and substance abuse. *Biological Psychiatry*, *56*(10), 738–748. doi:10.1016/j.biopsych.2004.05.008 PMID:15556118

LLerena, A., de la Rubia, A., Peñas-Lledó, E. M., Diaz, F. J., & de Leon, J.LLerena. (2003). Schizophrenia and tobacco smoking in a Spanish psychiatric hospital. *Schizophrenia Research*, *60*(2-3), 313–317. doi:10.1016/S0920-9964(02)00508-X PMID:12591592

Making a Difference: Interim Status Report of the McKinney Research Demonstration Program for Homeless Mentally Ill Adults. (1995). Retrieved December 18, 2015, from https://aspe.hhs.gov/report/performance-improvement-1995/making-difference-interim-status-report-mckinney-research-demonstration-program-homeless-mentally-ill-adults

Maniglio, R. (2009). The impact of child sexual abuse on health: A systematic review of reviews. *Clinical Psychology Review*, *29*(7), 647–657. doi:10.1016/j.cpr.2009.08.003 PMID:19733950

Maremmani, A. G. I., Rovai, L., Bacciardi, S., Rugani, F., Pacini, M., Pani, P. P., & Maremmani, I. (2013). The long-term outcomes of heroin dependent-treatment-resistant patients with bipolar 1 comorbidity after admission to enhanced methadone maintenance. *Journal of Affective Disorders*, *151*(2), 582–589. doi:10.1016/j.jad.2013.06.054 PMID:23931828

McCreadie, R. G.Scottish Comorbidity Study Group. (2002). Use of drugs, alcohol and tobacco by people with schizophrenia: Case-control study. *The British Journal of Psychiatry*, *181*(4), 321–325. doi:10.1192/bjp.181.4.321 PMID:12356659

McHugo, G. J., Drake, R. E., Burton, H. L., & Ackerson, T. H. (1995). A scale for assessing the stage of substance abuse treatment in persons with severe mental illness. *The Journal of Nervous and Mental Disease, 183*(12), 762–767. doi:10.1097/00005053-199512000-00006 PMID:8522938

Mercer-McFadden, C., Drake, R. E., Brown, N. B., & Fox, R. S. (1997). The community support program demonstrations of services for young adults with severe mental illness and substance use disorders, 1987–1991. *Psychiatric Rehabilitation Journal, 20*(3), 13–24. doi:10.1037/h0095368

Miller, W., & Rollnick, S. (1991). *Motivational Interviewing: Preparing People to Change Addictive Behavior*. New York: Guilford.

Mills, K. L., Teesson, M., Ross, J., & Peters, L. (2006). Trauma, PTSD, and substance use disorders: Findings from the Australian National Survey of Mental Health and Well-Being. *The American Journal of Psychiatry, 163*(4), 652–658. doi:10.1176/ajp.2006.163.4.652 PMID:16585440

Minkoff, K. (1989). An integrated treatment model for dual diagnosis of psychosis and addiction. *Hospital & Community Psychiatry, 40*(10), 1031–1036. PMID:2807203

Morgan, C. J. A., & Curran, H. V. (2008). Effects of cannabidiol on schizophrenia-like symptoms in people who use cannabis. *The British Journal of Psychiatry, 192*(4), 306–307. doi:10.1192/bjp.bp.107.046649 PMID:18378995

Morse, G. A., Calsyn, R. J., Allen, G., Tempelhoff, B., & Smith, R. (1992). Experimental comparison of the effects of three treatment programs for homeless mentally ill people. *Hospital & Community Psychiatry, 43*(10), 1005–1010. PMID:1398563

Mroziewicz, M., & Tyndale, R. F. (2010). Pharmacogenetics: A tool for identifying genetic factors in drug dependence and response to treatment. *Addiction Science & Clinical Practice, 5*(2), 17–29. PMID:22002450

Mueller, T. I., Lavori, P. W., Keller, M. B., Swartz, A., Warshaw, M., Hasin, D., & Akiskal, H. (1994). Prognostic effect of the variable course of alcoholism on the 10-year course of depression. *The American Journal of Psychiatry, 151*(5), 701–706. doi:10.1176/ajp.151.5.701 PMID:8166311

Mueser, L. (2005). Psychosocial interventions for adult with severe mental illness and co-occurring substance use conditions: A review of specific interventions. *Journal of Dual Diagnosis, 1*, 57. doi:10.1300/J374v01n02_05

Murthy, P., & Chand, P. (2012). Treatment of dual diagnosis disorders. *Current Opinion in Psychiatry, 25*(3), 194–200. doi:10.1097/YCO.0b013e328351a3e0 PMID:22395768

Osher, F. C., & Kofoed, L. L. (1989). Treatment of patients with psychiatric and psychoactive substance abuse disorders. *Hospital & Community Psychiatry, 40*(10), 1025–1030. PMID:2807202

Patton, G. C., Coffey, C., Carlin, J. B., Degenhardt, L., Lynskey, M., & Hall, W. (2002). Cannabis use and mental health in young people: Cohort study. *British Medical Journal (Clinical Research Ed.), 325*(7374), 1195–1198. doi:10.1136/bmj.325.7374.1195 PMID:12446533

Petrakis, I. L., O'Malley, S., Rounsaville, B., Poling, J., McHugh-Strong, C., & Krystal, J. H. (2004). Naltrexone augmentation of neuroleptic treatment in alcohol abusing patients with schizophrenia. *Psychopharmacology, 172*(3), 291–297. doi:10.1007/s00213-003-1658-9 PMID:14634716

Ray, R. (1989). Alcohol diagnosis and phenomenology. *Proceedings of the Indo-US symposium on alcohol and drug use.* NIMHANS publication No 20 Bangalore.

Regier, D. A., Farmer, M. E., Rae, D. S., Locke, B. Z., Keith, S. J., Judd, L. L., & Goodwin, F. K. (1990). Comorbidity of mental disorders with alcohol and other drug abuse. Results from the Epidemiologic Catchment Area (ECA) Study. *Journal of the American Medical Association, 264*(19), 2511–2518. doi:10.1001/jama.1990.03450190043026 PMID:2232018

Ridgely, M. S., Osher, F. C., & Goldman, H. H. (1987). Chronic Mentally Ill Young Adults With Substance Abuse Problems: A Review of Research, Treatment, and Training Issues. In *Report of the Task Force on Chronic Mentally Ill Young Adults With Substance Problems*. Baltimore, MD: University of Maryland, Department of Psychiatry.

Ries, R. K., Sloan, K. L., & Miller, N. S. (1997). Concept, diagnosis and treatment of dual diagnosis. [Philadelphia: W.B. Saunders.]. *Current Psychiatric Therapies, II*, 173–180.

Salloum, I. M., Cornelius, J. R., Daley, D. C., Kirisci, L., Himmelhoch, J. M., & Thase, M. E. (2005). Efficacy of valproate maintenance in patients with bipolar disorder and alcoholism: A double-blind placebo-controlled study. *Archives of General Psychiatry, 62*(1), 37–45. doi:10.1001/archpsyc.62.1.37 PMID:15630071

Salokangas, R. K., Vilkman, H., Ilonen, T., Taiminen, T., Bergman, J., Haaparanta, M., & Hietala, J. (2000). High levels of dopamine activity in the basal ganglia of cigarette smokers. *The American Journal of Psychiatry, 157*(4), 632–634. doi:10.1176/appi.ajp.157.4.632 PMID:10739427

Sansone, R. A., Watts, D. A., & Wiederman, M. W. (2014). Borderline personality symptomatology and legal charges related to drugs. *International Journal of Psychiatry in Clinical Practice, 18*(2), 150–152. doi:10.3109/13651501.2013.847107 PMID:24059849

Sareen, J., Chartier, M., Kjernisted, K. D., & Stein, M. B. (2001). Comorbidity of phobic disorders with alcoholism in a Canadian community sample. *Canadian Journal of Psychiatry, 46*(8), 733–740. PMID:11692976

Schäfer, I., & Fisher, H. L. (2011). Childhood trauma and psychosis - what is the evidence? *Dialogues in Clinical Neuroscience, 13*(3), 360–365. PMID:22033827

Sideli, L., Mule, A., La Barbera, D., & Murray, R. M. (2012). Do child abuse and maltreatment increase risk of schizophrenia? *Psychiatry Investigation, 9*(2), 87–99. doi:10.4306/pi.2012.9.2.87 PMID:22707958

Sokhlet, S., & Sharma, S. G. (1998). A study of psychiatric morbidity among heroin addicts. *Indian Journal of Psychiatry, 40*, 18–19.

Sørensen, H. J., Jepsen, P. W., Haastrup, S., & Juel, K. (2005). Drug-use pattern, comorbid psychosis and mortality in people with a history of opioid addiction. *Acta Psychiatrica Scandinavica, 111*(3), 244–249. doi:10.1111/j.1600-0447.2004.00445.x PMID:15701109

Stohler, R., & Rossler, W. (2005). Dual Diagnosis. The evolving conceptual framework. Bibl Psychiatr., 172, 1-10. doi:doi:10.1159/isbn.978-3-318-01002-2 doi:10.1159/isbn.978-3-318-01002-2

Strakowski, S. M., DelBello, M. P., Fleck, D. E., Adler, C. M., Anthenelli, R. M., Keck, P. E., & Amicone, J. (2005). Effects of co-occurring alcohol abuse on the course of bipolar disorder following a first hospitalization for mania. *Archives of General Psychiatry*, *62*(8), 851–858. doi:10.1001/archpsyc.62.8.851 PMID:16061762

Strakowski, S. M., DelBello, M. P., Fleck, D. E., Adler, C. M., Anthenelli, R. M., Keck, P. E., & Amicone, J. (2007). Effects of co-occurring cannabis use disorders on the course of bipolar disorder after a first hospitalization for mania. *Archives of General Psychiatry*, *64*(1), 57–64. doi:10.1001/archpsyc.64.1.57 PMID:17199055

Taiminen, T. J., Salokangas, R. K., Saarijarvi, S., Niemi, H., Lehto, H., Ahola, V., & Syvalahti, E. (1998). Smoking and cognitive deficits in schizophrenia: A pilot study. *Addictive Behaviors*, *23*(2), 263–266. doi:10.1016/S0306-4603(97)00028-2 PMID:9573430

Tiet, Q. Q., & Mausbach, B. (2007). Treatments for patients with dual diagnosis: A review. *Alcoholism, Clinical and Experimental Research*, *31*(4), 513–536. PMID:17374031

Todd, J., Green, G., Harrison, M., Ikuesan, B. A., Self, C., Baldacchino, A., & Sherwood, S. (2004). Defining dual diagnosis of mental illness and substance misuse: Some methodological issues. *Journal of Psychiatric and Mental Health Nursing*, *11*(1), 48–54. doi:10.1111/j.1365-2850.2004.00683.x PMID:14723639

Torrens, M., Fonseca, F., Mateu, G., & Farre, M. (2005). Efficacy of antidepressants in substance use disorders with and without comorbid depression. A systematic review and meta-analysis. *Drug and Alcohol Dependence*, *78*(1), 1–22. doi:10.1016/j.drugalcdep.2004.09.004 PMID:15769553

Torrey, E. F. (1994). Violent behavior by individuals with serious mental illness. *Hospital & Community Psychiatry*, *45*(7), 653–662. PMID:7927289

van Laar, M., van Dorsselaer, S., Monshouwer, K., & de Graaf, R. (2007). Does cannabis use predict the first incidence of mood and anxiety disorders in the adult population? *Addiction (Abingdon, England)*, *102*(8), 1251–1260. doi:10.1111/j.1360-0443.2007.01875.x PMID:17624975

van Os, J., Bak, M., Hanssen, M., Bijl, R. V., de Graaf, R., & Verdoux, H. (2002). Cannabis use and psychosis: A longitudinal population-based study. *American Journal of Epidemiology*, *156*(4), 319–327. doi:10.1093/aje/kwf043 PMID:12181101

Voruganti, L. N., Heslegrave, R. J., & Awad, A. G. (1997). Neuroleptic dysphoria may be the missing link between schizophrenia and substance abuse. *The Journal of Nervous and Mental Disease*, *185*(7), 463–465. doi:10.1097/00005053-199707000-00008 PMID:9240366

Wenger, T., Moldrich, G., & Furst, S. (2003). Neuromorphological background of cannabis addiction. *Brain Research Bulletin*, *61*(2), 125–128. doi:10.1016/S0361-9230(03)00081-9 PMID:12831997

Wilcox, H. C., Conner, K. R., & Caine, E. D. (2004). Association of alcohol and drug use disorders and completed suicide: An empirical review of cohort studies. *Drug and Alcohol Dependence*, *76*(Suppl), S11–S19. doi:10.1016/j.drugalcdep.2004.08.003 PMID:15555812

Wild, T. C., el-Guebaly, N., Fischer, B., Brissette, S., Brochu, S., Bruneau, J., & Mun, P. (2005). Comorbid depression among untreated illicit opiate users: Results from a multisite Canadian study. *Canadian Journal of Psychiatry*, *50*(9), 512–518. PMID:16262105

Wilson, C. S., Bennett, M. E., & Bellack, A. S. (2013). Impact of Family History in Persons With Dual Diagnosis. *Journal of Dual Diagnosis*, *9*(1), 30–38. doi:10.1080/15504263.2012.744937 PMID:23538687

Wilson, D. R. (2010). Health consequences of childhood sexual abuse. *Perspectives in Psychiatric Care*, *46*(1), 56–64. doi:10.1111/j.1744-6163.2009.00238.x PMID:20051079

Zammit, S., Allebeck, P., Andreasson, S., Lundberg, I., & Lewis, G. (2002). Self reported cannabis use as a risk factor for schizophrenia in Swedish conscripts of 1969: Historical cohort study. *BMJ (Clinical Research Ed.)*, *325*(7374), 1199. doi:10.1136/bmj.325.7374.1199 PMID:12446534

Ziedonis, D. M., & Trudeau, K. (1997). Motivation to quit using substances among individuals with schizophrenia: Implications for a motivation-based treatment model. *Schizophrenia Bulletin*, *23*(2), 229–238. doi:10.1093/schbul/23.2.229 PMID:9165633

Zimberg, S. (1999). A dual diagnosis typology to improve diagnosis and treatment of dual disorder patients. *Journal of Psychoactive Drugs*, *31*(1), 47–51. doi:10.1080/02791072.1999.10471725 PMID:10332638

KEY TERMS AND DEFINITIONS

Bipolar Disorder and Substance Use: Individuals who end up developing bipolar disorder have a substance use disorder prior to the first appearance of their bipolar symptoms. The potential for the bipolar disorder may already exist, but it doesn't manifest until after the substance abuse has already been occurring.

Comorbidity in Mental Illness: Comorbidity referred as the overlap of two or more psychiatric disorders.

Schizophrenia and Substance Use: The combination of mental illness and substance use disorder is often called "concurrent disorders" or "co-occurring disorders", and in the United States, "dual diagnosis". People living with schizophrenia and other psychotic disorders tend to use substances that are affordable, easily accessible and readily available, such as alcohol, cannabis and nicotine. Prescription drugs like tranquilizers and sleep medication may also be misused.

Substance Use Disorder: The psychiatric disorders manifested by the excessive use of substances like: cannabis, caffeine, alcohol, nicotine, opioids, inhalants, cocaine, hallucinogens, phencyclidine (PCP), steroids, and sedative hypnotics substance use disorders are complicated conditions that are governed by features both i.e., neurobiological aspect and behavioural features of disorders.

Substance Use Disorder in Mentally Ill in India: Consumption of different substances during the episode of psychiatric illness are showing a rising trend and rapidly recognized in India.

Section 3
Chronic Mental Illness:
Family and Global Burden

Chapter 7
Understanding and Management of Caregivers' Stress and Burden of Person with Obsessive Compulsive Disorder

Shikha Soni
NIMHANS, India

Poornima C.
NIMHANS, India

P. C. Ashfak Ahamed
NIMHANS, India

ABSTRACT

The objective of the chapter is to understand the processes involved in care giving for those with a Chronic Mental Illness and to develop an effective intervention incorporating methods and strategies that aims at reducing caregiver stress and burden. OCD is a neurobiological disorder characterized by the presence of symptoms such as obsessions and compulsions. Literature is reviewed on prevalence, intervention and tools that can assess caregiver stress and burden in OCD. Accommodation and Expressed emotion plays key roles in interpersonal relationships that exist in the families of those afflicted with mental illness and may affect the treatment. Psycho education found to be helpful in educating the family about all the relevant aspects of OCD and to determine their role as a caregiver in order to deal with the illness in an effective way. Family intervention beyond the scope of psycho-education programme is required to prepare caregivers to take on the role of care giving more effectively.

DOI: 10.4018/978-1-5225-0519-8.ch007

A positive attitude may not solve all your problems, but it will annoy enough people to make it worth the effort. – Herm Albright

INTRODUCTION

The concept of *Burden of care* due to the mental illness emerged following the evolution of the deinstitutionalization of the mental hospitals and was first acknowledged by Grad and Sainbusry, who defined the caregiver burden as the physical, psychological, or emotional, social and financial problems that can be experienced by caregivers while caring for their mentally ill relative (Grad & Sainsbury, 1963).Being the principal caregiver to a mentally ill family member is a stressor that often creates high level of burden and contributes many stressful symptoms in caregivers itself. Caring for a mentally ill can be strenuous and a difficult task and involves adequate knowledge and support on part of the caregivers to support.

Family and the Burden of Care

Burden on the family refers to the consequences for those in close contact with a severely disturbed person with mental health problems. Some authors further distinguish between objective and subjective burden. *Objective burden* relates to the patient's symptoms, behavior, and socio demographic characteristics, and factors such as changes in household routine, family or social relations, work, leisure time, and physical health. *Subjective burden* is the mental health and subjective distress among family members (Reine, Lancon, Simeoni, Duplan, & Auquier, 2003). From the 1970s to 1980s, the term caregiver burden has been used to describe the adverse consequences of mental disorders for family caregivers. In recent years, the view of caregiving burden has been broadened to involve the physical, psychological, social, and financial problems experienced by families caring for a relative with a chronic or mental illness. This view has been accepted by the global community (WFMH, 2010)

Caregiver Stress

Providing the direct care or simply called "Caregiving" brings to mind caring for someone who is chronically ill or caring for a small child. If caregiving is planned well, it can be fulfilling and healthy. On the other side "dark side of caregiving" includes anger, frustration, exhaustion etc. Many times when it comes as a crisis and one is not prepared for it, often ends up feeling the darker side of caregiving. Being thrown into the role of caregiving unexpectedly and without the opportunity to equip oneself emotionally will be very difficult. Becoming a caregiver gradually will give the time to develop caregiving skills. To determine the best options for the person with mental illness, the whole family should be involved in the decision making process.

According to Webster's Dictionary, stress is a physical, chemical, or emotional factor that causes bodily or mental tension. It is a reaction to changes that require adjustments orresponses and our stress level will depend upon how we respond to these adjustments. Stress is the way human beings react both physically and mentally to changes, events, and situations in their lives. People experience stress in different ways and for different reasons. The reaction is based on the perception of an event or situation. Stress as a condition or feeling experienced when a person perceives that demands exceed the personal and social resources the individual is able to mobilize. Stress is an unpleasant external forces or an emotional response. Early on in your caregiving experience you will notice increased stress. Accepting a caregiver role will cause you to redefine your life. Recognizing the changes that come with this adapting to the new role, yet still having expectations of life returning to normal during the caregiving period, will cause immense stress.

Warning Signs of Caregiver Stress

It is very crucial to understand what is causing the stress in your life. It is only by being conscious of what is affecting a person negatively that then the person will be able to avoid being overwhelmed at every turn of event. Sometimes when they have no choice to become caregiver they can become angry, impatient and questions of fairness of circumstances. Many times they are not able to recognize the beginning indications of stress. Overtime the constant physical and emotional demands can take a toll. Changes in our behavior or mental health can be signals that they are living with too much stress. Thus Jolly (1996) listed certain warning signs of caregiver stress are:

- **Physical:** Headaches, appetite or weight changes, feeling tired all the time, changes in sleep habits, muscle aches, getting sick often, stooped posture, sweaty palms, neck pain, weight gain or loss.
- **Emotional:** Anger, sadness or crying spells, irritability or short temper, worry or anxiety, discouragement, trouble relaxing, emptiness or loss of direction, looking for magic solutions, inability to concentrate, frequent mood swings.
- **Behavioral:** Increased use of drugs or alcohol, trouble concentrating, avoiding decisions, low productivity, forgetfulness, boredom, over-reacting, acting on impulse, changing jobs often.
- **Relationships:** Problems with marriage or children, intolerance of others, fewer contact with friends, nagging, lowered sex drive, loneliness, resentment.

Caregiver Burnout

"Caregiver burnout is a state of physical, emotional and mental exhaustion that may be accompanied by a change in attitude, from positive and caring to negative and unconcerned. Burnout can occur when caregivers don't get the help they need, or if they try to do more than they are able physically and financially" Chronic stresses will reduce the quality of caregiving and the rapport with the loved one will suffer and as you struggle to cope, your physical and mental health may deteriorate.

Many people with mental illness must rely on family and friends for support and to help them in their daily activities. Globally caregiver lay an important and ever-expanding role as developments in medical care find new ways to help control illness while health and social services systems are resources challenged.

THE ROLE OF OCD IN CAREGIVER'S STRESS

Obsessive-compulsive disorder (OCD) is chronic and disabling disorder characterized by symptoms of obsessions and compulsions that are distressing to the individuals. It ranks 10th in the World Health Organization's list of leading causes of disability (WHO, 1999).

The prevalence of OCD ranges from 1 to 3% in the general population (Mohammadi et al., 2004) women tend to have a later onset of OCD symptoms than men (Narayanaswamy et al.,2012). Men seem to have a higher frequency of sexual, religious and symmetry/exactness obsessions, in addition to checking, ordering/ arranging and hoarding compulsions, while obsessions related to contamination and washing/ cleaning compulsions appear to be more common among women (deMathis et al., 2008). Many OCD adult sufferers find themselves living at home with parents or other family members because of the debilitating nature of OCD. A retrospective study of adult patients admitted over a 7-month period in 2007 at Menninger Clinic OCD Treatment program confirms many of these difficulties (Björgvinsson et al.,2008). Approximately 81% of adults lived at home with family, despite only 14% of them being married. Although most were unemployed (86%), many also required help with daily living tasks such as grooming and cleaning (62%). In addition, most sufferers (75%) reported a significant disruption in social activities and indicated the cost of treatment and the loss of wages were a significant financial burden on family (77%). These data suggest that OCD presents ongoing challenges to both the patient and the family system. Marital problems, family conflict, isolation, and financial strain are common results of the stress that OCD places on both the sufferer and the family.

In addition, because of the nature of the symptoms, family members frequently get drawn into obsessive-compulsive rituals and are forced to accommodate a great deal (Cooper, 1996). The burden on caregivers may be especially large in developing countries like India, where family members take care of person with mentally ill because of the lack of adequate formal community mental health services (Giel et al., 1983).

The lifetime prevalence of OCD has been reported to be 0.8% to 3.2% in the general population (Bobes et al., 2001). OCD has negative effects on social relations, quality of life (QoL) and occupational functioning of the patients. The disorder affects not only the patient but also the family members who live with the patient. This high level of burden experienced by the caregivers is possibly due to the accommodation the family members have to make specifically in relation to the obsessive–compulsive symptomatology. The difficulties encountered by the family members are in the form of disrupted personal and social lives, anger/frustration/fatigue, depression and family conflicts (Kalra, Kamath, Trivedi, & Janca, 2008). Often the sufferer and the caregivers are experiencing similar feelings of hopelessness and exasperation. The nature of OCD symptoms leaves no family untouched, since the rituals usually influence family interactions in various ways.

For families who are already confronted with a range of day to day problems that affect all aspects of their lives, a member with severe mental illness may have a significant impact on the entire family system (Saunders, 2003) Caregiver burden is the first of all linked with personality and mood of the caregiver himself (da Silva et al., 2013; Houet, Ke, Su, Lung., & Huang, 2008). The stress of dealing with a family member suffering from mental illness is inversely proportional to a healthy personality and a great resilience (Lautenschlager, Kurz, Loi., & Cramer, 2013).Caregiver burden in mental disorder is strictly linked with severity of the symptoms and the presence of problematic behaviors (Ohaeri, 2003). Caring for someone with these pathologies can result in considerable consequences for the caregivers that usually are also family members(Grover & Dutt, 2011;Torres, Hoff, Padovani, & Ramos-Cerqueira, 2012). Results showed that family members are less satisfied with their overall quality of life and are significantly distressed as a result of having a family member with mental disorder (Foldemoet al., 2005; Martens & Addington, 2001). Greater burden and lower quality were predicted by three fundamentals parameters which are duration and severity of mental illness, decreased tangible social support with restriction of caregiver social life and negative feelings of caregiver such as shame, embarrassment, guilt and self-blame (Grover & Dutt, 2011). Studies have been done on the motivational aspects of caregivers and how they can serve as protective factor. Among a study, caregivers reported common negative impacts but also beneficial effects such as feelings of gratification, love and pride. But still there are not known a lot about role played by these motivational factors.

THE ROLE OF FAMILY IN PATIENTS WITH OCD

Families of sufferers with OCD had known firsthand how debilitating the disorder can be. The OCD has a substantial effect on sufferer's quality of life. Persons with OCD did not choose to have the disorder nor does their caregiver take on more accountability solely out of obligation as caregiving is defined as assuming the extra responsibilities associated with the onset of the mental health problem. It is important to note that most of these are performed out of love and concern, even necessity, for someone caregiver cares deeply about. Often the sufferer and caregivers are experiencing similar feelings of hopelessness and exasperation. The nature of OCD symptoms leaves no family untouched, since the rituals usually influence family interactions in various ways. The natural tendency for a family member is to soothe a loved one when they are in distress. To minimize anxiety and conflict, caregivers may "put up with" or accommodate the sufferers' symptoms by changing family routines and schedules and altering normal family activities. Additionally, families of OCD sufferers face challenges that other families with relatives that have severe non-OCD psychiatric problems do not. OCD caregivers may become involved in the core symptoms of the disorder, beyond altering schedules and avoiding activities, by helping or even carrying out the rituals for the sufferer. Family may participate in this in the concealment to protect both the family and the sufferer from embarrassment and rejections from those outside of a trusted circle of friends and relatives. Thus sufferer may offer a proclamation to family members not to reveal anything about the illness. While family member often want to respect the privacy, these vows of secrecy weather imposed by sufferers or the family adds to increased burden on everyone involved. When OCD occurs in the family, either in childhood or adulthood, the dynamics of the family changes, so that the caring often appears to be one sided. As symptoms of the OCD worsen and some sufferer becomes more focused on their fears and may require more assistance from caregivers, this creates a discrepancy in attention in the various relationships. As the nature of the anxiety and fears reveals it puts people on guard and thus narrows their attention. Intense fear takes up the space including the family life. Tis shift in attention ads to the burden of caregivers as family life become more and more focused on the OCD. Kuipers et al. (1997) researchers from King's College of London Institute of Psychiatry, have outlined a number of factors that seem to play a role in the experience of burden. They include the type and severity of symptoms, the beliefs about the disorder, the coping skills of the caretaker, and the availability of social support networks. Misunderstandings or misinformation about the nature of OCD will likely increase the feeling of burden for caregivers. Such misunderstanding or misinformation includes blaming oneself or the sufferer for the disorder, expecting the disorder will spontaneously disappear, or assuming that the sufferer can no longer handle any responsibilities. Many people experience some level of shock or confusion when encountering the symptoms of OCD or when they learn about the diagnosis of OCD, particularly because of the often bizarre and frightening nature of the obsessions or the peculiar and nonsensical nature of the rituals. Having limited resources and ability to cope with the onset and progression of OCD will also influence the experience of a caregiver's burden.

Is There a Ray of Hope?

Hope is an important factor in the ability to adapt and cope with stressful events. It involves a positive attitude towards a desired outcome that is worth the effort. It is related to the expectation they have towards a desired future that it is valuable and worthwhile, as well as probable and possible. Most caregivers take up the role in the absence of any significant knowledge about the illness. The role and demands are incorporated within the ongoing day to day family responsivities. They develop their own different kinds of strategies to cope with the stress. A lot of trial and error might be involved in the way to try and cope with the stress.

COPING WITH CAREGIVER BURDEN

Thus caregivers tend to generate certain coping strategies in order to deal with the stress. The coping strategies can be broadly divided into three categories: Appraisal focused, Emotion focused and Problem focused. The Appraisal focused coping involves attempts to understand the illness and present a search for meaning. Emotion focused coping involves managing and maintaining emotions and maintaining one's emotional equilibrium. Problem focused coping involves confronting the problem and reconstructing it as manageable ones. Thus using such coping strategies caregiver appraise the illness and then use a variety of adaptive tasks and coping skills which in turn determine the amount of stress experienced and expressed. It is important to understand the caregiver's coping mechanism for tacking their burden because it affects caregiver's day to day functioning. This burden becomes a constant source of stress and how the caregiver cope with it affects the course of the illness. The efficacy of the caregiver is affected by the burden and coping methods which also influences the caregiver physical and mental health. The emotion focused coping has been reported to be associated with the perception of higher burden, whereas predominantly problem focused and fewer emotion focused coping strategies lead to reduced perception of burden. Caregiver's positive evaluation of their coping strategies is associated with reduced distress levels and positive attitude toward the patient (independent of symptoms and levels of burden). Problem solving coping has been reported to be associated with better functioning (Credoet, Parkar, & Kamath, 2006).

GOING DEEP INTO THE MINDS OF CAREGIVERS

Caregiver felt that the patient was and will not accept by the society and will face rejection and isolation for rest of their life. They end up saying "People don't come to our house. Even Close relatives are reluctant to come". Many stereotypes and stigmas pay role because of which the burden of not telling about the illness to anyone and hiding it from the society is even higher. Thus the social discrimination and the prejudice expressed by the caregivers deeply affects the stress experienced by them thus it is not only the patient but the whole family faces the problem. Caregivers generally felt that society does not understand and support the patients suffering with mental illness ads up to their amount of stress and burden experienced as a caregiver. Different areas which can be affected within the family are:

1. *Affects the family functioning adversely.* The day to day activities of the family are affected including children's study, adult's daily chores, social activities etc.
2. *Adverse effects on caregiver's occupation.* They often remain worried at their work place about the patient and is anyone taking care of the patient in caregiver's absence.
3. *Maintain adherence to treatment and meeting treatment expenses.* Noncompliance with treatment can be major concern for the caregiver as the symptoms might increase if the treatment is stopped thus adding up to the burden of care. They are not able to devote time to their jobs and thus affecting their earnings.
4. *Effects of caregiving on their mental and physical health.* They too become frustrated and chances of developing secondary depression are higher. It can have adverse effects on caregiver's role.

ACCOMMODATION IN OCD

Accommodation can be defined as any type of familial response that is significantly related to obsessive compulsive symptomatology. It includes behaviours such as feeling obliged to assist a relative with obsessive compulsive disorder when he or she is performing a ritual or respecting the rules the obsessive-compulsive disorder imposes on the patient and at the opposite side, interfering with the rituals or actively opposing them.

Accommodation may not suggest a helping response or action but can also include antithetic behaviours that maybe directed towards the patient such as allowing living areas to become unreasonably cluttered due to hoarding tendencies or maintaining high standards of cleanliness at home in order to reduce fear of contamination. Providing excessive reassurance to reduce unfounded fears such as answering repetitive questions regarding irrational fears, or facilitating avoidance of feared objects or situations by performing rituals on the patients' behalf and modifying family routines and rituals such as changing meal times in order to accommodate compulsions are also considered to be part of the accommodation process.

A model given by Van Noppen and colleagues (1990) on the familial responses to OCD symptoms which may be dependent on symptom severity as seen on YBOCS ratings, duration of the illness, functional impairment of the patient and well as the family's anger and frustration towards the patient. These responses towards the patient can be seen as two opposite poles of a spectrum.

Family accommodation is present in families with pediatric OCD and it affects the first degree relatives, namely parents and siblings of the OCD probands. Studies show that there is a high correlation between symptom severity and the level of accommodation in families and outcomes in treatment, mainly outcomes in behavior therapy. Clinical care in pediatric OCD should also include measuring, monitoring, and tracking this phenomenon to provide family-based interventions in such cases. Another aspect of family accommodation and pediatric OCD is the presence of comorbid externalizing disorders as seen from the prevalence of disruptive and aggressive behaviors directed towards caregivers. Parental psychopathology and parental styles are other variables that play a role in the levels of parental accommodation (Lebowitz et al., 2012).

Figure 1. Describing the familial responses to OCD symptoms which are divided into 3 broad categories: enmeshed or accommodating families, antagonistic families and split families

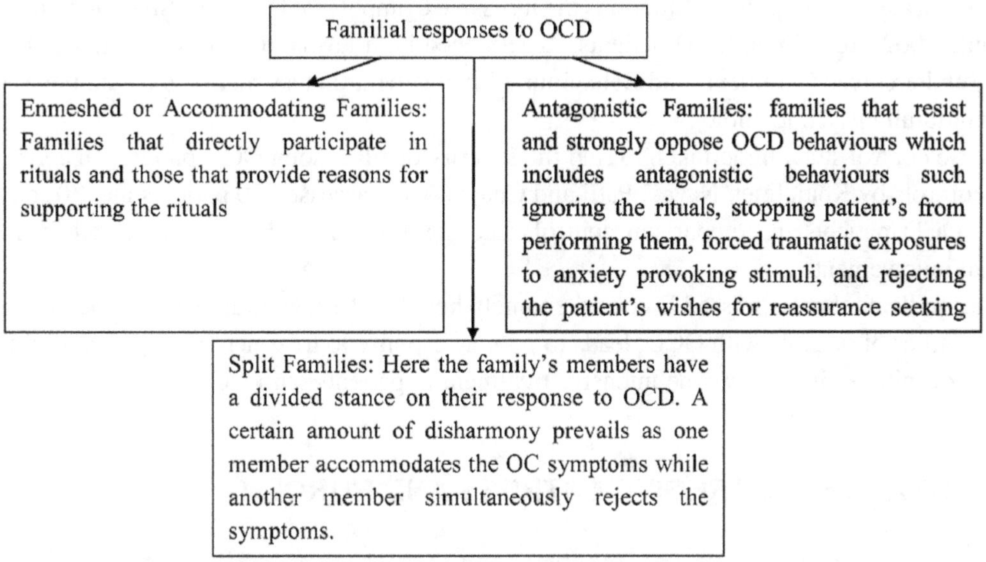

Romantic Partners and Spouses' accommodation in OCD has rarely been the focus of research; however, Boeding et al., (2013) have studied symptom accommodation in romantic partners of adults with OCD, and found that there was a high correlation between symptom severity and partner accommodation. Partners' of OCD patients reported low levels of relationship satisfaction than that reported by patients at pre-treatment and post-treatment partner accommodation seems to have led to poorer outcomes in therapy.

Higher the symptoms severity and higher the levels of accommodation shown by caregivers of patients with OCD. When parents, children and spouses are compared, romantic partners and spouses showed the highest level of accommodation which could be explained as their inability to see their partner in distress. In terms of outcome of behaviour therapy and its association with accommodation, poorer outcomes in treatment were linked with greater accommodation shown by caregivers.

EXPRESSED EMOTIONS IN OCD

Expressed emotion is an umbrella term used to describe various phenomena that occurs in the pattern of family interactions between caregivers and those afflicted with mental illness. Its represents the key aspects of the interpersonal relationship that exist in these families and includes; measurements of criticism, hostility, warmth, overprotection, over-involvement, and positive comments.

In a prospective study on Expressed Emotion in families of OCD and Agoraphobic patients by Chamblesset and Steketee (1999) the dropout rates were higher in patients whose relatives were hostile and emotionally overinvolved as assessed on the Camberwell Family Interview (CFI). Hostility and criticism also lead to poorer target ratings and low score on the Social Adjustment Scale. Better outcome was seen on behavioural avoidance test in families that were no hostile and noncritical. The use of psychotropic medication, contact with the relative, type of relationship with the patient and diagnosis had no effect on EE outcome measures.

In an India study on Expressed Emotions in Obsessive Compulsive Disorder (Shanmugiah, Varghese, & Khanna, 2002), found that OCD patients, experienced high levels of expressed emotions which included both Perceived Comments and Behavioural Involvement that seemed to indicate the presence of significant family psychopathology.

In a case control study undertaken to find the severity of EE among OCD patients in comparison to normal controls by Koujalgiet, Nayak, Patil and Chate (2014) assessed 30 patients and 30 sex matched controls. OCD patients in comparison controls had significantly increased perceived criticism and emotional involvement

Studies indicate that Expressed Emotions, namely hostility, behavioural over involvement and criticism in families of patients with OCD, leads to poorer response to treatment along with increased rates of relapse despite having undergone intensive treatment in patients with OCD.

TOOLS TO ASSESS CAREGIVER STRESS AND BURDEN

In order to caregiver burden and stress and to identify the area that is most affected by the chronic mental illness and to plan out suitable intervention strategies, tools are applied. The tools to assess stress and burden in OCD caregivers can be broadly divided into 2 categories

- Tools specific to assess accommodation in OCD (as accommodation was found to be source of caregiver stress and burden).
- Tools to assess caregiver stress and burden in chronic mental illnesses but can be applied on caregivers of patients with OCD.
- Tools to assess Expressed Emotion.

Tools Specific to Assess Accommodation in OCD

- **The Family Accommodation Scale for Obsessive Compulsive Disorder (FAS):** by Calvocoressi et al. (1999) was created to investigate the family accommodation construct, as seen in families of patients with OCD. It consists of 13 items, out of which the first 9 items include two types of accommodation: items 1-5 for participation in rituals and items 6-9 for modification in family functionality. The level of family accommodation is indicated by total scores ranging from 0-36, since each answer varies from0-4. The tenth item indicates stress levels experienced by the caregiver when he/she accommodates for the OC symptoms and the possible consequences for not accommodating is measured by items 11- 13. Mild family accommodation is indicated by a score of 9 on the scale, 10-18 is indicative of Moderate Accommodation; 19-27 is severe, while 28-36 is indicative of very severe accommodation.

Tools to Assess Caregiver Stress and Burden in Chronic Mental Illnesses but Can Be Applied on Caregivers of Patients with OCD

1. **The Burden Assessment Schedule (BAS):** By Thara, Kamath, and Kumar (1998): is a 40 item measure that assesses both objective and subjective burden of caregivers of chronic mentally patient. Stepwise ethnographic exploration was used in the development of the 40 items of this scale.
2. **Brief Measures of Secondary Role and Intrapsychic Strain Scale:** Pearlin and Schooler, (1990), in this scale there are three domains of Secondary Role Strains: Family Conflict (three subscales, 12 items); Job-Caregiving Conflict (5 items); and Economic Strains (3 items). Items are rated on 4-point scales (e.g. Strongly Agree to Strongly Disagree) without a specific time-frame, with Sample item (Job-Caregiving Conflict).
3. **The Perceived Benefits of Caregiving Scale:** Includes 11 items, and was developed by Beach, Schulz, Yee and Jackson (2000). Response options that have been used include a Yes/No format, and a 5-point Agree/Disagree scale.
4. **The Caregiver Reaction Scale:** (CRS; Qualls & Kenny, 2008) is a new scale that was adapted for use in a clinical setting from the research instrument used to develop a model of caregiver burden and competence developed by (Pearlin & Schooler, 1990). The measure includes subscales that assess feelings of role captivity, overload, relational deprivation, competence, personal gain, coping, family beliefs and conflict, job conflicts and financial disruption.
5. **The Zarit Burden Interview (ZBI):** Zarit, Stephens, Townsend and Greene (1980) it assesses the objective and subjective burden perceived by caregivers of psychiatric patients and originated as a 29-item questionnaire and is a popular caregiver self-report measure used by many aging agencies, the revised version contains 22 items. It assesses common problem areas such caregiver's physical health, emotional well-being, financial status, social relationships and the caregiver's relationship with the patient.
6. **Caregiver Self-Assessment Questionnaire:** This 18-item, caregiver self-report measure was devised by the American Medical Association as a means of helping physicians assess the stress-levels of family caregivers accompanying chronically ill older adult patients to their medical visits.
7. **The Self-Reporting Questionnaire (SRQ):** A screening measure for common mental and emotional suffering which indicates the presence of psychological morbidity in caregivers. There are 24 items in this questionnaire and the answer format is Yes/No (score 1 and 0, respectively). It has been divided into 2sections: the first 20 questions assess the presence of neurotic disorders while the rest of questions assess the presence of psychotic disorders. The duration of these symptoms should have been present during the previous one-month period. Cutoff scores of 7/8 for women and 5/6 for men can be used or the total score can be used as a continuous measure (Hardin et al. (1980)).
8. **Caregiver Burden Inventory:** It is used to measure caregiver burden as it relates to time, developmental comparison with peers, physical health, social relationships, and emotional health. it has 5 items for each:
    a. Time-dependence burden;
    b. Developmental burden;
    c. Physical burden;
    d. Social burden (5-point scale) and 4 items for emotional burden (5-point scale)
9. **Caregiver Burden Scale:** Measures caregiver burden at the end of life. It has 18 items (4-point scale)
10. **Caregiver Distress Activities:** Measures the effort made by the caregiver to decrease the symptoms of stress that result from caregiving. It has 8 items (4-point scale)

11. **Caregiver Strain Index:** Measures caregiver strain using yes/no response scales. It has 12 items (2-point scale)
12. **Caregiver Stress Effects:** Measures aspects of family life that are negatively affected by caregiving role, as well as restrictions in caregiver activities as a result of the caregiving role. It has 8 items for negative changes in elder, caregiver and family relationships and 5 items for restrictions in caregivers' activities
13. **Caregivers' Stress Scale:** Measures 15 domains: cognitive status, problematic behaviour, overload, relational deprivation, family conflict, job-caregiving conflict, economic strains, role captivity, loss of self, caregiving competence, personal gain, management of situation, management of meaning, management of distress, and expressive support. It has Series of 15 scales (3-point, 4-point, 5-point scales)
14. **Care-Related Strain:** Measures the stress felt by a caregiver as a result of having a relative in a nursing home. It has 7 items (4-point scale)
15. **Cost of Care Index:** Measures different aspects of burden including personal and social restrictions, emotional health, worthiness of caregiving, relationship with care recipient, and economic costs. It has 4 items for each:
    a. Personal and social restrictions;
    b. Physical and emotional health;
    c. Value investment in caregiving;
    d. Perception of the care recipient as a provocateur;
    e. Economic costs (4-point scales)
16. **Family Strain Scale:** Measures subjective burden related to emotional/psychological effect, changes in living in living patterns, and changes in relationships/health. It has 5 items
17. **Novel Caregiver Burden:** Measures strain, isolation, disappointment, and emotional involvement. It has 20 items (4-point scale).
18. **Measures of Strain:** Measures 3 domains: difficulty of caregiving (threat to family well-being), negative consequences of caregiving, and perceptions of negative consequences of caregiving on the family. It has 3 items for appraised difficulty of caregiving (4-point scale). And 3 items for negative consequences of caregiving (2-point scale) and 2 items for perceptions of negative consequences of caregiving on the family (2-point scale).
19. **Montgomery Burden Interview:** Two scales are used to assess both objective and subjective burden. The objective scale focuses on privacy, time, personal freedom, amount of money available, amount of energy, amount of vacation activities, recreational activities, relationships with other family members, and health. The subjective scale focuses on attitudes and emotional reactions toward caregiving. It has 9 items for objective scale (5-point scale) and 13 items for subjective scale ('rarely or never' to 'most of the time').
20. **Perceived Caregiver Burden Scale:** Measures caregiver burden in terms of perceptions and feelings about caregivers' physical and emotional health, family relationships, social life, work, and finances. It has 31 items (4-point scale).
21. **Perceived Caregiver Burden Scale, Revised:** Measures caregiver burden in terms of perceptions and feelings about caregivers' physical and emotional health, family relationships, social life, work, and finances. It has 13 items (4-point scale).
22. **Perceived Burden Scale:** Measures extent to which caregivers believe that changes have occurred because of problems or concerns with caregiving. It has 22 items (5-point scale).

23. **Perceived Stress Scale:** Measures the degree to which situations are perceived as stressful. It has 14 items (5-point scale).
24. **Relatives' Stress Scale:** Measures the reaction to caregiving of relative carers of elderly patients with senile dementia living in the community. Focuses on 3 domains: personal distress in relation to the care recipient, life upset as a result of caregiving, and negative feelings toward the care recipient. It has items (5-point scale).
25. **Screen for Caregiver Burden:** Measures objective and subjective burden relating to occurrence of care demands and distress associated with them. It has 25 items (5-point scale).
26. **Zarit Burden Interview:** Measures caregiver appraisal of the impact of caregiving. It has 22 items (5-point scale).

270 Short Form Zarit Burden Interview: Shorter version of the Zarit Burden Interview designed to measure impact of caregiving. It has 12 items (5-point scale).

Tools to Assess Expressed Emotion

1. **Family Emotional Involvement and Criticism Scale (FEICS):** This is a 14 item scale on which the items are clubbed to derive two subscales: Perceived Criticism (PC) and Intensity of Emotional Involvement (EI). The standardization of the scale was done on 83 respondents by Shields, Franks, Harp, McDaniel, and Campbell, (1992) at a Family Medicine Centre. There are 7 items on each subscale and are scored on a Likert scale ranging from0-5(minimum 0 to a maximum of 35 on each scale.
2. **Camberwell Family Interview (CFI):** Leff and Vaughn (1985): It is a semi-structured interview conducted in the absence of the patient, with the key relatives of the patient (parents or spouse) and is usually recorded and coded later and is considered the gold-standard measure for expressed emotion in families with mental illness. There areas that are covered in the interview are the onset of the illness prior to symptom exacerbation and hospitalization, participation of the patient in routine household activities, level of tension and irritability at home, and the daily routines of the family members including those of the patient. The interview duration can range from 1 to 2 hours. There are 5 subscales in the CFI: Criticism, Hostility, Emotional Over involvement, Warmth and Positive remarks, though Criticism, hostility and emotional over involvement are usually more commonly assessed in the study of expressed emotions. The classification of family members as being high or low on expressed emotion is based on the ratings on these scales.
3. **The Five Minute Speech Sample (FMSS):** Magna et al. (1986): family members are required to talk about their thoughts and feelings towards the patient for a period of five minutes without much interruption. It measures the frequency of positive comments made by the caregivers with regards to the patient. The speech is usually recorded and is later coded to assess the level of overall expressed emotion, over involvement and criticism.
4. **Level of Expressed Emotion Scale (LEE):** Cole and Kazarian (1993): is a self-report, used to assess the emotional environment in the patients' relationships. It comprises of 4 subscales: Intrusiveness, Emotional Response, Attitude towards Illness, and Tolerance and Expectations. The 60 items are rated in a true-false format and it provides score that ascertain the overall level of EE as well as scores for the 4 subscales.

5. **Perceived Criticism (PC):** Hooley and Teasdale (1989): in this scale patients are asked to rate how critical they thought they relatives are towards them, as well as how critical they felt towards their relative and indicate their preference on a 5-point Likert type scale. of this scale

PSYCHOLOGICAL INTERVENTION FOR CAREGIVER STRESS AND BURDEN

There is a dearth of literature on the intervention for caregiver stress and burden in OCD. The objective of the intervention should not aim at improving care-giving standards or improve the quality of life of the patients, but should aim at preventing the incidence of mental illness in the caregivers.

There are sufficient studies in terms of caregiver stress and burden and interventions in conditions as medical conditions. And among psychiatric disorders there are innumerable studies on caregiver stress and burden in organic conditions such as dementia (Alzheimer's disease), schizophrenia, and mood disorders. Studies on caregiver stress and burden in anxiety disorders may be present but not on OCD specifically.

Psycho-Education and Stress Management: Individualized as well as Group Based Programs

Psychoeducation is the act of imparting disease-related information to the patient or the patient's significant others (Michalak, Yatham, & Lam RW, 2004). It can also be defined as "a mutual process that attempts to improve a patient's illness management skills through bidirectional sharing of relevant information (Callahan & Bauer, 1999).

Family Psychoeducation a process by which knowledge of the illness is imparted to the family members or caregivers of the patient afflicted with a mental illness, and with continual assistance, it helps to modify their attitudes and behaviour towards the patient. It helps in the formulation and implementation of coping skills and other preferred interactions between the affected member and their caregivers.

Objectives of Psychoeducation

Psychoeducation refers to the education offered to individuals with a mental health condition and their families to help empower them and deal with their condition in an optimal way:

1. To educate the family about all the relevant aspects of OCD such as defining it as a neurobiological disorder this information will enable families to understand the illness in an objective way and care more effectively for their affected family member. It helps therapists determine the family's perception of the illness, and how their beliefs influence their behaviour and how amenable they are to seeing the illness from a different perspective.
2. To impart information about the disorder, its causes, symptom typology, age on onset, course of the illness, prognosis and types of treatment available.
3. Clarify doubts, misconceptions the family members may have had regarding the illness.
4. To reassure the family that there is hope for the affected member to get better.
5. To motivate the caregivers to comply with the medication as prescribed by the psychiatrist and assist the patient with homework assignments and exposure tasks given by the psychologist, as part of CBT intervention.

6. Engage and maintain the family in treatment to ensure the patient comes for regular follow up.
7. To reduce specific caregiver involvement in the performance of rituals and reduce perceived burden due to the disorder by allowing the caregivers to share their feelings and emotions, helping the accept patient's realistic limitations and dealing with the expectations from the treatment.

Various coping strategies have been used by the caregivers to come out of the stress of care giving. Focusing on the positive emotions like developing the faith in God, helping others with similar problem, hope for a better future also taking regular guidance from the experts. Engaging oneself in the activities liked by them will help in deviating one's focuses from the ongoing stress and leading to burnout. Carrying out daily activities like the way it used to be before adapting the role of a caregiver is also equally important. Problem solving skills to be taught to the caregivers for managing the problem and also the patient's behavior and increasing their access to social support and community resources would also help in dealing with stress and burden.

Acceptance of the illness as the way it is would also help caregivers to peacefully come in terms of the current ongoing situation. Accepting the fact that the illness is a long term and is now the part of one's current situation would lead to develop healthy relation with oneself.

A number of initiatives have taken place both in the voluntary sector and as well as the government sector. Voluntary sector as well as the efforts has been made by number of mental health professionals for the welfare of the family of mentally ill patients. Many nongovernmental organizations (NGOs) have been working in the area of providing community support to persons with mental illness and their caregivers.

From previous studies on psych educational and support groups for obsessive compulsive disorder and their significant others by Tynes and colleagues (1992), data obtained from self-report evaluation forms suggests that 10-week time-limited combined psych educational and support groups for patients as well their caregivers were found to be helpful to both groups. Informal lectures on topics such as types of OCD symptoms, relationship between OCD and other Axis I and Axis II disorders, neurobiological and learning basis of OCD, treatment compliance to medication and behavior therapy. Groups consisted of 15 to 25 members and the intervention comprised of informal lectures lasting approximately 45 minutes followed by 30 to 45-minute discussion on the presented topic.

Multifamily Behaviour Therapy is the behavior therapy intervention that is provided to spouses/partners, parents, children or any primary giver of an OCD patient. Van Noppenet, Steketee, McCorkle, & Pato, 1997) researched on group-based behavioural treatment: group (GBT) for OCD patients and multifamily (MFBT) for caregivers of OCD patients, multifamily behavioural therapy treatment participants showed clinically significant improvements, however, group treatments showed large effects comparable to those reported for a more intensive individual behavioral treatment. A partially manualized GBT was delivered by behavior therapy co-therapy teams to seventeen patients (10women and 7 men) diagnosed with OCD in 3 different groups of ten 2-hour sessions. Ratings on YBOCS reduced significantly at posttest and at 1-year follow-up, as did measures of overall functioning on the Sheehan Disability Scale at posttest and follow-up. In the MFBT group a cohort of 19 patients (14 women and 5 men) were treated with MFBT that included spouses/partners and parents of patients with OCD, who were further assigned to one of the three co-therapy. Two groups received ten 2-hr sessions and one received twelve 2-hr sessions. YBOCS scores reduced significantly at posttest and at 1-year follow-up, with corresponding gains in disability scores. When both forms of treatment were compared it was found that similar proportions of subjects were reliably changed at posttest and follow-up respectively, but more MFBT than GBT participants were clinically significantly improved.

Based on the IOWA model given by Black and Blum (1992) support groups were set up for patients afflicted with OCD. Support groups as adjuncts to the treatment for various conditions have existed for many years but in terms of OCD, research is still in its infancy. Patient groups have existed to provide services such as Psychoeducation and emotional support, however this program has now been extended to include caregivers of OCD patients as well. Conjoined Psychoeducation and support groups for OCD patients and their family members, with the aim of providing psychological support to patients and caregivers have proven to be beneficial in the treatment of OCD.

CONCLUSION

Today Caregiving has evolved over the years from various institutions to the community support groups. Various psychological variables affect the caregiving of the patient. These issues have to be discussed and resolved with caregiver who leads to increase of the stress and burden of care. Caregiving is one of the significant issue in the treatment of the illness thus there is a need to understand these psychological issue which help in the better management of the patient.

REFERENCES

Beach, S. R., Schulz, R., Yee, J. L., & Jackson, S. (2000). Negative and positive health effects of caring for a disabled spouse: Longitudinal findings from the caregiver health effects study. *Psychology and Aging*, *15*(2), 259–271. doi:10.1037/0882-7974.15.2.259 PMID:10879581

Bjorgvinsson, T., Wetterneck, C. T., Powell, D. M., Chasson, G. S., Webb, S. A., Hart, J., & Stanley, M. A. (2008). Treatment outcome for adolescent obsessive-compulsive disorder in a specialized hospital setting. *Journal of Psychiatric Practice*, *14*(3), 137–145. doi:10.1097/01.pra.0000320112.36648.3e PMID:18520782

Black, D. W., & Blum, N. S. (1992). Obsessive-compulsive disorder support groups: The Iowa model. *Comprehensive Psychiatry*, *33*(1), 65–71. doi:10.1016/0010-440X(92)90082-2 PMID:1555412

Bobes, J., Gonzalez, M. P., Bascaran, M. T., Arango, C., Saiz, P. A., & Bousono, M. (2001). Quality of life and disability in patient with obsessive-compulsive disorder. *European Psychiatry*, *16*(4), 239–245. doi:10.1016/S0924-9338(01)00571-5 PMID:11418275

Boeding, S. E., Paprocki, C. M., Baucom, D. H., Abramowitz, J. S., Wheaton, M. G., Fabricant, L. E., & Fischer, M. S. (2013). Let me check that for you: Symptom accommodation in romantic partners of adults with obsessive–compulsive disorder. *Behaviour Research and Therapy*, *51*(6), 316–322. doi:10.1016/j.brat.2013.03.002 PMID:23567474

Callahan, A. M., & Bauer, M. S. (1999). Psychosocial interventions for bipolar disorder. *The Psychiatric Clinics of North America*, *22*(3), 675–688. doi:10.1016/S0193-953X(05)70102-7 PMID:10550862

Calvocoressi, L., Mazure, C. M., Kasl, S. V., Skolnick, J., Fisk, D., Vegso, S. J., & Price, L. H. et al. (1999). Family accommodation of obsessive-compulsive symptoms: Instrument development and assessment of family behavior. *The Journal of Nervous and Mental Disease*, *187*(10), 636–642. doi:10.1097/00005053-199910000-00008 PMID:10535658

Chambless, D., & Steketee, G. (1999). Expressed emotion and behavior therapy outcome: A prospective study with obsessive-compulsive and agoraphobic outpatients. *Journal of Consulting and Clinical Psychology*, *67*(5), 658–665. doi:10.1037/0022-006X.67.5.658 PMID:10535232

Cole, J. D., & Kazarian, S. S. (1993). Predictive validity of the Level of Expressed Emotion (LEE) Scale: Readmission follow-up data for 1, 2, and 5-year periods. *Journal of Clinical Psychology*, *49*(2), 216–218. doi:10.1002/1097-4679(199303)49:2<216::AID-JCLP2270490214>3.0.CO;2-G PMID:8098049

Cooper, M. (1996). Obsessive-compulsive disorder: Effects on family members. *TheAmerican Journal of Orthopsychiatry*, *66*(2), 296–304. doi:10.1037/h0080180 PMID:8860758

Creado, D. A., Parkar, S. R., & Kamath, R. M. (2006). A comparison of the level of functioning in chronic schizophrenia with coping and burden in caregivers. *Indian Journal of Psychiatry*, *48*(1), 27–33. doi:10.4103/0019-5545.31615 PMID:20703411

da Silva Gdel, G., Jansen, K., Barbosa, L. P., Branco Jda, C., Pinheiro, R. T., Magalhães, P. V., & da Silva, R. A. et al. (2013). Burden and related factors in caregivers of young adults presenting bipolar and unipolar mood disorder. *TheInternational Journal of Social Psychiatry*, *60*(4), 396–402. doi:10.1177/0020764013491740 PMID:23828767

de Mathis, M. A., do Rosario, M. C., Diniz, J. B., Torres, A. R., Shavitt, R. G., Ferrao, Y. A., & Miguel, E. C. et al. (2008). Obsessive-compulsive disorder: Influence of age at onset on comorbidity patterns. *European Psychiatry*, *23*(3), 187–194. doi:10.1016/j.eurpsy.2008.01.002 PMID:18329252

Foldemo, A., Gullberg, M., Ek, A. C., & Bogren, L. (2005). Quality of life and burden in parents of outpatients with schizophrenia. *Social Psychiatry and Psychiatric Epidemiology*, *40*(2), 133–138. doi:10.1007/s00127-005-0853-x PMID:15685405

Giel, R., de Arango, M. V., Hafeiz Babikir, A., Bonifacio, M., Climent, C. E., Harding, T. W., & Wig, N. N. et al. (1983). The burden of mental illness on the family. Results of observations in four developing countries. A report from the WHO collaborative study on strategies for extending mental healthcare. *Acta Psychiatrica Scandinavica*, *68*(3), 186–201. doi:10.1111/j.1600-0447.1983.tb06998.x PMID:6637556

Grad, J., & Sainsbusy, P. (1963). Mental illness and the family. *Lancet*, *281*(7280), 544–549. doi:10.1016/S0140-6736(63)91339-4 PMID:13949711

Grover, S., & Dutt, A. (2011). Perceived burden and quality of life of caregivers in obsessive–compulsive disorder. *Psychiatry and Clinical Neurosciences*, *65*(5), 416–422. doi:10.1111/j.1440-1819.2011.02240.x PMID:21851450

Harding, T. W., De Arango, V., Baltazar, J., Climent, C. E., Ibrahim, H. H. A., Ladrido-Ignacio, L., & Wig, N. N. (1980). Mental disorders in primary health care: A study of their frequency and diagnosis in four developing countries. *Psychological Medicine*, *10*(02), 231–241. doi:10.1017/S0033291700043993 PMID:7384326

Hooley, J. M., & Teasdale, J. D. (1989). Predictors of relapse in unipolar depressives: Expressed emotion, marital distress, and perceived criticism. *Journal of Abnormal Psychiatry*, *98*(3), 229–235. doi:10.1037/0021-843X.98.3.229 PMID:2768657

Houet, S. Y., Ke, C. L., Su, Y. C., Lung, F. W., & Huang, C. J. (2008). Exploring the burden of the primary family caregivers of schizophrenia patients in Taiwan. *Psychiatry and Clinical Neurosciences*, *62*(5), 508–514. doi:10.1111/j.1440-1819.2008.01843.x PMID:18950369

Jolly, C. D. (1996). *Stress taking charge: All about stress*. Retrieved April 30, 2003, from Iowa State University Extension, Department of Human Development and Family Studies Web site: http://www.extension.iastate.edu/Publications/PM1660A.pdf

Kalra, H., Kamath, P., Trivedi, J. K., & Janca, A. (2008). Caregiver burden in anxiety disorders. *Current Opinion in Psychiatry*, *21*(1), 70–73. doi:10.1097/YCO.0b013e3282f2dfca PMID:18281843

Koujalgi, S. R., Nayak, R. B., Patil, N. M., & Chate, S. S. (2014). Expressed emotions in patients with obsessive compulsive disorder: A case control study. *Indian Journal of Psychological Medicene*, *36*(2), 138–141. doi:10.4103/0253-7176.130972 PMID:24860213

Lautenschlager, N. T., Kurz, A. F., Loi, S., & Cramer, B. (2013). Personality of mental health caregivers. *Current Opinion in Psychiatry*, *26*(1), 97–101. doi:10.1097/YCO.0b013e32835997b3 PMID:23041793

Lebowitz, E. R., Woolston, J., Bar-Haim, Y., Calvocoressi, L., Dauser, C., Warnick, E., & Leckman, J. F. et al. (2012). Family accommodation in pediatric anxiety disorders. *Depression and Anxiety*, *30*(1), 47–54. doi:10.1002/da.21998 PMID:22965863

Leff, J. P., & Vaughn, C. E. (1985). *Expressed emotion in families*. New York: Guilford Press.

Magan˜a, A. B., Goldstein, J. M., Karno, M., Miklowitz, D. J., Jenkins, J., & Falloon, I. R. (1986). A brief method for assessing expressed emotion in relatives of psychiatric patients. *Psychiatry Research*, *17*(3), 203–212.

Martens, L., & Addington, J. (2001). The psychological well-being of family members of individuals with schizophrenia. *Social Psychiatry and Psychiatric Epidemiology*, *36*(3), 128–133. doi:10.1007/s001270050301 PMID:11465784

Michalak, E. E., Yatham, L. N., & Lam, R. W. (2004). The role of psychoeducation in the treatment of bipolar disorder: A clinical perspective. *Clinical Approaches in Bipolar Disorder*, *3*, 5–11.

Mohammadi, M. R., Ghanizadeh, A., Rahgozar, M., Noorbala, A. A., Davidian, H., Afzali, H. M., & Tehranidoost, M. et al. (2004). Prevalence of obsessive-compulsive disorder in Iran. *BMC Psychiatry*, *4*(2). PMID:15018627

Narayanaswamy, J. C., Viswanath, B., Cherian, A. V., Bada Math, S., Kandavel, T., & Janardhan Reddy, Y. C. (2012). Impact of age of onset of illness on clinical phenotype in OCD. *Psychiatry Research*, *200*(2-3), 554–559. doi:10.1016/j.psychres.2012.03.037 PMID:22503329

Ohaeri, J. U. (2003). The burden of caregiving in families with a mental illness: A review of 2002. *Current Opinion in Psychiatry*, *16*(4), 457–465. doi:10.1097/01.yco.0000079212.36371.c0

Pearlin, L. I., Mullan, J. T., Semple, S. J., & Skaff, M. M. (1990). Caregiving and the stress process: An overview of concepts and their measures. *The Gerontologist*, *30*(5), 583–594. doi:10.1093/geront/30.5.583 PMID:2276631

Qualls, S. H., & Kenny, M. (2008). *Caregiver Reaction Scale*. Unpublished assessment.

Reine, G., Lancon, C., Simeoni, M. C., Duplan, S., & Auquier, P. (2003). Caregiver burden in relatives of persons with schizophrenia: An overview of measure instruments. *L'Encéphale*, *29*(2), 137–147. PMID:14567165

Saunders, J. C. (2003). Families living with severe mental illness: A literature review. *Issues in Mental Health Nursing*, *24*(2), 175–198. doi:10.1080/01612840305301 PMID:12554427

Shanmugiah, A., Varghese, M., & Khanna, S. (2002). Expressed emotions in obsessive compulsive disorder. *Indian Journal of Psychiatry*, *44*(1), 14–18. PMID:21206875

Shields, C. G., Franks, P., Harp, J. J., McDaniel, S. H., & Campbell, T. L. (1992). Development of the Family Emotional Involvement and Criticism Scale (FEICS)- A self report scale to measure Expressed Emotions. *Journal of Marital and Family Therapy*, 18.

Thara, R., Kamath, S., & Kumar, S. (1998). Women with schizophrenia and broken marriages-doubly disadvantaged? Part II: Family perspective. *The International Journal of Social Psychiatry*, *49*(3), 233–240. doi:10.1177/00207640030493009 PMID:14626366

Torres, A. R., Hoff, N. T., Padovani, C. R., & Ramos-Cerqueira, A. T. (2012). Dimensional analysis of burden in family caregivers of patients with obsessive–compulsive disorder. *Psychiatry and Clinical Neurosciences*, *66*(5), 432–441. doi:10.1111/j.1440-1819.2012.02365.x PMID:22834662

Tynes, L. L., Salins, C., Skiba, W., & Winstead, D. K. (1992). A psychoeducational and support group for obsessive-compulsive disorder patients and their significant others. *Comprehensive Psychiatry*, *33*(3), 197–201. doi:10.1016/0010-440X(92)90030-T PMID:1591912

Van Noppen, B., Steketee, G., McCorkle, B. H., & Pato, M. (1997). Group and multifamily behavioral treatment for obsessive compulsive disorder: A pilot study. *Journal of Anxiety Disorders*, *11*(4), 431–446. doi:10.1016/S0887-6185(97)00021-2 PMID:9276786

World Federation of Mental Health (WFMH). (2010). *Caring for the caregiver: Why your mental health matters when you are caring for others*. Woodbridge, VA: WFMH.

World Health Organization. (1999). *The 'Newly Defined' Burden of Mental Problems. Fact Sheet No. 217*. Geneva: World Health Organization.

Zarit, S. H., Reever, K. E., & Bach-Peterson, J. (1980). Relatives of the impaired elderly: Correlates of feelings of burden. *The Gerontologist*, *20*(6), 649–655. doi:10.1093/geront/20.6.649 PMID:7203086

KEY TERMS AND DEFINITIONS

Accommodation: Any type of familial response that is significantly related to obsessive compulsive symptomatology.

Burnout: A type of psychological stress. Caregiver burnout is a state of physical, emotional and mental exhaustion that may be accompanied by a change in attitude, from positive and caring to negative and unconcerned.

Coping: Expending conscious effort to solve personal and interpersonal problems, and seeking to master, minimize or tolerate stress or conflict.

Criticism: The expression of disapproval of someone or something on the basis of perceived faults or mistakes.

Expressed Emotions: The critical, hostile, and emotionally over-involved attitude that relatives have toward a family member with a disorder.

Hostility: Seen as form of emotionally charged angry behavior. In everyday speech it is more commonly used as a synonym for anger and aggression.

Objective Burden: It relates to the patient's symptoms, behavior, and socio demographic characteristics, and factors such as changes in household routine, family or social relations, work, leisure time, and physical health.

Over Involvement: An excessive or unusually great involvement.

Proxy Compulsions: Asking others to carry out compulsions on behalf of the patient.

Psychoeducation: The education offered to individuals with a mental health condition and their families to help empower them and deal with their condition in an optimal way.

Psychological Intervention: Actions performed to bring about change in people.

Subjective Burden: The mental health and subjective distress among family members.

Chapter 8
Predictors of Expressed Emotion, Caregiver's Burden, and Quality of Life in Chronic Mental Illness

Pratima Kaushik
Amity University, India

Tej Bahadur Singh
Central University of South Bihar (CUSB), India

ABSTRACT

In the present study we intend to assess if the expressed emotion perceived by the patients with schizophrenia and bipolar disorder has any effect on their quality of life. Is the burden experienced by the caregivers, has any effect up on their quality of life? To explore these issues, regression was employed to estimate the quantitative effect of the causal variables upon the variable that they influence and the "statistical significance" of the estimated relationships. This study consisted of 120 participants. 30 patients with Schizophrenia Bipolar disorder and two caregiver groups. Administration of tests was done on individual basis. FEICS was administered to assess EE perceived by the patients. WHOQOL (BREF) scale was used to assess quality of life of patients. BAS was given to assess caregiver's burden. For the assessment of data regression analysis was calculated.

INTRODUCTION

Families play important role in supporting people with long-term mental illness such as schizophrenia, and bipolar affective disorder are severe and disabling. The caregiving role is often not without difficulties, and is associated with considerable personal costs. In schizophrenia and bipolar affective disorder, many family members experience significant stress and subjective burden as a consequence of their caregiving roles. Not only is such stress affects the well-being of the relatives and compromise their long-term ability to support the patient, but it may also have an impact on the course of the illness

DOI: 10.4018/978-1-5225-0519-8.ch008

itself and on outcomes for the patient. Although the symptoms of schizophrenia and bipolar disorder may be controlled by medication, the course of illness is often marked by relapses or exacerbations of these phenomena. There are also long-term impairments in functioning which includes under activity, lethargy, poor motivation, general mental slowing, cognitive deficits, restricted emotions, or elation, and marked interpersonal difficulties. Due to a wide-range of problems, the illness makes considerable emotional, practical and financial demands on those who are close to the sufferer- typically the parents or the spouse or siblings. These demands are likely to persist over long, and advice, help and support may not be readily available.

This chapter aims to examine the predictors of expressed emotion, caregiver's burden and quality of life with schizophrenia and bipolar affective disorder and their caregivers. For better understanding detailed explanation of these constructs is done below.

EXPRESSED EMOTION

Expressed emotion is a reliable psychosocial predictor of relapse in the patients with various psychiatric disorders. It is described as the extent to which one expresses critical, hostile, and over-involved attitudes about the patient. Positive aspects of the expressed emotion may also be measured in the form of positive remarks, and warmth. However, it is the dimensions of criticism, hostility and emotional over involvement that is used to determine high and low levels of expressed emotion across cultures. Brown, Morick, Carstairs, & Wing (1962) attempted to look into the dimensions of expressed emotion:

1. Critical comments,
2. Hostility,
3. Emotional over involvement,
4. Emotional warmth, and
5. Positive remarks.

These dimensions are overlapping in nature. The above factors have been explained as follows: *Critical Comments* refers to the fault finding attitude in a particular relative towards the patient that is reflected consistently while talking about the patient. *Hostility* is defined as the generalization of the criticism i.e., criticizing the person on the account of his illness and blaming him for the disorder or rejection of the patient as a person or a combination of generalization and rejection. *Emotional over Involvement* (EOI) involves exaggerated emotional responses, usually self- sacrificing and devoted behavior, over protection that is inappropriate considering the patient's age and inability to maintain a boundary between the subject's existence and the patient's. *Warmth* refers not to the general quality in the respondent's personality, but to an emotion expressed specifically about the patient. *Positive Remark* is a statement which expresses praise, approval or appreciation of the behavior or personality of the patient.

Levels

There are three levels of expressed emotion. Description of these is mentioned below:

- **High Expressed Emotion:** Those who are decided to have high expressed emotion are very critical and hostile. They do not know other ways to help and support the ill family member. They feel that the illness is internal and can be controlled by the person will change his/ her behavior is through criticism which actually causes the relapse (Miklowitz, Goldstein, Nuechterlein, & Synder, 1998).
- **Low Expressed Emotion:** Low expressed emotion relatives are more conservative with their criticism. The family is more accepting of the disorder than those of high expressed emotion.
- **Perceived Expressed Emotion:** Another way to measure the amount of expressed emotion that is prevalent in a household is the one that involves measuring expressed emotion from the *point of view of the patient.*

Several studies have pointed out to the significance of family environmental stress for depressive, disorders in youth, with studies indicating that family stress in associated with poorer outcome (McCauley et al., 1993) and poor response to treatment (Birmaher et al., 2000). Patients living within high expressed emotion have environments may be at risk for relapse only if they are aware of the relative's critical behavior (Hooley, 1986). Patients' and relatives' appraisals of loss were strongly correlated, particularly high emotional over involvement relationships. Longer duration of untreated psychosis was associated with high critical comments (Peatterson, Birchwood, & Cochrane, 2005). The Schizophrenia and Bipolar patients are considered as having poor relationship with everyone including family members. In a naturalistic study Kim and Miklowitz (2004) reported that levels of expressed emotion in relatives are consistent predictors of relapse among bipolar and other mood disordered patients.

Gomez-de-Regil, Kwapil, and Barrantes-Vidal, (2014) studied relatives' self-report on expressed emotion, burden, quality of life, psychological distress and illness perception. Patients' functional status and relatives' psychological distress were significantly associated with expressed emotion, burden and quality of life. Patients' clinical status and relatives' illness perception were most strongly related to expressed emotion and burden. Relatives' psychological distress and illness perception dimensions predicted both burden and quality of life, over and above patients' clinical and functional status. Results underscore the relatives' need of support to overcome their own distress and concerns about the illness, for the psychological well-being of both patients and relatives.

QUALITY OF LIFE

In the scientific literature, the term quality of life refers to psychological well- being, social and emotional functioning, functional performance, life satisfaction, social support etc. The study of quality of life and the focus on patient's subjective sense of well- being is a fairly new phenomenon that has attracted professional attention only within the past two decades. The concept of life quality has long been considered an important aspect of mental health because of increasing awareness of the multidimensionality of the treatment outcome and the importance of patient satisfaction in health care, especially the interest in quality of life in psychiatry has been stimulated by the deinstitutionalization of psychiatric patients as well as a parallel interest in understanding the scope of their daily lives. Quality of life of persons with severe mental illness would be substantial and sustained due to its negative impact on the illness. Studies also showed that individuals with severe mental illness living in long term institutional set up had poorer quality of life than those living in the community (Hasson, Ofayon, Karvetz, & Roe, 2006). Mental illness in the home can affect not only the quality of family life but also the health of the family members. The marital relationship may suffer. Family patterns and responsibilities get altered and may be highly constrained by the sick member. Subjective quality of life in people with severe mental illness is only to a lesser extent related to external life conditions. Major determinants are psychopathology, especially symptoms of depression and anxiety, and aspects of social network (Ritsner et al., 2003; Young, 2004).

Many researchers attempted to study poor quality of life in severe mental illness like schizophrenia and bipolar disorder, despite significant improvement with pharmacological treatment (Solanki, Singh, Midha, & Chugh, 2008). An investigation revealed that depressive mood and uncooperativeness were negatively influence self-esteem (Kunikata, Mino, & Nakajima, 2005; Brissos, Balanza-Martinez, Dias, Carit, & Figueira, 2011). Greater symptom severity and worse insight were significantly associated with worse functioning in all QOL domains. Symptom severity may exert a greater influence on social functioning than on subjective quality of life. The cyclical nature of bipolar disorder, with its many remissions and symptom rich periods of exacerbation, affects an individual's physical, emotional, social and functional well-being and significantly impact their overall quality of life (Vojta, Kinosian,Glick, Altshuler, & Bauer, 2001). Patients with chronic mental illness and their caregivers described a wide variety of factors that influenced quality of life, including the adverse effects of medication, occupation, level of education, physical functioning, environment, health care factors, leisure activities, routine and sexuality. They show significant functional impairment, often has a negative impact on the performance of work related, leisure, and interpersonal activities (Calabrese, Hirschfeld, & Reed, 2003).

Numerous studies on the correlates and predictors of quality of life in Schizophrenia and Bipolar patients have been performed. The psychopathological symptoms especially negative and general psychopathology (Addington, Coldham, Jones, & Addington, 2003; Brown, Clarke, & Gervin, 2000; Priebe et al., 2006) duration of untreated psychosis (DUP), pre-morbid social adjustment (Brown et al., 2000), social support and demographic variables (age, gender) negatively affect quality of life. The subjective quality of life of Schizophrenia patients is described as associated with depression, anxiety, negative, and rarely positive symptoms (Bechdolf et al., 2003; Sim, Mahendram, Siris, Heckers, & Chong, 2004). Other studies have related to the role of social support (Caron, Mercier, Diaz, & Martin, 2005), stress related factors (Ritsner et al., 2003; Bechdolf et al., 2003; Sierra, Livianos, & Rojo, 2005). A study done by Awad and Voruganti (2007) suggested that misdiagnosis in associated with poorer quality of life than major depressive disorder or diagnosed bipolar disorder, which are recognized as having a considerable impact on quality of life. In a naturalistic longitudinal study Ritsner et al. (2003) determined predictors of perceived quality of life and explored changes that occurred regarding quality of life among Schizophrenias and Bipolar patients.

Long-Term caregiving has been found to be associated with a variety of negative outcomes. Caregivers, who are women, and those who are spouse, have higher rates of psychological morbidity, perhaps because of the increased stresses inherent in being married to a person with schizophrenia or bipolar disorder (Jungburer, Mory, & Angermeyer, 2004; Angermeyer, Kilian, Wilms, & Wittmund, 2006). Caregivers who cohabitate are more likely to be depressed or psychologically stressed than those living apart (Awadalla, Ohaeri, Salih, & Tawfiq, 2005). The stress spouses are exposed to during acute episodes of illness, spouses also experience chronic burdens in their everyday life which can severely affect their living situation and well-being: insecurity and ambivalence in the relationship with the patient, changes regarding intimacy and familiarity, shifts in role distribution, lack of opportunity for relaxing activities, sorrow and fears regarding the further course of the illness, impairment of health and financial strains (Jungbauer & Angermeyer, 2004).

Caregivers of schizophrenia group reported higher burden than care givers of affective disorder followed by mental retardation. Overall, caregivers reported high burden and significantly reduced quality of life in the domains of physical health, social relationships and environment. In particular, schizophrenia group of caregivers reported higher levels of burden and reduced quality of life in psychological and environmental domains (Narasipuram & Kasimahanti, 2012).

CAREGIVER'S BURDEN

Families have been the mainstay of caregiving for persons with mental illnesses. The caregivers take care of the day-to-day needs of the patients, monitoring the mental state, identify the early signs of illness, relapse and deterioration, and help the patient in accessing services. They also supervise treatment and provide emotional support to the patient. Caregivers bear with the behavioral disturbances of the ill family members and sometimes can also be a target of the patient's abusive or violent behavior. They have to curtail on their social and leisure activities, and sometimes have to take leave from their jobs. In addition, they have to meet the financial needs of the ill member besides meeting the treatment costs. The continuous stress of caregiving may adversely affect the physical and mental health of the caregivers (Chadda, 2014). This is the reason why Caregiver's Burden has occupied a prominent position. It is the area of great concern for the professionals because of the fact that it influences/affects the treatment as well as outcome of any treatment program. The existence of a burden indicates the breakdown of reciprocal arrangements that people maintain in their relationships. Thus, one person ends up doing more than his fair share of work. This may result in taking on a greater proportion or number of shared tasks, but it may also restrict their activities outside the relationship. This change in pattern, when assessed against approximate norms, gives a fair idea of the burden experienced. Hoeing and Hamilton (1969) made a distinction between two types of burden: 'objective and subjective burden'. If the burden experienced by the subject internally and sometimes it is not reflected in the activities and behavior. It is the '*subjective burden*' of a member of the household in relation to a particular problem behavior. While '*objective burden*' is reflected by the behavior and activities of the caregivers. Authors further subdivide objective burden into two categories:

Type 1: This consisted of certain specific effects on the life or the household. This was grouped under 4 main areas, namely:

1. Financial effects on the household;
2. Effects on the health of any member of the household;
3. Effects on children;
4. Effects on family routine.

Type 2: Objective burden was based on the occurrence of certain abnormal behavioral traits in the patient (e.g., danger to self and others) which could be assumed to cause distress.

Burdensome events reported by several caregivers included perception of patients as danger to themselves or others and problems frequently arose with neighbors as a result of the patients' behavior. Many relatives complained of disturbed nights, and reported that practical problems caused fewer difficulties than the patient's strange fancies or dumb apathy. The burden on families' ranges from economic difficulties to emotional reaction to the illness, the stress of coping with disturbed behavior, the disruption of household routine and the restriction of social activities (WHO, 2001). The families of chronic mentally ill patients are required not only to provide physical and emotional support, but also to bear the negative impact of stigma and discrimination. Narendra, Bhattacharjee, Nishant, Sanjay, and Nizamie, (2011) suggested that caregivers of adolescents with chronic mental illness experienced higher level of burden of care, and less social support from their respective social networks. Several studies examined the role of gender, and reported that relatives of male patients with schizophrenia frequently experience more social dysfunction and disabilities than those of female patients (Awad & Voruganti, 2008).

The chronic burdens of everyday living can profoundly reduce the quality of life and the subject's satisfaction with the partnership (Singh, Verma,Verma, & Chaudhary, 2009). Caregiver burden is associated with depression, which affects patient recovery by adding stress to the living environment. Sub-syndromal depressive symptoms are common in this phase of the illness, resulting in severe and widespread impairment of function (Ogilive, Morant, & Goodwin, 2005; Davenport, 2008). The onset of bipolar disorder in an adult child presents potentially lifelong care giving challenges for the parents. Parents may provide decades of extended care giving challenges for the adult son or daughter who is suffering from bipolar disorder when debiting symptoms produce ongoing obstacles to social and occupational functioning and independent living. This chronic care giving role may cause stress for parents and threaten their physical and mental health. Due to the cyclical nature of bipolar disorder, parents of adult children with bipolar disorder show a wear and tear affect over time (Aschbrenner, Greenberg, & Seltzer, 2008). Caring for a relative with bipolar disorder is associated with reports of high caregiver burden, symptoms of depression, poor physical health, negligence of the caregiver's own health needs, elevated health service use, low use of social supports, and financial strain. High burden caregivers reported more physical health problems, depressive symptoms, health risk behavior and health service use, and less social support than less burdened caregivers. They also provided more financial support to their bipolar relative (Perlick et al., 2008). Studies have also revealed violent behavior in acute mania and suicide threats or attempts in depressive episodes as the most troubling characteristics of illness. Patients listed poor judgment in mania and hopelessness and poor concentration in depression as the troubling characteristics of illness causes considerable burden among caregivers The most frequently experienced psychological problems were relationship problems, including interpersonal conflicts with family & friends, marital difficulties, job & school related problems, physical health problems and alcohol and substance abuse (Hirshfeld, Lewis, & Vornik, 2003).

Most of the caregivers show a highest level of subjective burden in the area of patient's behavior such as hyperactivity, irritability, sadness and withdrawal. Regarding the patient's role performance, the most worrying aspects were those associated with the patient's work or study and social relationships. Most key relatives of Schizophrenia and Bipolar patients frequently report emotional, social, physical and financial burden associated with caring process of their patients. Numerous studies have explored the existence of burden among primary caregivers and family members of Schizophrenia patients. Burden of care in schizophrenia correlates with patients' illness variables (Dyck, Short & Vitaliano, 1999), availability of caregiver's recourses as well as coping skills (Magliano, Fiorillo, De Rosa, Malangone, & Maj, 2005). Burden was significantly associated with several psychosocial resources and dispositions of the relatives. Multivariate linear regression analysis indicated that expressed emotion, emotion-focused coping strategies and generalized negative stress response are the most relevant predictors of burden (Moller- Leimkuhler, 2008).

Previous research suggests that certain patient factors may increase family burden. These factors include the severity of patient's symptoms, length of time in the hospital, number of hospitalizations, the length of time the patient has been ill, and the level of social functioning (Magliano et al., 2005). Symptom type (positive or negative symptoms) has also received attention as a factor related to family burden, although studies have yielded equivocal results. Social support, age and education level are also related to level of burden (Magliano et al., 1998). Research suggests that level of burden is reduced when family members have a more positive attitude toward the patient, when there is an increase in social support and fewer hospitalizations as well as improved social functioning for the patient (Magliano et al., 2003; Saunders, 2003; Zergaw, Hailemariam, Alem, & Kebede, 2008; Heru & Rayan, 2008). Spouses of persons with mental disorder show lower subjective well-being and increased symptoms of anxiety and depression compared to spouses of index persons without mental disorder (Idstad, Ask, & Tambs,, 2010; Grandón, Jenaro, & Lemos, 2008). Swapna et al. (2012) mentioned that caregivers of bipolar disorder and alcohol dependence experienced high level of burden. In bipolar disorder patients burden was experienced during the episode. The burden and the quality of life are worse for caregivers who care for patients with both physical and mental diseases. The sons and daughters, differently from the parents, experience greater burden of required time and a lower quality of life (Kate, Grover, Kulhara, & Nehra, 2013; Salvatore et al., 2014). In general, it is the poor functioning of the patient due to symptoms, which leads to more severe burden.

The aim of the present study was to understand how actually the construct of expressed emotion and caregivers' burden operate in different demographic conditions are determining relapse and poor quality of life. The present study was designed mainly to assess the burden on the families of a particular group of patients namely those with schizophrenia and bipolar disorder. Moreover, this is also a dearth of studies delineating the association of expressed emotion and burden of care and its effect on quality of life with the nature and severity of psychopathology in India. Therefore focusing on these issues, the present study has been designed as an attempt to develop meaningful insight into what and how the constructs of caregiver's burden, expressed emotion and quality of life operate in Indian context thereby influencing the course of schizophrenia and bipolar affective disorder.

The objectives of the present research were to:

1. Study the construct of expressed emotion, quality of life, and caregiver burden in relation to chronic mental illness,
2. Examine the relationship expressed emotion and burden experienced by their caregivers of schizophrenia and bipolar disorder,
3. Analyze the relationship of expressed emotion and quality of life among schizophrenia and bipolar patients,
4. Elucidate upon caregivers' overall burden and their quality of life,
5. Assess quality of life of married caregivers and burden experienced by them.

The study was intended to assess if the expressed emotion perceived by the patients with schizophrenia and bipolar disorder has any effect on their quality of life. Is the burden experienced by the caregivers, due to tiresome and unending duty to care patients, has any effect up on their quality of life? To explore these issues, regression was employed to estimate the quantitative effect of the causal variables upon the variable that they influence and the "statistical significance" of the estimated relationships.

METHODS

This study consisted of 120 participants from Psychiatry OPD, GTB hospital, Dilshad Garden, Delhi, India. Two patients group i.e. 30 patients with Schizophrenia and 30 patients with Bipolar disorder and two caregiver groups i.e. 30 caregivers working with Schizophrenia and 30 caregivers working with Bipolar disorder. Patients who are fulfilling ICD-10 criterion for definite diagnosis of schizophrenia and bipolar affective disorder and patient were diagnosed by a senior psychiatrist. Age range included was between 15-45 years. Patients had minimum primary education and patients of both genders were included. Patients were without any co-morbid medical and psychological illness. Patients with organicity (such as delirium, dementia, substance abuse, amnesic syndrome, epilepsy, head injury, etc.) were not included in the study. Caregivers were first-degree caregivers, who have spent two years of minimum time with patient. Caregiver's had minimum education of primary level. Spouse as a caregiver, were included in the study. Caregivers who are suffering from physical illness and second and third degree relatives were not included in the study.

The socio- demographic conditions of schizophrenic and bipolar affective patients is as followed: Average age of the patients ranged between 24- 35 years. 63% of patients were male and 36.6% of patients were female in bipolar patients and schizophrenics respectively. 70% of patients with schizophrenia and bipolar disorder were form urban locality. 60% of the patients were married, 35% were unmarried and 5% of the patients were divorced. 63.3% of the schizophrenics were married, 30% were unmarried and 6.6% were divorced, on the other hand, 56.6% of bipolar patients were married, 40% were unmarried and 3.3% of divorced. Average educational status ranged from 9th -12th. 36.6% of the patients were employed while, 63.3% were unemployed. On an average they earned Rs. 6000- Rs. 15000. Illness experience ranged from 2-10 years in bipolar patients was 56.6% and in schizophrenics it was 73.3%.

The socio-demographic details of primary caregivers of schizophrenics and bipolar affective patients suggested: Average age of the caregivers ranged from 25-50 years in both the groups. 58.3% of total caregivers were male, while remaining 41.6% were female. Educational status of the caregivers of both the group ranged from 9th-12th grade. While discussing occupational status of the caregivers, 35% of them were working at government sector, while 31.6% of the caregivers are housewife, 15% of them have their own business. 40% of caregivers do not earn anything. 51.6% get income of Rs. 3000- 15,000. All the caregivers were staying with the patients and had daily contact with them.

Administration of tests was done on individual basis. FEICS was administered to assess Expressed Emotion perceived by the patients. WHOQOL (BREF) scale was used to assess quality of life of patients and their caregivers. BAS was given to assess caregiver's burden. Brief description of tools is mentioned below:

- **Burden Assessment Schedule (BAS):** By (Thara, Padmavati, Kumar, & Srinivasan, 1998): It attempts to assess objective and subjective burden of primary caregiver of chronic mentally ill patients on five factors namely; impact on well-being; on marital relationship, on relationship with others; appreciation for caring; and perceived severity of the disease, on 3-point scale. The validity has been established by comparing it with family Burden Schedule of Pai and Kapur (1981).
- **Family Emotional Over Involvement and Criticism Scale (FEICS):** By (Shields, Franks, Harp, Campbell, & McDaniel, 1992): This test is a measure of subjective expressed emotion from the perspective of the patient. This is a 14 items, 5-point rating scale measuring the two factors analogues to the components of expressed emotion 'Perceived Criticism' and 'Intensity of Emotional Over involvement'.

Table 1. Regression analysis to determine the association between the expressed emotion score perceived by patients on FEICS and patient's quality of life on WHOQOL (BREF)

Patient Group	Dependent Variables	Physical Health	Psychological Health	Social Relationships	Environment	R Square (F-Ratio)
	Independent Variables	β coeff (t-Value)	β coeff (t-Value)	β coeff (t-Value)	β coeff (t-Value)	
BPAD	EOI	-0.3 (1.01)	-0.63 (2.05)*	0.4 (1.7)	0.8 (3.28)*	0.34 (3.35, df=4)
	CC	-0.01 (0.05)	0.2 (0.04)	0.2 (0.6)	-0.3 (1.07)	0.07 (0.5, df=4)
SCHIZ	EOI	0.63 (3.01)*	-0.3 (1.34)	-0.1 (0.46)	0.4 (1.6)	0.4 (4.01, df=4)
	CC	-0.43 (2.05)*	0.03 (0.13)	0.15 (0.7)	-0.42 (1.9)	0.4 (3.9, df= 4)**

BPAD- Bipolar Affective Disorder, SCHIZ- Schizophrenia, EOI- Emotional Over Involvement, CC- Critical Comments, (**)- significant at 0.01 level, (*)- Significant at 0.05 level

- **World Health Organization Quality of Life Scale BREF (WHO-QOL-BREF, Orley et al., 1998):** It is a 26 item self-administered generic questionnaire and a shorter version of the WHO-QOL-100 item scale (WHO-QOL Group, 1998). It covers four domains namely: physical health, psychological health, social relationship and environment.

Unstructured open-ended interview was conducted in clinical setting. Written consent was taken followed by questionnaire was assessed and results were analyzed with suitable statistics.

RESULTS

In the study authors intend to assess if the expressed emotion perceived by the patients with schizophrenia and bipolar disorder has any effect on their quality of life? Is the burden experienced by the caregivers, due to tiresome and unending duty to care patients, has any effect up on their quality of life? To explore these issues, regression was employed to estimate the quantitative effect of the causal variables upon the variable that they influence and the "statistical significance" of the estimated relationships.

Multiple linear regression analysis was conducted to estimate the association between expressed emotion perceived by the patients and their quality of life. In Table 1 show expressed emotion dimensions, emotional over- involvement (EOI) and critical comments (CC) were independent variables and quality of life domains, physical health; psychological health, social relationships, and environment were dependent variables. The two patient groups were bipolar affective disorder (BPAD), and schizophrenia (SCHIZ).

Association between Expressed Emotion and Quality of Life of Patients

Emotional over-involvement perceived by bipolar patients was significantly negatively associated with psychological health (β coeff= -0.63, t-value= 2.05, significant at 0.05 level), and significantly positively associated with environment domain of quality of life (β coeff= -0.8, t-value= 3.28, significant at 0.01 level). Thus, suggesting that high critical comment predicts low quality of life of bipolar patients.

Emotional over-involvement perceived by the Schizophrenia patients is significantly positively associated with physical health (β coeff= 0.63, t-value= 3.01, significant at 0.05 level), suggesting that it is moderately associated with physical health domain of quality of life. Similarly critical comments perceived by the Schizophrenia patients is significantly negatively associated with physical health (β coeff= -0.43, t-value= 2.05, significant at 0.05 level), suggests that it is moderately associated with physical health domain of quality of life. Critical comment perceived by Schizophrenia patients is also negatively associated with environment domain of quality of life at moderate level.

Previous studies suggest that psychological and social rather than psychopathology predict perceived quality of life of patient with severe mental illness including bipolar disorder and schizophrenia. Results of multiple regression analysis confirmed this assumption: for both groups of patients, changes in psychological and social factors contributed substantially more in long-term changes in perceived quality of life when compared to psychopathology. These findings are consistent with cross- sectional results (Ritsne & Endcott, 2000). The fact that psychological and social factors have stronger predictive value as compared with psychopathologic factors does not seem to actually be paradoxical since psychological and social factors and psychopathology present two different realities that coexist within the mentally ill individual: internal (psychological) as well as external (clinical) worlds (Ritsner, & Ponizovsky, 2002). The psychological reality expressing the subjective experience of disease or suffering may be accessible only through patient self-report (primary factors), while clinical reality is presented through psychopathologic symptoms that can be ascertained by clinician observation of behavior and interview using observer- based scales (secondary factors). Primary factors are closet to the individual and determine his or her perception of quality of life and health status. Therefore, it is suggested that secondary clinical factors influence subjective QOL via primary psychological factors.

Association between Expressed Emotion Perceived by Patients and Burden Experienced by Their Caregivers

Several studies suggest that expressed emotion originates from family members and that they have ingrained negative behaviors that place stress on the relative with mental illness, subsequently precipitating relapse (Leff & Vaughn, 1985).

Table 2. Regression analysis to determine the association between the expressed emotion score perceived by patients on FEICS and caregiver's experience of burden on BAS

Patient Groups	BPAD		Schiz	
Dependent Variable	EOI	CC	EOI	CC
Independent Variable	β coeff (t-Value)	β coeff (t-Value)	β coeff (t-Value)	β coeff (t-Value)
Appreciation of caregiving	-0.3 (1.4)	0.34 (2.08)*	-0.3 (0.75)	0.09 (0.31)
R square (F- ratio)	0.15 (1.18,df=4)	0.42 (4.5**,df=4)	0.23 (1.84, df= 4)	0.4 (3.85**,df=4)

BPAD- Bipolar Affective Disorder, SCHIZ- Schizophrenia, EOI- Emotional Over Involvement, CC- Critical Comments, (**)- significant at 0.01 level, (*)- Significant at 0.05 level

Multiple linear regression analysis was conducted to estimate the association between expressed emotion perceived by the patients and burden experienced by their caregivers. In Table 2 show expressed emotion dimensions, emotional over- involvement (EOI) and critical comments (CC) were dependent variables and factors of burden, impact on general well-being, appreciation of caregiving, impact on relation with others and perceived severity of illness were independent variables. The two patient groups were bipolar affective disorder (BPAD), and schizophrenia (SCHIZ) and their respective caregivers.

Critical comments perceived by bipolar patients were positively significantly associated with appreciation of caregiving (β coeff= 0.34, t-value= 2.08, significant at 0.05 level) suggesting that critical comments perceived by bipolar patients is moderately associated with appreciation of caregiving factor of burden experienced by their caregivers. Emotional over-involvement perceived by Schizophrenia patients was strongly positively associated with impact on general well- being and negatively moderately associated with perceived severity of illness. Several researchers have identified factors that adversely influence the experiences of careers – psychological and emotional distress; physical illness; disruption of the family, and social and sexual relationships; curtailment of social activities; and financial hardship. The chronic burden of caregiving to a patient with schizophrenia is likely to generate negative emotions and their expression. Expressed emotion (EE) comprises critical or emotionally over-involved attitudes and behaviors (McGlashan, 1994).

Chakrabarti, Kulahara and Verma (1992); Perlick, Clarkin, and Sirey (1999); Dore and Romans (2001) reported that a high burden level on relatives of bipolar disorder patients which has been reported and recent studies have shown that caregivers' burden may influence the clinical outcome of bipolar disorder (Perlick, Rosenheck, & Clarkin, 2001, 2004; Hooley (1986) suggested that family members are more critical of a mentally ill relative if they believe the individual has control over his or her own behavior. As a result, criticism assumes more of the form of social control and coercion because it is based on the belief that the behavior of the consumer is within his or her control. Scazufca and Kuipers (1996) reported that high expressed emotion relatives of patients with schizophrenia had higher levels of burden of care than low expressed emotion relatives. Furthermore, relatives reporting high burden had more negative perceptions of the patients' functioning than those who reported lower burden and these perceptions were not necessarily related to the patients' actual deficits.

Similarly, variables that previous studies have found to predict burden [symptoms severity, whether the patient lives with the caregiver or caregiver stigma] (Perlick et al., 2001; Perlick, 1999; Gallagher & Mechanic, 1996; Carpentier, 1992; Struening et al., 2001) and critical comments and emotional over involvement [the caregiver's relationship to the patient] (Goldstein, Rea, & Miklowitz, 1996). Schizophrenia patients' perceptions of parental characteristics have been found to predict high expressed emotion and relapse. Parker, Fairley, Greenwood, Jurd, & Silove (1982); Warner & Atkinson (1988) reported that patients who perceived their parents to be low in care (ie, indifferent or rejecting) or high in protection (ie, controlling, intrusive, and infantilizing) had a more severe course of illness compared with patients who rated their parents as high in care and low in protection. According to Warner and Atkinson (1988), low care and high protection is considered analogous to high EE. Kazarian, Malla, Cole, & Baker, (1990) found that relatives rated high EE-criticism were perceived by patients as being more intrusive, having less tolerance, and having higher expectations. (Kanter, Lamb, & Loeper, 1987) asserts that expressed emotion emanates from patient behavior and somatology, which, in turn, prompts relatives to react to patient with negative behavior. While Strachan, Leff, and Goldstein (1986) reported that patient and family member behaviors as part of an essentially interactive process with both parties being integral in generating expressed emotion.

Table 3. Regression analysis to determine the association between the caregiver's quality of life scores on WHOQOL (BREF) and caregiver's experience of overall burden on BAS

Caregiver Group	Independent Variable	Overall Burden		R Square (F- Ratio)
	Dependent Variables	β Coeff	t-Value	
Caregivers of BPAD	Physical health	-0.3	1.63	0.08 (2.7, df=1)
	Psychological health	-0.4	2.32*	0.16 (5.4*,df= 1)
	Environment	-0.21	1.18	0.5 (1.4, df=1)
Caregivers of SCHIZ	Physical health	-0.52	3.26*	0.27 (10.7*,df=1)
	Psychological health	-0.6	3.6**	0.31 (12.57**,df=1)
	Environment	-0.51	3.14**	0.3, (9.9*,df= 1)

BPAD- Bipolar Affective Disorder, SCHIZ- Schizophrenia, (**)- significant at 0.01 level, (*)- Significant at 0.05 level

Association between Caregivers' Overall Burden and Quality of Life

Multiple linear regression analysis was conducted to estimate the association between caregivers' overall burden and their scores on quality of life domains. In Table 3 show quality of life domains, physical health, psychological health, social relationships and environment were dependent variables and overall burden was independent variables. The two groups included caregivers of bipolar affective disorder (BPAD), and Schizophrenia (SCHIZ) patients.

Overall burden experienced by caregivers of bipolar patients was significantly negatively associated with psychological health (β coeff= -0.4, t-value= 2.32, significant at 0.05 level), suggesting that caregiver burden puts its negative effect on their psychological health.

Overall burden experience by caregivers of Schizophrenia patients was significantly negatively associated with physical health (β coeff= -0.52, t-value= 3.26, significant at 0.05 level), it suggests that burden experienced by caregivers puts its negative effect on their physical health. It suggests that burden experienced by caregivers of Schizophrenia patient puts its negative effect on their physical health. Psychological health is also significantly negatively associated with over all burden experienced by Schizophrenia patients (β coeff= -0.6, t-value= 3.6, significant at 0.01 level), suggests that psychological health of caregivers of bipolar patients is negatively affected by the burden experienced by them. Thus, burden experienced by caregivers of Schizophrenia patient puts its negative effect on their psychological health. Overall burden was significantly negatively associated with environment domain of quality of life (β coeff= -0.51, t-value= 3.14, significant at 0.01 level), it suggests that burden experienced by the caregivers of Schizophrenia patients put its negative effect on their perception of environment. It suggests that caregiver's burden puts it negative effect on their environment.

Burden on relatives of patients with schizophrenia has been found associated with an important reduction in their QOL, causing damage in caregiver's health condition (Fadden, Bebbington, & Kuipers, 1987; Kuipers, Leff, & Lam, 1992; Gutiérrez-Maldonado, Caqueo-Urizar, & Kavanagh, 2005; Raune, Kuipers, & Bebbington, 2004) reported that the only significant predictors of caregivers' QOL were caregivers' appreciation of the patients' QOL and caregiver state of health. The salutary effect of the caregiver's positive appreciation of the patient and the caregiving role on subjective burden and QOL has been robustly predicted by the findings from expressed emotion (EE) research.

Caregiver's burden puts it negative effect on their environment. Martens and Addington (2001) observed that family members are significantly stressed as a result of having one of them with schizophrenia. Ivarsson, Sidenvall, and Carlsson (2004) agreed that burden on a family caregiver is complex and includes many areas, such as daily life, worries, and social pressure. In addition, empirical evidence confirms that caring for a patient with schizophrenia generates economic burden on the family.

Caregivers' health was highly deteriorated. Stress problems, anxiety, and depression were observed in several studies (Magliano et al., 1998; Ohaeri, 2001; Jungbaurer et al., 2002; Woldhaus et al., 2002; Lee et al., 2006; Chien, Chan, & Morrissey, 2007; Awadh et al., 2008; Ochoa et al., 2008, Grandon et al., 2008; Hanzawa et al., 2008). Interestingly, Dyck, Short, Vitaliano, (1999) found that caregivers catch infectious diseases. This could have occurred due to deterioration in the caregiver's immune system.

FUTURE RESEARCH DIRECTION

The present study is a cross-sectional assessment, poses limitations as variables such as dysfunction of the patient pose a lot of difficulties in interpretation of results. A longitudinal assessment might have solved some of this problem. Further, a hospital based cross- sectional design neglects a large number of patient and their caregiver non seeking services from the place of the study. The minimum duration of illness has been taken as 2 years mainly to make the same homogenous. This however, leaves out the considerations of burden in acute onset of illness. Study done in the future should this aim to rectify some of the methodological limitations of this study. A large sample of patients, longitudinal assessment of burden and more in-depth analysis of the determinants will certainly be able to answer a lot of questions posed by the study.

CONCLUSION

Family caregivers of persons with mental illnesses are a key support system in our country as well as in most of the nonwestern world. In a country like India where the resources to care for patients with mental illness are limited, family is seen as a significant source of support without knowledge or preparation for caring role. Most caregivers feel burdened when caring for relatives with major psychiatric disorders, as these disorders are unpredictable and long-lasting. In order to keep the patients stable and maintain function, family members need to supervise medication compliance, urge patient self-care and protect them from possible harm. It is evident from the studies that families are affected in a number of ways: family life is disorganized, household routines are upset, and family members face physical and mental health problems. In addition to the impact on the caregivers' lives, an increased care burden has been associated with greater use of health services, psychotropic drugs and higher expressed emotion toward the patients, which may eventually lead to patient relapse. Not only caregivers but the patients with schizophrenia and bipolar disorder report disturbed quality of life. Due to long lasting illness, patients complain about difficulties in their physical health, social relationships and other environmental factors. In the absence of adequate mental health infrastructure, the family caregivers take multiple roles at providing care for persons with mental illnesses. The family caregivers suffer substantial burden as a result of the caregiving role and need help from the mental health professionals. It is very important for the mental health professionals to identify the needs of the family caregivers, the stresses faced by them and introduce suitable interventions, so as to reduce the burden as well as help in developing healthy coping strategies.

REFERENCES

Addington, J., Coldham, E. L., Jones, T., & Addington, K. D. (2003). The first episode of psychosis: The experience of relatives. *Acta Psychiatrica Scandinavica*, *108*(4), 285–289. doi:10.1034/j.1600-0447.2003.00153.x PMID:12956829

Angermeyer, M. C., Kilian, R., Wilms, H. U., & Wittmund, B. (2006). Quality of life of spouses of mentally ill people. *The International Journal of Social Psychiatry*, *52*(3), 278–285. doi:10.1177/0020764006067186 PMID:16875199

Aschbrenner, A.K., Greenberg, J.S., & Seltzer, M. M. (2008). The long- term impact of parenting and adult child with bipolar disorder. *Research that Matters,* 17-20.

Awad, G., & Voruganti, L. (2008). The Burden of Schizophrenia on Caregivers. *PharmacoEconomics*, *26*(2), 149–162. doi:10.2165/00019053-200826020-00005 PMID:18198934

Awadalla, W. A., Ohaeri, J. U., Salih, A. A., & Tawfiq, A. M. (2005). Subjective quality of life of family caregivers of community living Sudanese psychiatric patients. *Social Psychiatry Epidemiology*, *40*(9), 755–763. doi:10.1007/s00127-005-0947-x PMID:16151598

Bechdolf, A., Maier, S., Knost, B., & Wagner, M. (2003). A psychological early intervention program for the prepsychotic prodromal state. A case report. *Der Nervenarzt*, *74*, 436–439. doi:10.1007/s00115-002-1322-3 PMID:12966818

Birmaher, B., Brent, D. A., Kolko, D., Baugher, M., Bridge, J., Holder, D., & Ulloa, R. E. et al. (2000). Clinical outcome after short term psychotherapy for adolescents with major depressive disorder. *Archives of General Psychiatry*, *57*(1), 29–86. doi:10.1001/archpsyc.57.1.29 PMID:10632230

Brissos, S., Balanzá-Martinez, V., Dias, V. V., Carita, A. I., & Figueira, M. L. (2011). Is personal and social functioning associated with subjective quality of life in schizophrenia patients living in the community? *European Archives of Psychiatry and Clinical Neuroscience*, *261*(7), 509–517. doi:10.1007/s00406-011-0200-z PMID:21384166

Browne, G. M., Morick, E., Carstairs, G., & Wing, J. (1962). Influence of family life on the course of Schizophrenia illness. *British Journal of Preventive & Social Medicine*, *16*, 55–68.

Browne, S., Clarke, M., & Gervin, M. (2000). Determinants of quality of life at first presentation with schizophrenia. *The British Journal of Psychiatry*, *176*(2), 173–176. doi:10.1192/bjp.176.2.173 PMID:10755056

Calabrese, J. R., Hirschfeld, R. M., Reed, M., Davies, M. A., Frye, M. A., Keck, P. E. Jr, & Wagner, K. D. et al. (2003). Impact of bipolar disorder on a U.S. community sample. *The Journal of Clinical Psychiatry*, *64*(4), 425–432. doi:10.4088/JCP.v64n0412 PMID:12716245

Caron, J., Mercier, C., Diaz, P., & Martin, A. (2005). Socio-demographic and clinical predictors of quality of life in patients with schizophrenia or schizo-affective disorder. *Psychiatry Research*, *137*(3), 203–213. doi:10.1016/j.psychres.2005.07.002 PMID:16298428

Carpentier, N., Lesage, A., & Goulet, J. (1992). Burden of care of families not living with young Schizophrenia relatives. *Hospital & Community Psychiatry*, *43*, 38–43. PMID:1544645

Chadda, R. K. (2014). Caring for the family caregivers of persons with mental illness. *Indian Journal of Psychiatry*, *56*(3), 221–227. doi:10.4103/0019-5545.140616 PMID:25316932

Chadda, R. K., Singh, T. B., & Ganguly, K. K. (2007). Caregiver burden and coping: A prospective study of relationship between burden and coping in caregivers of patients with schizophrenia and bipolar affective disorder. *Social Psychiatry and Psychiatric Epidemiology*, *42*(11), 923–930. doi:10.1007/s00127-007-0242-8 PMID:17700975

Chakraborty, S., Kulahara, P., & Verma, S. K. (1992). Extent and determinants of burden among families of patients with affective disorders. *Acta Psychiatrica Scandinavica*, *86*(3), 247–252. doi:10.1111/j.1600-0447.1992.tb03261.x PMID:1414422

Chien, W. T., Chan, S. W., & Morrissey, J. (2007). The perceived burden among Chinese family caregivers of people with schizophrenia. *Journal of Clinical Nursing*, *16*(6), 1151–1161. doi:10.1111/j.1365-2702.2007.01501.x PMID:17518890

Davenport, L. (2008). Patient depression predicts bipolar disorder caregiver burden. *Acta Psychiatrica Scandinavica*, *118*, 49–56. doi:10.1111/j.1600-0447.2008.01201.x PMID:18582347

Davenport, L. (2008). Quality of life reduced in euphoric bipolar disorder. *Perspectives in Psychiatric Care*, *44*, 275–284. PMID:18826466

Dore, G., & Romans, S. E. (2001). Impact of bipolar affective disorder on family and partners. *Journal of Affective Disorders*, *67*(1-3), 147–158. doi:10.1016/S0165-0327(01)00450-5 PMID:11869762

Dyck, D. G., Short, R., & Vitaliano, P. P. (1999). Predictors of burden and infectious illness in schizophrenia caregivers. *Psychosomatic Medicine*, *61*(4), 411–419. doi:10.1097/00006842-199907000-00001 PMID:10443748

Fadden, G., Bebbington, P., & Kuipers, L. (1987). The burden of care: The impact of functional psychiatric illness on the patient's family. *The British Journal of Psychiatry*, *150*(3), 285–292. doi:10.1192/bjp.150.3.285 PMID:3311267

Gallagher, S. K., & Mechanic, D. (1996). Living with the mentally ill: Effects on the health and functioning of other members. *Social Science & Medicine*, *42*(12), 1691–1701. doi:10.1016/0277-9536(95)00296-0 PMID:8783431

George, & Lakshmi. (2007). The burden of schizophrenia on caregivers: A review. *PharmacoEconomics*, *26*, 149–162. PMID:18198934

Goldstein, M. J., Rea, M., & Miklowitz, D. J. (1996). Family factors related to the course and outcome of bipolar disorder. In M. J. Mundt, K. Goldstein, & K. Hahlweg et al. (Eds.), *Interpersonal Factors in the Origin and Courses of Affective Disorder*. Washington, DC: American Psychiatric Press.

Gómez-de-Regil, L., Kwapil, T. R., & Barrantes-Vidal, N. (2014). Predictors of expressed emotion, burden and quality of life in relatives of Mexican patients with psychosis. *Journal of Psychiatric and Mental Health Nursing*, *21*(2), 170–179. doi:10.1111/jpm.12071 PMID:23551489

Grandon, P., Jenaro, C., & Lemos, S. (2008). Primary caregivers of schizophrenia outpatients: Burden and predictor variables. *Psychiatry Research*, *158*(3), 335–343. doi:10.1016/j.psychres.2006.12.013 PMID:18280584

Gutierrez-Maldonado, J., Caqueo-Urizar, A., & Kavanagh, D. J. (2005). Burden of care and general health in families of patients with schizophrenia. *Social Psychiatry and Psychiatric Epidemiology*, *40*(11), 899–904. doi:10.1007/s00127-005-0963-5 PMID:16245190

Hanzawa, S., Tanaka, G., Inadomi, H., Urata, M., & Ohta, Y. (2008). Burden and doping strategies in mothers of patients with schizophrenia in Japan. *Psychiatry Journal of Clinical Neurosciences*, *62*(3), 256–263. doi:10.1111/j.1440-1819.2008.01791.x PMID:18588584

Hasson-Ohayon, I., Kravetz, S., Roe, D., David, A. S., & Weiser, M. (2006). Insight into psychosis and quality of life. *Comprehensive Psychiatry*, *47*(4), 265–269. doi:10.1016/j.comppsych.2005.08.006 PMID:16769300

Heru, A. M., & Ryan, C. E. (2008). Burden, reward and family functioning of caregivers for relatives with mood disorders: 1 year follow-up. *Journal of Affective Disorders*, *83*, 221–225. doi:10.1016/j.jad.2004.04.013 PMID:15555717

Hirschfeld, R., Lewis, L., & Vornik, L. A. (2003). Perception and Impact of bipolar disorders how far have we really come? Results of the National Depressive and Manic-Depressive association 2000 survey of Individuals with bipolar disorder. *The Journal of Clinical Psychiatry*, *64*, 161–174. doi:10.4088/JCP.v64n0209 PMID:12633125

Hoeing, J., & Hamilton, M. (1969). *The Degeneration of Mentally Ill*. London: Routledge and Kegan Paul.

Hooley, J. M. (1986). An introduction to expressed emotion measurement and research. In M. J. Goldstein, I. Hand, & K. Hahlweg (Eds.), *Treatment of schizophrenia: family assessment and intervention* (pp. 25–34). Berlin: Springer- Verlag. doi:10.1007/978-3-642-95496-2_3

Idstad, M., Ask, H., & Tambs, K. (2010). Mental disorder and caregiver burden in spouses: The Nord-Trøndelag health study. *Bio Med Central Public Health*, *26*, 34–51. PMID:20796279

Ivarsson, A. B., Sidenvall, B., & Carlsson, M. (2004). The factor structure of the Burden Assessment Scale and the perceived burden of caregivers for individuals with severe mental disorders. *Scandinavian Journal of Caring Sciences*, *18*(4), 396–401. doi:10.1111/j.1471-6712.2004.00298.x PMID:15598247

Jungbauer, J., Wittmund, B., Dietrich, S., & Angermeyer, M. C. (2004). The disregarded caregivers: Subjective burden in spouses of schizophrenia patients. *Schizophrenia Bulletin*, *30*(3), 665–675. doi:10.1093/oxfordjournals.schbul.a007114 PMID:15631259

Kanter, J., Lamb, R., & Loeper, C. (1987). Expressed emotion in families: A critical review. *Hospital & Community Psychiatry, 338*, 374–380. PMID:3552930

Kate, N., Grover, S., Kulhara, P., & Nehra, R. (2013). Caregiving appraisal in schizophrenia: A study from India. *Social Science & Medicine, 98*, 135–140. doi:10.1016/j.socscimed.2013.09.005 PMID:24331891

Kazarian, S. S., Malla, A. K., Cole, J. D., & Baker, B. (1990). Comparisons of two expressed emotion scales with the Camberwell Family Interview. *Journal of Clinical Psychology, 46*(3), 306–309. doi:10.1002/1097-4679(199005)46:3<306::AID-JCLP2270460310>3.0.CO;2-2 PMID:2347936

Kim, E.Y., & Miklowitz., & D.J. (2004). Expressed emotion as a predictor of outcome among bipolar patients undergoing family therapy. *Journal of Affective Disorders, 82*, 343–352. PMID:15555685

Kuipers, L., Leff, J., & Lam, D. (1992). *Family Work for Schizophrenia: A Practical Guide*. London: Gaskell.

Kunikata, H., Mino, Y., & Nakajima, K. (2005). Quality of life of Schizophrenia patients living in the community: The relationships with personal characteristics, objective indicators and self-esteem. *Psychiatry and Clinical Neurosciences, 59*(2), 163–169. doi:10.1111/j.1440-1819.2005.01352.x PMID:15823162

Lee, T., Yang, Y., Chen, P., Hung, N., Lin, S., Chang, F., & Cheng, S. (2006). Different dimensions of social support for caregivers for patient with schizophrenia: Main effect and stress-buffering models. *Psychiatric Journal of Clinical Neurosciences, 60*(5), 546–550. doi:10.1111/j.1440-1819.2006.01556.x PMID:16958936

Leff, J., & Vaughn, C. (1985). *Expressed emotion in families*. New York: The Guilford Press.

Magliano, L., Fadden, G., Madianos, M., De Almeida, J. M., Held, T., Guarneri, M., & Maj, M. et al. (1998). Burden on the families of patients with schizophrenia: Results of the BIOMED I study. *Social Psychiatry and Psychiatric Epidemiology, 33*(9), 405–412. doi:10.1007/s001270050073 PMID:9766166

Magliano, L., Fiorillo, A., De Rosa, C., Malangone, C., & Maj, M. (2005). Family burden in long-term diseases: A comparative study in schizophrenia vs. physical disorders. *Social Science & Medicine, 61*(2), 313–322. doi:10.1016/j.socscimed.2004.11.064 PMID:15893048

Magliano, L., Marasco, C., Fiorillo, A., Malangone, C., Guarneri, M., & Maj, M. (2003). The impact of professional and social network support on the burden of families of patients with schizophrenia in Italy. *Acta Psychiatrica Scandinavica, 106*(4), 291–298. doi:10.1034/j.1600-0447.2002.02223.x PMID:12225496

Martens, L., & Addington, J. (2001). The psychological well-being of family members of individuals with schizophrenia. *Social Psychiatry and Psychiatric Epidemiology, 36*(3), 128–133. doi:10.1007/s001270050301 PMID:11465784

McCauley, E., Myers, K., Mitchell, J., Calderon, R., Schloredt, K., & Treder, R. (1993). Depression in young people; initial presentation and clinical course. *Journal of the American Academy of Child and Adolescent Psychiatry, 32*(4), 714–722. doi:10.1097/00004583-199307000-00003 PMID:8340290

McGlashan, T. H. (1994). Psychosocial treatments of schizophrenia: The potential of relationships. In N. C. Andreasen (Ed.), *Schizophrenia: From mind to molecule*. Washington, DC: American Psychiatric Press.

Miklowitz, D., Goldstein, M. J., Nuechterlein, K. H., & Synder, K. S. (1998). Family factors and the course of BPAD. *Archives of General Psychiatry*, *45*, 225–231. doi:10.1001/archpsyc.1988.01800270033004 PMID:3341878

Mishra, M., Trivedi, J.K., & Sinha, P.K. (2005). Burden of care of key relatives of chronic depressives. *SAARC Psychiatric Foundation Souvenir, 56*.

Möller-Leimkühler, A. M., & Obermeier, M. (2008). Predicting caregiver burden in first admission psychiatric patients: 2 year follow up results. *European Archives of Psychiatry and Clinical Neuroscience*, *258*(7), 406–413. doi:10.1007/s00406-008-0818-7 PMID:18574613

Narasipuram, S., & Kasimahanti, S. (2012). Quality of life and perception of burden among caregivers of persons with mental illness. *Applied Journal of Psychological Medicine*, *13*, 99–103.

Narendra, K. S., Bhattacharjee, D., Nishant, G., Sanjay, K. M., & Nizamie, S. H. (2011). Perceived burden and social support of caregivers in early onset psychosis and epilepsy: A comparative study. *Malaysian Journal of Psychiatry*, *20*, 2.

Ochoa, S., Vilaplana, M., Haro, J., Villalta-Gil, V., Martínez, F., Cruz, M., & Autonell, J. et al. (2008). Do needs, symptoms, or disability of outpatients with Schizophrenia influence family burden? *Social Psychiatry and Psychiatric Epidemiology*, *43*(8), 612–618. doi:10.1007/s00127-008-0337-x PMID:18340397

Ogilvie, A. D., Morant, N., & Goodwin, G. M. (2005). The burden on informal caregivers of people with bipolar disorder. *Bipolar Disorders*, *7*(s1), 25–32. doi:10.1111/j.1399-5618.2005.00191.x PMID:15762866

Ohaeri, J. U. (2001). Caregiver burden and psychotic patients' perception of social support in a Nigerian setting. *Social Psychiatry and Psychiatric Epidemiology*, *36*(2), 86–93. doi:10.1007/s001270050294 PMID:11355450

Orley, J., Saxena, S., & Herrman, H. (1998). Quality of life and mental illness: Reference from perspective of the WHOQOL. *The British Journal of Psychiatry*, *172*(4), 291–293. doi:10.1192/bjp.172.4.291 PMID:9715330

Parker, G., Fairley, M., Greenwood, J., Jurd, S., & Silove, D. (1982). Parental representations of Schizophrenias and their association with onset and course of schizophrenia. *The British Journal of Psychiatry*, *141*(6), 573–581. doi:10.1192/bjp.141.6.573 PMID:7159804

Patterson, P., Birchwood, M., & Cochrane, R. (2005). Expressed emotion as an adaptation to loss: Prospective study in Ist- episode psychosis. *The British Journal of Psychiatry*, *187*(48), s59–s64. doi:10.1192/bjp.187.48.s59 PMID:16055810

Perlick, D., Clarkin, J. F., Sirey, J., Raue, P., Greenfield, S., Struening, E., & Rosenheck, R. (1999). Burden experienced by care-givers of persons with bipolar affective disorder. *The British Journal of Psychiatry*, *175*(1), 56–62. doi:10.1192/bjp.175.1.56 PMID:10621769

Perlick, D., Rosenheck, R. A., Clarkin, J. F., Raue, P., & Sirey, J. (2001). Impact of family burden and patient symptom status on clinical outcome in bipolar affective disorder. *The Journal of Nervous and Mental Disease*, *189*(1), 31–37. doi:10.1097/00005053-200101000-00006 PMID:11206662

Perlick, D. A., Rosenbeck, R. A., Clarkin, J. F., Maciejewski, P. K., Sirey, J., Struening, E., & Link, B. G. (2004). Impact of family burden and affective response on clinical outcome among patients with bipolar disorder. *Psychiatric Services (Washington, D.C.), 55*(9), 1029–1035. doi:10.1176/appi.ps.55.9.1029 PMID:15345763

Perlick, D. A., Rosenheck, R. A., Milkowitz, D. J., Kaczynski, R., Link, B., & Ketter, S. G. (2008). Caregiver burden and health in bipolar disorder: A Cluster analytic approach. *The Journal of Nervous and Mental Disease, 196*(6), 484–491. doi:10.1097/NMD.0b013e3181773927 PMID:18552626

Perlick, D. A., Rosenheck, R. A., Milkowitz, D. J., Kaczynski, R., Link, B., Ketter, T., & Sachs, G. et al. (2008). Caregiver burden and health in bipolar disorder: A Cluster analytic approach. *The Journal of Nervous and Mental Disease, 196*(6), 484–491. doi:10.1097/NMD.0b013e3181773927 PMID:18552626

Priebe, S., Roeder-Wanner, U.-U., & Kaiser, W. (2006). Quality of life in Ist admitted Schizophrenia patients: A follow up study. *Psychological Medicine, 30*(1), 225–230. doi:10.1017/S0033291798008253 PMID:10722193

Raune, D., Kuipers, E., & Bebbington, P. E. (2004). Expressed emotion at first episode-psychosis: Investigating a career appraisal model. *The British Journal of Psychiatry, 184*(4), 321–326. doi:10.1192/bjp.184.4.321 PMID:15056576

Ristner, M., Modai, I., & Endicott, J. (2000). Differences in quality of life domains and psychopathologic and psychosocial factors in psychiatric patients. *The Journal of Clinical Psychiatry, 61*(11), 880–889. doi:10.4088/JCP.v61n1113 PMID:11105747

Ristner, M., Modai, I., & Ponizovsky, A. (2002). Assessing psychological distress in psychiatric patients: Validation of the Talbieh Brief Distress Inventory. *Comprehensive Psychiatry, 43*(3), 229–234. doi:10.1053/comp.2002.30800 PMID:11994843

Ritsner, M., Kurs, R., Gibel, A., Hirschmann, S., Shinkarenko, E., & Ratner, Y. (2003). Predictors of quality of life in major payshosis: A naturalistic follow- up study. *The Journal of Clinical Psychiatry, 64*, 308–315. doi:10.4088/JCP.v64n0313 PMID:12716273

Salvatore, S., Amelia, R., Marco, L., & Carmela, M. (2014). Caregiver's Burden and Quality of Life: Caring for Physical and Mental Illness. *International Journal Psychological Research, 7*, 30–39.

Saunders, J. (2003). Families living with severe mental illness: A literature review. *Issues in Mental Health Nursing, 24*(2), 175–198. doi:10.1080/01612840305301 PMID:12554427

Scazufca, M., & Kuipers, E. (1996). Links between expressed emotion and burden of care in relatives of patients with schizophrenia. *The British Journal of Psychiatry, 168*(5), 580–587. doi:10.1192/bjp.168.5.580 PMID:8733796

Shields, C. G., Franks, P., Harp, J. J., Campbell, T. L., & McDaniel, S. H. (1992). Development of the Family Emotional Involvement and Criticism, Scale (FEICS): A self-report scale to measure EE. *Journal of Marital and Family Therapy, 18*, 395–407. doi:10.1111/j.1752-0606.1992.tb00953.x

Sierra, P., Livianos, L., & Rojo, L. (2005). Quality of life for patients with bipolar disorder: Relationship with clinical and demographic variables. *Bipolar Disorders*, *7*(2), 159–165. doi:10.1111/j.1399-5618.2005.00186.x PMID:15762857

Sim, K., Mahendram, R., Siris, S. G., Heckers, S., & Chong, S. A. (2004). Subjective quality of life in first episode schizophrenia spectrum disorders with comorbid depression. *Psychiatry Research*, *15*(2), 141–147. doi:10.1016/j.psychres.2004.07.007 PMID:15590041

Singh, A. R., Verma, A. N., Verma, P. K., & Chaudhary, S. (2009). Subjective burden on spouses of schizophrenia patients. *Industrial Psychiatry Journal*, *18*(2), 97–100. doi:10.4103/0972-6748.62268 PMID:21180485

Solanki, R. K., Singh, P., Midha, A., & Chugh, K. (2008). Schizophrenia: Impact on quality of life. *Indian Journal of Psychiatry*, *50*(3), 181–186. doi:10.4103/0019-5545.43632 PMID:19742235

Strachan, A. M., Leff, J. P., Goldstein, M., Doane, J. A., & Burtt, C. (1986). Emotional attributes and direct communication in the families of Schizophrenias: A cross national replication. *The British Journal of Psychiatry*, *149*(3), 279–287. doi:10.1192/bjp.149.3.279 PMID:3779290

Struening, E. L., Perlick, D. A., Link, B. G., Hellman, F., Herman, D., & Sirey, J. A. (2001). Stigma as a barrier to recovery. The extent to which caregivers believe most people devalue consumers and their families. *Psychiatric Services (Washington, D.C.)*, *52*(12), 1633–1638. doi:10.1176/appi.ps.52.12.1633 PMID:11726755

Swapna, B., Sudarshan, S. Y., & Shamshad, B. (2012). Burden on caregivers in Bipolar disorder and Alcohol. *International Journal of Biosocial and Medical Research*, *3*, 1992–1997.

Thara, R., Padmavati, R., Kumar, S., & Srinivasan, L. (1998). Instrument to assess burden on caregivers of chronic mentally ill. *Indian Journal of Psychiatry*, *40*, 21–29. PMID:21494438

Vojta, C., Kinosian, B., Glick, H., Altshuler, L., & Bauer, M. S. (2001). Self-reported quality of life across mood states in bipolar disorder. *Comprehensive Psychiatry*, *42*(3), 190–195. doi:10.1053/comp.2001.23143 PMID:11349236

Warner, R., & Atkinson, M. (1988). The relationship between Schizophrenia patients' perceptions of their parents and the course of their illness. *The British Journal of Psychiatry*, *153*(3), 344–353. doi:10.1192/bjp.153.3.344 PMID:3250671

Wolthaus, J., Dingemans, P., Schene, A., Linszen, D., Wiersma, D., Bosch, R., & Hijman, R. (2002). Caregiver burden in recent - onset schizophrenia and spectrum disorders: The influence of symptoms and personality traits. *The Journal of Nervous and Mental Disease*, *190*(4), 241–247. doi:10.1097/00005053-200204000-00005 PMID:11960085

World Health Organization, World Health Report. (2001). *Mental Health: New Understanding, New Hope*. WHO.

Young, K. W. (2004). Quality of life of people with long- term psychiatric illness living in residential home. *International Journal of Psychosocial Rehabilitation*, *9*, 133–145.

Zergaw, A., Hailemariam, D., Alem, A., & Kebede, D. (2008). A longitudinal comparative analysis of economic and family caregiver burden due to bipolar disorder. *Bipolar Disorders*, *11*, 191–198. PMID:19588042

KEY TERMS AND DEFINITIONS

Bipolar Affective Disorder: Bipolar disorder is a serious, long-term (chronic) condition where you have 'lows' (periods of depression) and 'highs' (periods of mania or hypomania).

Caregiver Burden: A multidimensional response to the negative appraisal and perceived stress resulting from taking care of an ill individual.

Chronic Mental Illness: People with chronic mental illness are significantly functionally impaired by the illness for an indefinite period of time (diagnosis, disability, duration).

Expressed Emotion: Expressed emotions are the attitude that the relatives or family member show towards the sick or ill person. The key elements of expressed emotion are criticism, hostility, and emotional over involvement.

Predictors of Chronic Mental Illness: The public health significance of any trait/ factor depends heavily on its ability to *predict* future adverse outcomes with an effect size large enough to be of practical importance. In case of chronic mental illness, there are certain factors/ conditions such environment, caregiver burden response, perception of expressed emotion by patient which affect the future outcome/ relapse/ prognosis of any mental illness.

Psychopathology: The study of psychological and behavioral dysfunction occurring in mental disorder or in social disorganization. It includes the dimensions such as: social, behavioral, thought and emotions.

Quality of Life: Quality of Life is individuals' perception of their position in life in the context of the culture and value systems in which they live and in relation to their goals, expectations, standards and concerns. It is measured by person's physical health, psychological state, level of independence, social relationships, personal beliefs and their relationship to salient features of their environment.

Schizophrenia: A long-term mental disorder of a type involving a breakdown in the relation between thought, emotion, and behavior, leading to faulty perception, inappropriate actions and feelings, withdrawal from reality and personal relationships into fantasy and delusion, and a sense of mental fragmentation.

Chapter 9
Global Burden of Mental Disorders:
Quality of Care and Unmet Needs for Treatment of Chronic Mental Illness

Meghamala S. Tavaragi
DIMHANS, India

Sushma C.
DIMHANS, India

ABSTRACT

Mental disorders are an important cause of long-term disability and dependency. It accounts for over 15% of the disease burden in developed countries, which is more than the disease burden caused by all cancers. Mental illness is a leading cause of suffering, economic loss and social problems. The burden of mental disorders is likely to have been underestimated because of inadequate appreciation of the connectedness between mental illness and other health conditions. Mental disorders increase risk for communicable and non-communicable diseases, and contribute to unintentional and intentional injury, and comorbidity complicates help-seeking, diagnosis, and treatment, and influences prognosis. Consequently, health professionals have trivialized the issue of mental illness. It is essential that researchers and public health professionals work together to resolve the enormous public health crisis presented by mental disorders. In short, we must "mainstream" mental health.

INTRODUCTION

The WHO proposition that there can be "no health without mental health" has also been endorsed by the Pan American Health Organization, the EU Council of Ministers, the World Federation of Mental Health, and the UK Royal College of Psychiatrists. Mental disorders are an important cause of long-term disability and dependency. Mental health is more than the mere lack of mental disorders. The positive dimension of mental health is stressed in WHO's definition of health as contained in its constitution:

DOI: 10.4018/978-1-5225-0519-8.ch009

"Health is a state of complete physical, mental and social well-being and not merely the absence of disease or infirmity." Concepts of mental health include subjective well-being, perceived self-efficacy, autonomy, competence, intergenerational dependence and recognition of the ability to realize one's intellectual and emotional potential. It has also been defined as a state of well-being whereby individuals recognize their abilities, are able to cope with the normal stresses of life, work productively and fruitfully, and make a contribution to their communities. Mental health is about enhancing competencies of individuals and communities and enabling them to achieve their self-determined goals. Mental health should be a concern for all of us, rather than only for those who suffer from a mental disorder (World Health Organization [WHO], 2003).

DEFINING CHRONIC MENTAL ILLNESS

1. Who Is Chronically Ill?

Individuals who, through no fault of their own or their families, suffer from one of several diseases affecting the brain, the most complex of human organs. The causes remain unknown, but are probably multiple. There is no cure, but we do have effective treatment. In addition to having a brain disease, people with chronic mental illness (serious mental illness) are (by definition) significantly functionally impaired by the illness for an indefinite period of time (diagnosis, disability, duration). At least 1% of the population are chronic mentally ill. The problems of victims and their families are compounded by stigma, one of the cruellest and most prevalent forms of bigotry that exists.

- **Symptoms of Chronic Mental Illness:** Acute, "positive" symptoms (at least one of these usually present, at least during an exacerbation of illness):
  - Distorted perceptions; loss of contact with reality;
    - Delusions.
    - Hallucinations.
  - Disordered, disorganized and confused thinking.
  - Unstable and inappropriate emotions.
  - Bizarre behavior; impaired judgment.
- Residual ("negative") or deficit symptoms (several of these usually present most of the time):
  - Vulnerability to certain kinds of stress.
  - Extreme dependency (sometimes combined with hostility).
  - Difficulty with interpersonal relationships.
  - Deficient coping skills.
  - Poor transfer of learning; fear of new situations.
  - Restricted emotional response and lack of enjoyment.
  - Reduced speech and impaired abstract thinking.
  - Reduced ability to pay attention; slowness.
  - Apathy; lack of motivation; phobic avoidance of situations.
  - Sensitivity to over- (and under-) stimulation (Goldman, 1998).

- **"Normal" Reactions to Chronic Illness:** These reactions are common in anyone who realizes they have a serious, chronic (incurable) illness, and may progress through stages (like the mourning process). Some of these characteristics are often present and can be mis-diagnosed as positive or negative symptoms.
  - General stress response ("fight, flight, fright").
  - Grief; denial and impatience (lack of acceptance).
  - Anger and striking out.
  - Guilt and self-blame.
  - Depression; hopeless, helpless feelings; demoralization.
  - Regression to earlier levels of functioning.
  - Preoccupation with "self" (apparent disinterest in others).
  - Interruption of normal development (immaturity).
- **Social Breakdown Syndrome:** This includes loss of normal role functioning and varying degrees of extrusion (or exclusion) from normal family/community functioning. Characteristics are similar to the negative symptoms of chronic mental illness and also resemble institutionalization syndrome. Social breakdown syndrome can be a side effect of any treatment that removes the client/patient from his/her usual social environment (or excuses him from usual role expectations) (e.g., prolonged hospitalization or too much "overprotection" on the part of clinical staff and/or family members) (Goldman, 1998).

2. Chronically Mentally Ill Law and Legal Definition

Chronically mentally ill is a term used to describe a major mental disorder based on a diagnosis by a licensed medical health professional which shows that such a person has serious problems in the areas of work, family and also has frequent variations in his/her thinking or mood. The following is an example of a federal statute defining chronically mentally ill. "Chronically mentally ill means a condition of schizophrenia or major affective disorder or post-traumatic stress disorder (PTSD), based on a diagnosis from a licensed mental health professional, with at least one documented hospitalization for this condition sometime in the last 2 years or with documentation of a formal assessment on a standardized scale of any serious symptomology or serious impairment in the areas of work, family relations, thinking, or mood."

3. Chronic Mental Illness Is Difficult to Define

Before deinstitutionalization, the criterion for chronicity was current or prior hospitalization (Bachrach, 1988). Present definitions emphasize three criteria: duration, diagnosis, and disability (Bachrach, 1988).

- First, chronic illness is distinguished by its gradual onset, indefinite duration, threat of relapse, and lack of return to prodromal functioning. Acute illness, in contrast, has an abrupt onset and finite duration (Anderson, cited in Wintersteen,1986).
- The second criterion is diagnosis, which is made on the basis of psychiatric symptoms, such as depressed mood, hallucinations, or delusions. A diagnosis of schizophrenia implies chronicity, almost by definition, because of its generally poor prognosis.

- The third criterion is disability. In addition to the severe psychiatric symptoms suffered in CMI, secondary disabilities are also present that lead to considerable financial, social, vocational, and personal impairment (Gregory, Andrew, Ryan, & Stephanie, 1993).

Because CMI is characterized by chronic deficits in personal and social functioning, many people with CMI are unable to perform the basic activities of daily living. Many are unemployed, are dependent on welfare services for survival, and lack adequate health care. In addition, the chronically mentally ill must also deal with stigma and discrimination. These factors combine to make them "one of the most needy and disadvantaged groups of society" (Shadish, Lurigio, & Lewis, 1989).

4. "Chronically Mentally Ill Adult" or "Adult Who Is Chronically Mentally Ill"

This means an adult who has a mental disorder and meets at least one of the following criteria:

1. Has undergone two or more episodes of hospital care for a mental disorder within the preceding two years; or
2. Has experienced a continuous psychiatric hospitalization or residential treatment exceeding six months' duration within the preceding year;
3. Has been unable to engage in any substantial gainful activity by reason of any mental disorder which has lasted for a continuous period of not less than twelve months. "Substantial gainful activity" shall be defined by the department by rule consistent with Public Law 92-603, as amended (Washington state legislature Definitions, Effective until, 2016).

GLOBAL BURDEN OF MENTAL DISORDERS

Mental disorders make a substantial independent contribution to the burden of disease worldwide (WHO, 1992 - 94). WHO's 2005 estimates of the global burden of disease provide evidence on the relative effect of health problems worldwide (Murray, & Lopez, 1996,&Mathers & Loncar 2006).Non-communicable diseases are rapidly becoming the dominant causes of ill health in all developing regions except sub-Saharan Africa (Mathers,& Loncar, 2006).The Global Burden of Disease report has revealed the scale of the contribution of mental disorders, by use of an integrated measure of disease burden, the disability-adjusted life-year, which is the sum of years lived with disability and years of life lost (Mathers, & Loncar, 2006).The report showed that neuropsychiatric conditions account for up to a quarter of all disability-adjusted life-years, and up to a third of those attributed to non-communicable diseases, although the size of this contribution varies between countries according to income level (Mathers, & Loncar, 2006).The neuropsychiatric conditions that contribute the most disability-adjusted life-years are mental disorders, especially unipolar and bipolar affective disorders, substance-use and alcohol-use disorders, schizophrenia, and dementia. Neurological disorders (such as migraine, epilepsy, Parkinson's disease, and multiple sclerosis) make a smaller but still significant contribution. Of the non-communicable diseases, neuropsychiatric conditions contribute the most to overall burden (Mathers & Loncar, 2006) more than either cardiovascular disease or cancer.

Mental disorders are an important cause of long-term disability and dependency. WHO's 2005 report attributed 31.7% of all years lived-with-disability to neuropsychiatric conditions: the five major contributors to this total were unipolar depression (11.8%), alcohol-use disorder (3.3%), schizophrenia (2.8%), bipolar depression (2.4%), and dementia (1.6%) (Mathers & Loncar, 2006). However, the interaction between mental disorder and disability is more complex and extensive than the WHO report suggests. Only 40 000 deaths were attributed to mental disorders (mainly unipolar and bipolar depression, schizophrenia, and post-traumatic stress disorder) and 182 000 to use of drugs and alcohol (Mathers & Loncar, 2006).These numbers are almost certainly underestimated, since the report attributes death by suicide to intentional injury(Mathers & Loncar, 2006).Every year, about 800 000 people commit suicide, 86% of whom are in low-income and middle-income countries, and more than half of whom are aged between 15 and 44 years. Even these figures might be under-estimated, since official statistics in low-income and middle-income countries are not reliable. For example, studies in south India that used surveillance with validated verbal autopsy showed that rates of suicide were ten times greater than the official national estimates (Aaron, Joseph, & Abraham, 2004; Prasad, Abraham, & Minz, 2006), that suicide was the leading cause of death in 10–19 year olds; and that suicides accounted for a quarter of all deaths in boys and up to three-quarters of all deaths in young women (Aaron, Joseph, & Abraham, 2004).A systematic review of psychological autopsy case-control studies identified mental disorders (depression, schizophrenia and other psychoses, and alcohol-use and substance-use disorders) as important proximal risk factors for suicide, with a median prevalence of mental disorder of 91% in suicide completers, and a population-attributable fraction of 47–74% (Cavanagh, Carson, Sharpe, & Lawrie, 2003).Findings from psychological autopsy studies in India and China were similar (Vijayakumar & Rajkumar, 1999; Phillips et al., 2002).Therefore, prevention, identification, and appropriate management of mental health problems is an important element of suicide prevention.

The burden of mental disorders is likely to have been underestimated because of inadequate appreciation of the connectedness between mental illness and other health conditions. Because these interactions are protean, there can be no health without mental health. Mental disorders increase risk for communicable and non-communicable diseases, and contribute to unintentional and intentional injury. Conversely, many health conditions increase the risk for mental disorder, and comorbidity complicates help-seeking, diagnosis, and treatment, and influences prognosis. Health services are not provided equitably to people with mental disorders, and the quality of care for both mental and physical health conditions for these people could be improved. As many as 450 million people worldwide are estimated to be suffering at any given time from some kind of mental or brain disorder, including behavioural and substance abuse disorders. In the World Health Report 2001 that we devote to mental health, we bring updated figures which show that four of the ten leading causes of disability worldwide are neuropsychiatric disorders, accounting for 30.8% of total disability and 12.3% of the total burden of disease. This latter figure is expected to rise to 15% by the year 2020 (Ministerial Round Tables, 2001). The 1990 WHO report indicated that 5 of the 10 leading causes of disability were psychiatric conditions. Psychiatric and neurologic conditions account for 28% of all years lived with disability, but only 1.4% of all deaths and 1.1% of years of life lost. Thus, psychiatric disorders, while traditionally not regarded as a major epidemiological problem, are shown by consideration of disability years to have a huge impact on populations.

Today, about 450 million people suffer from a mental or behavioural disorder. According to WHO's Global Burden of Disease 2001, 33% of the years lived with disability (YLD) are due to neuropsychiatric disorders, a further 2.1% to intentional injuries. Unipolar depressive disorders alone lead to 12.15% of years lived with disability, and rank as the third leading contributor to the global burden of diseases.

Four of the six leading causes of years lived with disability are due to neuropsychiatric disorders (depression, alcohol-use disorders, schizophrenia and bipolar disorder). Neuropsychiatric conditions account for 13% of disability adjusted life years (DALYs), intentional injuries form 3.3% and HIV/AIDS for another 6%. These latter two have a behavioural component linked to mental health. Moreover, behind these oft-repeated figures lies enormous human suffering.

- More than 150 million persons suffer from depression at any point in time;
- Nearly 1 million commit suicide every year;
- About 25 million suffer from schizophrenia;
- 38 million suffer from epilepsy; and
- More than 90 million suffer from an alcohol- or drug-use disorder.

The number of individuals with disorders is likely to increase further in view of the ageing of the population, worsening social problems and civil unrest.

This growing burden amounts to a huge cost in terms of human misery, disability and economic loss (WHO, 2003)

- As many as 450 million people suffer from a mental or behavioural disorder.
- Nearly 1 million people commit suicide every year.
- Four of the six leading causes of years lived with disability are due to neuropsychiatric disorders (depression, alcohol-use disorders, schizophrenia and bipolar disorder).
- One in four families has at least one member with a mental disorder. Family members are often the primary caregivers of people with mental disorders. The extent of the burden of mental disorders on family members is difficult to assess and quantify, and is consequently often ignored. However, it does have a significant impact on the family's quality of life.In addition to the health and social costs, those suffering from mental illnesses are also victims of human rights violations, stigma and discrimination, both inside and outside psychiatric institutions (WHO, 2003). Mental illness is a leading cause of suffering, economic loss and social problems. It accounts for over 15% of the disease burden in developed countries, which is more than the disease burden caused by all cancers (Prince et al., 2007). In the EU at least 83 million people (27%) suffer from mental health problems (16.7 million in the UK) (Wittchen & Jacobi, 2005). The most common mental health problem is depression which is experienced by 8–12% of the adult population (Ustun, Ayuso–Mateos, Chatterji, Mathers, & Murray, 2004). In addition, about 10% (nearly 850,000) of children and young people aged between 5–16 years have mental health problems (Green, McGinnity, Meltzer, Ford, & Goodman, 2005).

BURDEN OF SPECIFIC MENTAL ILLNESS

Depression

- According to the World Health Organization, unipolar depression was the third most important cause of disease burden worldwide in 2004. Unipolar depression was in "eighth place in low-income countries, but at first place in middle- and high-income countries" (WHO, 2008).

- In a nationally representative face-to-face household survey, 6.7% of U.S. adults experienced a major depressive episode in the past 12 months (Kessler, Chiu, Demler, Merikangas, & Walters, 2005).
- Significantly greater percentages of lifetime major depression have been reported among women (11.7%) than men (5.6%) (Ford, & Erlinger, 2004).
- Examining ethnic differences reveals lifetime percentages of depression of 6.52% among whites and 4.57% among blacks and 5.17% among Hispanics (Oquendo, Lizardi, Greenwald, Weismann, & Mann, 2004).

Anxiety

- Anxiety disorders, which include panic disorder, generalized anxiety disorder, post-traumatic stress disorder, phobias, and separation anxiety disorder, are the most common class of mental disorders present in the general population (Kessler et al., 2009).
- The estimated lifetime prevalence of any anxiety disorder is over 15%, while the 12-month prevalence is more than 10% (Kessler et al., 2009).
- Prevalence estimates of anxiety disorders are generally higher in developed countries than in developing countries (Kessler, Aguilar-Gaxiola., & Philip, 2009).
- Most anxiety disorders are more prevalent in women than in men (McLean, Asnaani, Litz, & Hofmann, 2011).
- One study estimated the annual cost of anxiety disorders in the United States to be approximately $42.3 billion in the 1990s, a majority of which was due to non-psychiatric medical treatment costs. This estimate focused on short-term effects and did not include the effect of outcomes such as the increased risk of other disorders (Greenberg et al., 1999).

Bipolar Disorder

- The National Comorbidity Study reported a lifetime prevalence of nearly 4% for bipolar disorder. Bipolar disorder is more common in women than men, with a ratio of approximately 3:2. The median age of onset for bipolar disorder is 25 years, with men having an earlier age of onset than women (Andreasen & Black, 2006).
- In an insured population, 7.5% of all claimants with behavioral health care coverage filed a claim, of which 3.0% had bipolar disorder (Peele, Xu, &Kupfer, 2003). Persons with bipolar disorder incurred $568 in annual out-of-pocket expenses—more than double the expenses incurred by all claimants. Annual insurance payments were greater for medical services for persons with bipolar disorder than for patients with other behavioral healthcare diagnoses (Peele, Xu, &Kupfer, 2003).
- The inpatient hospitalization rate of bipolar patients (39.1%) was greater than the 4.5% characterizing all other patients with behavioral health care diagnoses.
- Bipolar disorder has been deemed the most expensive behavioral health care diagnosis (Peele, Xu, & Kupfer, 2003), costing more than twice as much as depression per affected individual (Laxman, Lovibond, & Hassan, 2008). Total costs largely arise from indirect costs and are attributable to lost productivity, in turn arising from absenteeism and presenteeism (Laxman & Hassan, 2008).

- For every dollar allocated to outpatient care for persons with bipolar disorder, $1.80 is spent on inpatient care, suggesting early intervention and improved prevention management could decrease the financial impact of this illness (Peele & Kupfer, 2003).

Schizophrenia

- Worldwide prevalence estimates range between 0.5% and 1%. Age of first episode is typically younger among men (about 21 years of age) than women (27 years). Of persons with schizophrenia, by age 30, 9 out of 10 men, but only 2 out of 10 women, will manifest the illness (Andreasen & Black, 2006).
- Persons with schizophrenia pose a high risk for suicide. Approximately one-third will attempt suicide and, eventually, about 1 out of 10 will take their own lives (Andreasen & Black, 2006).
- A Canadian study found that the direct health care and non-health care costs of schizophrenia were estimated to be 2.02 billion Canadian dollars in 2004. This, combined with a high unemployment rate due to schizophrenia and an added productivity and morbidity and mortality loss of 4.83 billion Canadian dollars, yielded a total cost estimate of 6.85 billion in U.S. and Canadian dollars (Goeree, Farahati, Pyne, & Tarride, 2005).
- The economic burden of schizophrenia is particularly great during the first year following the index episode, relative to the third year onwards. This finding suggests the need for improved monitoring of persons with schizophrenia upon initial diagnosis (Nicholl, Akhras, Diels, & Schadrack, 2010).

ECONOMIC BURDEN MENTAL ILLNESS

The economic burden of mental illness is a world-wide problem. Mental health problems comprise 5 of the 10 leading causes of disability and 10.5% of global burden of disease (Murray, & Lopez, 1996, & 1999). Mental illness imposes a huge burden on individuals, families and society (Centre for Mental Health, 2010). The cost of illness incurred by individuals, employers and governments is enormous and includes:

- Direct healthcare costs (services and materials used in prevention, diagnosis and treatment);
- Indirect healthcare costs (other resources);
- Indirect costs (value of the output lost because of inability to work due to illness);
- Intangible costs (can be valued as quality-adjusted life years; QALY) (Andlin-Sobocki, Jonsson, Wittchen, & Olesen, 2005).

In England alone, mental illness costs over £105.2 billion a year, through the costs of medical or social care, production output losses, and a monetary valuation of the intangible human cost of disability, suffering and distress (Centre for Mental Health, 2010.). In Scotland, the total cost of mental illness is £8.6 billion, which is equivalent to about 9% of its GDP; in Northern Ireland the cost is £2.8 billion, and in Wales £7.2 billion a year. The overall prevalence of mental illness is similar in England and Scotland, but estimates are about 25% higher in Wales and Northern Ireland (Northern Ireland Association for Mental Health & Sainsbury Centre for Mental Health. 2007; Singleton, Bumpstead, O'Brien, Lee, & Meltzer, 2001; Scottish Association for Mental Health & Sainsbury Centre for Mental Health, 2007).

GLOBAL BURDEN ASSESMENT SCALES

The GBD uses several metrics to determine health loss:

- Years of Life Lost due to premature mortality (YLLs),
- Years Lived with Disability (YLDs), and
- Disability-Adjusted Life-Years (DALYs).

Years of life lost (YLL) are calculated by multiplying the number of deaths in each age group by a reference life expectancy at that age – so a disease that kills many young people will generate a greater YLL than a disease that kills older people. Years lived with disability (YLD) are calculated by multiplying the prevalence of a consequence of an illness by its disability weight. Disability weights are based largely on surveys of the general population – to determine how much disability is accounted for by blindness, for example, compared with being unable to walk. Disability adjusted life years (DALY) are the sum of the above two numbers – representing the entire amount of healthy life years lost due to premature death and impaired function caused by an illness (Horowitz, 2013; Christopher & Murray, 2013).

Results of Mental Illnesses

Years of Life Lost (YLL): Self-harm, overwhelmingly related to mental health issues, has remained the number 8 cause of years of life lost in the UK from 1990 to 2010 in all age groups, and the number 2 cause in the 20-54-year-old group. The years of life lost due to drug use disorders have increased by 577% for all age groups, and 812% for those 20-54, who have also experienced a 230% increase in alcohol use disorders.

- **Years lived with disability (YLD):** Mental illnesses were the second greatest contributor to years lived with disability in 2010, with six out of the top twenty causes of years lived with disability being mental health disorders – major depression (third largest cause overall), anxiety, drug use, alcohol use, schizophrenia and bipolar disorder.
- **Disability Adjusted Life Years (DALYs):** The report showed that almost every mental health disorder increased its burden of disease.Mental and behavioural disorders accounted for 1.65 million disability adjusted life years in 1990, increasing to 1.94 million in 2010 (an increase of 17%). As a point of comparison the number one cause of DALYs is cardiovascular disease which in the same period decreased by 39%. There are few good news stories in the mental health section – almost every mental health disorder increased its burden of disease:
    - Alcohol use disorders increased the number of disability adjusted life years by 56.1%,
    - Unipolar depression increased by 9%,
    - Eating disorders increased by 53.9%,
    - Opioid drug use increased by 56.3% and
    - Schizophrenia increased by 14% (Horowitz, 2013; Christopher & Murray, 2013).

DISABILITY ASSESMENT SCALE

WHO Composite International Diagnostic Interview [CIDI] (Kessler & Ustun, 2004). The CIDI is a state-of-the-art fully structured research diagnostic interview designed to be used by trained lay interviewers who do not have any clinical experience. CIDI includes a disorder specific measure of role impairment that is administered in exactly the same fashion for each mental disorder assessed in the surveys and for each of the physical disorders assessed for comparison purposes in the surveys. This measure is known as the Sheehan Disability Scales (SDS). The SDS is a widely used self-report measure of condition-specific role impairment that consists of four questions, each asking the respondent to rate on a 0–10 scale the extent to which a particular disorder "interfered with" activities in one of four role domains during the month in the past year when the disorder was most severe. The four domains include:

1. "Your home management, like cleaning, shopping, and taking care of the (house/apartment)" (home);
2. "Your ability to work" (work);
3. "Your social life", social); and
4. "Your ability to form and maintain close relationships with other people" (close relationships).

The 0–10 response options were presented in a visual analogue format with labels for the response options None (0), Mild (1–3), Moderate (4–6), Severe (7–9), and Very Severe (10) (Kessler, Aguilar-Gaxiola, Ustun, & Philip, 2009)

DISABILITY IN INDIA

According to Census 2001there are 2.19 crore people with disabilities in India, who constitute 2.13% of the total population. Of these, 9,40,643 are in Karnataka state, with 92,631 being mentally disabled. 75% of all persons with disabilities live in rural areas, 49% are literates and only 34% are employed Chaudhury, Dekaand Chetia (2006) were found more people with schizophrenia in the rural areas and with dementia in the urban areas, with mood and anxiety disorders approximately evenly distributed. They also found that 64% of patients with schizophrenia, around 30% with mood disorders, 16.7% of anxiety disorders, had a disability of more than 40% on the IDEAS scale. Singh and Nizamie (2004) found that only 6% of the guardians of mentally retarded were aware of the persons with disabilities (PWD) Act. They also reported poor awareness and underutilization of disability benefits. Hence, in practice, disability benefits are still elusive for persons with mental disorders.99.4% of the disabled in rural areas had not availed any benefits other than disability pension, which was statistically very highly significant (χ^2 =151.73; P<0.001). 62% of urban disabled were already residing in rehabilitation centers/custodial care centers. 47.6% of persons with a disability of more than 70% were not availing any benefits other than the disability pension, which is statistically very highly significant with χ^2=16.311 and P<0.001.

In India, majority of the 125 million mental ill require intensive rehabilitation services (Thara, 2005). The transient nature of the disabilities of mental illnesses and the nature of the socio-occupational impairment posed a challenge for the measurement of the disability. As this was the major hurdle in including mental illnesses into the government's social welfare benefits under the Persons with Disability Act of 1995(www.acmiindia.org), the Rehabilitation Committee of the Indian Psychiatric Society developed the

Indian disability evaluation and assessment scale [IDEAS] (Thara, 2005), which is now recommended by the Government of India to measure psychiatric disability (The Rehabilitation Committee of the Indian Psychiatric Society, 2002). The disabled are eligible for the following welfare schemes from the government (Karnataka State Mental Health Rules, 2007; National Policy for Persons with Disabilities, 1993; Ministry of Social Justice and Empowerment (Disabilities Division), Government of India; 2007; Ministry of Social Justice and Empowerment, Government of India, 2009; Directorate of Welfare of Disabled and Senior Citizens, Government of Karnataka. 2008).

1. Disability pension/unemployment pension,
2. Disabled person's scholarship,
3. Insurance scheme for the mentally challenged,
4. Adhara scheme helping to set up small shops,
5. Telephone booth,
6. Free education up to 18 years,
7. Free legal aid,
8. Aids and appliances (for multiple disabilities),
9. 3% Job reservation (only cerebral palsy included),
10. Concessional bus passes,
11. Railway concession.

UNMET NEEDS

Within this panorama, the care of those suffering from chronic serious mental disorder, and probably the care of depression and identifying and meeting the treatment gap in their needs, becomes the most central public mental health problem. A WHO study that adopted a global perspective sought to discover not only the prevalence of the most frequently encountered SMDs(serious mental disorders) but also the relative weight of unmet need (Demyttenaere, Bruffaerts, & Posada, 2004). The European data showed that, within the EU, the Netherlands has the highest percentage of people with untreated SMD, half of the total (49.8%). Outside the EU, in Ukraine, only one in five of those with SMD are in treatment (19.7%). Moreover, the paper showed that, while many people with discomfort below the threshold of SMD receive treatment, others with SMD do not. A publication entitled The Treatment Gap in Mental Health reviewed a number of studies that gave very worrying data on countries in all continents and concluded that the mean rate of people with schizophrenia who do not receive treatment was 32% (Kohn, Saxena, Levav, & Saraceno, 2004).

Another survey in six EU countries estimated that 3.1% of the adult population had an unmet need for mental health care, and that one in five of those who sought treatment did not receive it. This represents around 6.6 million adults in a population of 213 million. It was also shown that the groups that show a higher risk of unmet need included young people, retired people and homemakers, as well as those-with long-term mental disorders, usually SMD (Alonso, Codony, & Kovess, 2007). Many psychiatric diagnoses lead to vulnerability, particularly a diagnosis of schizophrenia. Although statistics based on reliable studies state that 30–50% of those who suffer schizophrenia recover completely, the negative side is that 50–70% of those with the disorder develop a chronic illness. The terms psychoses, long-term mental disorders and SMD, and others, are used somewhat imprecisely to define a wide group of clinical conditions within the schizophrenia spectrum, which require continuing care for a long time or sometimes indefinitely. A significant proportion of this group remains uncared for, either because they fail to adhere to therapy or because of structural flaws in the services that should care for them. When the deinstitutionalization policy was implemented and conventional psychiatric hospitals closed, they were not replaced by alternative community resources, contrary to policy recommendations. This combination of factors turned people with schizophrenic disorders into a very vulnerable and increasingly conspicuous group, and those with more severe signs of the illness became more likely to be admitted to social, forensic and prison settings.

International bodies have shown their concern by starting to develop policies to protect vulnerable groups. Strategies and guidelines aimed at the prevention of mental health problems and designed specifically to meet the needs of certain vulnerable groups should be formulated and promoted at national, regional and local levels with clear objectives linked to resources and should: offer continuity of care, be community oriented, be flexible, and ensure access to services and offer a wide range of professional skills. They should be linked to housing, provision of health and social services, accommodation and social security policies which are crucial to community care and to the implementation of mental health policy (Council of Europe, 1998). In other words, it recommends positive discrimination by cutting across social and health policies oriented towards continuous care and the social integration of this vulnerable group, and the provision of emergency care 24 hours a day and 7 days a week in community-based treatment settings. Beyond any theoretical considerations, as expected, staffing and care resources are also related to the treatment gap. Patel points out that the dramatically low ratio of psychiatric resources to mental health patient need in low- and middle-income countries is one of the principal reasons to explain the large treatment gap for people with mental disorders in these settings (Patel, 2009).He suggests that, in such countries, psychiatrists should play a leadership role in addressing health mental health needs by advocating and increasing the delivery of mental health care through non-psychiatric professionals (Patel, 2009). In many countries, general practitioners would be the core professionals delivering day-to-day mental health care.

There is an urgent need for policy makers to afford public health priority to the treatment gap in SMD. Along these lines is the Spanish Government initiative launched in 2006 called Strategy in Mental Health of the National Health System (Strategy in Mental Health of the National Health System, 2007.). It includes, among other specific objectives for care of the mentally ill, the following objectives specifically related to SMD:

1. The establishment of guidelines for the management of psychiatric emergencies and crisis situations, collaborating with the different sectors involved.
2. An increase in the percentage of patients with SMD included in a rehabilitation programme.
3. An increase in the percentage of families with SMD patients who receive a specific family intervention programme, to improve their capacity to face the crisis and prevent relapses.
4. The provision of adequate general health care to SMD patients.
5. The Ministry of Health and Consumer Affairs to develop with the Autonomic Communities a collaborative model with the Justice Bodies and Penitentiary Institutions to improve the care of mentally disordered people subjected to the Penal Code and the Under Age Law, assuring continuity and equity of care with the rest of the population.

6. Establishment in each of the territorial health organisations, access to all relevant therapeutic and rehabilitation interventions or programmes, to address the needs of the population, assuring continuity of assistance through an integrated network of services, where the general hospitals will be included, and in co-ordination with primary care.
7. Establishment of an individualized care plan for mentally disordered people in treatment.
8. The availability, in the mental health teams in the community and in relation to serious prolonged mental disorders, of an organized system to avoid abandonment and facilitate engagement, which includes home care, as well as multisectorial management and co-ordination of the care process.

In conclusion there is still a lot to be learned in understanding the problem of the treatment gap. Even in the wealthiest countries in Europe with a high level of human resources and beds in psychiatric and general hospitals, the treatment gap for those with SMD is almost 50%.

Where Are the Failures?

The need for research in this field has been summarized by researchers in Washington University in the USA: One of the most critical issues in mental health services research is the gap between what is known about effective treatment and what is provided to consumers in routine care. Concerted efforts are required to advance implementation science and produce skilled implementation researchers (Proctor, Landover, & Aarons, 2009). Co-coordinating efforts between secondary and tertiary care mental health services and primary care is a must, and 24 hours a day, 7 days a week community based treatment for SMD should be guaranteed.

Long-Term Adverse Effects of Mental Disorders

Mental disorders are known to have much earlier ages-of-onset (AOO) than most chronic physical disorders. WMH analyses show that early-onset mental disorders are significant predictors of the subsequent onset and persistence of a wide range of physical disorders (Ormel et al., 2007). This is part of a larger pattern of associations between early-onset mental disorders and a wider array of adverse life course outcomes that might be conceptualized as societal costs of these disorders, including reduced educational attainment, early marriage, marital instability, and low occupational and financial status (Kessler et al., 2009).

Short-Term Adverse Effects of Mental Disorders

A considerable amount of research has been carried out to quantify the magnitude of the short-term societal costs of mental disorders in terms of healthcare expenditures, impaired functioning, and reduced longevity, but most of this work has been done in the US (Greenberg, McGinnity, Meltzer, Ford, & Goodman, 2005; Greenberg et al., 1999). The magnitude of the cost estimates in these studies is staggering. For example, Greenberg et al. (1999) estimated that the annual total societal costs of anxiety disorders in the US over the decade of the 1990s exceeded $42 billion. This estimate excludes the indirect costs of early-onset anxiety disorders through adverse life course outcomes described in the previous section (e.g., the effects of child adolescent anxiety disorders in predicting low educational attainment and consequent longterm effects on lower income) and through increased risk of other disorders (e.g., anxietydisorders predicting the subsequent onset of cardiovascular disorder) and focuses exclusively on such short-term effects as healthcare expenditures and days out of role (Kessler, Aguilar-Gaxiola, Ustun, &Philip, 2009).

QUALITY OF CARE OF CHRONIC MENTALLY ILL

In addition to suffering from the severe psychiatric symptoms of chronic mental illness (CMI), people with this type of disorder suffer from a variety of secondary disabilities and face societal obstacles that interfere with their ability to maximize their personal, social, and vocational potentials. Following the deinstitutionalization of long-term psychiatric patients in recent decades, many different understandings of the etiology, treatment, and management of CMI have evolved, including those derived from the biological, vulnerability, cognitive, case management, rehabilitation, and psychoeducational models. Because psychologists are trained in a wide range of psychological theories and a broad repertoire of applications, they have unique contributions to make within each model, particularly, as discussed here, to prevent, treat, and manage CMI through research, assessment, and intervention. Because CMI is characterized by chronic deficits in personal and social functioning, many people with CMI are unable to perform the basic activities of daily living. Many are unemployed, are dependent on welfare services for survival, and lack adequate health care. In addition, the chronically mentally ill must also deal with stigma and discrimination. These factors combine to make them "one of the most needy and disadvantaged groups of society" (Shadish, Lurigio, & Lewis, 1989; Gregory, Andrew, Ryan, & Stephanie, 1993)

Prevention: There is a critical need for psychologists to become more active in the prevention of mental health problems. In preventing CMI, regardless of the model that is assumed, a first step forward is building better understandings of the conditions affecting the nature, onset, and course of chronic mental illness (Albee, Bond, & Monsey, 1992). Obviously, psychologists are well prepared to make substantial contributions in these areas. In order to better specify the breadth of the area of prevention and the roles that psychologists can assume, they drew upon a useful framework characterizing prevention as primary, secondary, or tertiary (Caplan, 1964).

- Primary prevention refers to broad efforts to decrease the incidence of CMI, or number of new occurrences, through individual and community change.
- Secondary prevention refers to decreasing the prevalence or number of cases of CMI at any given time. This is accomplished through screening aimed at the early detection of mental illness and providing crisis intervention with high-risk groups.
- Tertiary prevention refers to decreasing the short- and long-term severity of symptoms of individuals already affected by CMI. In practice, tertiary prevention interventions appear to be very much like treatment. However, whereas the principal aim of treatment is to remedy present occurrences of the illness, the aim of tertiary prevention is to prevent or reduce the severity of future occurrences of the illness.

Over the long term, primary prevention efforts appear to promise the best payoff, although they are generally the most difficult to implement. Such programs in the area of CMI could focus on preventing individuals from developing CMI by helping them become competent, healthy persons, characterized by their psychological and physical wellness. Primary prevention programs, Cowen (1986) suggested, would have two thrusts: a systems-level strategy, which would reduce the stress individuals experience while providing them with ample personal opportunities for development, and a person-centered strategy, which would strengthen individuals' abilities to effectively cope with whatever stressors they faced. Thus, primary prevention efforts would be broad-based, directed at alleviating social problems associated with the onset of CMI, such as poverty, and, at the same time, fostering the development of personal competencies in both healthy and "at-risk" individuals.

- To illustrate the role of psychologists in primary prevention, they use the vulnerability model as an example. The vulnerability model recognizes the interaction of both biological and psychosocial factors in the onset of CMI. Psychologists could, perhaps, have the greater impact by intervening with psychosocial factors. This could consist of a twofold approach. First, psychologists could work to alleviate, where possible, the stressful conditions in the environment that contribute to the onset of CMI. Second, psychologists could work to promote the mental health of the population at large and to increase peoples' resiliency in the face of stressful conditions that cannot be eliminated.
- Interventions at the level of secondary prevention generally require less time and money to develop and thus are more readily implemented by psychologists. To illustrate the role of psychologists in secondary prevention, we again use the vulnerability model as a framework. Psychologists can identify people at risk for developing CMI and attempt to reduce stress that might contribute to the onset of a disorder by providing education, treatment, and support in crises. In addition, psychologists can increase the competence of people at risk through skills training and other means, enabling them to better cope with stress and thus avoid the onset of exacerbation of symptoms of mental illness.
- Interventions at the level of tertiary prevention generally require the least change in professional practice to implement, partly because the roles of psychologists in such interventions are much like the roles they already play in treatment. Using the vulnerability model to illustrate, psychologists engaging in tertiary prevention, besides treating current symptoms, would try to prepare patients to better cope with future stress. For example, they might teach patients skills they could use to reduce the impact of future stressors or strengthen patients in ways that make them more resilient (Gregory, Andrew, Ryan, &Stephanie, 1993).
- **Coping and Adaptation:** This is the hoped for and very possible outcome of treatment, rehabilitation, family support and self-help.
- Acceptance and hope; curiosity about the illness and its treatment, and/or efforts to be "like everyone else."
- "Responsible patient hood" and active collaboration with treatment and rehabilitation.
- Compensatory changes; lifestyle modifications (including more realistic goals and expectations).
- Full participation in life ("love" and "work").

TREATMENT AND REHABILITATION

In general, patients/clients need:

- Individualized treatment.
- Continuity of care (includes continuity of relationships with staff as well as smooth transition between, and coordination among, programs and treatment components).
- Patient education about the illness and its treatment (leading to informed consent; responsible patient role).
- Safe and comfortable surroundings with adequate privacy and desired amount of contact with others.
- Contingency plans for crises (to avoid "walking on eggshells").
- Involvement, support and education of family and/or significant others (with elimination of guilt!).
- An approach which identifies and builds on strengths.
- Outreach, or help and support provided in "natural" settings.
- A gradual, realistic, "step-wise", long term approach, recognizing various phases and stages of illness and recovery.
- To deal constructively and positively with stigma (starting with self-stigmatization, then family stigma, and finally stigma from broader social network). This often involves working through grief and mourning process.

THE BIO-PSYCHO-SOCIAL APPROACH

Biological Needs

- Psychiatric care with appropriate MEDICATION by a physician (and treatment team) who understands the illness and its treatment.
- Careful monitoring of intended effects and side effects.
- Identification of new physical and mental/emotional problems as they emerge.
- Attention to both active (positive) and deficit (negative) symptoms.
- Elimination of toxic chemicals and unnecessary drugs (alcohol, caffeine, marijuana, "cold" medicine, etc.).
- Early detection of "danger signals" and symptom monitoring by patient and others.
- Adequate rest and regular, planned, aerobic exercise.
- A balanced, nutritional diet.

Psychological Needs

- A therapeutic alliance with a person (or "team") which involves "titrated" support (varying degree of support depending on need), respect, reality orientation.
- Dealing with "normal" reactions to serious illness.
- Being actively, comfortably and usefully busy.

- A balance between over- and under-stimulation (everyone has a "window" of optimal stimulation; this tends to be constricted in serious mental illness).
- A relaxed (non-"rat race") atmosphere.
- A regular daily routine (including evenings, weekends and holidays).
- Substitution of responsible adult behavior for inappropriate behavior (behavioral approach using natural consequences, with some similarity to "tough love" concept. This should be done in an empathic and supportive way).
- Minimization of handicap; emphasis on strengths; independence as tolerated.
- If alcohol/drug uses a problem, appropriate attention to dependencies should be integrated with other treatment.

Social Needs

- Learning "survival skills"; psychosocial and occupational rehabilitation.
- Communication and problem solving skills for patient and significant others.
- Construction of supportive social network; prevent or reverse social breakdown syndrome.
- Instrumental help with daily living (money management, transportation, housing, etc.) (Goldman, 1998)

RECOMMENDATIONS

Health care reform should encourage better management of chronic, long-term illnesses, including severe mental illnesses.

- Health care reform should include effective strategies for meeting the needs of people with all forms of long-term, chronic illnesses, including those with severe mental illnesses.
- These strategies should recognize that, in addition to typical medical services, individuals may need a mix of other supports to maximize the likelihood of recovery and to improve their ability to function and care for themselves in the community.
- Delivery-system innovations designed specifically to improve chronic-care management—including medical homes, electronic records, patient registries and other programs—should be encouraged through incentives.
- Behavioral health intervention should be available and incorporated into all programs for people with chronic physical illnesses.

The service needs of people with severe mental illnesses must be recognized and addressed:

- Benefit packages should include coverage of an appropriate array of evidence based and best practices in mental healthcare, including rehabilitation for individuals with severe mental illnesses.
- Case management to link individuals to other support services (housing, transportation, etc.) should be the norm.
- Private and public plans should coordinate to ensure that there is one person or entity responsible for each individual's overall care.

Financing policies should encourage improved management of long-term chronic illnesses:

- Payment mechanisms should enable flexibility in service delivery so as to encourage providers to accept responsibility for the total care of the individual; this might include case rates, capitation or other forms of bundled payment.
- Providers who treat people with more severe disorders should be compensated for the extra time it will take to serve a population with higher needs. Payment should reflect the intensity of care. For example, a system based on three levels would allow for a basic payment rate for those with mild or moderate disorders, a second level of rates for those with more complex needs (this might include people with, for example, significant limitations from bipolar disorder) and a third tier of rates for those with severe mental illnesses, including schizophrenia

CONCLUSION

Mental disorders are an important cause of long-term disability and dependency. 450 million people suffer from a mental or behavioural disorder. Nearly 1 million people commit suicide every year. Four of the six leading causes of years lived with disability are due to neuropsychiatric disorders (depression, alcohol-use disorders, schizophrenia and bipolar disorder). One in four families has at least one member with a mental disorder. The economic burden of mental illness is a world-wide problem. Mental health problems comprise 5 of the 10 leading causes of disability and 10.5% of global burden of disease. Mental illness imposes a huge burden on individuals, families and society. The cost of illness incurred by individuals, employers and governments is enormous. Hence first aim is to critically appraise the way that the burden of disability and premature mortality is apportioned, in WHO's estimates of global burden of disease, between underlying conditions within groups of disorder, and, specifically, to assess whether these estimates account for the full contribution of mental disorder to mortality and disability. Second aim is to review available evidence for interactions between mental disorders and other health conditions (such as medically unexplained somatic symptoms, communicable diseases, maternal and perinatal conditions, non-communicable diseases, and injuries). Third aim is to discuss the implications of these links for the future orientation of health policies, health systems, and services. And finally Health care reform should include effective strategies for meeting the needs of people with all forms of long-term, chronic illnesses, including those with severe mental illness.

REFERENCES

Aaron, R., Joseph, A., & Abraham, S. (2004). Suicides in young people in rural southern India. *Lancet, 363*(9415), 1117-8.

Albee, G. W., Bond, L. A., Monsey, T., & Cook, V. (Eds.). (1992). Improving children's lives: Global perspectives on prevention. In *Primary Prevention of Psychopathology* (vol. 14, pp. 279-295). Thousand Oaks, CA: Sage Publications, Inc.

Alonso, J., Codony, M., & Kovess, V. (2007). Population level of unmet need for mental healthcare in Europe. The British Journal of Psychiatry, 190(4), 299–306. PubMed PMID:17401035

Andlin-Sobocki, P., Jonsson, B., Wittchen, H. U., & Olesen, J. (2005). Cost of disorders of the brain in Europe. European Journal of Neurology, 12(1), 1–27. doi:10.1111/j.1468-1331.2005.01202.x PubMed doi:10.1111/j.1468-1331.2005.01202.x PMID:15877774

Andreasen, N. C., & Black, D. W. (2006). Introductory Textbook of Psychiatry (4th ed.). Washington, DC: American Psychiatric Publishing.

Bachrach, L. L. (1988). Defining chronic mental illness: A concept pape. Hospital and Community, 398, 383–288.

Caplan, C. (1964). Principles of Preventive Psychiatry. New York: Basic Books, Inc.

Cavanagh, J. T., Carson, A. J., Sharpe, M., & Lawrie, S. M. (2003). Psychological autopsy studies of suicide: A systematic review. Psychological Medicine, 33(3), 395–405. doi:10.1017/S0033291702006943 PubMed doi:10.1017/S0033291702006943 PMID:12701661

Centre for Mental Health. (2010). Economic and social costs of mental health problems in 2009/10. London: Author.

Chaudhury, P. K., Deka, K., & Chetia, D. (2006). Disability associated with mental disorders. Indian Journal of Psychiatry, 48(2), 95–101. doi:10.4103/0019-5545.31597 PubMed doi:10.4103/0019-5545.31597 PMID:20703393

Christopher, J.L., & Murray, M.D. (2013). *UK health performance: findings of the Global Burden of Disease Study 2010*. Academic Press.

Council of Europe. (1998). *Recommendation NO R (98) 11 on the organisation of health care services for the chronically ill (Adopted by the Committee of Ministers at the 641st meeting of the Ministers' Deputies)*. Author.

Cowen, R. (1968). A new type of delthyrial cover in the Devonian brachiopod Mucrospirifer. Palaeontology, 11, 317–327.

Demyttenaere, K., Bruffaerts, R., & Posada, V. J. (2004). Prevalence, Severity, and Unmet Need for Treatment of Mental Disorders in the World Health Organization World Mental Health Surveys. *JAMA, 291*(21), 2581-90.

Directorate of Welfare of Disabled and Senior Citizens, Government of Karnataka. (2008).

Disability-adjusted life year (DALY). (2016). From *Wikipedia, the free encyclopedia*. Retrieved from https://en.wikipedia.org/wiki/Disability-adjusted_life_year

Ford, D. E., & Erlinger, T. P. (2004). Depression and C-reactive protein in US adults: Data from the third National Health and Nutrition Survey. Archieves of International Medicine, 168, 284–290. PubMed PMID:15136311

Goeree, R., Farahati, F., Burke, N., Blackhouse, G., O'Reilly, D., Pyne, J., & Tarride, J. E. (2005). The economic burden of schizophrenia in Canada in 2004. Current Medical Research and Opinion, 21(12), 2017–2028. doi:10.1185/030079905X75087 PubMed doi:10.1185/030079905X75087 PMID:16368053

Goldman, C. R. (1998). *Handout.* Retrieved 04 January, 2016. Available at www.karunadu.gov.in/welfareofdisabled/Documents/RTI.pdf

Green, H., McGinnity, A., Meltzer, H., Ford, T., & Goodman, R. (2005). *Mental health of children and young people in Great Britain 2004.* Academic Press.

Greenberg, P. E., Sisitsky, T., Kessler, R. C., Finkelstein, S. N., Berndt, E. R., Davidson, J. R., . . . Fyer, A. J. (1999). The economic burden of anxiety disorders in the 1990s. The Journal of Clinical Psychiatry, 60(7), 427–435. doi:10.4088/JCP.v60n0702 PubMed doi:10.4088/JCP.v60n0702 PMID:10453795

Gregory, B.S., Andrew, I.S., Ryan, L.D., & Stephanie, D. M. (1993). *The International Journal of Psychosocial Rehabilitation.* The Role of Psychologists in the Treatment, Management, and Prevention of Chronic Mental Illness.

Horowitz, M. (2013). *The burden of disease due to chronic illnesses, especially mental health illnesses is rising in the UK.* Academic Press.

Karnataka State Mental Health Rules. (2007). Retrieved from karhfw.gov.in/Karnataka_state_mental_health_authority.pdf

Kessler, R. C., & Ustun, T. B. (2004). The World Mental Health (WMH) Survey Initiative version of the World Health Organization (WHO) Composite International Diagnostic Interview (CIDI). [Pubmed Abstract Full Text]. International Journal of Methods in Psychiatric Research, 13(2), 93–121. doi:10.1002/mpr.168 PubMed doi:10.1002/mpr.168 PMID:15297906

Kessler, R. C., Chiu, W. T., Demler, O., Merikangas, K. R., & Walters, E. E. (2005). Prevalence, severity, and comorbidity of 12-month DSM-IV disorders in the National Comorbidity Survey Replication. Archives of General Psychiatry, 62(6), 617–627. doi:10.1001/archpsyc.62.6.617 PubMed doi:10.1001/archpsyc.62.6.617 PMID:15939839

Kessler, R.C., Aguilar-Gaxiola, S., Alonso, J., Chatterji, S., Lee, S., Johan Ormel, T.J., ... Philip, S. W. (2009). *The global burden of mental disorders: An update from the WHO World Mental Health (WMH) Surveys.* Academic Press.

Kohn, R., Saxena, S., Levav, I., & Saraceno, B. (2004). The treatment gap in mental health. Bulletin of the World Health Organization. PubMed PMID:15640922

Laxman, K. E., Lovibond, K. S., & Hassan, M. K. (2008). Impact of bipolar disorder in employed populations. The American Journal of Managed Care, 14(11), 757–764. PubMed PMID:18999910

Mathers, C.D., & Loncar, D. (2006). *Projections of global mortality and burden of disease from 2002 to 2030.* doi: 10.1371/journal.pmed.00304424.

McLean, C. P., Asnaani, A., Litz, B. T., & Hofmann, S. G. (2011). Gender differences in anxiety disorders: Prevalence, course of illness, comorbidity and burden of illness. Journal of Psychiatric Research, 45(8), 1027–1035. doi:10.1016/j.jpsychires.2011.03.006 PubMed doi:10.1016/j.jpsychires.2011.03.006 PMID:21439576

Ministerial Round Tables. (2011). *54th World Health Assembly Mental Health, A call for Action by World Health Ministers.* Author.

Ministry of Social Justice and Empowerment (Disabilities Division). Government of India. (2007). Retrieved, 23 February, 2016 from http://socialjustice.nic.in/incentdd.php

Ministry of Social Justice and Empowerment. Government of India. (2009). *Annual report.* Retrieved 4 January, 2016, from http://socialjustice.nic.in/annualreports.php

Murray, C. J. L., & Lopez, A. D. (1996). The Global Burden of Disease: A Comprehensive Assessment of Mortality and Disability From Diseases, Injuries and Risk Factors in 1990 and Projected to 2020. Boston: Harvard School of Public Health, World Health Organization, World Bank.

Murray, C. J. L., & Lopez, A. D. (1999). Global burden of disease. Geneva: World Health Organisation.

National Policy for Persons with Disabilities. (1993). Government of India. Handbook on Disability Rehabilitation. New Delhi: National Information Centre on Disability Rehabilitation, Ministry of Social Justice and Empowerment.

Nicholl, D., Akhras, K. S., Diels, J., & Schadrack, J. (2010). Burden of schizophrenia in recently diagnosed patients: Healthcare utilization and cost perspective. Current Medical Research and Opinion, 26(4), 943–955. doi:10.1185/03007991003658956 PubMed doi:10.1185/03007991003658956 PMID:20163295

Northern Ireland Association for Mental Health and The Sainsbury Centre for Mental Health Counting the Cost. (2007). *The Economic and Social Costs of Mental Health Problems in Northern Ireland.* Northern Ireland Association for Mental Health & Sainsbury Centre for Mental Health.

Oquendo, M. A., Lizardi, D., Greenwald, S., Weissman, M. M., & Mann, J. J. (2004). Rates of lifetime suicide attempt and rates of lifetime major depression in different ethnic groups in the United States. Acta Psychiatrica Scandinavica, 110(6), 446–451. doi:10.1111/j.1600-0447.2004.00404.x PubMed doi:10.1111/j.1600-0447.2004.00404.x PMID:15521829

Ormel, J., Von Korff, M., Burger, H., Scott, K., Demyttenaere, K., Huang, Y. Q., & Kessler, R. (2007). Mental disorders among persons with heart disease - results from World Mental Health surveys. General Hospital Psychiatry, 29(4), 325–334. doi:10.1016/j.genhosppsych.2007.03.009 PubMed doi:10.1016/j.genhosppsych.2007.03.009 PMID:17591509

Patel, V. (2009). The future of psychiatry in low- and middleincome countries. Psychological Medicine, 39(11), 1759–1762. doi:10.1017/S0033291709005224 PubMed doi:10.1017/S0033291709005224 PMID:20162837

Peele, P. B., Xu, Y., & Kupfer, D. J. (2003). Insurance expenditures on bipolar disorder: Clinical and parity concerns. The American Journal of Psychiatry, 160(7), 1286–1290. doi:10.1176/appi.ajp.160.7.1286 PubMed doi:10.1176/appi.ajp.160.7.1286 PMID:12832243

Phillips, M.R., Yang, G., Zhang, Y., Wang, L., Ji, H., & Zhou, M. (2002). Risk factors for suicide in China: a national case-control psychological autopsy study. *Lancet, 360*(9347), 1728-36.

Prasad, J., Abraham, V. J., & Minz, S. (2006). Rates and factors associated with suicide in Kaniyambadi Block, Tamil Nadu, South India, 2000–2002. The International Journal of Social Psychiatry, 52(1), 65–71. doi:10.1177/0020764006061253 PubMed doi:10.1177/0020764006061253 PMID:16463596

Prince, M., Patel, V., Saxena, S., Maj, M., Maselko, J., & Phillips, M.R. (2007). No health without mental health. *Lancet, 370*(9590), 859-77.

Proctor, E. K., Landsverk, J., Aarons, G., Chambers, D., Glisson, C., & Mittman, B. (2009). Implementation research in mental health services: An emerging science with conceptual, methodological, and training challenges. Administration and Policy in Mental Health, 36(1), 24–34. doi:10.1007/s10488-008-0197-4 PubMed doi:10.1007/s10488-008-0197-4 PMID:19104929

Scottish Association for Mental Health & Sainsbury Centre for Mental Health. (2007). Glasgow, UK: Scottish Association for Mental Health.

Shadish, W. R., Jr., Lurigio, A. J., & Lewis, D. A. (1989). After deinstitutionalization: The present and future of mental health long-term care policy. The Journal of Social Issues, 45(3), 1–15. doi:10.1111/j.1540-4560.1989.tb01551.x doi:10.1111/j.1540-4560.1989.tb01551.x

Singh, A., & Nizamie, S. H. (2004). Disability: the concept and related Indian legislations. *Mental Health Reviews*. Retrieved February 23, 2016 from http://www.psyplexus.com/mhr/disability_india.html

Singleton, N., Bumpstead, R., O'Brien, M., Lee, A., & Meltzer, H. (2001). Psychiatric Morbidity among people living in private households in 2000. London: The Stationary Office.

Strategy in Mental Health of the National Health System. (2007). *Ministry of health and consumer affairs. Ministry of health and consumer affairs*. Publications center paseo del prado.

Thara, R. (2005). Measurement of psychiatric disability. The Indian Journal of Medical Research, 121, 723–724. PubMed PMID:16037616

The Rehabilitation Committee of the Indian Psychiatric Society. (2002). IDEAS (Indian Disability Evaluation and Assessment Scale) - A scale for measuring and quantifying disability in mental disorders. Indian Psychiatric Society.

Ustun, T. B., Ayuso–Mateos, J. L., Chatterji, S., Mathers, C., & Murray, C. J. (2004). Global burden of depressive disorders in the year 2000. The British Journal of Psychiatry, 759–763. PubMed PMID:15123501

Vijayakumar, L., & Rajkumar, S. (1999). Are risk factors for suicide universal? A case-control study in India. Acta Psychiatrica Scandinavica, 99(6), 407–411. doi:10.1111/j.1600-0447.1999.tb00985.x PubMed doi:10.1111/j.1600-0447.1999.tb00985.x PMID:10408261

Washington State Legislature Definitions. (2016). *Definitions*. Retrieved on 04 January, 2016 from http://apps.leg.wa.gov/rcw/default.aspx?cite=24.06.005

Wintersteen, R. T. (1986). Rehabilitating the chronically mentally ill: Social work's claim to leadership. Social Work, 31, 332–337.

Wittchen, H. U., & Jacobi, F. (2005). Size and burden of mental disorders in Europe: A critical appraisal of 27 studies. European Neuropsychopharmacology, 21, 655–679. doi:10.1016/j.euroneuro.2011.07.018 PubMed doi:10.1016/j.euroneuro.2011.07.018 PMID:15961293

World Health Organization. (1992–94). *International Statistical Classification of Diseases and Related Health Problems*. WHO.

World Health Organization. (2003). The burden of mental disorders is expected to rise significantly over the next 20 years: Are we doing enough to address the growing mental health challenges. WHO.

World Health Organization. (2008). The Global Burden of Disease: 2004 Update. Geneva, Switzerland: WHO Press.

KEY TERMS AND DEFINITIONS

Burden: A source of great worry or stress.

Chronicity (of an Illness): Persisting for a long time or constantly recurring.

Disability: A condition that damages or limits person's abilities.

Economic Loss: Financial loss due to illness.

Mental Health: Defined as state of well-being in which every individual realizes his or her own potential, can cope with the normal stresses of life, can work productively and fruitfully, and is able to make a contribution to her or his community.

Rehabilitation: A process of helping a person who suffered an illness to restore lost skills and so regain maximum self-sufficiency.

Section 4
Chronic Mental Illness:
Disabilities and Legal Issues

Chapter 10
Disability in Schizophrenia:
The Psychosocial and Neurocognitive Perspective

Akash Mahato
Amity University, India

Susmita Halder
Amity University, India

ABSTRACT

Schizophrenia is considered to be the paradigmatic illness of psychiatry. The illness is characterized by marked disturbances and abnormalities in the domains of thought, perception, speech, emotion and behavior. The expression of the symptoms varies across patients and over time, but the cumulative effect of the illness is always severe and usually long lasting. Schizophrenia often takes a chronic course and patients exhibit difficulty re-attaining their optimum level even after resolution of clinical symptoms. Disability though is associated with many illnesses, with arguably the disability associated with chronic mental illness and schizophrenia in particular is more difficult to cope up with due to the associated stigma and care burden. The chapter focuses on different aspects of disability in schizophrenia with specific emphasis on neurocognitive and psychosocial functioning and their correlation in schizophrenia, with support from research by the author and relevant literature.

INTRODUCTION

Every illness has its own impact on the human body and brain. They can restrict the person from executing certain tasks for a certain period of time and are certainly stressful. In acute illness, the impact is short lived and patients recover fully; however, in chronic conditions the impact may persist for considerable longer period of time or lifelong taking a toll on patients overall functioning. The impact is also different when one compares physical illnesses and mental illness. One major reason behind this could be heterogeneity in etiology of mental illness, and diverse manifestation of symptoms in mental illness unlike physical illness, where etiology is more or less specified and so is the manifestation of symptoms. The

DOI: 10.4018/978-1-5225-0519-8.ch010

heterogeneity and non-uniformity of symptoms in schizophrenia make every patient unique, demanding a customized therapeutic approach. The illness brings gross impairment in a person's ability of his or her self-care, occupational functioning; ability to relate with family, friends and other people and involve in premorbid activities of interest. The impairment generally happens after onset of the illness, but there are evident literature suggesting a prelude of these impairments even before onset of florid symptoms.

Defining Disability

Defining disability is a complex task, although there have been comprehensive attempts to define disability. The conventional notion of disability in common mass revolves around physical disability, blindness and hearing impairment, but disability is evident in many illness conditions including mental illness, where a person may appear physically fit, but could be severely disabled. Worldwide researchers, policy makers and health care providers have tried to incorporate different dimensions of disability and shift from the medical model to the more inclusive social model while defining disability. The World Health Organization (WHO) describes disability as an umbrella term covering impairments, activity limitations, and participation restrictions; and as a reflection of interaction of the person's limitations and the society he or she lives in (WHO, 2001).

The Nature of Disability in Schizophrenia

If we consider the components of functioning and disability as per the International Classification of Functioning, (WHO, 2001), that are: Body functions, Body structures, Impairments, Activity, Participation, Activity limitations, Participation restrictions and Environmental factors; majority of schizophrenia patients will have impairment in the above domains barring body structures. Patients with schizophrenia have a heterogeneous manifestation of symptoms, and the resultant disability is seen as mild to gross disability in personal, social and occupational functioning. Research studies documenting disability in schizophrenia conventionally take into account tools that measure disability in the domains of personal area, social functioning and occupational functioning.

How Does It Translate to Real World Functioning?

A patient with schizophrenia may have difficulty in initiating as well as maintaining conversation. He may not be that apt in remembering address or phone numbers told verbally. He could be lacking in showing adequate emotional warmth and reciprocation in social situations. At work place he may not be his previous best and have difficulty following instructions, take prompt decisions. They may look disoriented with blank face. People eventually lose job unless not secured. Even at home, he may not be that prompt in activities and may need persuasion to engage in daily routine activities. Depending on the severity of symptoms, a patient with schizophrenia may need an accompanying person always to monitor him whenever stepping out of home. Any or all of these manifestations could be present in a patient with schizophrenia. In one of the early prospective studies from India on disability in schizophrenia; Thara and Rajkumar (1993) mentioned stable course of disability in schizophrenia which was not related to relapse. The findings revealed disability in the domain of personal, social, occupational and global disability; however disability in occupational domain was significantly higher.

Psychosocial Functioning in Schizophrenia

The term can be put close to a person's psychological wellbeing, subjective as well as objective; occupational functioning and social functioning. Diminished psychosocial functioning is synonymous to disability, or poor adjustment, coping or quality of life; which is evident in literature, through assessment of this abstract term by measures of disability in parallel with quality of life, coping and adjustment measures. Psychosocial functioning of an individual is an index of how he or she fares in individual and other social situations, which comes across in daily living. Although normal individual's too experience some decline in their psychosocial functioning across life, but mostly it is situational and temporary and unlike of mentally ill persons, especially in schizophrenia where a gross decline in their psychosocial functioning is observed.

Impaired psychosocial functioning in schizophrenia is mainly observed in domains of occupation, social interaction and communication, family and health. This may sound simple, but is harsh on caregivers who find the patient lacking motivation to carry his or her daily self-care activities, need to be pushed for maintaining his work, reminded and even forced to take prescribed drugs. On top of this, the patient could be unpredictable in his behaviour and could be blaming family members because of poor insight. Impairment in psychosocial functioning in schizophrenia is so evident that research studies have focused more on documenting the causes of it. However, it is worth to measure these impairments that are evident in schizophrenia (Brissos, Molodynski, Vasco Videira Dias, & Figueira, 2011; Goreishizadeh, Mohagheghi, Farhang, & Alizadeh, 2012).

In a study comprising 130 schizophrenia patients, the patients were found no different than normal control on activities of daily living; however, they had performed poorly in activities of Intermediate activities of daily living; mental health; work area; quality of social interaction; and social areas (Mahato, 2011). This particular finding that the subjects were no different in activities of daily life, but significantly differed in intermediate activities of daily life; suggest that schizophrenia patients needed guided supervision and coaxing to come to normal level of functioning, in spite of minimal clinical symptoms. In a comprehensive meta-analytic review, Switaj et al. (2012) reviewed 104 studies concerning psychosocial difficulties in schizophrenia in accordance to the International Classification of Functioning, Disability and Health (ICF). The results revealed that in the domain of activities and participation, the most widely investigated psychosocial difficulty were difficulties in relationships with others (31%), and employment (20%). Other psychosocial difficulties reported were: disability and functioning (38%), quality of life and well-being (23%), global psychosocial functions (9%), looking after one's health (11%), participating in social activities (11%) and skills (10%).

NEUROCOGNITIVE FUNCTIONING IN SCHIZOPHRENIA

Patients of schizophrenia apparently may appear normal and devoid of active symptoms, but could be significantly different from healthy controls when compared over performance on neuropsychological tests. There is evident literature suggesting impaired neuro- cognitive functioning in schizophrenia, which arguably is also the basis of impaired psychosocial functioning in schizophrenia patients. Studies regarding impairment in neurocognitive functions in schizophrenia are presented with a contentious picture. Certain studies have estimated percentage of schizophrenia patients who do not have a cognitive deficit varying from 27% (Palmer et al., 1997) to 55% (Bryson, Silverstein, Nathan, & Stephen,

1993). However more recent studies in the field document that cognitive deficits are found almost in all patients of schizophrenia (Keefe & Harvey, 2012) with evidences of impairment in several cognitive domains two standard deviations below the healthy control mean (Harvey & Keefe, 1997; Heinrichs & Zakzanis, 1998; Saykin et al., 1991)

The cognitive deficits are mostly seen in the domains of executive functions, information processing and attention, learning and memory, psychomotor activity, speech and abstraction. Global literature suggests and supports cognitive impairment in these domains. However, depending on the domain assessed, population and other variables, there could be minor variations. Heinrichs and Zakzanis (1998) in a review of 204 studies, inferred that schizophrenia is characterized by a broadly based cognitive impairment, with varying degrees of deficit in all ability domains measured by standard clinical tests. The domains reported were global and selective verbal memory, nonverbal memory, bilateral and unilateral motor performance, visual and auditory attention, general intelligence, spatial ability, executive function, language, and inter-hemispheric tactile-transfer test performance.

Another recent meta-analytic study (Reichenberg, 2010) summarizes cognitive impairment in schizophrenia in domains of general intellectual ability, attention, executive functions, declarative and working memory, processing speed, Language, perception, visuo-spatial ability, and motor speed. This is important to note that the pattern of cognitive impairment in schizophrenia is similar to that seen in affective psychosis, but the degree of impairment is worse in schizophrenia compared to bipolar disorder and psychotic major depression (Barch & Sheffield, 2014; Bora, Yucel., & Pantelis, 2009), thus the subsequent disability too is ought to be worse than these conditions. Studies from the Indian subcontinent too support the notion of cognitive impairment in schizophrenia. The cognitive domains reported to be impaired are similar to that of western literature (Nizamie, Nizamie., & Shukla, 1992; Srinivasan, Thara & Tirupati, 2005; Halder, Mahato, & Jahan, 2015; Trivedi et al., 2007) to name a few. Certain group of studies cites neurocognitive impairment as a consequence of schizophrenic illness; on the other hand, others have found these neurocognitive impairments evident even before florid onset of symptoms of schizophrenia or in the prodromal phase (Keefe, 2014; Harvey, 2009; Caspi et al., 2003).

Although cognitive impairment is not a formal symptom in the any of the classificatory systems (either DSM or ICD); they are gradually now being seen as an integral part of schizophrenia to the extent that, many researchers imply cognitive impairment as the core the disorder (Elvevag & Goldberg, 2000). Recent developments in the field have seen researchers looking at the prospect of including cognitive impairment as diagnostic criteria of schizophrenia and even proposals been made (Keefe & Fenton, 2007; Keefe, 2008). The importance of neurocognitive functioning in schizophrenia doubles as it is like double disability for the patients. The patients are significantly different compared to normal population on various cognitive assessment tasks. On top of that these tasks are related to functionality level of the patients too.

FACTORS THAT AFFECT PSYCHOSOCIAL FUNCTIONING IN SCHIZOPHRENIA

A host of factors appear to affect psychosocial functioning in schizophrenia. The relative degree of their impact is though variable, researchers agree on the following factors often implicated:

1. Clinical symptoms and affective states,
2. Motivation,
3. Neurocognitive impairment.

Clinical Symptoms

Clinical symptoms of schizophrenia are conventionally described in terms of positive and negative symptoms. It would be very obvious that when a person is having florid symptoms like hallucinations or delusions, he or she would be unable to interact appropriately with people around and could be very confined guided by his or her own abnormal ideas. Subsequently social roles are bound to be unfulfilled. In particular, positive symptoms have been found impacting health adjustment, and Activities of Daily Life of schizophrenia patients, while negative symptoms are more related with occupational adjustment as well as functionality of the schizophrenia patients (Mahato, 2011; Shamsi et al., 2011; Hunter & Barry, 2012; Lin et al., 2013). However, research also suggests that schizophrenia patients have impairment in social competence even when these clinical symptoms are under control or in remission stage (Harvey, 2011). It is important to understand affective state in schizophrenia; as social interaction often is very anxiety provoking and thus individuals avoid interacting with others. They avoid take self-initiation and their subjective normal mood may not be appropriate objectively for social interaction.

Motivational Factors

While clinical symptoms have an impact on social functionality of schizophrenia patients; Individuals with schizophrenia have been found to actively avoid social interaction even after amelioration of symptoms, thus highlighting motivation as a detrimental factor. Underlying this lack of motivation could be past experience of critical comments, feeling of rejection and failure as well as guilt feelings. Patients may fail to cope with prolonged medication and feel hopeless regarding full recovery. Some with better level of insight may be guilt ridden for bringing trouble to family. Majority, if not all schizophrenia patients are subject to critical comments at home as well as workplace. So even if they are willing to improve their social interaction; the past experience could comatose them back. Certain individuals with schizophrenia may continue with their non-productive lifestyle because of conditioned behaviour.

NEUROCOGNITIVE IMPAIRMENT AND PSYCHOSOCIAL FUNCTIONING

While it is understood that all behaviour are moderated by the brain; daily functioning is bound to get impaired in event of cognitive impairment. Schizophrenia patients display gross decline in their activities of daily living and is evidently related to neurocognitive functioning.

Activities of Daily Living

Individuals with schizophrenia face varying degree of difficulty in taking proper self-care. The degree may vary across schizophrenia subtype, but overall figures suggest significant numbers of such patients. Right from maintaining a structured daily routine, waking up timely, cleaning, taking food and most importantly taking medications often require supervision from care givers. Schizophrenia patients could also have difficulty in doing house hold chores, shopping, driving and several other tasks.

Occupational Functioning and Employment

This is a major domain in which schizophrenia patient's fare poorly compared to healthy individuals. Impaired attention and concentration levels are implicated in poor occupational functioning. There could be differences in literature findings across cultures, and these differences generally happen due to the difference of work nature of the individuals assessed and subjective reporting. Individuals with schizophrenia not only find it difficult to sustain their employment, but also find it very difficult to get one. From Indian perspective, where agriculture is a major occupation, individuals with schizophrenia though are not at risk of losing job, but their productivity is certainly reduced. There are several semi-skilled or unskilled occupations which may not require fine motor skills, but do require sustained attention which have an impact on occupational functionality in diminished state. A host of Indian studies infer that impaired cognitive functioning is not related to occupational functioning in Indian subjects and attribute this to better social and familial support (Srinivasan & Tirupati, 2005; Krishnadas, Moore, Nayak., & Patel, 2007; Mahato, 2011). In one of the longest follow up studies in India, employment rates were found as high as 75% at 20 year follow up (Thara, 2004). The same study at 25 years' follow-up reported that out of 24 males, 13 were unemployed, 11 were gainfully employed and supporting themselves and their families. Strong family support in the sample was evident, as nearly 32% of the sample supported themselves financially, while in 36% it was the spouse, 17% parents, and the rest by other relatives (Thara, 2012).

Communication and Social Skills

Thought, language and speech abnormalities are evident during active psychotic phase in schizophrenia. A substantial number of patients show difficulty in regaining the premorbid fluency and clarity in their thought and speech functions. The speech could be coherent, but with delayed reaction time, reduced productivity with monotonous tone and lacking content. Patients could also be lacking behind in showing appropriate emotions, salutations, and initiation to interact with others, even for their daily needs. Some may hesitate to start conversation even for important issues due to anxiety of prolonged talk. This has a direct impact on familial relationship of the patient. While direct care givers may have certain level of insight of patient's behaviour, others may find the patients behaviour repulsive. Emotional apathy shown by the patient also has adverse effect on his/ her marital relations. A contrasting picture is seen in this context where male patients usually are taken care of by their wives, but women patients are at risk of separation or send back to their parental home.

Decision Making

Impaired cognitive abilities are linked to problem solving and decision making capabilities in schizophrenia. Under remission or remitted patients capable of handling their daily chores independently, may find it difficult to handle complex social situations and take prompt decisions. Thus they are trouble free when under supervision, but could be at same functionality level as of a borderline intellect person.

Participation in Community and Leisure Activities

Community and leisure activity participation is just another domain in which schizophrenia patient's fare poorly. Impaired neurocognitive functions in terms of poor attention, executive functions, working memory and language are implicated for this in varying degree across different studies documented below.

SUPPORTIVE FINDINGS

Findings of a study (Mahato, 2011) comprising 130 non- chronic schizophrenia patients from a tertiary care mental hospital from India, which gives a comprehensive view of neurocognitive factors affecting psychosocial functioning in schizophrenia. In the study, neurocognitive and psychosocial functioning of the schizophrenia patients was assessed and compared with normal controls. Neurocognitive functions were assessed using the Wechsler Adult Intelligence Scale-Revised (WAIS-R), Wisconsin Card Sorting Test (WCST) and the Stroop Neuropsychological Screening Test. Psychosocial functioning was assessed across the domains of:

1. Global adjustment (Family, Health, Social, Emotions, Occupation and Sex),
2. Functional status (Activities of Daily Living),
3. Mental Health,
4. Work,
5. Social and Quality of Social Interaction.

Measures used were Global Adjustment Scale, and Functional Status Questionnaire. The findings are relevant from another aspect that the samples were non chronic patients with illness duration of less than two years. Major findings of the study are Social functionality was found significantly correlated with semantic knowledge and verbal fluency, as assessed on Wechsler Adult Intelligence Scale-R (WAIS-R) (McClure et al., 2007; Bowie et al., 2008). Set shifting capability assessed through Stroop test had significant correlation with Intermediate activity of daily life, Mental Health and Work functionality of the schizophrenia patients (Bowie, Reichenberg, Patterson, Heaton., & Harvey, 2006; Leifker, Bowie & Harvey., 2009; Lepage, Bodnar., & Bowie, 2014). Executive functions as assessed on Wisconsin card sorting test (WCST) were significantly correlated with emotion, mental health and work areas of the schizophrenia patients (Hofer et al., 2005; Tabares et al., 2008; Puig et al., 2008). Overall, High predictive value of executive functions, verbal memory, verbal expression, attention, set shifting; problem solving and abstract thinking was indicated for better functioning in social and emotion areas (Green, Kern, Braff., & Mintz, 2000; Addington & Addington, 2000). Better Psychological functioning and emotional adjustment were most reliably predicted by executive functions, verbal memory, problem solving, abstract thinking and general intelligence (Velligan, Bow-Thomas., & Mahurin, 2000). Impaired Occupational functionality and adjustment in the schizophrenia patients could not be explained by cognitive functions in this study, which is in contrast to western literature, but gets support from Indian studies (Krishnadas et al., 2007; Srinivasan & Tirupati, 2005).

INDIRECT DISABILITIES

It is important to stress that schizophrenia often takes a chronic course. A significant proportion of patients fail to regain their premorbid functionality and require long term medication and supervision in daily life activities. This limiting of optimum functionality is not limited to the patient himself, rather also impact caregivers and family members of the patient and is like an indirect disability to them. Managing schizophrenia patients often involves situations beyond control of caregivers.

Mental Health Care Resources

Availability of mental health care resources across the world does not present a very happy picture. The WHO study of worldwide country mental health resources reveal a majority of mentally ill people unable to receive basic treatment (W.H.O, Project ATLAS; 2000-2001). Among 96.9% of all member states of the WHO covering 99.3% of the world's population, it was found that 41% of countries do not have a mental health policy. 25% of countries have no legislation on mental health and 37% of countries do not have mental health community care facilities. Further, more than 25% of countries do not have access to basic psychiatric medication at the primary care level and shockingly 70% of the world's population has access to less than one psychiatrist per 100,000 people.

In Indian context, the Persons with Disability Act 1995, includes mental illness as one of the disabling conditions along with six other conditions that are blindness, low vision, leprosy cured, hearing impairment, locomotor disability and mental retardation. The act is about to be replaced with the rights of persons with disabilities bill, 2014 and covers 19 disability conditions. The bill proposes reservation benefits in education, employment and preference in government schemes for persons with at least 40% disability. It also confers right to friendly access to all public buildings, hospitals, transport modes and polling stations etc. (PRS legislative research, 2014). As of now, the Mental Health Act, 1987 is the prevailing law to dealing with mentally ill persons. Even this act is sought to be replaced by the Mental Health Care bill (Govt. of India[GoI], 2012), that was cleared by Indian cabinet in June 2013, but yet to be approved by the parliament. The bill has tried to overcome the shortcomings of the previous act and provide better and equal provisions for mentally ill people in terms of treatment guidelines, admission policies, right to consent for treatment, provision of medical insurance at par with physical illness etc. to name a few. More importantly the bill defines "mental illness" as a disorder of mood, thought, perception and memory, causing significant distress to a person or impairs his ability to meet demands of daily life.

Cost Factor

Treatment in mental illness like schizophrenia could be a costly affair, considering prolonged medication regime, consultancy and visits to mental health care centers. Many countries including India don't have a comprehensive public health insurance policy. General health insurances otherwise don't cover psychiatric illness; thus treatment is a costly affair. High and recurrent treatment cost could be a risk for poor and improper drug compliance. Care givers may skip medications for certain duration or continue the same drugs without follow-up, risking relapse of symptoms. There is very less literature that speaks on treatment cost as factor for drug compliance, but definitely an issue in country like India, where a large section of clients rely on discounted or free medication from government based hospitals, but fail to continue the treatment once switching to private practitioners.

Care Burden

Caring for a mentally ill patient could be challenging task. It is very distressing for caregivers who are boggled by unpredictable behaviour of the patient, at risk of assault by them and many a times at dark regarding the prognosis of the illness of their patient. This poses as a risk of developing significant stress and depressive symptoms in caregivers and adds to another dimension of disability in schizophrenia. Treatment of schizophrenia should essentially include giving psychoeducation to caregivers regarding nature and symptoms of schizophrenia.

Stigma

Stigma in mental illness, particularly schizophrenia is talked about a lot, but remains a big barrier. It's a disability to not only the patients, but also to caregivers. Stigma in psychotic illnesses like schizophrenia could be multifaceted, like patients being stigmatized by outside people as well as their caregivers. At the same time caregivers too are stigmatized by the society they live in. The biggest impact of stigma is upon seeking proper treatment, as family members try to hide and hesitate to consult mental health professionals. In certain instances, family members try to consult culturally accepted faith healing practices which prolongs the untreated duration and exacerbate the symptoms further. In clinical practice it has been noticed miserably, that at times the patients, especially women are married off without informing the in-laws. The patient either takes medicines covertly or relapses without medication. Family members also deny regarding their wards illness before marriage fearing breaking of the marriage alliance without concerning treatment of the patient. Evidence of psychotic illness dissuades other people to initiate or maintain social relationship or marital alliance among families. This maintains the vicious circle of stigma in the society towards mental illness like schizophrenia. The stigma remains even after the patient has recovered, and affects patient's employment status, both present and future. Thus stigma poses to be one of the biggest social disabilities in patients with schizophrenia.

ASSESSMENT OF DISABILITY IN SCHIZOPHRENIA AND ISSUES

The dimensions of disability in schizophrenia or in psychotic illness are so vast that it is virtually impossible to incorporate all of them in a single tool. The term is often used synonymously with occupational functioning, daily functioning, psychosocial difficulty and community functioning. This is evident from the use of same or similar tools to assess these different but synonymous constructs in different studies. Literature also suggest of studies e.g. Swartz et al. (2007) where psychosocial functioning has been considered solely as quality of life and accordingly measured by Quality of Life scale scores. While it is a good for researchers to use different tools to assess different functionality aspects in schizophrenia, it becomes difficult when a same tool is used to assess different functionality aspects and can lead to different interpretation from a same research. Global organizations like the World Health Organization (W.H.O) have developed framework for conceptualization, definition, classification and measurement of disability in the form of International Classification of Functioning [ICF] (W.H.O, 2001). The W.H.O Disability Assessment Schedule 2.0 (WHODAS 2.0) is another instrument developed by the WHO that is grounded in the conceptual framework of ICF and used across all diseases including mental illness like schizophrenia (WHO, 2001). It directly corresponds to dimensions of activity and participation of the ICF and includes items on Cognition, mobility, self-care, getting along, life activities and participation.

All across the world caregivers of schizophrenia seek for certification for the illness of their wards, that may be used for various welfare purposes and the protocol to issue disability certificates may vary from country to country. From Indian perspective, the Indian Disability Evaluation and Assessment Scale (IDEAS) is a government approved scale for certification of mental illnesses including schizophrenia. Developed by the Rehabilitation Committee of the Indian Psychiatric Society (IPS, 2002) and field tested across nine centres, the scale has good internal consistency and criterion validity compared with the Schedule for Assessment of Psychiatric Disability, standardized in India (Mohan, Tandon, Kalra., & Trivedi, 2005).

Researchers have cautioned regarding changes in disability score while certifying disability in mental illness as severity and manifestation of symptoms in mental illness like schizophrenia could be transient and heterogeneous, and unlike other disabilities where locomotion and access may be the prime concern; social and work functioning are more important in disability due to mental illness (Thara, 2005). One important issue is the subjective perspective of disability in schizophrenia. The objective perception of disability is usually measured through functionality level of the individual, but the subjective perception could be different and include perceived illness burden and impressions of the quality of life. Psychosocial support to the patient will definitely be vital factor in perception of disability in schizophrenia patient and lend support to environmental forces acting upon the patient.

CONCLUSION

Schizophrenia is a grossly disabling disease and the disability is quite different from disabilities seen in other illness. The heterogeneity of the symptoms of schizophrenia, the chronic course followed by the illness and reduced functionality of the individual even after remission of symptoms make schizophrenia a unique psychiatric illness. The disability in schizophrenia is mostly observed in occupational, social and interpersonal domains and has been closely related with neurocognitive impairment in schizophrenia. Minor differences in research findings may be evident regarding domains of impairment in schizophrenia, especially work and occupational area that can be explained by the difference of tools used, population included and family support to patients. However, studies have the same opinion on predictive value of neurocognitive functions in different psychosocial functions in schizophrenia. Considering the importance of neurocognitive functioning and its role in psychosocial functioning of schizophrenia patients, further research is required which could help in formulating better management plan and reduce the disability. Apart from this, researchers and policy makers should also consider about other indirect disabilities arising from environmental and social factors.

REFERENCES

Addington, J., & Addington, D. (2000). Neurocognitive and social functioning in schizophrenia: A 2.5 year follow-up study. *Schizophrenia Research*, *44*(1), 47–56. doi:10.1016/S0920-9964(99)00160-7 PMID:10867311

Barch, D. M., & Sheffield, J. M. (2014). Cognitive impairments in psychotic disorders: Common mechanisms and measurement. *World Psychiatry; Official Journal of the World Psychiatric Association (WPA)*, *13*(3), 224–232. doi:10.1002/wps.20145 PMID:25273286

Bora, E., Yucel, M., & Pantelis, C. (2009). Cognitive functioning in schizophrenia, schizoaffective disorder and affective psychoses: Meta-analytic study. *The British Journal of Psychiatry*, *195*(6), 475–482. doi:10.1192/bjp.bp.108.055731 PMID:19949193

Bowie, C. R., Leung, W. W., Reichenberg, A., McClure, M. M., Patterson, T. L., Heaton, R. K., & Harvey, P. D. (2008). Predicting schizophrenia patients' real-world behavior with specific neuropsychological and functional capacity measures. *Biological Psychiatry*, *63*(5), 505–511. doi:10.1016/j.biopsych.2007.05.022 PMID:17662256

Bowie, C. R., Reichenberg, A., Patterson, T. L., Heaton, R. K., & Harvey, P. D. (2006). Determinants of real-world functional performance in schizophrenia subjects: Correlations with cognition, functional capacity, and symptoms. *The American Journal of Psychiatry*, *163*(3), 418–425. doi:10.1176/appi.ajp.163.3.418 PMID:16513862

Brissos, S., Molodynski, A., Vasco Videira Dias, V. V., & Figueira, M. L. (2011). The importance of measuring psychosocial functioning in schizophrenia. *Annals of General Psychiatry*, *10*(1), 18. doi:10.1186/1744-859X-10-18 PMID:21702932

Bryson, G. J., Silverstein, M. L., Nathan, A., & Stephen, L. (1993). Differential rate of neuropsychological dysfunction in psychiatric disorders: Comparison between the Halstead-Reitan and Luria-Nebraska batteries. *Perceptual and Motor Skills*, *76*, 305–306. PMID:8451141

Caspi, A., Reichenberg, A., Weiser, M., Rabinowitz, J., Kaplan, Z., Knobler, H., & Davidson, M. et al. (2003). Cognitive performance in schizophrenia patients assessed before and following the first psychotic episode. *Schizophrenia Research*, *65*(2-3), 87–94. doi:10.1016/S0920-9964(03)00056-2 PMID:14630301

Elvevag, B., & Goldberg, T. E. (2000). Cognitive impairment in schizophrenia is the core of the disorder. *Critical Reviews in Neurobiology*, *14*(1), 1–21. doi:10.1615/CritRevNeurobiol.v14.i1.10 PMID:11253953

Goreishizadeh, M. A., Mohagheghi, A., Farhang, S., & Alizadeh, L. (2012). Psychosocial Disabilities in Patients with Schizophrenia. *Iranian Journal of Public Health*, *41*(5), 116–121. PMID:23113186

Govt. of India. (2012). *Draft Mental Health Care Bill.* Retrieved from http://mohfw.nic.in/WriteReadData/l892s/6420662643DRAFT%20THE%20MENTAL%20HEALTH%20CARE%20BILL.pdf

Green, M. F. (1996). What are the functional consequences of neurocognitive deficits in schizophrenia? *The American Journal of Psychiatry*, *153*(3), 321–330. doi:10.1176/ajp.153.3.321 PMID:8610818

Green, M. F., Kern, R. S., Braff, D. L., & Mintz, J. (2000). Neurocognitive deficits and functional outcome in schizophrenia: Are we measuring the "right stuff"? *Schizophrenia Bulletin*, *26*(1), 119–136. doi:10.1093/oxfordjournals.schbul.a033430 PMID:10755673

Halder, S., Mahato, A., & Jahan, M. (2015). Cognitive profile of paranoid schizophrenia on LNNB. *The international. Journal of Indian Psychology*, *2*(3), 174–181.

Harvey, P. D. (2009). When Does Cognitive Decline Occur in the Period Prior to the First Episode of Schizophrenia? *Psychiatry*, *6*(7), 12–14. PMID:19724764

Harvey, P. D. (2011). Mood Symptoms, Cognition, and Everyday Functioning in Major Depression, Bipolar Disorder, and Schizophrenia. *Innovations in Clinical Neuroscience*, *8*(10), 14–18. PMID:22132366

Harvey, P. D., & Keefe, R. S. E. (1997). Cognitive impairment in schizophrenia and implications of atypical neuroleptic treatment. *CNS Spectrums*, *2*, 1–11.

Heinrichs, R. W., & Zakzanis, K. K. (1998). Neurocognitive deficit in schizophrenia: A quantitative review of the evidence. *Neuropsychology*, *12*(3), 426–445. doi:10.1037/0894-4105.12.3.426 PMID:9673998

Hofer, A., Baumgartner, S., Bodner, T., Edlinger, M., Hummer, M., Kemmler, G., & Fleischhacker, W. W. et al. (2005). Patient outcomes in schizophrenia II: The impact of cognition. *European Psychiatry*, *20*(5-6), 395–402. doi:10.1016/j.eurpsy.2005.02.006 PMID:16171654

Hunter, R., & Barry, S. (2012). Negative symptoms and psychosocial functioning in schizophrenia: Neglected but important targets for treatment. *European Psychiatry*, *27*(6), 432–436. doi:10.1016/j.eurpsy.2011.02.015 PMID:21602034

Indian Psychiatric Society. (2002). *IDEAS (Indian Disability Evaluation and Assessment Scale) - A scale for measuring and quantifying disability in mental disorders.* Retrieved from http://www.indianjpsychiatry.org/cpg/cpg2009/article3.pdf

Keefe, R. S. E. (2008). Should cognitive impairment be included in the diagnostic criteria for schizophrenia? *World Psychiatry; Official Journal of the World Psychiatric Association (WPA)*, *7*(1), 22–28. doi:10.1002/j.2051-5545.2008.tb00142.x PMID:18458774

Keefe, R. S. E. (2014). The Longitudinal course of cognitive impairment in schizophrenia: An examination of data from premorbid through post treatment phases of illness. *The Journal of Clinical Psychiatry*, *75*(2suppl 2), 8–13. doi:10.4088/JCP.13065su1.02 PMID:24919165

Keefe, R. S. E., & Fenton, W. S. (2007). How Should DSM-V Criteria for Schizophrenia Include Cognitive Impairment? *Schizophrenia Bulletin.* Retrieved from schizophreniabulletin.oxfordjournals.org/content/early/2007/06/13/schbul.sbm046. full.pdf

Keefe, R. S. E., & Harvey, P. D. (2012). Cognitive Impairment in Schizophrenia. In M. A. Geyer & G. Gross (Eds.), Handbook of Experimental Pharmacology: Vol. 213. *Novel Antischizophrenia Treatments* (pp. 11–37). Springer-Verlag Berlin Heidelberg. doi:10.1007/978-3-642-25758-2_2

Krishnadas, R., Moore, B. P., Nayak, A., & Patel, R. R. (2007). Relationship of cognitive function in patients with schizophrenia in remission to disability: A cross-sectional study in an Indian sample. *Annals of General Psychiatry*, *6*(1), 19. http://www.annals-general-psychiatry.com/content/6/1/19 doi:10.1186/1744-859X-6-19 PMID:17663763

Leifker, F. R., Bowie, C. R., & Harvey, P. D. (2009). Determinants of everyday outcomes in schizophrenia: The influences of cognitive impairment, functional capacity, and symptoms. *Schizophrenia Research*, *115*(1), 82–87. doi:10.1016/j.schres.2009.09.004 PMID:19775869

Lepage, M., Bodnar, M., & Bowie, C. R. (2014). Neurocognition: Clinical and Functional Outcomes in Schizophrenia. *Canadian Journal of Psychiatry*, *59*(1), 5–12. PMID:24444318

Lin, C. H., Huang, C. L., Chang, Y. C., Chen, P. W., Lin, C. Y., Tsai, G. E., & Lane, H. Y. (2013). Clinical symptoms, mainly negative symptoms, mediate the influence of neurocognition and social cognition on functional outcome of schizophrenia. *Schizophrenia Research*, *146*(1-3), 231–237. doi:10.1016/j.schres.2013.02.009 PMID:23478155

Mahato, A. (2011). *A correlational study of neurocognitive factors and psychosocial functioning in schizophrenic patients.* (Unpublished Doctoral dissertation). RINPAS, Ranchi University, Ranchi, India.

McClure, M. M., Bowie, C. R., Patterson, T. L., Heaton, R. K., Weaver, C., Anderson, H., & Harvey, P. D. (2007). Correlations of functional capacity and neuropsychological performance in older patients with schizophrenia: Evidence for specificity of relationships? *Schizophrenia Research*, *89*(1-3), 330–338. doi:10.1016/j.schres.2006.07.024 PMID:16982175

Mohan, I., Tandon, R., Kalra, H., & Trivedi, J. K. (2005). Disability assessment in mental illnesses using Indian Disability Evaluation Assessment Scale (IDEAS). *The Indian Journal of Medical Research*, *121*, 759–763. PMID:16037620

Nizamie, A., Nizamie, S. H., & Shukla, T. R. (1992). Performance on Luria - Nebraska Neuropsychological Battery in Schhizophrenic Patients. *Indian Journal of Psychiatry*, *34*, 321–330. PMID:21776138

Palmer, B. W., Heaton, R. K., Paulsen, J. S., Kuck, J., Braff, D., Harris, M. J., & Jeste, D. V. et al. (1997). Is it possible to be schizophrenic yet neuropsychologically normal? *Neuropsychology*, *11*(3), 437–446. doi:10.1037/0894-4105.11.3.437 PMID:9223148

PRS Legislative Research. (2014). *Legislative brief. The Rights of Persons with Disabilities Bill.* Retrieved March 12, 2015, from http://www.prsindia.org/uploads/media/Person%20with%20Disabilities/Legislative%20Brief%20%20-%20Disabilities%202014.pdf

Puig, O., Penades, R., Gasto, C., Catalan, R., Torres, A., & Salamero, M. (2008). Verbal memory, negative symptomatology and prediction of psychosocial functioning in schizophrenia. *Psychiatry Research*, *158*(1), 11–17. doi:10.1016/j.psychres.2007.04.017 PMID:18001844

Reichenberg, A. (2010). The assessment of neuropsychological functioning in schizophrenia. *Dialogues in Clinical Neuroscience*, *12*(3), 383–392. PMID:20954432

Saykin, A. J., Gur, R. C., Gur, R. E., Mozley, P. D., Mozley, L. H., Resnick, S. M., & Stafiniak, P. et al. (1991). Neuropsychological function in schizophrenia. Selective impairment in memory and learning. *Archives of General Psychiatry*, *48*(7), 618–624. doi:10.1001/archpsyc.1991.01810310036007 PMID:2069492

Shamsi, S., Lau, A., Lencz, T., Burdick, K. E., DeRosse, P., Brenner, R., & Malhotra, A. K. et al. (2011). Cognitive and symptomatic predictors of functional disability in schizophrenia. *Schizophrenia Research*, *126*(1-3), 257–264. doi:10.1016/j.schres.2010.08.007 PMID:20828991

Srinivasan, L., Thara, R., & Tirupati, S. N. (2005). Cognitive dysfunction and associated factors in patients with chronic schizophrenia. *Indian Journal of Psychiatry*, *47*(3), 139–143. doi:10.4103/0019-5545.55936 PMID:20814455

Srinivasan, L., & Tirupati, S. (2005). Relationship between cognition and work functioning among patients with schizophrenia in an urban area of India. *Psychiatric Services (Washington, D.C.)*, *56*(11), 1423–1428. doi:10.1176/appi.ps.56.11.1423 PMID:16282262

Swartz, M. S., Perkins, D. O., Stroup, T. S., Davis, S. M., Capuano, G., Rosenheck, R. A., & Lieberman, J. A. et al. (2007). Effects of antipsychotic medications on psychosocial functioning in patients with chronic schizophrenia: Findings from the NIMH CATIE Study. *The American Journal of Psychiatry*, *164*(3), 428–436. doi:10.1176/ajp.2007.164.3.428 PMID:17329467

Switaj, P., Anczewska, M., Chrostek, A., Sabariego, C., Cieza, A., Bickenbach, J., & Chatterji, S. (2012). Disability and schizophrenia: A systematic review of experienced psychosocial difficulties. *BMC Psychiatry*, *12*(1), 193. doi:10.1186/1471-244X-12-193 PMID:23137171

Tabares-Seisdedos, R., Balanza-Martínez, V., Sanchez-Moreno, J., Martinez-Aran, A., Salazar-Fraile, J., Selva-Vera, G., & Vieta, E. (2008). Neurocognitive and clinical predictors of functional outcome in patients with schizophrenia and bipolar I disorder at one-year follow-up. *Journal of Affective Disorders*, *109*(3), 286–299. doi:10.1016/j.jad.2007.12.234 PMID:18289698

Thara, R. (2004). Twenty-year course of schizophrenia: The Madras Longitudinal Study. *Canadian Journal of Psychiatry*, *49*, 564–569. PMID:15453106

Thara, R. (2005). Measurement of psychiatric disability. *The Indian Journal of Medical Research*, *121*, 723–724. PMID:16037616

Thara, R. (2012). Twenty-five years of schizophrenia: The Madras Longitudinal Study. *Indian Journal of Psychiatry*, *54*(2), 134–137. doi:10.4103/0019-5545.99531 PMID:22988319

Thara, R., & Rjkumar, S. (1993). Nature and course of disability in schizophrenia. *Indian Journal of Psychiatry*, *35*(1), 33–35. PMID:21776165

Trivedi, J. K., Goel, D., Sharma, S., Singh, A. P., Sinha, P. K., & Tandon, R. (2007). Cognitive functions in stable schizophrenia & euthymic state of bipolar disorder. *The Indian Journal of Medical Research*, *126*, 433–439. PMID:18160747

Velligan, D. I., Bow-Thomas, C. C., Mahurin, R. K., Miller, A. L., & Halgunseth, L. C. (2000). Do specific neurocognitive deficits predict specific domains of community function in schizophrenia? *The Journal of Nervous and Mental Disease*, *188*(8), 518–524. doi:10.1097/00005053-200008000-00007 PMID:10972571

World Health Organization. (2001). *Project Atlas: Mapping mental health resources around the world.* Retrieved March 12, 2015, from http://www.who.int/ whr/2001/media_centre/en/ whr01_fact_sheet3_en.pdf

World Health Organization. (2001). *International Classification of Functioning*. Geneva: Disability and Health.

KEY TERMS AND DEFINITIONS

Disability: Disability is an umbrella term covering impairments, activity limitations, and participation restrictions; and a reflection of interaction of the person's limitations and the society he or she lives in that is secondary to some illness or bodily condition.

Neurocognitive Impairment: The impairment of cognitive functions of a person following a neurological illness, mental illness and drug use or brain injury. Most common cognitive domains are attention, memory and executive functions.

Psychosocial Functioning: Psychosocial functioning is a multidimensional construct and generally indicated by an individual's effective functioning in the domains of personal well-being, occupation, daily living activities, social relations and interactions. The impact of mental illness on psychosocial functioning is highly documented.

Schizophrenia: Schizophrenia is a psychiatric illness characterized by abnormalities in thought, perception, language and speech. The symptoms are manifested variably in combination of hallucinations, delusions, impaired reality contact and abnormal behaviour.

Chapter 11
Chronic Mental Illness in Prisons: Global Scenario

Meghamala S Tavaragi
Dharwad Institute of Mental Health and Neurosciences, India

ABSTRACT

It has been known that psychiatric disorders are highly prevalent among prisoners. Many people with identifiable psychiatric illness do conflict with the law, often by no fault of their own but because of symptoms of their psychiatric illness and end up in jails. Poor communication between the prison, court, and hospital systems hinders the assessment and management of the mentally disordered offender, and medical intervention can actually delay release from custody. In conclusion Prisons are detrimental to mental-health, and the standards of psychiatric care are significantly lower than those for the general public. Certain remedial measures are to be implemented for a better future of prison and community because ultimately these prisoners will be released from prison and become a part of community. Beginning of reforms is the immediate need as a long journey ahead.

INTRODUCTION

Mental Health and Prison

Mental disorders occur at high rates in all countries of the world. An estimated 450 million people worldwide suffer from mental or behavioural disorders (World Health Report,. 2001). These disorders are especially prevalent in prison populations (Brinded, 2001; Brugha, 2005; Holley, Arboleda, & Love, 1995).The disproportionately high rate of mental disorders in prisons is related to several factors: the widespread misconception that all people with mental disorders are a danger to the public; the general intolerance of many societies to difficult or disturbing behavior, the failure to promote treatment, care and rehabilitation, and above all, the lack of, or poor access to, mental health services in many countries. Many of these disorders may be present before admission to prison, and may be further exacerbated by

DOI: 10.4018/978-1-5225-0519-8.ch011

the stress of imprisonment. However, mental disorders may also develop during imprisonment itself as a consequence of prevailing conditions and also possibly due to torture or other human rights violations. Prisons are bad for mental health. There are factors in many prisons that have negative effects on mental health, including: overcrowding, various forms of violence, enforced solitude or conversely, lack of privacy, lack of meaningful activity, isolation from social networks, insecurity about future prospects (work, relationships etc), and inadequate health services, especially mental health services, in prisons. The increased risk of suicide in prisons (often related to depression) is, unfortunately, one common manifestation of the cumulative effects of these factors. Prisons are sometimes used as dumping grounds for people with mental disorders. In some countries, people with severe mental disorders are inappropriately locked up in prisons simply because of the lack of mental health services. People with substance abuse disorders or people who, at least in part due to a mental disorder, have committed minor offences are often sent to prison rather than treated for their disorder. These disorders therefore continue to go unnoticed, undiagnosed and untreated.

It has been known that psychiatric disorders are highly prevalent among prisoners (Coid, 1984). Many people with identifiable psychiatric illness do conflict with the law, often by no fault of their own but because of symptoms of their psychiatric illness and end up in jails. Such symptoms include impaired judgment, lack of impulse control, suspiciousness, disinhibition, paranoia, inability to trust others, delusions and hallucinations. It is quite likely that act of incarceration may well exacerbate underlying psychiatric conditions. The effect of such incarceration may well be so severe as to precipitate mental abnormality in vulnerable individuals (Coid, 1984). Different levels of stress during incarceration give rise to different incidence of psychiatric morbidity among remand prisoners (Anderson et al., 2000).

PRISONS AND PRISONER STATISTICS IN WORLD

More than 10.1 million people are held in penal institutions throughout the world, mostly as pre-trial detainees/remand prisoners or as sentenced prisoners. Almost half of these are in the United States (2.29m), Russia (0.81m) or China (1.65m sentenced prisoners). In addition, more than 650,000 are in 'detention centres' in China; if these are included the overall Chinese total is over 2.3 million and the world total more than 10.75 million. The United States has the highest prison population rate in the world, 743 per 100,000 of the national population, followed by Rwanda (c. 595), Russia (568), Georgia (547), U.S. Virgin Is. (539), Seychelles (507), St Kitts & Nevis (495), British Virgin Is. (468), Belize (439), Dominica (431), Bermuda (428), Grenada (423) and Curacao (422). However, more than half the countries and territories (54%) have rates below 150 per 100,000. The world population at mid-2010 was estimated at 6.9 billion (United Nations); if set against the world prison population of 10.1 million this would produce a world prison population rate of 146 per 100,000 (156 per 100,000 if set against a world prison population of 10.75 million).

Prison population rates vary considerably between different regions of the world, and between different parts of the same continent, for example:

1. In Africa the median rate for western African countries is 47.5 whereas for southern African countries it is 219.
2. In the Americas the median rate for South American countries is 175 whereas for Caribbean countries it is 357.5.

3. In Asia the median rate for south central Asian countries (mainly the Indian sub-continent) is 42 whereas for eastern Asian countries it is 155.5.
4. In Europe the median rate for western European countries is 96 whereas for the countries spanning Europe and Asia (e.g. Russia & Turkey) it is 228.
5. In Oceania (including Australia and New Zealand) the median rate is 135.

Prison populations are growing in all five continents. Updated information on countries included in previous editions of the World Prison Population List shows that prison populations have risen in 78% of countries (in 71% of countries in Africa, 82% in the Americas, 80% in Asia, 74% in Europe and 80% in Oceania (Walmsley, 2005).

There are over 10 million prisoners worldwide (Fazel & Seewald, 2012), a population that has been growing by about 1 million per decade. In 2008, the USA had the largest number of people imprisoned at 2.3 million and the highest rate per head of population (at 756 per 100 000 people compared with a median of 145 per 100 000 worldwide), and China, Russia, Brazil and India had more than a quarter of a million prisoners each ((Fazel & Seewald, 2012), It has been widely reported that prisoners have elevated rates of psychiatric disorders compared with the general population, including for psychosis, depression, personality disorder and substance misuse, which are risk factors for elevated suicide rates (Baillargeon, Penn, Thomas, Temple, & Murray, 2009; Fazel, Cartwright, Norman-Nott, & Hawton, 2008) premature mortality on release from prison (Kariminia et al., 2007) and increased reoffending rates (Fazel, & Yu, 2011; Baillargeon, Binswanger., & Murray, 2009).

PRISONS AND PRISONER STATISTICS IN INDIA

During the ancient times, 'Prisons' were considered as a 'House of Captives' where the prisoners were held for deterrent and retributory punishment. Determined and sustained efforts of the thinkers and human right activists in this field led to progressive transformation of the concept of 'deterrence and retribution' into 'reformation and rehabilitation'. Therefore, under the modern correctional philosophy prisons are now considered as correctional institutions where the prisoners are sent after punishment for their reformation and rehabilitation. Prisons have now been considered as a 'community', reflecting the multifaceted socio-cultural, socio-economic and socio-political scenario of the society as a whole. Prisoners of all sections of society are confined in prisons and conscious efforts are being made to provide such conditions to the prisoners in prisons as are conducive to their physical as well as mental treatment and care, and to maintain their human dignity, as also visualized by Indian father of the Nation, Mahatma Gandhi. Mahatma Gandhi had visualized crime and prisons in therapeutic context and observed that 'Crime is the outcome of a disease mind and jail must have an environment of hospital for their treatment and care'. This principle has become a State Policy in India and efforts have all along been made to protect all basic rights of prisoners to maintain their human dignity during the period of their incarceration. In India, prison is State subject. Thus, States have the primary role, responsibility and authority w. r. t. prison laws, rules and regulations.

Prison Statistics of India – 2012

Total number of jails in the country are 1,394, Central jails-127, District jails-340, Sub jails-806, Women jails-20, Open jails-46, Borstal schools-21, Special jails-31 and Other jails-3. Total capacity of jails in the country is 3,43,169. Central jails-1,46,648 (42.7%), District jails-1,26,110 (36.7%), Sub jails-48,474 (14.1%). Women jails-4,817 (1.4%), Open jails-4,028 (1.2%), Borstal schools-2,438 (0.7%), Special jails-10,331 (3.0%) and other jails-323 (0.1%). Total number of jail inmates as on 31.12.2013 is 3,85,135; Male-3,68,184 (95.6%), Female-16,951 (4.4%). Occupancy rate in 2010-115.1%, 2011-112.1%, 2012-112.2%.

1. Convicts are 1,27,789 (33.2% of total inmates), Male-1,22,776 (96.1% of total convicts), Female-5,013 (3.9% of total convicts).
2. Under trials are 2,54,857 (66.2% of total inmates), Male-2,43,055 (95.4% of total under trials), Female-11,802 (4.6% of total under trials).
3. Detenues are 1,922 (0.5% of total inmates), Male-1,832 (95.3% of total detenues), Female-90 (4.7% of total detenues) others-567 (0.1% of total inmates).

The highest number of 80,311 inmates (77,148 male and 3,163 female) were reported from Uttarϖ Pradesh (20.9%) followed by Madhya Pradesh 33,959 (32,778 male and 1,181 female), Bihar 28,550 (27,622 male and 928 female), Maharashtra 24,509 (23,171 male and 1,338 female) and Punjab 23,219 (21,944 male and 1,275 female) at the end of the year 2012. Chhattisgarh reported the highest overcrowding in prisons (252.6%) followed by Delhi (193.8%). A total of 344 women convicts with their 382 children and 1,226 women under trials with their 1,397 children were lodged in various prisons in the country at the end of 2012. A total of 4,470 inmates having mental illness out of 3,38,135 inmates, accounting for 1.2% of total inmates, were lodged in various jails during 2012. Prison population is number of prisoners kept in prison at any given point of time. The prison population keeps changing because of addition of new prisoners and release of the old ones (Prison Statistics India, 2012).

STATISTICS OF INCIDENCE AND PREVALENCE OF MENTAL ILLNESS IN PRISONS ACROSS THE WORLD

Country Wise

1. According to a new report from the Treatment Advocacy Center (TAC), a nonprofit advocacy organization, the United States has fully returned to the 18th-century model of incarcerating the mentally ill in correctional institutions rather than treating them in health care facilities like any other sick people. In 2012, there were roughly 356,268 inmates with severe mental illnesses in prisons and jails, while only 35,000 people with the same diseases were in state psychiatric hospitals (Mencimer, 2014).
2. The failure to treat the mentally ill properly in hospitals is directly related to recent violent crimes. In case of Virginia, where the largest mental institution is the largest state prison and the state's jails hold three times more people with serious mental illnesses than the state hospitals do. The problem is so bad that in 2011, a Virginia Beach sheriff offered to transfer part of his jail budget to

the mental-health system to try to get some of the sick people out of his institution and into proper care (Brownell, 2014).

3. The United States has the highest rate of adult incarceration among the developed countries, with 2.2 million currently in jails and prisons. Those with mental disorders have been increasingly incarcerated during the past three decades, probably as a result of the deinstitutionalization of the state mental health system. Correctional institutions have become the *de facto* state hospitals, and there are more seriously and persistently mentally ill in prisons than in all state hospitals in the United States. A study by Doris and Lauren (2006) the U.S. Department of Justice found that more than half of all prison and jail inmates have a mental health problem compared with 11 percent of the general population, yet only one in three prison inmates and one in six jail inmates receive any form of mental health treatment (Tanay, 2007).
4. According to the Bureau of Justice Statistics, 56 percent of state prisoners and 45 percent of federal prisoners have symptoms or a recent history of mental health problems (Doris & Lauren, 2006). Prisoners have high rates of mental illness-including such serious disorders as schizophrenia, bipolar disorder, and major depression-that are two to four times higher than members of the general public.
5. The numbers are staggering: over the past 15 years, the number of mentally ill people in prison in California has almost doubled (California Department of Corrections and Rehabilitation report [CDCRR], 2014). Today, 45 percent of state prison inmates have been treated for severe mental illness within the past year. The Los Angeles County Jail is "the largest mental health provider in the county," according to the former official in charge of the facility (Los Angeles Times, 2010). As usual, what started in California spread throughout the country.In 1971 there were 20,000 people in California prisons; by 2010 the population had increased to 162,000 people, of which 45 percent are estimated to be mentally ill (CDCRR, 2014).
6. South Africa has a rapidly growing prison population and has the most prisoners amongst all African countries. It also has the world's seventh highest number of prisoners, outranking countries with up to nearly five times its population. In the continent of Africa, South Africa has the highest ratio of prisoners to total population; 348 prisoners for every 100, 000 people. International studies have consistently shown a high prevalence of mental disorders among prisoners.

Butler et al. (1997) in New South Wales, Australia screened both sentenced and reception prisoners and found that 43% of those prisoners screened had at least one of the following mental diagnoses: psychosis, anxiety or affective disorders in the past 12 months.

Study in Canada comparing the prevalence of mental disorders in prisoners and the community found a very high rate of Axis 1 disorders among prisoners. Prisoners had a 91.7% lifetime prevalence of psychiatric disorders while 76.7% showed symptoms in the past six months. This study also found a high rate of comorbidity with substance use disorders (Naidoo & Mkize, 2012). Prison population in Durban, South Africa, one of the largest prisons in the Southern hemisphere.193 prisoners were interviewed using the Mini Neuro-psychiatric Interview, a screening questionnaire and a demographic questionnaire. The study demonstrated that 55.4% of prisoners had an Axis 1 disorder. The commonest disorder being substance and alcohol use disorders (42.0%). 23.3% of prisoners were diagnosed with current psychotic, bipolar, depressive and anxiety disorders. 46.1% were diagnosed with antisocial personality disorder (Naidoo & Mkize, 2012).

PERCENTAGE PREVALENCE OF VARIOUS PSYCHIATRIC ILLNESSES IN PRISONS: INTERNATIONAL PERSEPECTIVE

Indian Scenario

Somsundram (1997) studied 53 criminal patients admitted to the Government Mental Hospital. It was found that 40 of them suffered from schizophrenia, 10 from affective disorders (3 mania and 7 depression), 1 epilepsy and 2 temporary insanity. The criminal patients who were inpatients in the Government Mental Hospital Madras during 1972 were taken into consideration by Somsundram (1974). Only guilty but insane (19) out of total 79 inpatients were studied and he found that 18 were schizophrenic. Jha (1968) studied case records of criminal patients admitted in Ranchi Mansik Arogyashala and found 338 schizophrenic patients out of 1011 criminal patients admitted there during the years 1925 to 1963 giving an incidence of 33%. Singh and Verma (1976) in an Indian Prison study, studied 50 consecutive subjects convicted of murder or attempt to murder and imprisoned at Central Jail Amritsar from January 1970 onwards. Fifteen (30%) of the subjects were found to have no evidence of psychiatric illness. The most common diagnosis was anxiety neurosis in 4 (8%) and depressive reaction in 8 (16%) cases. Psychopathic personality disorder was found in 8 (16%) cases, schizophrenia in 2 (4%), sexual deviation in 2 (4%), alcohol addiction in 6 (12%) and opium dependence in 5 (10%). Mohan and Dhar (2001) assessed 120 under trials as per ICD-10 and 9% were diagnosed having different psychiatric disorder. Twenty-eight percent suffered from schizophrenic psychosis, 13% from MDP, 14% from anxiety state and depression, 9% from malingering and 7% from seizure disorder in the assessed number of under trials. Pre-existing psychiatric illness before committing major crime was detected in 35% of under trials referred.

Distribution of total sample according to total period of stay among prisoners with and without psychiatric illness (*N*=500). Among prisoners without psychiatric illness, 39.90% stayed for 3–6 years, 22.83% stayed for 1–3 years, 16.54% stayed for 6–9 years, 12.86% stayed for less than 1 year, 4.72% stayed for 9–12 years and 3.15% stayed for >12 years see the Table 1, (Sandeep, Paramjit, & Aseem, 2011). A study commissioned by the National Commission for Women in the Central Prison, Bangalore (Murthy et al., 1998), found higher rates of symptoms of common mental disorder among under trials compared to convict prisoners. Common symptoms were unhappiness (73% versus 43%), worrying (65% versus 29%), poor sleep and appetite (65% of under trials). In the recent Prison Mental Health Study (Math et

Table 1. Distribution of total sample according to total period of stay among prisoners with and without psychiatric illness (N=500) age

Duration of Stay (in Years)	Prisoners with Psychiatric Illness		Prisoners without Psychiatric Illness	
	No	%	No	%
<1	8	6.72	49	12.86
1-3	15	12.61	87	22.83
3-6	57	47.90	152	39.90
6-9	30	25.21	63	16.54
9-12	5	4.20	18	4.72
>12	4	3.36	12	3.15
	119	100.0	381	100.0

Table 2. Prevalence of common mental disorders among prisoners in Central Prison, Bangalore

Disorder	Lifetime Diagnosis %	Current Diagnosis %
Panid disorder	1.0	0.9
Agoraphobia	0.3	0.2
Social Phobia	1.8	0.6
Obsessive compulsive disorder	-	0.1
Post traumatic stress disorder	-	0.3
Generalised anxiety disorder	-	0.3
Hypochondriasis	-	0.1
Body dysmorphic disorder	-	0.8
Somatisation	2.1	1.7
Pain disorder	-	5.4

(Suresh, Pratima, Rajani, Naveen & Madhusudhan, 2011)

al., 2011), of 197 women who were interviewed for psychiatric morbidity, 2.5% had dysthymia (minor depression), 4.6% had specific phobia, 1.5% social phobia and one person had a panic disorder. Among the entire prison population evaluated for this study (5024), lifetime and current rates of dysthymia were 2.9% and 2.5% respectively. Prevalence of major depressive disorders was relatively higher. Similarly in another study done by Suresh, Pratima, Rajani, Naveen, and Madhusudhan (2011) Prevalence of common mental disorders among prisoners in Central Prison, Bangalore, was shown in Table 2.

World Scenario

1. Steadman, Fabisiak, Dvoskin, and Holohean (1987) studied a random sample of 3332 inmates representing 9.4% of New York's general prison population as well as 352 of the 360 inmates in the prison's mental health units. They found that 8% of the sample had severe psychiatric functional disabilities that clearly warranted some type of mental health intervention, and another 16% had significant mental disabilities that required periodic services (specific diagnoses were not given). Agbahowe, Fabisiak, Dvoskin and Holohean (1998) conducted a study to find prevalence of psychiatric morbidity among convicted inmates at a medium security prison in Nigeria. They assessed 100 inmates and found schizophrenia in 2, major depression in 2, recurrent mild depression in 21, generalized anxiety disorder in 8 and somatization disorder in 1. Maden, Swinton and Gunn (1992) did retrospective, self-report survey of pre-arrest drug use in a representative sample of 1751 men serving a prison sentence. Reported drugs used were cannabis (34%), opiates (9%), amphetamines (9%) and cocaine (5%), including 1% 'Crack' users. Pre-arrest injecting was reported by 11% of inmates. Drug dependence was reported by 11%, including 7% dependent on opiates, 2% on amphetamines and 1% on cocaine. Mason, Birmingham and Grubin (1997) concluded that of 548 newly remanded prisoners studied, 57% men were using illicit drugs and 33% met DSM-IV drug misuse or dependence criteria. Thirty two percent met misuse or dependence criteria for alcohol.
2. Prisoners have a higher incidence of mental health problems, in particular, neurotic disorders, compared to the general population (Marshall & Orr, 1999). In male prisoners, the prevalence of any neurotic disorder in the week before the study was, 59% in remand and 40% in sentenced pris-

oners. In female prisoners, 76% and 63% of remanded and sentenced prisoners respectively had a neurotic disorder. Estimates of mental health morbidity in UK local prisons, HMP Littlehey and HMP Whitemoor, show a high prevalence of personality and neurotic disorders of 64% and 40% respectively. This translates to a heavy burden of illness, with about 723 inmates with personality disorders and 452 with neurotic disorders in the two prisons. The prevalence rates for self-harm and suicide (7%) were also high (Joint Strategic Needs Assessment, 2008). The Office of National Statistics survey was carried out in 131 of the 133 English and Welsh prisons. Of 51,834 remanded and sentenced males, 5% were interviewed as the initial sample. 6,500 of that sample group had personality disorders, 55% had neurotic disorders, 60% showed hazardous drinking in the year prior to incarceration and 10% had psychiatric disorders. 62% of sentenced women and up to 81% of those on remand reported sleep problems. 54% of women prisoners reported symptoms of depression.

Women prisoners were about twice as likely as men to suffer from post-traumatic stress than male prisoners (Singleton et al, 1998). Eating disorders presented in over 6% of women in the sample who were diagnosed with anorexia. Rates for bulimia were higher, at 14% for the whole sample (15% for remand and 14% for sentenced prisoners). 59% of remand and 40% of sentenced male prisoners in England and Wales had a neurotic disorder, the corresponding figures for women were 76% and 63%. Sixty percent of the women who took part in the study had mental disorders; 35% had diagnoses of personality disorder; none had psychotic disorders (such as schizophrenia for example); 35% had current neurotic disorders (such as depression, anxiety disorders and phobias), nearly all of whom were depressed; 13% had been drinking alcohol at hazardous levels in the year prior to imprisonment, and 36% had been abusing or were dependent on drugs in the year prior to imprisonment. None of the participants reported using alcohol or drugs in prison (Suresh, Pratima, Rajani, Naveen & Madhusudhan, 2011).

3. The overall prevalence of 3.7% of male and female prisoners with a psychotic illness, and 11.4% with major depression have not materially changed since a 2002 review based on 56 publications of mental illness (Fazel, & Danesh, 2002).
4. There were five publications since 2001 that reported rates of comorbidity in prisoners (Assadi et al., 2006; Bermu´ dez, Romero Mendoza, Rodrı´guez Ruiz, Durand-Smith & Saldı´var Herna´ ndez., 2007; Butler & Allnutt., 2003; Duffy, Linehan & Kennedy, 2006, & Piselli, Elisei, Murgia, Quartesan & Abram, 2009).These rates ranged from 20.4 to 43.5% in those with any mental disorder who had comorbid substance misuse, from 13.6 to 95.0% in prisoners with psychotic illnesses with comorbid substance misuse, and 9.2 to 82.5% in individuals with mood disorders and major depression with concurrent substance misuse.
5. A systematic review of 62 surveys of the incarcerated population from 12 Western countries showed that, among the men, 3.7 percent had psychotic illness, 10 percent major depression, and 65 percent a personality disorder, including 47 percent with antisocial personality disorder. Among the women, 4 percent had psychosis, 12 percent major depression, and 42 percent a personality disorder. In addition, a significant number suffered from anxiety disorders, including post-traumatic stress disorder (PTSD), organic disorders, short- and long-term sequelae of traumatic brain injury (TBI), suicidal behaviors, distress associated with all forms of abuse, attention deficit hyperactivity disorder (ADHD), and other developmental disorders, including mental retardation and Asperger's syndrome. Approximately 70 percent had primary or comorbid substance abuse disorders (Tanay, 2007).

6. The suicide rate in prisons is almost 15 times higher than in the general population: in 2002 the rate was 143 per 100,000 compared to 9 per 100,000 in the general population. (The National Service Framework For Mental Health: Five Years On, Department of Health, 2004; Samaritans Information Resource Pack (Mental health foundation-Mental Health Statistics: Prisons).

CAUSES AND EXCERBATION OF PSYCHIATRIC ILLNESS IN PRISON

1. Prisons have high percentage of mentally ill prisoners (Fazel & Danesh, 2002; Assadi et al., 2006; Birmingham, Mason, & Grubin, 1996; Baillargeon, Binswanger, Penn, Williams, & Murray, 2009; James & Glaze, 2006). Firstly, mentally ill persons are more frequently than others involved in crime due to symptoms like impaired judgment, lack of impulse control, suspiciousness, loss of inhibitions, paranoid ideas, inability to trust others, delusions, and hallucinations and most of them are less smart, so easily caught by police. Secondly, prisoner's living conditions in prison make them more susceptible to psychiatric disorders. Because conditions in prison are not conducive to good mental health, prisoners with mental illness are at risk of experiencing deterioration in their mental state. In 2004, Anderson (Andersen, 2004) pointed in a review that psychiatric morbidity including, schizophrenia is higher and perhaps increasing in prison populations compared with general populations and also with dependence syndromes being the most frequent disorders. He further added that early phase of imprisonment is a vulnerable period with a moderately high incidence of adjustment disorders and twice the incidence in solitary confinement compared with non solitary confinement. Finally, he concluded that there is a growing population of mentally ill prisoners being insufficiently detected and treated.
2. The level of confinement and isolation experienced by some prisoners is detrimental to mental health and people with a pre-existing psychiatric disorder deteriorate, and others who are vulnerable can become psychiatric patients. Long stay of prisoners in prison may be a contributing factor in high number of psychiatric prisoners and vice versa psychiatric persons more involved in unlawful activities and further easily caught by police. Cause for poor mental health of prisoner is overcrowding, very few recreational and intellectual activities and sometimes unnecessary prolongation of under trial period due to lengthy judicial system of hearings (Vinod Kumar & Usha Daria, 2013).
3. Without the necessary care, mentally ill prisoners suffer painful symptoms and their conditions can deteriorate. They are afflicted with delusions and hallucinations, debilitating fears, or extreme mood swings. They huddle silently in their cells, mumble incoherently, or yell incessantly. They refuse to obey orders or lash out without apparent provocation. They beat their heads against cell walls, smear themselves with feces, self-mutilate, and commit suicide. Doing time in prison is hard for everyone. Prisoners struggle to maintain their self-respect and emotional equilibrium in facilities that are typically tense, overcrowded, fraught with the potential for violence, cut off from families and communities, and devoid of opportunities for meaningful education, work, or other productive activities. But life in prison is particularly difficult for prisoners with mental illnesses that impair their thinking, emotional responses, and ability to cope. They are more likely to be exploited and victimized by other prisoners. They are less likely to be able to adhere to the countless formal and informal rules of a strictly regimented life and often have higher rates of rule-breaking than other prisoners (Mental Illness, Human Rights, and US Prisons, 2009)

4. Supermaximum Security Prisons and Isolation: When mentally ill prisoners break the rules, officials punish them as they would any other prisoner, even when their conduct reflects the impact of mental illness (Fellner, 2006). If lesser sanctions do not curb the behavior, officials "segregate" the prisoners from the general prison population, placing them in supermaximum security ("supermax") prisons or in segregation units within regular prisons. Once isolated, continued misconduct-often connected to mental illness-can keep them there indefinitely. A disproportionate number of the prisoners in segregation are mentally ill (Lovell, 2008; Maureen, O'Keefe, & Marissa, 2007). Prison officials across the country have increasingly embraced long-term segregation to manage and/or to discipline prisoners who are perceived to be dangerous, but also those who are seen as difficult or disturbing. Supermax prisons such as Tamms Correctional Center in Illinois or segregation units in other prisons constitute the modern day variant of solitary confinement. Prisoners are confined 23 to 24 hours a day in small cells that frequently have solid steel doors. They live with extensive surveillance and security controls, the absence of ordinary social interaction, abnormal environmental stimulus, a few hours a week of "recreation" alone in caged enclosures, and little, if any, educational, vocational, or other purposeful activities. They are handcuffed and frequently shackled every time they leave their cells.

Prolonged confinement under such conditions can be psychologically harmful to any prisoner, with the nature and severity of the impact depending on the individual, the duration, and the specific conditions (for example, access to natural light, radio, or books). It can provoke anxiety, depression, anger, cognitive disturbances, perceptual distortions, obsessive thoughts, paranoia, and psychosis (Jeffrey & Dvoskin, 2006). But the risk of harm is particularly grave for prisoners who already have serious mental illnesses. The stress, lack of meaningful social contact, and unstructured days can exacerbate symptoms of illness or provoke a reoccurrence. Suicides occur proportionately more often in segregation units than elsewhere in prison. All too frequently, mentally ill prisoners decompensate in isolation, requiring crisis care or psychiatric hospitalization. Many simply will not get better as long as they are isolated. According to one federal judge, putting mentally ill prisoners in isolated confinement "is the mental equivalent of putting an asthmatic in a place with little air.

5. A comprehensive review of national and international research clearly demonstrates that inmate suicide arises from a complex array of inter-related and self-reinforcing risk factors. These risk factors include mental illness, substance abuse, prior serious suicide attempts, chronic stresses of incarceration (i.e., family separation, solitary confinement, intimidation, and victimization), acute psychosocial stressors (i.e., parole setback, death of a loved one, rape), and staff errors or oversights (Daniel, 2006).

TREATMENT AND INTERVENTION STRATEGIES

1. A synthesis of the available literature on the management of common mental disorders in prison populations suggests the following approaches in order to address these disorders effectively:
    a. Assessment for common mental disorders at the point of entry into prison and during imprisonment, particularly during crisis points.

b. Admission procedures in individual receiving prisons can be good, but if information from the community or sending prisons is poor or non-existent then the health care professional has to rely on information given by the prisoner. This could be scant or misleading due to the stigma attached to mental health issues.
c. Reception is a vital stage for prisoners as they pass into the care and control of the prison Service who take on responsibility for their safety and welfare. The importance of receiving accurate and detailed information about each prisoner, from the courts, other/ prisons, probation, and health services cannot be over-stated.
d. Good practice in reception includes:
   i. Screening everyone carefully
   ii. Excellent communication between different groups in the prison
   iii. Continuous availability of mental health specialist care.
e. One of the central concerns about the initial screening is the extent to which it relies on self-reported problems.

2. A second concern is the level of training required accurately to assess mental health problems.
3. A third concern is an imbalance between assessment and treatment (Kimmett & Dora, 2009).
4. Induction into prisoners needs to be phased and counselled regarding the life style, rules, regulations and rights of the prisoners.
5. Violence inside prison needs to be kept under check.
6. Prisoner education and information about common mental disorders.
7. Training peers and prison staff to provide support in individual and group settings.
8. Counselling through trained volunteers.
9. Non pharmacological measures to handle sleep problems, psychological symptoms of pain.
10. Adequate recreational activities.
11. Training in problem solving.
12. Counselling.
13. **Family Therapy:** Family contact can reduce the feelings of isolation and stress caused by imprisonment. Prisons can more effectively meet the needs of prisoners for emotional support, and respond to families in a more consistent way, by:
    a. Further development of family contact development officers ensuring that families are kept well-informed.
    b. Involving them in key processes such as sentence planning and suicide prevention. 3. Conferring responsibility for family relations to a specific, accountable person, to coordinate the work with families
    c. Initiating a family relations working group, with a remit that parallels the work of race relations management teams (Kimmett & Dora, 2009).
14. Cognitive Behavior Therapy.
15. Professional help using psychotherapeutic methods to validate the distressing experiences, reframing of symptoms, support and counselling.
16. Relaxation techniques such as meditation, yoga, prayers, etc.
17. Stress management programmes (Suresh et al., 2011).

Simple measures, including having policies and guidelines for the transfer of severely mentally ill people to psychiatric hospitals, training of prison staff and discharge planning, may improve these rates (Torrey, Kennard, Eslinger, Lamb, & Pavle, 2010).

SHORT COMINGS OF TREATMENT AND INTERVENTON STRATGIES

Privatization

Because of ever-increasing health care costs, staff expense, lack of qualified health care professionals to work in prisons, lack of visionary correctional leadership (with exceptions), and ever-increasing litigation, more and more states have privatized the mental health and medical services. Contractors range from small private vendors for mental health services with various agreements for staffing and services to large private correctional health care companies providing both medical and mental health care.

There are no studies to indicate which model is best suited to deliver adequate, reasonable, and cost-effective mental health and psychiatric services in correctional systems: services directly provided by the state; large private vendors providing both medical and mental health services; separate small or large specialist mental health vendors; public medical institutions exclusively; or medical school-private vendor partnership. Appelbaum, Manning and Noonan (2002) have delineated the advantages of the university-state-corporation partnership in Massachusetts. In this model, the state correctional program receives enhanced quality of services, recruitment of high-quality professionals and expansion of training programs, while the medical school expands its revenue source while providing much needed public service as well as opportunities to engage in correctional research (Appelbaum & Noonan, 2002).

The profit motive may trump quality and compromise ethics standards and practice. Profit-oriented service providers tend to keep certain key staff positions unfilled or partially filled and encourage less expensive treatment approaches and medications, potentially jeopardizing patient care. Although the experience of private vendors indicates that they are more successful in recruiting professionals, including psychiatrists and psychologists, the correctional system still lags behind other provider systems in attracting qualified personnel. Departments of corrections should develop operational and performance criteria and benchmarks for evaluating vendor compliance. Conducting regular objective and impartial audits with well-designed and valid audit tools would hold the vendors accountable and at the same time help them to take timely corrective action. Once the contract is awarded to a service provider, such entities are become full partners with the state. Communication between the state and the service providers is essential. Key elements of success include establishing credibility and trust. This element should be mutual, in that both entities respect what is agreed on and do not deviate from the established contractual expectations and compliance indicators.

The Open Formulary vs. Restricted Formulary Controversy

Pharmaceutical costs are a significant component of the overall mental health care costs in corrections, and they generally increase about 15 to 20 percent annually. As a result, prescription drugs often become the target of aggressive cost-cutting by private health care providers. A commonly used tactic to control cost is to establish a restricted formulary of older generation psychotropics and generic agents that are less expensive and then insist that the psychiatrist preferentially prescribe medications from this restricted formulary instead of the newer, generally more expensive medications that are often included in the non-formulary list. Control and cost-containment measures are mediated via a concurrent non-formulary review process that is time consuming both for the psychiatrist provider and the psychiatrist reviewer. The reviewer who is employed by the service provider organization is placed in a situation in which he or she must manage the psychopharmacologic practice consistent with accepted standards while trying to control costs to make a profit, sometimes at the expense of quality care.

Newer medications improve the quality of life of offenders. More importantly, they help to reduce overall health care costs by reducing long-term hospitalization, emergency admissions to psychiatric units, and indirect costs associated with transportation of offenders to DMH facilities. According to the "Massachusetts Biotechnology Council White Paper Executive Summary" (MBC, 2004) on drug costs: Given that prescription drug costs (10%) are a fraction of health care spending in the U.S. (compared with hospital and physician care: 32 v. 22% respectively), targeting pharmaceuticals to restrain health care cost is questionable as a significant saving mechanism and may in fact cost the health care system dollars if it involves restricting access (MBC, 2004). The irony that cost-saving measures can in fact increase the cost of care may be true of the correctional system as well. Instituting practice parameters and guidelines for prescription practice, stringent peer review, and proper quality-assurance activities, including monitoring long- and short-term side effects should be the preferred method of cost stabilization and control.

Suicide Prevention in Prisons

Suicide is the third leading cause of death in U.S. state and federal prisons, exceeded only by natural causes and AIDS. Comprehensive suicide-prevention programs in prisons are of increasing importance to mental health professionals, correctional administrators, health care providers, legislators, attorneys, and others as they seek to rehabilitate offenders and avoid the multimillion-dollar lawsuits that often arise from inmate suicides. A comprehensive review of national and international research clearly demonstrates that inmate suicide arises from a complex array of inter-related and self-reinforcing risk factors (Daniel, 2006).These risk factors include mental illness, substance abuse, prior serious suicide attempts, chronic stresses of incarceration (i.e., family separation, solitary confinement, intimidation, and victimization), acute psychosocial stressors (i.e., parole setback, death of a loved one, rape), and staff errors or oversights.

Responsibility for suicide prevention in corrections has traditionally been placed squarely on mental health staff. Experience has shown that their efforts may be doomed to failure in the absence of adequate support and involvement of administrators and custodial staff. These correctional employees have joint responsibility for ensuring the health and safety of prison inmates, and they are increasingly held liable, individually and collectively, when they fail in this duty. Best practice in suicide prevention, outlined in the World Health Organization's updated resource guide (Konrad, Daigle, & Daniel, 2007), calls for a state-of-the-art collaborative effort of administrators, medical and mental health clinicians, and custodial staff to identify at-risk inmates and intervene appropriately.

Pharmacological Treatment for Substance Abuse

Inmates being released from prison are particularly vulnerable to serious relapse from the effects of drugs and alcohol within the first month of release (Binswanger, Stern, & Deo, 2007). While in prison, most inmates receive minimal medical treatment for substance abuse, except for detoxification. Long-term relapse prevention is limited to self-help groups, like Alcoholics Anonymous, and therapeutic communities. The overt acute symptoms of withdrawal dissipate within a few days of incarceration. Upon release, substance-abusing offenders return to a cue-rich environment of past drug use that can trigger a powerful rekindling of the addiction. This familiar environment results in the manifestation of physical symptoms similar to acute withdrawal, known as conditioned abstinence, first observed by Abraham Wikler (1973). Conditioned abstinence can occur even before release, when patients recall past drug use, and has been shown in laboratory studies in which exposure of former drug users to drug paraphernalia triggered intense cravings akin to acute drug withdrawal, even though patients had not used drugs for months.

Offenders with an established history of drug or alcohol abuse should be treated with anti-craving and relapse-prevention medications two to four weeks before release, and the medication regimen should be continued 30 to 60 days after release. Although there are no medications that treat cocaine, methamphetamine, and marijuana abuse, medications such as naltrexone (Cornish, Metzger, & Woody, 1997) and acamprosate are effective for opioids and alcohol. Naltrexone tablets and the recently approved monthly injection may be well-suited to the correctional setting, unlike methadone. Naltrexone is likely to generate less controversy and problems because it has virtually no potential for abuse or diversion. The availability of newer pharmacotherapy agents to treat addictions ranging from smoking to alcoholism should be aggressively utilized to reduce the unacceptable rate of recidivism.

RECOMMENDATIONS

What Can Be Done?

The detection, prevention and proper treatment of mental disorders, together with the promotion of good mental health, should be both a part of the public health goals within prison, and central to good prison management. Even in countries with limited resources, steps can be taken that will improve the mental health of prisoners and prison staff, and these steps can be adapted to the cultural, social, political and economic context within that country.

- **Divert People with Mental Disorders towards the Mental Health System:** Prisons are the wrong place for many people in need of mental health treatment, since the criminal justice system emphasizes deterrence and punishment rather than treatment and care. Legislation can be introduced which allows for the transfer of prisoners to general hospital psychiatric facilities at all stages of the criminal proceedings (arrest, prosecution, trial, imprisonment). For people with mental disorders who have been charged with committing minor offences, the introduction of mechanisms to divert them towards mental health services before they reach prison will help to ensure that they receive the treatment they need and also contribute to reducing the prison population. The imprisonment of people with mental disorders due to lack of public mental health service alternatives should be strictly prohibited by law.
- **Provide Prisoners with Access to Appropriate Mental Health Treatment and Care:** Access to assessment, treatment, and (when necessary) referral of people with mental disorders, including substance abuse, should be an integral part of general health services available to all prisoners. The health services provided to prisoners should, as a minimum, be of an equivalent level to those

in the community. This may be achieved by providing mental health training to prison health workers, establishing regular visits of a community mental health team to prisons, or enabling prisoners to access health services outside the prison setting. Those requiring more specialist care for example, can be referred to specialist mental health providers where inpatient assessment and treatment can be provided. Primary health care providers in prisons should be provided with basic training in the recognition and basic management of common mental health disorders.

- **Provide Access to Acute Mental Health Care in Psychiatric Wards of General Hospitals:** When prisoners require acute care they should be temporarily transferred to psychiatric wards of general hospitals with appropriate security levels.
- **Ensure the Availability of Psychosocial Support and Rationally Prescribed Psychotropic Medication:** Prisoners, through appropriately trained health care providers - should have the same access to psychotropic medication and psychosocial support for the treatment of mental disorders as people in the general community.
- **Provide Training to Staff:** Training on mental health issues should be provided to all people involved in prisons including prison administrators, prison guards and health workers. Training should enhance staff understanding of mental disorders, raise awareness on human rights, challenge stigmatizing attitudes and encourage mental health promotion for both staff and prisoners. An important element of training for all levels of prison staff should be the recognition and prevention of suicides. In addition, prison health workers need to have more specialized skills in identifying and managing mental disorders.
- **Provide Information/Education to Prisoners and Their Families on Mental Health Issues:** Prisoners and their families should receive information and education on the nature of mental disorders, with a view to reducing stigma and discrimination, preventing mental disorders and promoting mental health. Information can help prisoners and their families better understand their emotional responses to imprisonment and provide practical strategies on how to minimize the negative effects on their mental health and inform them as to when and how to seek help for a mental disorder.
- **Promote High Standards in Prison Management:** The mental health of all prisoners, including those with mental disorders, will be enhanced by appropriate prison management that promotes and protects human rights. Attention to areas such as sanitation, food, meaningful occupation, and physical activity, prevention of discrimination and violence, and promotion of social networks are essential.
- **Ensure that the Needs of Prisoners Are Included in National Mental Health Policies and Plans:** National mental health policies and/or plans should encompass the mental health needs of the prison population. Where, policies and plans fail to do *so* it may be necessary to advocate for their inclusion. Whenever a mental health policy or plan is being developed, prisons (staff and prisoners) should be included as stakeholders in the development process.
- **Promote the Adoption of Mental Health Legislation That Protects Human Rights:** All prisoners, including those with mental disorders, have the right to be treated humanely and with respect for their inherent dignity as human beings. Furthermore, conditions of confinement in prisons must conform to international human rights standards. Mental health legislation can be a powerful tool to protect the rights of people with a mental disorder, including prisoners, yet in many countries mental health laws are outdated and fail to address the mental health needs of the prison population (WHO Resource Book on Mental Health, Human Rights and Legislation; WHO, 2005

& WHR, 2001).The development of legal provisions that address these needs can help to promote the rights of prisoners, including the right to quality treatment and care, to refuse treatment, to appeal decisions of involuntary treatment, to confidentiality, to protection from discrimination and violence, and to protection from torture and other cruel, inhuman and degrading treatment (including abusive use of seclusion, restraints and medication, and non-consensual scientific or medical experimentation), among others. Legislation should provide prisoners with mental disorders with procedural protections within the criminal justice system equivalent to those granted other prisoners. The protections, through legislation, of other basic rights of prisoners, such as acceptable living conditions, adequate food and access to the open air, meaningful activity, and contact with the family are also important and can further contribute to the promotion of good mental health. Independent inspection mechanism such as mental health visiting boards can also be established through legislation, to inspect prisons as well as other mental health facilities in order to monitor conditions for people with mental disorders.

- **Encourage Inter-Sectoral Collaboration:** Many problems and issues can be solved by bringing relevant Ministries and others together to discuss the needs of prisoners with mental health disorders. Different stakeholders should meet to discuss mental health in prisons and to plan an inter-sectoral response (WHO Resource Book on Mental Health, Human Rights and Legislation).
- **Social Reintegration:** Often understood as the support given to offenders during their reentry into society following imprisonment. A broader definition, however, encompasses a number of interventions undertaken following an arrest to divert offenders away from the criminal justice system to an alternative measure, including a restorative justice process or suitable treatment. It includes imposing community-based sanctions rather than imprisonment in an attempt to facilitate the social reintegration of offenders within the community, rather than subjecting them to the marginalizing and harmful effects of imprisonment. For those who are sentenced to imprisonment, it includes correctional programs in prison, and aftercare interventions (World Drug Report, 2006). In recent years, the post-release, community-based component of these interventions has been variously referred to as "aftercare", "transitional care", "reentry" or "reentry support", reintegration, or resettlement. Some post-release interventions may begin while the offender is still incarcerated with the intent of facilitating post-release adjustment.

Programs to Support and Assist for Mentally Ill Offenders

Offenders afflicted by mental illness encounter particular problems upon release into the community. These offenders may experience extreme social isolation and, as well, are often at risk for a co-occurring substance abuse disorder. As well, these offenders may encounter particularly difficulties in finding suitable accommodation and securing employment. And, it is likely that most of these offenders will require further medical and therapeutic services and assistance with money management. These factors, in combination with noncompliance of treatment orders, may make these individuals a risk not only to themselves, but to others as well (Hartwell & Orr, 1999).

The unique challenges faced by mentally ill offenders upon release require the development of a community-based treatment model of continuing care to address the risks, needs, and vulnerabilities of this offender group. Community-based treatment models of continuing care may reduce the risk to the public, for the individual offenders and reduce future correctional system involvement for these individuals, in addition to providing a diversion program from the traditional justice system (Griffiths, 2004;

Hartwell & Orr, 2004). Research has identified continuity of care as an essential component of effective mental health treatment for mentally ill persons who are involved in the criminal justice system. This includes multidisciplinary case management for psychiatric treatment and social services, e.g. housing, food, help with disability benefits, and vocational training.

Forensic mental health professionals have identified the core components of any intervention designed to assist mentally ill offenders to successfully re-enter the community, these include;

1. A focus on stabilizing the offender's illness;
2. Enhancing their independent functioning;
3. Maintaining their internal and external controls so as to minimize the likelihood they will act violently and commit new offences;
4. Establishing a liaison between treatment staff and the justice system;
5. Providing structure in the offender's daily life;
6. Using authority comfortably;
7. Managing the offender's violence and impulses;
8. Integrating treatment and case management;
9. Obtaining therapeutic living arrangements; and,
10. Working with the offender's family to determine if they are a reliable source of social support (Griffiths, Dandurand, & Murdoch, 2007).

CONCLUSION

The psychiatric morbidity among prison inmates is substantially higher than in the general population. Most inmates have a number of defined problem areas, with substance use, depression and anxiety disorders most prevalent. The high rate of common psychiatric disorders argues for the use of improved psychiatric screening instruments, improved assessment and treatment capacities in the prison and an increased number of psychiatric inpatient facilities to care for the inmates who are too unwell to be treated in the prison. The burden of psychiatric illness in this vulnerable and marginalized population poses a serious challenge. For remedial measures to be taken identification of magnitude of problem, preventable causes and treatment with proper compliance and follow-up is needed. Mental disorders are highly stigmatized conditions that many people want to keep private because of their embarrassment or fear of discrimination. Certain remedial measures are to be implemented for a better future of prison and community because ultimately these prisoners will be released from prison and become a part of community. Beginning of reforms is the immediate need as a long journey ahead.

REFERENCES

Agbahowe, S. A., Ohaeri, J. U., Ogunlesi, A. O., & Osahon, R. (1998). Prevalence of psychiatric morbidity among convicted inmates in a Nigerian prison community. *East African Medical Journal*, *75*(1), 19–26. PMID:9604530

Andersen, H. S. (2004). Mental health in prison populations. A review – With special emphasis on a study of Danish prisoners on remand. *Acta Psychiatrica Scandinavica, 424*(s424), 5–59. doi:10.1111/j.1600-0447.2004.00436_2.x PMID:15447785

Anderson, H. S., Sestoft, D., Lillebaek, T., Gabrielsen, G., Hemmingsen, R., & Kramp, P. (2000). A longitudinal study of prisoners on remand: Psychiatric prevalence, incidence and psychopathology in solitary vs non-solitary confinement. *Acta Psychiatrica Scandinavica, 102*(1), 19–25. doi:10.1034/j.1600-0447.2000.102001019.x PMID:10892605

Appelbaum, K. L., Manning, T. D., & Noonan, J. D. (2002). A university-state-corporation partnership for providing correctional mental health services. *Psychiatric Services (Washington, D.C.), 53*(2), 185–189. doi:10.1176/appi.ps.53.2.185 PMID:11821549

Assadi, S. M., Noroozian, M., Pakravannejad, M., Yahyazadeh, O., Aghayan, S., Shariat, S. V., & Fazel, S. (2006). Psychiatric morbidity among sentenced prisoners: Prevalence study in Iran. *The British Journal of Psychiatry, 188*(2), 159–164. doi:10.1192/bjp.188.2.159 PMID:16449704

Baillargeon, J., Binswanger, I. A., Penn, J. V., Williams, B. A., & Murray, O. J. (2009). Psychiatric disorders and repeat incarcerations: The revolving prison door. *The American Journal of Psychiatry, 166*(1), 103–109. doi:10.1176/appi.ajp.2008.08030416 PMID:19047321

Baillargeon, J., Penn, J. V., Thomas, C. R., Temple, J. R., Baillargeon, G., & Murray, O. J. (2009). Psychiatric disorders and suicide in the nation's largest state prison system. *The Journal of the American Academy of Psychiatry and the Law, 166*(1), 103–109. doi:10.1176/appi.ajp.2008.08030416 PMID:19535556

Bermu´dez, C.E., Romero Mendoza, M.P., Rodrı´guez Ruiz, E.M., Durand-Smith, A.L., & Saldı´var Herna´ndez, G.J. (2007). *Female depression and substance dependence in the Mexico City penitentiary system*. Academic Press.

Binswanger, I. A., Stern, M. F., & Deo, R. A. (2007). Release from prison: A high risk of death for former inmates. *Cross Ref Medline, 356*, 157–165. PMID:17215533

Birmingham, L., Mason, D., & Grubin, D. (1996). Prevalence of mental disorder in remand prisoners: Consecutive case study. *British Medical Journal, 313*(7071), 1521-4.

Brinded, P. M., Simpson, A. I. F., Laidlaw, T. M., Fairley, N., & Malcolm, F. (2001). Prevalence of psychiatric disorders in New Zealand prisons: A national study. *The Australian and New Zealand Journal of Psychiatry, 35*(2), 166–173. doi:10.1046/j.1440-1614.2001.00885.x PMID:11284897

Brownell, B. (2014). *Crime and Justice, Health Care, Human Rights, Prisons, op Stories, There Are 10 Times More Mentally Ill People Behind Bars Than in State Hospitals*. Academic Press.

Brugha, T., Singleton, N., Meltzer, H., Bebbington, P., Farrell, M., Jenkins, R., & Lewis, G. et al. (2005). Psychosis in the community and in prisons: A report from the British National Survey of psychiatric morbidity. *The American Journal of Psychiatry, 162*(4), 774–780. doi:10.1176/appi.ajp.162.4.774 PMID:15800152

Butler, T., & Allnutt, S. (2003). *Mental Illness among New South Wales Prisoners*. NSW Correction Health Service.

Butler, T. K., Males, J. J., Robinson, L. P., Wechsler, A. W., Sutton, G. L., Cheng, J., & McClellan, K. et al. (1997). Six-year review of Acanthamoeba keratitis in New South Wales, Australia: 1997-2002. *Clinical & Experimental Ophthalmology, 33*(1), 41–46. doi:10.1111/j.1442-9071.2004.00911.x PMID:15670077

California Department of Corrections and Rehabilitation Report. (2014). *Unless otherwise noted, all data in this report were provided by the For purposes of this report, "mental illness" is defined as a condition that qualifies for placement in the prison's Mental Health Delivery System within the last year*. Academic Press.

Coid, J. (1984). How many psychiatric patients in prison? *The British Journal of Psychiatry, 145*(1), 78–86. doi:10.1192/bjp.145.1.78 PMID:6743949

Cornish, J. W., Metzger, D., Woody, G. E., Wilson, D., McLellan, A. T., Vandergrift, B., & O'Brien, C. P. (1997). Naltrexone pharmacotherapy for opioid dependent federal probationers. *Journal of Substance Abuse Treatment, 14*(6), 529–534. doi:10.1016/S0740-5472(97)00020-2 PMID:9437624

Daniel, A. E. (2006). Preventing suicide in prison: A collaborative responsibility of administrative, custodial, and clinical staff. *The Journal of the American Academy of Psychiatry and the Law, 34*(2), 165–175. PMID:16844795

Doris, J. J., & Lauren, E. G. (2006). *Mental Health Problems of Prison and Jail Inmates*. Bureau of Justice Statistics.

Duffy, D., Linehan, S., & Kennedy, H.G. (2006). *Psychiatric morbidity in the male sentenced Irish prisons population*. Academic Press.

Fazel, S., Cartwright, J., Norman-Nott, A., & Hawton, K. (2008). Suicide in prisoners: A systematic review of risk factors. *The Journal of Clinical Psychiatry, 69*(11), 1721–1731. doi:10.4088/JCP.v69n1107 PMID:19026254

Fazel, S., & Danesh, J. (2002). Serious mental disorder in 23 000 prisoners: a systematic review of 62 surveys. Severe mental illness in 33 588 prisoners worldwide: systematic review and meta regression analysis. *Lancet, 359*(9306), 545–550. doi:10.1016/S0140-6736(02)07740-1 PMID:11867106

Fazel, S., & Seewald, K. (2012). Severe mental illness in 33,588 prisoners worldwide: Systematic review and meta-regression analysis. *The British Journal of Psychiatry, 200*(5), 364–373. doi:10.1192/bjp.bp.111.096370 PMID:22550330

Fazel, S., & Yu, R. (2011). Psychotic disorders and repeat offending: Systematic review and meta-analysis. *Schizophrenia Bulletin, 37*(4), 800–810. doi:10.1093/schbul/sbp135 PMID:19959703

Fellner, J. (2006). A Corrections Quandary. *Harvard Civil Rights-Civil Liberties Law, 29*, 773–789.

Griffiths, C. T., Dandurand, Y. V., & Murdoch, D. (2007). *The Social Reintegration of Offenders and Crime Prevention- The International Centre for Criminal Law Reform and Criminal Justice Policy*. ICCLR.

Hartwell, S. W., & Orr, K. (1999, September). The massachusetts forensic transition program for mentally ill offenders reentering the community. *Psychiatric Services (Washington, D.C.), 50*(9), 1220–1222. doi:10.1176/ps.50.9.1220 PMID:10478911

Holley, H. L., Arboleda, F. J., & Love, E. (1995). Lifetime prevalence of prior suicide attempts in a remanded population and relationship to current mental illness. *International Journal of Offender Therapy and Comparative Criminology*, *10*(2), 239–256.

James, D.J., & Glaze, L.E. (2006). *Mental health problems of prison and jails inmates*. U.S. Dept. of Justice: Office of Justice Programs.

Jeffrey, M., & Dvoskin, J. (2006). An overview of correctional psychiatry. *The Psychiatric Clinics of North America*, *29*, 773–789. PMID:16904511

Jha, B. K. (1968). A study of the nature of criminal offences of mental patients. *Indian Journal of Psychiatry*, *10*(1), 166–176.

Kariminia, A., Law, M., Butler, T., Corben, S. P., Levy, M. H., Kaldor, J. M., & Grant, L. (2007). Factors associated with mortality in a cohort of Australian prisoners. *European Journal of Epidemiology*, *22*(7), 417–428. doi:10.1007/s10654-007-9134-1 PMID:17668280

Kimmett, E., & Dora, R. (2009). *An independent review of unmet mental health need in prison*. Prison Reform Trust.

Konrad, N., Daigle, M. S., & Daniel, A. E. (2007). *Preventing suicide in jails and prisons*. Geneva: World Health Organization.

Kumar, V., & Daria, U. (2013). Psychiatric morbidity in prisoners. *Indian Journal of Psychiatry*, *55*(4), 366–370. doi:10.4103/0019-5545.120562 PMID:24459308

Los Angeles Times. (2010). Sheriff says proposed mental health cuts would burden L.A. jails. *Los Angeles Times.*

Lovell, D. (2008). Patterns of disturbed behavior in a supermax prison. *Criminal Justice and Behavior*, *35*(8), 985–1004. doi:10.1177/0093854808318584

Maden, A., Swinton, M., & Gunn, J. (1992). A survey of pre-arrest drug use in sentenced prisoners. *British Journal of the Addictions, 87*, 27-33.

Mason, D., Birmingham, L., & Grubin, D. (1997). Substance use in remand prisoners: A consecutive case study. *British Medical Journal*, *315*(7099), 8–21. doi:10.1136/bmj.315.7099.18 PMID:9233320

Massachusetts Biotechnology Council. (2004). *White paper executive summary on prescription drug cost, access and affordability*. Cambridge, MA: Author.

Maureen, L. (2007). Offenders with mental illness in the correctional system. *Journal of Offender Rehabilitation*, *45*(1-2), 81–104. doi:10.1300/J076v45n01_08

Mencimer, S. (2014). *Crime and Justice, Health Care, Human Rights, Prisons, Top Stories. There Are 10 Times More Mentally Ill People Behind Bars Than in State Hospitals*. Academic Press.

Mental Illness, Human Right, and US Prisons. (2009). *Human Rights Watch Statement for the Record to the Senate Judiciary Committee Subcommittee on Human Rights and the Law*. Author.

Mohan, C., & Dhar, V. (2001). Study of psychiatric status of Central Jail under trials at psychiatric hospitals, Government Medical College, Jammu. *Indian Journal of Psychiatry*, *43*, 59.

Naidoo, S., & Mkize, D.L. (2012). Prevalence of mental disorders in a prison population in Durban, South Africa. *African Journal of Psychiatry, 15*(1).

Piselli, M., Elisei, S., Murgia, N., Quartesan, R., & Abram, K. M. (2009). Co-occurring psychiatric and substance use disorders among male detainees in Italy. *International Journal of Law and Psychiatry*, *29*, 370–385. PMID:19237198

Prison Statistics India. (2012). *Prison Statistics India is the eighteenth in the series of annual publication*. The National Crime Records Bureau, Ministry of Home Affairs.

Report, W. H. (2001). *Mental Health: New Understanding, New Hope*. Geneva: World Health Organization.

Sandeep, K. G., Paramjit, S., Parshotam, D. G., Samta, G., & Aseem, G. (2011). Psychiatric morbidity in prisoners. *Indian Journal of Psychiatry*, *53*(3), 253–257. doi:10.4103/0019-5545.86819 PMID:22135446

Singh, G., & Verma, H. C. (1976). Murder in Punjab: A psychosocial study. *Indian Journal of Psychiatry*, *18*, 243–251.

Singleton, N., Meltzer, H., & Gatward, R. (1998). *Psychiatric Morbidity among Prisoners in England and Wales*. London: Stationery Office.

Somsundram, O. (1974). Crimes of persons with schizophrenia. *Indian Journal of Psychiatry*, *16*(2), 121–130.

Somsundram, O. (1997). Crimes of persons with affective disorders. *Indian Journal of Psychiatry*, *39*, 13–17. PMID:21584037

Steadman, H. J., Fabisiak, S., Dvoskin, J., & Holohean, E. J. (1987). Jr A survey of mental disability among state prison inmates. *Hospital & Community Psychiatry*, *38*(10), 1086–1090. PMID:3666699

Suresh, B. M., Pratima, M., Rajani, P., Naveen, K. C., & Madhusudhan, S. (2011). *Minds Imprisoned: Mental Health Care in Prisons. Publication, National Institute of Mental Health Neuro Sciences*. Bangalore: Common Mental Disorders in Prisons.

Tanay, E. (2007). Virginia Tech mass murder: A forensic psychiatrist's perspective. *The Journal of the American Academy of Psychiatry and the Law*, *35*, 152–153. PMID:17592159

Torrey, E., Kennard, A., Eslinger, D., Lamb, R., & Pavle, J. (2010). *More Mentally Ill Persons are in Jails and Prisons than Hospitals: A Survey of the States*. Treatment Advocacy Center.

Walmsley, R. (2005). *The World Female Imprisonment*. The International Centre for Prison Studies (ICPS).

Walmsley, R. (2009). *World Prison Population List* (8th ed.). King's College London International Centre for Prison Studies.

WHO. (2005). *Resource Book on Mental Health, Human Rights and Legislation*. World Health Organization.

Wikler, A. (1973). Dynamics of drug dependence: Implications of a conditioning theory for research and treatment. *Archives of General Psychiatry*, *28*(5), 611–616. doi:10.1001/archpsyc.1973.01750350005001 PMID:4700675

World Drug Report. (2006). Retrieved 9 February, 2016, from https://www.unodc.org/unodc/en/data-and-analysis/WDR-2006.html

KEY TERMS AND DEFINITIONS

Incarceration: Putting in prison or another enclosure.

Mental Health: Emotional, psychological and social well-being.

Mental Illness: Refers to wide range of mental health conditions –disorders that affect mood, thinking and behaviour.

Prison: Place were prisoners reside called a prison, jail or detention center.

Prisoners: All persons detained, incarcerated or imprisoned in a facility on the basis of, or allegation of, a criminal offence in prisons.

Chapter 12
Legal Aspects of Chronic Mental Illness

Raveesh B. N.
Dharwad Institute of Mental Health and Neurosciences, India

Barre Vijay Prasad
Dharwad Institute of Mental Health and Neurosciences, India

Meghamala S. Tavaragi
Dharwad Institute of Mental Health and Neurosciences, India

ABSTRACT

People with a chronic mental illness or disability have been identified as a group suffering multiple disadvantages. Law interacts with mental disorder to protect society from the dangerous consequences of mental disorder. The legal interaction with mental disorder includes both civil and criminal issues. A paradigm shift has given a new perspective to the care of mental disorders and has led to the review of mental health legislations worldwide in general, India in particular. This chapter will discuss the interaction of law and psychiatry, rights of persons with mental disorder and the gap in implementation of these laws.

INTRODUCTION

The mental health is a part of the general health and has a serious concern in the society. A person who suffers mental illness suffers not only for himself but also would bring about suffering for the people who are not only to the family but to the society at large. However, a person who suffers from such a mental illness cannot be neglected. They cannot be denied with the basic needs to level in a respectable manner. The doctrine of parens patriae allows the state to intervene and to act as a surrogate parent for those who are unable to care for themselves or who may harm themselves. The Mental Health enactments are promulgated with dual objects such as:

DOI: 10.4018/978-1-5225-0519-8.ch012

1. To have a concern for the rights and protection of people with mental disorder.
2. To have a concern for rights and protection of community to which the person with mental disorder belongs.

Mental illness has been recognized as one of the disabilities under Section 2 (i) of the Persons with Disabilities (Equal Opportunities, Protection of Rights and Full Participation) (PWD) Act, 1995. "Mental illness" has been defined under Section 2(q) of the said Act as any mental disorder other than mental retardation. As a socio-welfare measure, to ameliorate the condition of people suffering from mental disability the appropriate local government may frame such schemes to provide unemployment allowance, insurance and rehabilitative homes.

DISABILITY

The United Nations Convention on the Rights of Persons with Disabilities (UNCRPD) marks a "paradigm shift" in attitudes and approaches to persons with disabilities by treating them as "subjects" with rights, who are capable of claiming those rights. The concept of disability differs from society to society because of the attitude towards disability are deeply rooted in socio-cultural values. The term disability has been defined in many ways such as handicap, incapacitated, impaired, abnormal and inform and so on. The World Health Organisation (WHO) has defined it 'to mean any restriction or lack (resulting from an impairment) of ability to perform an activity in the manner or within the range considered normal for a human being'. The PWD Act (1995) socio-welfare legislation, for the first time recognised the mental illness as a disability. A person suffering not less than forty percent of any disability as certified by a medical authority would be a person with disability. A person having mental illness not less than forty percent would be a person with disability. Such a person having mental disability would be entitled to have a rehabilitation to reach and maintain the optimal intellectual, psychiatric or social functional level. Such a person shall not be discriminated and in fact should be provided with concession and encouragement in the areas of education, employment, transportation and access to public places, sports and cultural activities, medical acre financial benefits and property (Gautam, Jain, Batra, Sharma & Munshi, 2009).

People with a chronic illness or disability are particularly vulnerable to experiencing legal problems and have difficulty resolving these problems. People with a chronic illness or disability have increased vulnerability to experiencing a wide range of legal problems, including civil, criminal and family law problems (Coumarelos, Wei, & Zhou, 2006; Currie, 2007; Pleasence, Balmer & Buck, 2006; Pleasence, Buck, Balmer, O'Grady, Genn & Smith, 2004b). Furthermore, these surveys indicate that such people have lower resolution rates for their legal problems (Coumarelos et al., 2006; Curry, 2007).

In Oregon (United States), Dale (2000) found high levels of legal need among people with a mental disability, particularly for problems related to public benefits and family law. Dale also found high levels of legal need among with a physical disability, particularly concerning discrimination, wills and estates, consumer and health care matters. In Washington State, the Task Force on Civil Equal Justice Funding (2003) reported that people with physical disabilities had relatively high rates of consumer, health, estates and trusts issues, while people with mental disabilities had relatively high rates of legal issues related to housing, municipal services and public services.

The association of chronic illness or disability with legal problems may well be bi directional. For example, Pleasence et al. (2004a) cite studies indicating that housing related problems, homelessness, family problems and domestic violence can emerge for people with long-term physical or mental incapacity. They also cite studies suggesting that poor quality housing, relationship breakdown, domestic violence, unemployment, mortgage indebtedness and other debt problems can result in psychological or physical ill-health. The results of the English and Welsh Civil and Social Justice Surveys are also consistent with a two-way relationship between chronic illness or disability and legal problems. In addition to examining the incidence of legal problems among people with a chronic illness or disability, these surveys also examined whether stress-related illness and various other adverse consequences occurred after the legal problems were experienced. For example, examining housing rights problems, Pleasence and Balmer (2007) reported that such problems are not only associated with mental illness, but may also have a role in bringing about or exacerbating mental illness.

About half of those who reported that stress-related ill-health followed housing rights problems went onto receive medical treatment as a result. Furthermore, Pleasence, Balmer and Buck (2008) found that adverse health consequences reportedly followed over one-third of the legal problems experienced and led to a significant use of health services. Pleasence and Balmer (2007) report elevated incidence rates across many different types of legal problems for people with a mental illness relative to people with other illnesses or disabilities. Qualitative research in Australia further supports the idea that people with a mental illness are a vulnerable group who may experience a number of legal problems and face a range of barriers in accessing justice (Karras, McCarron, Gray, & Ardasinski, 2006). Mental health-related issues such as problems with mental health care and involuntary psychiatric hospitalization, were more likely to report health legal events overall.

Recent analyses of the English and Welsh Civil and Social Justice Survey data revealed higher rates of non-health related legal problems for people with a mental illness than for people with other chronic illnesses or disabilities (Pleasence & Balmer, 2007). Thus, the present findings and other recent findings are beginning to identify people with a mental illness as a particularly vulnerable group with special legal needs. The high use of non-legal professionals as first advisers for people from all walks of life is a common finding across recent legal needs surveys (Coumarelos et al., 2006; Genn, 1999; Pleasence et al., 2004b; 2006). This finding has provided impetus for the argument that non-legal professionals could be used to ‘sign post’ legal problems and act as ‘gateways’ into legal services (Balmer et al., 2006; Coumarelos et al., 2006; Pleasence et al., 2004b). The aim would be to equip non-legal professionals with the skills to be able to identify people who have legal problems and refer them to appropriate legal services.

People with all types of chronic illness or disability appear to have an increased propensity for experiencing multiple legal problems and a reduced ability for resolving these legal problems. Furthermore, given the health needs of this demographic group and their high use of non-legal advisers, the present findings add credence to the argument that the more effective coordination of legal services with non-legal services such as health services is likely to improve both health and justice outcomes for this group (Balmer et al., 2006; Pleasence et al., 2004b; 2008). Nonetheless, future research into the nature of the association of chronic illness or disability with legal needs has the potential to further inform the tailoring of legal services to meet the needs of people with different types of chronic illness or disability. Forinstance, such research could help identify the forms of coordination between legal and non-legal services that are likely to be particularly beneficial for people with different types of chronic illness or disability. Few of legal services for person suffering from mental illness, are mentioned below giving importance to Indian scenario.

INVOLUNTARY ADMISSION

Involuntary admission is a legal procedure used to compel an individual to receive inpatient treatment for a mental health disorder against his or her will (Dhanda, 2000). The legal justifications are that a person is imminently dangerous to self or others; is gravely disabled; or clearly needs immediate care and treatment (Nambi, 2014). The Mental Health Act 1987 provides following provisions;

Admission under Special Circumstances

It is an involuntary hospitalization when the mentally ill person does not or cannot express his willingness for admission. Admission is made, if a relative or a friend of the mentally ill person applies in writing for admission and the medical officer in-charge of the hospital is satisfied that the admission will be the interest of the mentally ill person. The duration of admission cannot exceed 90 days.

Admission through Reception Orders

1. Reception Order on Application

An application for a reception order may be made by the medical officer in-charge of a psychiatric hospital or nursing home or by the husband, wife or any other relative of the mentally ill person. This application for admission should accompany the medical certificates from two medical practitioners of whom one should be a Government doctor. On receipt of this application the magistrate may issue a reception order for admission after he is satisfied that the alleged person is suffering from mental illness.

2. Reception Orders on Production of a Mentally Ill Person before a Magistrate (Admission of a Dangerous Wandering Mentally Ill Person)

The police officer in-charge of a police station may take into protection any person found wandering at large whom he has reason to believe to be mentally ill. He should produce him before the nearest magistrate within 24 hours. The magistrate shall examine the person and assess his capacity to understand and if he is satisfied that the said person is a mentally ill person, the magistrate may pass a reception order, authorizing the detention of the said person as an inpatient in a psychiatric hospital, and later should the medical officer certify that such a person is a mentally ill person, he should be given care and treatment in a psychiatric hospital.

Every officer in charge of a police station, who has reason to believe that any mentally ill person is cruelly treated or is not under proper care and control by relatives or other persons, shall report this to a magistrate. This complaint to the magistrate can also be submitted by any individual. The magistrate may summon such relatives along with the patient and order the relative or other person to take care of the mentally ill person. If this relative willfully neglects to comply with this order he shall be punishable with a fine up to Rs 2,000. If there is no person legally bound to maintain this mentally ill person he can issue a reception order for admission to a psychiatric hospital.

3. Admission as an In-Patient for Inquisition

A district court holding an inquisition regarding any person who is found to be mentally ill, may direct such a person for admission in a psychiatric hospital. Inquisition is examination or investigation whether the person who is alleged to be mentally ill is of unsound mind and incapable of managing his affairs.

Application can be made by

1. A relative.
2. Advocate General.
3. Public Prosecutor, or
4. District Commissioner.

The magistrate will give notification and the order for an enquiry.

- **Communication Rights:** Patients should generally have free and open communication with the outside world by telephone or mail, but this right varies regionally to some degree. Some jurisdictions charge the hospital administration with a responsibility for monitoring the communications of patients. In some areas, hospitals are expected to make available reasonable supplies of paper, envelopes, and stamps for patient's use.
- **Least Restrictive Alternative:** The principle holds that patients have the right to receive the least restrictive means of treatment for the requisite clinical effect. Therefore, if a patient can be treated as an outpatient, commitment should not be used; if a patient can be treated on an open ward, seclusion should not be used.

CIVIL RIGHTS OF PATIENTS

Because of several clinical, public, and legal movements, criteria for the civil rights of persons who are mentally ill, apart from their rights as patients, have been both established and affirmed. Persons with mental disorders suffer certain disadvantages in their day-to-day life on account of their incapacity to take certain decisions independently. Even if they take such decisions, at the time when the said decisions were taken, whether they had understood the implications of the said action is an important question. The civil law broadly regulates the said aspects of power to hold and to alienate property as well as issues related to their marriage (Raveesh et al., 2013).

- **Right to Treatment:** Among the rights of patients, the right to the standard quality of care is fundamental. This right has been litigated in highly publicized cases in recent years under the slogan of right to treatment
- **Right to Refuse Treatment:** The right to refuse treatment is a legal doctrine that holds that, except in emergencies, persons cannot be forced to accept treatment against their will. An emergency is defined as a condition in clinical practice that requires immediate intervention to prevent death or serious harm to the patient or another person or to prevent deterioration of the patient's clinical state.

- **Right to Hold Property:** The ancient Hindu law had certain restrictions regarding the right of a person who is having disorder of mind to hold the property. The legislative step taken during 1928though had removed the disabilities of persons to hold the property; it did not remove the disability of a person with mental disorder. However, after 1956, the disqualification based on diseases, defect or deformity is not a bar to have property (Section 28 of Indian Succession Act 1956).
- **Testamentary Capacity:** Testamentary capacity of a person follows the soundness of mind. A person who cannot understand his/her act on account of intoxication or illness or from any other cause cannot make a Will (Section 59 Indian Succession Act 1956). However, a Will or testament made during the lucid interval (intervening periods of normalcy) would be a valid document. Similar is the situation in respect of a person who is a habitual drunkard but has made the testament when he/she is not under the influence of drunkenness. Letter of administration or probate cannot be granted to any person who has disordered mind (Section 236 & 223 of Indian Succession Act 1956). However, could be a legatee under a Will.
- **Contract Law:** Every person is competent to make contract, provided they have attained an age of majority and that he/she is of a sound mind. A genuine consent is very much necessary to have a valid contract. The Indian Contract Act for the said purposes has specifically envisaged that a person entering into the contract should not have any disorder of the mind at the time of making the contract. This is to ensure that he is capable of understanding it and is capable of forming a rational judgement as to its effect upon his interest (Section 12 Indian Contract Act 1872). A person who is having a disorder of mind but occasionally of sound mind can make a contract when he is of sound mind. Similarly, a person who is usually of sound mind but occasionally has a disorder of mind cannot make a contract when he is ill. A contract entered in to by a lawful guardian of a mentally ill person is valid. Also, the manager duly appointed under the Mental Health Act could enter in to a contract to bind award.
- **Partnership:** The relationship of partnership arises from contract and not from status (Section 5 Indian Partnership Act 1932). To become a member of a partnership firm the soundness of mental health is important. If a person of sound mental health, after becoming a partner suffers mental illness, then any other partner or other person who is found to be entitled may seek dissolution of partnership of such a person by filing an application before the District Court. On such application, after enquiry if it is noticed by the District Court that the person is mentally ill, then the District Court would appoint a manager. The manager so appointed by, as the district court may direct, shall join with other partners in disposing of the partnership property and shall do all such acts for carrying in to effect the dissolution of the partnership.
- **Transfer of Property:** Only the persons having competency to contract could effect a transfer of property. As a contract made by a person with mental disorder is void, so the transfer made by him would be void. However, if the person transfers a property during the lucid interval, then such a transfer would be valid (Section 5 Transfer of Property Act 1882). On behalf of a mentally ill under the Mental Health Act 1987, a manager appointed by the Court, with its prior approval could mortgage, charge or transfer by sale, gift, and exchange or otherwise transfer any of the immovable property of the person who has mental illness. However before granting the permission the court shall make such an inquiry to protect the interest of the person with mental disorder.

- **Stocks, Shares, and Securities:** Acquisition, holding and transfer of shares, stocks and securities by a person who is mentally ill are equally an important aspect in the commercial market. If a person who holds such valuables becomes mentally ill or the manager appointed for such mentally ill dies or himself becomes mentally ill, then for the purposes of effective regulation of these stocks/shares, the District Court may direct the company or Government concerned to make such transfer or to transfer the same and receive and pay over the dividends (Section 72 & 73 of Mental Health Act 1987).
- **Durable Power of Attorney:** A modern development that permits persons to make provisions for their own anticipated loss of decision-making capacity is called a durable power of attorney. The document permits the advance selection of a substitute decision maker who can act without the necessity of court proceedings when the signatory becomes incompetent through illness
- **Marriage and Mental Illness:** Most of the personal laws, barring Muslim law, disqualify a person with disorder of mind from getting married. There is almost a consonance in the legal field that at the time of marriage both bride and bridegroom should be of sound mind though there is a divergence about the degree of sanity required to make a person fit for marriage. The Hindu Marriage Act and Special Marriage Act both emphasize that neither party must be suffering from disorder of mind. However, if a marriage has taken place in respect of a person who has the infirmity then the marriage ipso facto (by that very fact) would not be void but is voidable at the instance of the other party. So it is up to the spouse of the mentally ill whether he/she can continue the married life with such a person. However, the framers of law have stated that the mental disorder shall be of such a kind or to such an extent as to render the person to be unfit for marriage and procreate the children (Nambi, 2008). Here a grey area would be the situation where both the parties are suffering from mental disorder to render them as mentally ill and are capable to procreate children.
- **Divorce:** A person having a severe disorder of mind or suffering continuously or intermittently from mental disorder of such kind and to such extent that he cannot be reasonably expected to live with his/her spouse would suffer a ground to have his marriage dissolved by a decree of divorce (Nambi, 2005).
- **Adoption:** The concept of adoption is a unique feature of Hindu personal law as far as India is concerned. The person giving in adoption must have age of discretion and must be of sound mind. Similarly, to take in adoption the soundness of mind is an essential prerequisite (Section 7 & 8 of Hindu Adoption and Maintenance Act 1956).
- **Abortion:** Prior to 1971, termination of pregnancy was considered an offence punishable under law and so also was treated as a taboo (Section 312 to 316 of IPC). Shantilal Shah Committee recommended among several aspects as to when the termination of pregnancy could be done. The committee recommended that where the pregnancy resulted from rape with a mentally retarded, serious mentally handicapped child being born or serious risk to the life of mother, the pregnancy could be terminated. To terminate pregnancy of a woman who has not attained the age of eighteen years or a woman more than eighteen years but mentally ill the consent of guardian in writing is a mandatory requirement and without such consent, no termination could be done.

Code of Civil Procedure and Persons with Mental Disorder

Separate provisions are made in Code of Civil Procedure (CPC) to regulate the proceedings relating to persons with mental disorder and minors. In respect of persons who are adjudged or not before or during the pendency of a suit, to be mentally ill or incapable of understanding by reason of mental illness, the procedure as contemplated in Rule 1 to 14 (except Rule 2A) of Order 32 shall be applied with such modifications as needed. Where a suit is to be brought by a person with disorder of mind, a next friend and where he is to be a defendant the suit must be defended by a guardian and item must sue on his behalf. Where a manager is appointed under the provisions of Mental Health Act to manage the property, no person other than the said Manager should act as a next friend of the person with mental disorder in respect of the property. The enquiry contemplated under the provisions of Order 32 is not similar to that of the enquiry under the Mental Health Act. Any appointment of guardian based on a medical certificate without examining the medical officer on oath and by conducting enquiry is not proper.

PRIVATE RIGHTS

Patients have several rights to privacy. In addition to confidentiality, they are allowed private bathroom and shower space, secure storage space for clothing and other belongings, and adequate floor space per person. They also have the right to wear their own clothes and to carry their own money.

ECONOMIC RIGHTS

Apart from special considerations related to incompetence, psychiatric patients generally are permitted to manage their own financial affairs. One feature of this fiscal right is the requirement that patients be paid if they work in the institution (e.g., gardening or preparing food). This right often creates tension between the valid therapeutic need for activity, including jobs, and exploitative labour. A consequence of this tension is that valuable occupational, vocational, and rehabilitative therapeutic programs may have to be eliminated because of the failure of legislatures to supply the funding to pay wages to patients who participate in these programs.

CRIMINAL LAW AND PEOPLE WITH MENTAL DISORDER

The common law jurisdiction in India recognizes defence of insanity against a charge of crime. This defence is different from other defences in so far as the result is concerned. If the defence is successful, it is not acquittal and release of accused but a special verdict which says that as they are not guilty by reasons of insanity, they need to be admitted and treated in a mental hospital. A person who has to stand criminal trial in a criminal court shall know as to what is happening against him and shall have full opportunity to contest the case. A special provision is envisaged in the Code of Criminal Procedure while dealing with a matter concerned with a person who is of unsound mind. In such of the cases, it is for the prosecution to establish that the said person is sane and capable of making defence. Act of a person with disorder of mind is not an offence is based on the famous dictum Rule of Mc'Naughten. The Courts in some of the cases looking at the facts and circumstances have held that the plea of insanity would be available and the act complained of would not constitute an offence (Section 83 of Indian Penal Code (IPC)). The rule of Mc'Naughten is being criticised heavily that in legal sphere the rule is being applied blindly (Sethi, 1984). The courts however, have continued to use the standard of over hundred years old. This is because law and medicine do not look at the individual with same perspectives.

CONCLUSION

People with mental illness are often subject to social isolation, poor quality of life and increased mortality. People with mental illness can have direct and indirect costs on the society. Disability legislation plays a very important role in upholding the rights of the mentally ill. The fundamental aim of this legislation is to protect, promote and fulfill the rights of the persons with disability. It also plays a vital role in dictating the terms and conditions of mental health care and protecting the human rights and fundamental rights of people with mental disorders. Reality is a far cry from what this legislation had proposed to achieve. The three pillars of our democracy- legislature, executive and judiciary continue to discriminate and ignore the human rights of persons with mental illness.

REFERENCES

Balmer, N., Pleasence, P., Buck, A., & Walker, H. (2006). Worried sick: The experience of debt problems and their relationship with health, illness and disability. *Social Policy and Society*, *5*(1), 39–51. doi:10.1017/S147474640500271X

Code of Civil Procedure. (1908). *Bare Act; Bare Act*. Lucknow: Eastern Book Company.

Code of Criminal Procedure Amendment Act. (2010). Bare Act; Eastern Book Company, Lucknow.

Convention on Rights of Person with Disability. (n.d.). Available online on website http://www.un.org/disabilities/countries.asp?id=166htm

Coumarelos, C., Wei, Z., & Zhou, A. (2006). *Justice made to measure: NSW Legal Needs Survey in disadvantaged areas*. Sydney: Law and Justice Foundation of NSW.

Currie, A. (2007). Civil justice problems and the disability and health status of Canadians. In P. Pleasence, A. Buck, & N. Balmer (Eds.), *Transforming lives: law and social process*. London: The Stationary Office.

Dale, D. M. (2000). The state of access to justice in Oregon, part 1: assessment of legal needs. Portland, OR: Oregon State Bar. Retrieved from http://www.nlada.org/DMS/Documents/1028902493.69/LegalNeedsreport.pdf

Dhanda, A. (2000). *Legal order and mental disorder*. New Delhi: Sage Publications.

Gautam, S., Jain, S., Batra, L., Sharma, R., & Munshi, D. (2009). Human rights and privileges of mentally ill persons. In S. Gautam & A. Avasthi (Eds.), *Forensic Psychiatry, Clinical Practice Guidelines for Psychiatrists in India* (pp. 82–112). New Delhi: Indian Psychiatric Society.

Genn, H. (1999). *Paths to justice: what people do and think about going to law*. Portland, OR: Hart Publishing.

Hindu Adoption and Maintenance Act. (1956). Bare Act; Eastern Book Company, Lucknow.

Indian Contract Act. (1872). *Bare Act*. Lucknow: Eastern Book Company.

Indian Partnership Act. (1932). *Bare Act*. Lucknow: Eastern Book Company.

Indian Penal Code. (1860). *Bare Act*. Lucknow: Eastern Book Company.

Karras, M., McCarron, E., Gray, A., & Ardasinski, S. (2006). *On the edge of justice: the legal needs of people with a mental illness in NSW*. Sydney: Law and Justice Foundation of NSW.

Nambi, S. (2005). Marriage, mental health and the Indian legislation. *Indian Journal of Psychiatry*, *47*(1), 3–14. doi:10.4103/0019-5545.46067

Nambi, S. (2008). *Legal aspects in Psychiatry – Indian Perspective*. Manashanthi Mental Health Care Publications.

Nambi, S. (2014). Forensic Psychiatry (Psychiatry & Law). Jaypee Brothers Medical Publishers.

Pleasence, P & Balmer, N. (2007). *Mental health and the experience of problems involving rights*. Academic Press.

Pleasence, P., & Balmer, N. (2007). Mental health and the experience of housing problems involving rights. *People, Place and Policy Online*, 2(1), 4–16. Retrieved from http://extra.shu.ac.uk/ppponline/issue_1_300108/documents/mental_health_housing_problems_rights.pdf

Pleasence, P., Balmer, N., & Buck, A. (2006). Causes of action: civil law and social justice (2nd ed.). London: Stationery Offifice. Retrieved from http:// www.lsrc.org.uk/publications/cofa2006.pdf

Pleasence, P., Balmer, N., & Buck, A. (2008). The health cost of civil-law problems: Further evidence of links between civil-law problems and morbidity, and the consequential use of health services'. *Journal of Empirical Legal Studies*, *5*(2), 351–373. doi:10.1111/j.1740-1461.2008.00127.x

Pleasence, P., Balmer, N., Buck, A., O'Grady, A., & Genn, H. (2004a). Civil law problems and morbidity'. *Journal of Epidemiology and Community Health*, *58*(7), 552–557. doi:10.1136/jech.2003.014076 PMID:15194714

Pleasence, P., Buck, A., Balmer, N., O'Grady, A., Genn, H., & Smith, M. (2004b). Causes of action: civil law and social justice. Stationery Office, Norwich.

Raveeshm, B. N., Anil, M. N., & Narendra, K. M. S. (2013). Law & Psychiatry in India: An Overview. *J Forensic Sci Criminol*, *1*, 203.

Sethi, B. B. (1984). Need for Growth of Forensic Psychiatry. *Indian Journal of Psychiatry*, *26*, 1–2. PMID:21965949

Task Force on Civil Equal Justice Funding. (2003). *The Washington State civil legal needs study*. Washington State Supreme Court. Retrieved from <http://www.lri.lsc.gov/pdf/03/030185_lglndstudy093003.pdf>

The Indian Succession Act. (1956). Bare Act; Eastern Book Company, Lucknow.

The Mental Health Act 1987 with Central and State Rules (1990). Delhi Law House, Delhi.

The persons with disability (equal opportunities, protection of rights and full participation Act (1995). Bare Act; Eastern Book Company, Lucknow.

Transfer of Property Act. (1882). *Bare Act.* Lucknow: Eastern Book Company.

KEY TERMS AND DEFINITIONS

Disability: The condition of being unable to do things in the normal way: the condition of being disabled.

Legal Services: Legal services are services that come within the meaning of the practice of law under the Legal Profession Act and services.

Mental Health: A mental illness is a health problem that significantly affects how a person thinks, behaves and interacts with other people. It is diagnosed according to standardised criteria.

Testamentary Capacity: Having the mental competency to execute a will at the time the will was signed and witnessed. To have testamentary capacity the author of the will must understand the nature of making a will, have a general idea of what he/she possesses.

Section 5

Chronic Mental Illness:
Children and Adolescents

Chapter 13
Psychosocial Intervention Studies for Street Children with Substance Abuse

Lakshmana G.
Central University of Karnataka, India

ABSTRACT

The chapter made an attempt to review the literature and describes various interventions available for street children. The current chapter enlists all the intervention activities carried out for this group. Method of the study followed web based literature review (secondary data) using pubmed, Ebsco, Psyinfo, like on by using key words such as street children, substance abuse, motivation, intervention like on. Totally about 300 studies had been found out which discussed about street children. Among them the reviewers had chosen important studies for review purpose. Studies were discussed under the subthemes of concept of street children, prevalence of street children, reasons for on the street, street life and ways of coping with stress, substance abuse among street children, intervention carried out with street children and substance abuse, suggestions and conclusion. Conclusion: The discussed psychosocial intervention in the chapter are well proven in the general population and effectively tried with street children.

INTRODUCTION

The present society which is the transitory from rural to the urbanization is facing lot of new challenges like HIV/AIDS, sanitation problem, environmental pollution, infrastructure along with many new types of social problems such as detached families, single parent families, street children, elderly people dislodgement from family are different from the traditional problems of racism, castism, gender discrimination, population escalation, poverty etc. Among all the present social problems providing various psychosocial interventions for single parents, detached families, street children, old age problems are the need of the hour and all the governments in the world are trying their level best to minimize these problems. Street children are more vulnerable and there is a huge need to address this issue. Children are the future

DOI: 10.4018/978-1-5225-0519-8.ch013

citizens of any country and if they are on the streets, they will not get the adequate love and affection, education, values etc which makes them to be the burden of the country. Hence, there is a great need to address the issues of street children.

The limited and insufficient studies done so far on street children show that, the problem is increasing at an alarming rate. It is worsened by some factors such as economic crisis, displacement caused by war and political instability, rapid and uncontrolled urbanization. Studies show that, there are a large number of children working in the cities and major towns. A number of factors push these children to work on the streets. In the developing countries like India, the problems are rural to urban migration, unemployment, broken families, parents scolding, beating, alcoholic parents, poverty, orphan, fought with parents, step mother problem, stolen money from home etc., whereas in the developed countries they are victims of alienation and systematic exclusion (BOSCO, 1998; World Health Organization [WHO], 1993; Agnelli, 1986).

Some children come to the streets seeking better lifestyle but the condition makes their life still shoddier. Studies show that, many of the children work on the streets in all the weather conditions without proper shelter and clothing. Many of them suffer from different illnesses, drop out of school or compromise their education itself. Furthermore, these children suffer from abuses by different people including employers and street gangs. Due to poverty, the children do not get proper food and their housing condition will be very poor. Due to various reasons, there is a high chance of these children vulnerable to all kind of exploitation. It may be physical, economical, emotional, psychological and sexual. Peer pressure and use of substances in streets among the street children is common and it is a part of the street life. In spite of living on the streets due to the nature of work they do and lack of protection, they are vulnerable to all kinds of high risk behaviours. Substance abuse is a major concern in these children and it is evident that, majority of the street children use some kind of psychoactive substance.

NEED AND SCOPE OF THE CHAPTER

This chapter made an attempt to review the literature and describes various interventions available for street children. The chapter enlists all the intervention activities carried out for this group. As treating this group is challenging, understanding this group and planning an intervention requires special knowledge. This chapter also bridges the gap and helps to the mental health professionals, activists, Non Govt. Organization [NGO] personnel to have comprehensive idea on available intervention activities for this group.

METHOD

The chapter followed web based literature review (secondary data) using pubmed, Ebsco, Psyinfo, and other search engines by using key words such as street children, substance abuse, motivation, intervention like on. Along with web based literature, other available secondary sources were also reviewed for the purpose. Totally about 300 studies had been found out which discussed about street children. Among them the reviewers had chosen important studies for review purpose. Studies were discussed under the subthemes of concept of street children, prevalence of street children, reasons for on the street, street life and ways of coping with stress, substance abuse among street children, intervention carried out with street children and substance abuse, suggestions and conclusion.

CONCEPT OF STREET CHILDREN

Many eminent scholars have tried to define the street children more comprehensively. Below are the few definitions.

According to Juvenile Justice (care and protection of children) Govt. Of India [GoI] act, 2000, a person who has not completed 18 years, living on the street in the presence of the family or absent of the family is a street child.

UNICEF (1998) has categorized the street children into three categories:

1. **Children on the Street:** These are those, who still have family connections of a more or less regular nature. Their focus in life is still the home. The child might even return every night to sleep at home, but spends most days and some nights on the streets because of poverty, overcrowding, sexual or physical abuse at home.
2. **Children of the Street:** These children are small in number. Children in this group see the street as their home and there they seek shelter, food and a sense of family among companions and although family ties exist that are remote.
3. **Abandoned Children:** These are those children whose ties with the home have broken. They are without the family.

PREVALENCE OF STREET CHILDREN

United Nations in 1999 estimated that, there were over 150 million street children in the world, of which 40 percent were permanently homeless. Consortium for Street Children, an organization (2011) compiled magnitude of the street children in the world by reviewing epidemiological studies and this report reports that; Every Child estimated that 100 – 150 million children live and/or work on the streets across the world (Every Child, 2008). Indian Embassy estimated that, 314,700 street children live in metros such as Bombay, Calcutta, Madras, Kanpur, Bangalore and Hyderabad. In Delhi alone, 1,00,000 street children were reported (Railway Children, 2008 (Consortium for Street Children, 2011). BOSCO in 1999 conducted a study which coated that, in Bangalore alone, around 65,000 street children were present.

Reasons for Being on the Street

Generally, the problem of street children cannot be related to a single cause or factor. Unlike the situation in other countries, where a single cause such as extreme poverty, civil wars, or natural disasters might be the leading cause, the problem of street children in India is multi-dimensional in which a combination of factors often leads to a single child ending up being on the street. The leading factors for street children existence are family break-up, Parental scolding and beating, addicted parents, step mother problem, orphan, poverty, natural and manmade disasters, famine, physical and social allure, exploitation by adults, dislocation through migration, urbanization, unemployment, overcrowding and lack of political will (Olley, 2006; Consortium for Street Children, 2011; BOSCO, 1998; WHO,1993;UNICEF, 1993,1998; Schurink & Tiba, 1993).

Nature of the Work of Street Children

Street children usually do the odd jobs of washing cars, selling paper tissues, other items on the streets, collecting plastic from wastes to recycling factories, shining shoes, carrying luggage, selling newspapers and prostitution. They work temporarily in shops, workshops or small factories informally when the jobs are available.

PROBLEMS OF STREET CHILDREN

Problems of street children could be listed under social, physical, psychological, drug use and legal problems. After thorough review, the following problems have been listed (Bal, Mitra, Mallick, Chakraborti, & Sarkar, 2010; Mathur et al., 2009; WHO, 2000; Altanis & Goddard, 2004; Ahmadkhaniha, Shariat, Torkaman-nejad, & Moghadam, 2007; Merill Merrill, Njord, Njord, Read, & Pachano, 2010).

Social Problems

The following are the important social problems of street children:

- Poverty and illiteracy among the children,
- Discrimination and lack of accessible resources in the community,
- Violent environment where they stay,
- Stigmatization in the society,
- Poor social support,
- Poor public awareness,
- Lack of willingness to help them by society members,
- Poor social responsibility in the society for societal cause,
- Early sexual exposure and having children.

Physical Problems

The following are the physical problems of street children:

- Lack of adequate nutrition,
- Injuries may be caused by intentionally and unintentionally sexual and reproductive health problems such as HIV/ AIDS,
- Common diseases such as tuberculosis, skin diseases, dental problems etc.

Psychological and Mental Problems

The following are the psychological and mental problems faced by street children:

- Transitory lifestyle leads to problems of isolation and loneliness,

- Stresses that they experience make them vulnerable to emotional problems, physical disorders, and learning difficulties,
- Pessimism about future,
- Emotional problems,
- Self harm behavior,
- Psychological problems such as depression, behavioral problems.

Drug Use and Legal Problems

Street children are susceptible for substance abuse either by force or course of stay on street makes them to use:

- Drug smuggling and gang activities,
- Police harassment,
- Inadequate safety for life and belongings,
- Transitory life style,
- No legal security for them,
- Misuse by antisocial elements,
- Poor laws which address their needs,
- Lack of supervision by adults,
- Lack of treatment options and unwilling to help them by service provider,
- Poor rehabilitation programs,
- Poor legal help for them.

Street children face multiple problems and the above mentioned problems show the severity of the various problems. They are vulnerable for all kinds of exploitation, poor policy and lack of programs made them to suffer more.

SUBSTANCE ABUSE AMONG STREET CHILDREN

Substance abuse among the street children is common and well known phenomena. The review of literature showed that, the substance abuse among the street children is common phenomena and studies reported that, about 25% to 90% of the street children use some kind of substance (WHO, 2000). The gateway theory is applicable with the street children and also that, they start with tobacco and slowly move onto other drugs. Once they are addicted, they face withdrawal symptoms in the form of irritability, psychomotor retardation, craving, anhedonia, dry mouth, sleep disturbances, increased lacrimation etc. Some children would have exposed to substances before they come onto the streets but majority would have not exposed to any kind of substances. Once they come onto the streets, though they are not using, the street gangs push them to use substances. Gradually, they also start using in order to join the groups. After sometime, the recreational use will become addiction and they will be caught in the hands of addiction. The magnitude of the problems indicates the need for intervention in greater manner and this will not be easy job.

Types of Drug Use

The review of literature shows that the following substances are abused by street adolescents:

- Inhalants.
- Solvents.
- Rugby (glue).
- Cough syrups.
- Marijuana and shabu.
- Nail varnish.
- Cocaine.
- Alcohol.
- Tobacco.
- Tablets.
- Injection.
- Opium.
- Cannabis (bhang, charas and ganja).
- Heroin (smack, brown sugar).
- Opioids.

The common substance being used by street children is tobacco, alcohol, inhalants, cannabis, opioids, Benzodiazepamsare the common drugs abused by street children depending upon local factors. Street children use smokeless as well as smoking form of tobacco. They use smokeless tobacco forms of gutkha, powdered tobacco, hans, pan parag, manikchand etc. They also use smoking form of tobacco like beedi and cigarette. The commonest inhalants were fluid (eraser fluid), paint thinner, glue (dendrites etc.), petroleum products etc. Among all the substances, inhalants are the most commonly used in world as well as in India (Lakshmana, Dhanasekara, & Prabhat, 2014).

Inhalants are known by a number of different names some of which refer to all inhalants, such as air blast, huff, medusa, spray and others that refer to a specific substance, such as amys (amyl nitrite), rush or white out (isobutyl nitrite), poppers (amyl or isobutyl nitrite), laughing gas or whippets (nitrous oxide) and tolly or Texas shoe shine (toluene) (Kilmer, Cronce, & Palmer, 2005). Inhalants can be sniffed or snorted directly from their original container or in the case of aerosols, directly dispensed into the mouth. Individuals may also engage in huffing or bagging. Huffing involves saturating a rag with the inhalant and then placing the rag directly over the nose and mouth, whereas bagging involves inhaling the substance from a plastic bag. Because the effects of most inhalants peak rapidly and dissipate within a few minutes (Cohen, 1984), individuals may engage in more covert means of using these substances in the presence of other people (Keriotis & Upadhyaya, 2000).

Impact of Inhalants Use

Most inhalants (i.e., volatile solvents and anesthetic gases) have a depressant effect on the central nervous system and induce feelings of euphoria and intoxication. While under the influence of these inhalants, individuals may appear inebriated, exhibiting impaired motor control, disinhibition, slurred speech and belligerent behaviour and may also experience hallucinations and delusions (Kurtzman, Otsuka, & Wahl,

2001, American Psychiatric Association [APA], 2000). Other negative effects of inhalants use include coughing, wheezing, dizziness, stupor, skin irritation around the nose and mouth (sniffer's rash), headache, tremor, muscle weakness, abdominal pain, nausea, vomiting, loss of consciousness and irregular heart rhythms leading to heart failure and death (American Psychiatric Association [APA], 2000). Use of inhalants by adolescents is troubling for reasons beyond the known physical consequences. Inhalant use in adolescence may increase the risk for the use of other substances in young adulthood. Various reports have noted tolerance to inhalants among heavy users (Kono et al., 2001; APA, 2000). Individuals may also develop dependence (APA, 2000) and experience symptoms typically associated with withdrawal such as craving, anxiety, irritability, restlessness, difficulty concentrating or paying attention and sleep disturbances. Additionally, individuals may experience increased heart rate, headache, hallucinations, excessive perspiration, shivering, tremors, nausea, diarrhea and fluctuations in appetite after discontinuation of inhalant use (Kono et al., 2001; Keriotis & Upadhyaya, 2000). Studies have been found that, 25% to 90% of street children use some kinds of psychoactive substances (WHO, 1993). In Bangalore about 70-80% of the street children abuse some kinds of drugs (Benegal et al., 1999). Majority of the studies are focused on the prevalence and extent of the problem. Only few studies are focused on the intervention. Intervention for these children is very challenging and necessary of the hour due to the extent of the problem (Bal, Mitra, Mallick, Chakraborti, & Sarkar, 2010; Njord, Merrill, Njord, Lindsay, & Pachano, 2010; Praharaj, Verma, & Arora, 2008).

INTERVENTION PROGRAMS

Western Studies

Conrod, Castellanos-Ryan, and Strang (2010) studied the efficacy of targeted coping skills interventions on illicit drug use in adolescents with personality risk factors for substance misuse. The brief interventions which involved two 90-minute group sessions were manualized and were carried out at the participant's schools. The manuals incorporated a psycho educational component, a motivational component and a cognitive behavioural therapy component and included real-life scenarios. Results revealed that, the number of drugs used (P0.01) and drug use frequency (P0.05) had been reduced than compared to controls over the 2-year period. Nalkur (2009a) study compared the street children former street children and school-going children (n = 183). Findings showed that, just after 1 year of rehabilitative care, former street children's priorities are more similar to school-going children's and thus rehabilitative care may be instrumental in enabling children to prioritize preparing for the future. Street children's emphasis on a safe place to sleep and adult support may reflect unmet basic needs. Xue (2009) study reported that, the actual number of urban street children may be even greater than reported statistics because reported statistics always based on past counts and estimates. Analysis revealed that, social exclusion was a major feature of the lives of the street children in China. Therefore, taking valid measures to eliminate the various forms of exclusion should provide guidelines for developing future policies and practices. The study also reported that, encouraging provisions by nongovernmental and the reform of educational opportunities were few important strategies to develop social work services for families with problems.

Pinzon-Rondon, Hofferth, and Briceno (2008) study revealed that, compared to the working children, the displaced children were more likely to be under 5 years old for having adult supervision and to beg. These children were less likely to have a social security affiliation. Compared to the displaced children, the homeless children were likely to be older to work for longer periods of hours, to be boys, to beg and were less likely to attend schools. The study reported that, different types of street children are existed and suggested that, different approaches for improving the lives of these three groups of children are needed. Lam and Cheng (2008) examined the effectiveness of the government-managed Protection and Education Centre for Street Children program in China based on a 7-months ethnographic study of street children in public streets at the centre in Shanghai. They findings were revealed that, most of the street children disliked the high security of the centre and many had rejected going home. So they tended to keep away from the centre even though it could provide them with lodging and food. It was suggested that, the policy for street children should be reviewed with the consideration given to the street children's family situations and the children's own thoughts and preferences. The programs at the Centre should be enriched and training of the staff should be provided. Moolla, Myburgh, and Poggenpoel (2008) reported that, the street children have negative attitude and fear towards law authority. Life skills facilitation and peer support program could assist the street children to interact with the police in healthier ways. Kudrati, Plummer and Yusuf (2008) suggested that, the street-based services to improve children's health and safety are urgently needed. Re-integration programs may help large number of children to voluntarily and permanently leave the streets. Schimmel (2008) reported that, in the developing countries, overwhelming emphasis has been paid to outreach programs for street children on providing them with their basic needs of food, shelter and clothing but often disregarding their psychological needs. This approach to the street children may help them in the short term but impedes the likelihood of their achieving a rehabilitation that is sustainable and that meets the full range of their needs in a holistic manner.

Fernandes and Vaughn (2008) reviewed the street children literature reported that, findings are limited in studies and available research reveals an urgent need for implementation of policies for the street children. They also reported that, programs for preventing substance misuse and delinquency are still missing the political and infrastructural support. This clearly showed that, our policy makers are not proactive in preventing this. Plummer, Mustafa and Nassrin Dafalla, (2007) reported that, services should be tailored to the particular needs of the street children, working children, abandoned children group by gender including the community-based prevention, street-based health and safety interventions and street child counseling and re-integration programs. Patterson (2007) examined the situational and demographic characteristics in a sample of 47 children missing person police reports obtained from a law enforcement agency to identify the service needs of runaway youth and their families. His showed that, runaways represented the only category of missing children contained in the data. The results support the need for a comprehensive integration between the social work research and practice and are used to provide recommendations for the service needs of runaway children and their families. Social work practice recommendations include:

1. Community campaigns,
2. Training, and
3. Increased collaboration between law enforcement and child welfare agencies.

Olley (2006) revealed that, implementing a life skill program to address these antisocial behaviours may help to increase the well-being of the street youths in developing countries in Africa. Dybicz (2005) reported that, most professional literature had concentrated solely on describing this population and the knowledge base on intervention strategies for the street children remains at a nascent stage of development. The resources of society through the governments needed to be addressed the issue of extreme poverty and the street children for any significant thing to occur in servicing the needs of this population. Life skills training programme (teaching skills including communication, decision making, stress and anxiety management) was effective in reducing smoking, alcohol and drug use and there was significant difference found in studies (Rakshit, 2004; Michale, 2001; Errecart et al., 1991; Botvin, Baker, Botvin, Filazzola, & Millman, 1984).

Veale and Dona (2003) highlighted and suggested the need for community based support for the children in alternative guardianship care and for policies to support the reintegration of male youths in post conflict welfare strategies as prevention strategies for street migration. Meyer, Madu, and Mako (2002) analyzed two hundred and sixteen (216) participants made up of 54 hardcore, 54 sheltered, 54 part-time street children and 54 non-street children (as control group). Findings were revealed that, hardcore and sheltered street children have a lower level of self-esteem than the control group. Hardcore street children also have a lower level of emotional stability than the control group. Psychologists, educators, social workers and other mental health professionals charged with the responsibility of designing rehabilitation programs for hardcore and sheltered street children should take the self-esteem into consideration while intervening. Browne and Falshaw (1998) reported that, 14 to 20% of children run away from home for at least one night and that 2% run away 10 times or more from home or a care setting. Their study proposed that, counselling should be a part of intervention with street children and counsellors should be available free to them.

Le Roux and Smith (1998) studied the public perceptions and reactions to the street children and they were reported that, no treatment program designed for street children can succeed unless the community is prepared to respect, protect and provide opportunities for them. This study also reported that the street children are abused in many parts of the world. Aidan (1997) studied the street children life stressors. The study reported that, most of them lived at home with both parents but a sizable minority lived on the streets with peers. Lack of proper homes, lack of employment by parent(s), lack of education, violence and hunger were the major stress reported by them. The study also pointed out that, changing national economy, growing urbanization and broken families were the major stressors and suggested to include positive coping to handle this in interventions. Rhodes and Jason (1988) study reported that, stress is a way, the person feels in response to real or perceived stressors. The more stress a child is under, the more likely he or she is to use the substance. The street children often have extremely stressful lives. The children face five types of stress and they are, major life events, enduring life strains, everyday problems, life transitions and adolescent development change (Rhodes & Jason, 1988). The modified stress model that is derived from original work of Rhodes et al. (1988) also ratify this (WHO, 1993).

INDIAN STUDIES

In India, the studies have been done with the street children. Majority of the studies discussed the need for an intervention with this population and only few studies were intervention studies. Merriman and Guerin (2007) studied the aspirations of Kolkata street children. The participants were 66 males (43.7%) and 85 females (56.3%), of which 51 (33.8%) were “on the streets” and 100 (66.2%) were “off the streets”. They were asked to draw a picture of the sort of person they wanted to be when they grew up and to write who the person was and what they were doing and why they were chosen. The most common occupations recorded were teacher (n = 48, 31.8%) and doctor (n = 29, 19.2%) and there was a majority of higher socio-economic status (SES) occupations with high Educational requirements.

Benegal et al., (2010) conducted a cross sectional study among 92 inhalant users and 128 non-users. Inhalants (96.0%) and tobacco (81.5%) were the most commonly used drugs of abuse in the last 30 days followed by the alcohol (38.0%), heroin (20.7%) and cannabis use (15.2%). The mean frequency of use of inhalants was 6.18±2.8 /day. Majority of inhalant users reported tolerance (66.3%) and withdrawal symptoms (65.2%). Around 72.8% inhalant users reported that they considered stopping/reducing use of drugs at some point of time in their life but only 41.3% were able to stop using the inhalants at some point of time in their lifetime.

PSYCHO-SOCIAL INTERVENTIONS USED WITH ADOLESCENTS

Psychosocial treatment for substance abuse is widely used in the world. It includes many types of treatment options. Modalities of delivering psychosocial therapies can be either therapist mediated or non-therapist mediated. They have been used extensively with adult population and tried with adolescents. The few models could be tried with street children also based on the needs.

Therapist Mediated

These can be of two types: Brief Interventions (BIs) and Extended Interventions (EIs).

1. **Brief Interventions (BIs):** BIs are characterized by involving 1-4 sessions. They improve staff efficiency and are generally cost effective. The main characteristics of BI are: keeping the goal of reduced or non-problem alcohol/drug use as opposed to abstinence; generally delivered by a non-specialist; generally directed at non-dependent rather than dependent individuals; addressing the person's motivation to change habits; being self-directed; and having certain key components/ingredients (feedback of risk involved, encouraging responsibility for change, advice, alternative options, enhancing self-efficacy). These interventions could be more effective with street children as they are mobile population and require less time. Based on the rapport, and if the children are staying in rehabilitation centre, the extended interventions are more suitable.
2. **Extended Interventions (EIs):** EIs are characterized by involving 5-12 sessions which are carried out either in a group or alone. The type of intervention delivered depends upon the aims of the treatment and can be relapse prevention programs, cognitive behaviour therapy, behavioural interventions, social skill training, supportive-expressive psychotherapy etc. Varied types of EIs have been found to have similar benefits where results being similar across both inpatients and outpatients. However, it has been seen that, it is necessary to address problems with psychiatric illness and lifestyle concurrent with drug/alcohol abuse.

Non-Therapist Mediated

These are essentially Self-Help Groups (SHGs); the commonest and popular ones being Alcoholic Anonymous (AA), Narcotic Anonymous (NA), Cocaine Anonymous etc. The SHG is a group of individuals with similar problems who meet voluntarily to help each other to help themselves.

The following are the important psychosocial interventions used for adolescents, which can be tried with street children and few studies tried few interventions.

- **Individual Psychotherapy and Group Psychotherapy:** In this, the common issues and strategies include setting the resolve to stop, teaching coping skills, changing reinforcement contingencies, fostering management of painful affects, improving interpersonal functioning and enhancing social support. The treatment goals are establishing abstinence, establishing stable functioning, preventing relapse, addressing psychological issues and managing care considerations.
- **Relapse Prevention:** This involves the specific techniques of exploring the positive and negative consequences of continued use, self-monitoring to recognize drug cravings early and identifying high-risk situations for use, developing strategies for coping with and avoiding high-risk situations and the desire to use. The central element involves anticipating the problems of patients that are likely to meet and helping them develop effective coping strategies.
- **Supportive-Expressive Psychotherapy:** This has two main components i.e. supportive techniques to help patients feel comfortable in discussing their personal experiences and expressive techniques to help patients identify and work through interpersonal relationship issues.
- **Individualized Drug Counselling:** This focuses directly on reducing or stopping the addict's illicit drug use. It also covers other related areas of impaired functioning like employment status, illegal activity, family/social relations, content and structure of the patient's recovery program. Through its emphasis on short-term behavioural goals, it also helps the patient to develop coping strategies, tools for abstaining from drug use and maintaining abstinence.
- **Motivation Enhancement Therapy:** This approach employs strategies to evoke rapid and internally motivated change in the client. The first treatment session focuses on providing feedback generated from the initial assessment battery to stimulate discussion regarding personal substance use and to elicit self-motivational statements. In subsequent sessions, the therapist monitors change, reviews cessation strategies being used, continues to encourage commitment to change or sustained abstinence and sometimes encourages the clients to bring a significant other to the sessions.
- **Behavioural Therapy for Adolescents:** Therapeutic activities include fulfilling specific assignments, rehearsing desired behaviours, recording and reviewing progress, with praise and privileges given for meeting assigned goals. Urine samples are collected regularly to monitor drug use. The therapy aims to equip the patient to gain three types of control viz. stimulus control, urge control and social control.
- **Multidimensional Family Therapy (MDFT) for Adolescent Family Members:** This is an outpatient family based drug abuse treatment for teenagers. Treatment includes individual and family sessions held in the clinic, home or with family members at the family court, school or other community locations. Here with street children, wherever possible we need to use family. Many times the family problems contribute for running away from home and staying on street. The problems need to be handled with the family.
- **Multi Systemic Therapy (MST):** This addresses factors associated with serious antisocial behaviour in children and adolescents who abuse drugs. These factors focus on the characteristics of the adolescent (favourable attitudes toward drug use), the family (poor discipline, family conflict, and parental drug abuse), peers (positive attitudes toward drug use), school (dropout, poor performance) and neighbourhood (criminal subculture).
- **Community Reinforcement Approach (CRA) Plus Vouchers:** This involves an intensive 24-week outpatient therapy. The treatment goals are two-fold i.e. to achieve abstinence long enough for patients to learn new life skills that will help sustain abstinence and to reduce alcohol con-

sumption for patients whose drinking is associated with drug use. Patients attend one or two individual counselling sessions per week where they focus on improving family relations, learning a variety of skills to minimize drug use, receiving vocational counselling and developing new recreational activities and social networks.

- **The Matrix Model:** This provides a framework for engaging stimulant abusers in treatment and helping them achieve abstinence. Patients learn about issues critical to addiction and relapse, receive direction and support from a trained therapist who become familiar with self-help programs and are monitored for drug use by urine testing. The program includes education for family members affected by the addiction.
- **Aftercare and Rehabilitation:** Aftercare suggests different things to different people and even treatment specialists are often unclear as to what the term means. In a basic sense, it simply refers to whatever follows a given form of treatment. But it can also be understood with reference to the process of recovery itself. Recovery is not just the cessation of drug use but it is also adjustment to a new way of life within the culture of the larger community. The challenges to such adjustment come from:
    - Persistent drug craving
    - Need for establishing a new social network
    - Need to derive satisfaction from drug-free activities and lifestyle finally
    - Dealing with the risk of relapse. Aftercare can be provided in the de-addiction clinic as follow-up patient visits or it can be provided by follow-up home visits.

PSYCHO-SOCIAL INTERVENTIONS TRIED WITH STREET CHILDREN

Motivation Interviewing

The review of literature had been carried out in this aspect and few studies tried to use this intervention among the street children. Baer et al. (2008) used Brief Motivational Interviewing dividing the BMI into four shorter sessions that were spread over a 4-week period design with homeless adolescents. A sample of 117 homeless youths was recruited from a nonprofit, faith-based drop-in center. Participants reported high use of several different substances, abstaining from alcohol and other drugs an average of 8.4 days in the prior month ($SD = 9.2$); 24% reported ever injecting drugs. Of 117 youths in the sample for analysis, 97 youths (82.9%) returned for one-month interview and 89 (76.1%) completed all the three interviews (first, second & third month). Homeless youths who received BMI reported greater reductions in one of the several measures of polysubstance use compared to those in the control condition. Peterson, Wells, Ginzler, and Garrett (2006) studied "Short-term effects of a brief motivational intervention to reduce alcohol and drug risk among homeless adolescents". Homeless adolescents (N = 285) recruited from drop-in centers at agencies and from street intercept were randomly assigned to either a brief motivational enhancement (ME) group or 1 of 2 control groups. The 1-session motivational intervention presented personal feedback about patterns of risks related to alcohol or substance use in a style consistent with motivational interviewing. Follow-up interviews were conducted at 1 and 3 months post intervention. Findings were shown that at the baseline, most youths were on the pre-contemplation stage of change when asked about the goals for abstaining from alcohol or drug use (77.6% and 84.5%, respectively). Less than 10% were in each of the other stages for both the alcohol and drug abstention. In contrast, when asked about goals for reducing alcohol or substance use, many fewer youths were in the pre-contemplation stage (50.3% for alcohol, 52.9% for drugs) and many more were in the preparation stage of change (34% for both alcohol and drugs). Relatively few were in the contemplation stage of change (7% for alcohol and 11% for drug) or action–maintenance stages (8.7% for alcohol and 3% for drugs).

Brands, Leslie, and Catz-Biro (2005) interviewed forty-nine heroin-using adolescents from four youth community agencies in Toronto. Although more than half of the sample had sought treatments for their substance use problems and were knowledgeable about the treatment options available. Many believed factors such as lack of housing, finances, and contact with drug-using acquaintances would hamper their rehabilitation. Treatment programs for these youth should include the assessment and treatment of co-morbid psychiatric disorders and the provision of comprehensive services including 'safe' housing, vocational guidance and financial supports.

Indian Studies

Lakshmana, Pandian, Kumar, and Marimuttu (2013) based on the needs assessment, developed intervention package for street children with substance abuse and tested its efficacy. They were used motivation enhancement and relapse prevention strategies with street children. The study followed the classical experimental design and by using the cluster sampling method, a total of 120respondents were recruited. The majority of the respondents were on pre-contemplation stage of motivation in both the control and experimental group at the baseline. Atthe end of the third month of intervention, 78.9 percent of the respondents in the control group were on pre-contemplation stage, whereas in the experimental group about 50percent were on the contemplation and 33.3 percent were on the action stage of motivation. Bal, Mitra, Mallick, Chakraborti and Sarkar (2010) suggested that, community-based intervention is necessary for rehabilitation of street children with substance abuse. Malhotra Sharma, Saxena, and Ingle (2007) qualitative study reported that, peer influence and media plays a vital role in initiating substance use. Consuming drugs was considered to be a sign of maturity and the best way to impress a girl. Some of the boys also mentioned that, drugs were the means of escaping an emotional stress or anxiety due to the death of a family member or loss of a girlfriend. Seth, Kotwal, and Ganguly (2005) reported that, the street children used multiple drugs, among them whitener fluid was common. They reported nearly one-third of the children never tried to quit whitener fluid inhalation. A few had tried to quit, but failed, some were in various stages of trying to give up this habit. However, a few questioned the need to quit. The majority did not get any support for quitting and only two participants received any support from their parents. A few were using the help of counsellors and thought their role to be an important one. Benegal, Bhushan, Seshadri and Karott (1999) study had used experimental brief intervention session consisted of a single viewing of an animated video film ["Gold- tooth "made by the Street Kids International] and two or three workbook sessions. Even though the studies goal is not on substance, large number of the children (78%) had stopped or reduced the use of solvent drugs. 95% of the children had talked to their friends about the program and 88% had told their friends about what they had learnt for handling the stress.

Group Work with Adolescents

Various studies proved that, Group work is an effective method to deal with adolescents and street children. Conrod, Castellanos-Ryan, and Strang (2010) studied the efficacy of targeted coping skills interventions on illicit drug use in adolescents with personality risk factors for substance misuse. The brief interventions which involved two 90-minute group sessions were manualized and were carried out at the participants' schools. The manuals incorporated a psycho educational component, a motivational component and a cognitive behavioural therapy component and included real-life scenarios shared by high-personality-risk British youth in specifically organized focus groups. The first sections of the manual involved guiding the participants to increase motivation for behavioural change. Psycho educational strategies were then used to teach participants about the target personality variable (hopelessness, anxiety sensitivity, impulsivity, or sensation seeking) and associated problematic, personality-specific coping behaviours like avoidance, interpersonal dependence, aggression, risky behaviours and substance misuse. The adolescents were then introduced to the cognitive behavioural therapy model and guided in breaking down a personal experience according to the cognitive behavioral therapy components of an emotional response. Their findings revealed that, the number of drugs used (P0.01) and drug use frequency (P0.05) reduced compared to controls over the 2-year period.

Malekoff (2007) presented a framework for thoughtful and self-reflective group work with adolescents. The organizing framework contains three overarching, interrelated and flexible components: attitudinal set, conceptual base/skill set and value base. Themes and concepts that are addressed to illustrate the framework include: staying in the mess, embracing your inner clumsiness, assuming a stance of uncertainty, becoming an itinerant educator, teaching-on-the-go, setting your ego aside, differentiating the words from the music, hanging out, shifting from a formal interviewing approach to a meandering conversational style, decentralizing authority using activities of everyday life and making waves. They were concluded that this flexible framework can be easily adapted for group work with any population.

Newbauer and Blanks (2001) study described a four-process outpatient group-therapy program based on Individual Psychology. They were discussed the effective components of boundaries, including offender responsibility, accountability, restitution and also discussed various types of denial put forth by offenders and how offender's parents are integrally part of the rehabilitation process. Their study concluded that, the group work is effective method with adolescent sexual offenders. Sharry and Owens (2000); Andrew (2007) presented five guidelines for group worker for working with adolescents. They are:

1. A sense of humor and willingness to check one's ego at the door;
2. An appreciation for paradox and the ability to differentiate between words and music;
3. Access to one's own early memories;
4. The capacity to relate to the whole person; and
5. Collegial support.

Motivational Interviewing Group with Adolescents

Peterson, Baer, Wells, Ginzler and Garrett (2006) studied "Short-term effects of a brief motivational intervention to reduce alcohol and drug risk among homeless adolescents". Homeless adolescents (N = 285) recruited from drop-in centers at agencies and from street intercept were randomly assigned to either a brief motivational enhancement (ME) group or 1 of 2 control groups. The 1-session motivational intervention presented personal feedback about patterns of risks related to alcohol or substance use in a style consistent with motivational interviewing. Follow-up interviews were conducted at 1 and 3 months post intervention. Their findings were revealed that the group work on motivational enhancement is effective.

Group Work with Street Children

Group work has been used with the street children to handle various issues in general and results were positive in this aspect. The few studies which tried to use group work with substance abusing street children proved and it can be used effectively with this group. Danielset al. (1999) in their study "Group work with homeless youngsters and their mothers" evaluated a group-counselling intervention among 8, 10–17 years old and their mothers (aged 33–38 yrs) living in a homeless shelter. The intervention was specifically designed to reduce familial conflicts by enhancing the participants' interpersonal problem-solving skills. Einar (1996) study demonstrated that care no longer supplied by the family is replaced within street children groups. The study suggested that, social group work should be included while doing the intervention with this population.

DISCUSSION

The above said psycho-social intervention have been extensively used with adult population and proven their efficacy. As studies clearly shows that pharmacotherapy is not yet available for substance use disorders among adolescents and street children. There are no practice guidelines to assist psychiatrists, general physicians, paediatricians and other clinicians in the management of adolescents with inhalant use disorders. The treatment approaches being used for this are mostly multi-component and multi-model. Psycho-social approaches are commonly being used for treatment of inhalant and other substance disorders among street children (Dhawan, Chopra, Ambekar, & Ray, 2015; Lakshmana et al., 2013). The psychosocial interventions described here have been proven with adult population and there is a need to adopt with street children. There is a need to integrate these interventions in community based activities by service providers. The intervention must be tailored to each individual and must have integrated various approaches. The eclectic model would fit with this population. NGOs, community based organizations, clinicians, health providers, government hospitals, should be interlinked. While treating this population, there is a need to integrate individual, group, community and allied services in to the process of treatment. There is a need to train service providers about the sensitivity of the population, skills required to handle the issues and reintegration with the family and community. Studies exclusively conducted with street children shows that psychosocial interventions bring desirable changes among this population (Lakshmana et al., 2013, 2014; Bal et al., 2010; Njord et al., 2010; Praharaj et al., 2008).

CONCLUSION

There is lack of literature related to intervention among the street children with the substance abuse. Gradually there is a shift from exploratory to descriptive and from descriptive to intervention studies in this area. Few studies talked about the street children efforts to quit or motivation and their past efforts to quit. Few researchers tried to use motivation enhancement therapy in groups as well as individually with the street children. These studies clearly indicate that, motivation among the street children to quit substance is very low; even though they try they will not get support from family, friends, and supervisors and from others. Once they are motivated, they will try to quit and if they have coping skills to cope with various kinds of problems effectively, they tackle the relapse or lapse. Barriers to health among the street children showed that, though the street children wanted to seek help for all kinds of problems but the present society is not equipped. In the health sector, they are seen as problem creators and there is no respect for them. Even if they approach, the attitude of health provider is questionable. The stigma is very high among the general practitioners, professionals and others. Due to this, even though they seek help, discrimination will be meted for them. Once they expose to these kind of attitude, other children will not approach for any kind of help. Another important factor is that, there is no system in the society to help them. The cost of treatment is unaffordable for them. Though non-government organizations are working for them, their resources are not affordable for the street children with substance abuse. Once the children decide to overcome from this problem, they do not know how to cope with craving and to say no to offer drugs. The above discussed psychosocial intervention are well proven in the general population and effectively tried with street children. The governments, nongovernmental organizations and other service providers should utilize the psychosocial intervention in their activities to bring change among street children with substance abuse.

REFERENCES

Agnelli, S. (1986). *Street Children: A growing urban tragedy* (1st ed.). London: George Weiden Field & Nicholson.

Ahmadkhaniha, H. R., Shariat, S. V., Torkaman-nejad, S., & Moghadam, M. M. H. (2007). The frequency of sexual abuse and depression in a sample of street children of one of deprived districts of Tehran. *Journal of Child Sexual Abuse*, *16*(4), 23–35. doi:10.1300/J070v16n04_02 PMID:18032244

Aidan, M. (1997). Stress and coping strategies among street children in Lusaka. *Journal of Psychology in Africa*, *2*(1), 24–33.

Altanis, P., & Goddard, J. (2004). Street children in contemporary Greece. *Children & Society*, *18*(4), 299–311. doi:10.1002/chi.797

American Psychiatric Association. (2000). Diagnostic and statistical manual of the mental disorders (4 TR ed.). Washington, DC: Author.

Andrew, M. (2007). A flexible organizing framework for group work with adolescents. Social Work with Groups. *A Journal of Community and Clinical Practice*, *30*(3), 85-102.

Baer, J. S., Beadnell, B., Garrett, S. B., Hartzler, B., Wells, E. A., & Peterson, P. L. (2008). Adolescent change language within a brief motivational intervention and substance use outcomes. *Psychology of Addictive Behaviors*, *22*(4), 570–575. doi:10.1037/a0013022 PMID:19071983

Baer, J. S., Garrett, S. B., Beadnell, B., Wells, E. A., & Peterson, P. L. (2007). Brief Motivational Intervention With Homeless Adolescents: Evaluating Effects on Substance Use and Service Utilization. *Psychology of Addictive Behaviors*, *21*(4), 582–586. doi:10.1037/0893-164X.21.4.582 PMID:18072842

Bal, B., Mitra, R., Mallick, A. H., Chakraborti, S., & Sarkar, K. (2010). Nontobacco substance use, sexual abuse, HIV, and sexually transmitted infection among street children in Kolkata, India. *Substance Use & Misuse*, *45*(10), 1668–1682. doi:10.3109/10826081003674856 PMID:20590379

Benegal, V., Bhushan, K., Seshadri, S. P., & Karott, M. (1999). *Drug Abuse Among Street Children in Bangalore*. Unpublished manuscript, Bangalore.

Benegal, V., Sheshadri, S. P., Chand, P. K., Pandian, D., Lakshmana, G., & Subodh, B. N. (2010).Inhalant use among street children in Bangalore (Project report). Bangalore: NIMHANS (Unpublished Document).

BienBOSCO. (1998). *In partnership for children*. Bangalore: Adithya.

Botvin, G. J., Baker, E., Botvin, E. M., Filazzola, A. D., & Millman, R. B. (1984). Alcohol abuse prevention through the development of personal and social competence: A pilot study. *Journal of Studies on Alcohol*, *45*, 550–554. doi:10.15288/jsa.1984.45.550 PMID:6521482

Brands, B., Leslie, K., Catz-Biro, L., & Li, S. (2005). Heroin use and barriers to treatment in street-involved youth. *Addiction Research and Theory*, *13*(5), 477–487. doi:10.1080/16066350500150624

Browne, K., & Falshaw, L. (1998). Street children and crime in the UK: A case of abuse and neglect. *Child Abuse Review*, *7*(4), 241–253. doi:10.1002/(SICI)1099-0852(199807/08)7:4<241::AID-CAR501>3.0.CO;2-0

Cohen, S. (1984). The Hallucinogens and the inhalants. *The Psychiatric Clinics of North America*, *7*, 681–688. PMID:6097885

Conrod, P. J., Castellanos-Ryan, N., & Strang, J. (2010). Brief, Personality-Targeted Coping Skills Interventions and Survival as a Non–Drug User Over a 2-Year Period During Adolescence. *Archives of General Psychiatry*, *67*(1), 85–93. doi:10.1001/archgenpsychiatry.2009.173 PMID:20048226

Consortium For Street Children. (2011). *Street Children Statistics*. Retrieved on 5 July 2011 from http://www.streetchildren.org.uk/reports/State%20of%20he%20World's%20Street%20Children-Violence.pdf

Daniels, J., D'Andrea, M., Omizo, M., & Pier, P. (1999). Group work with homeless youngsters and their mothers. *Journal for Specialists in Group Work*, *24*(2), 164–185. doi:10.1080/01933929908411428

Dhawan, A., Chopra, A., Ambekar, A., & Ray, R. (2015). Treatment seeking behavior of Inhalant using street children: Are we prepared to meet their treatment needs. *Indian Journal of Psychological Medicine*, *37*(3), 282–287. doi:10.4103/0253-7176.162918 PMID:26664076

Dybicz, P. (2005). Interventions for street children: An analysis of current best practices. *International Social Work*, *48*(6), 763–771. doi:10.1177/0020872805057083

Einar, H. (1996). Finding care on the street: Processes in the careers of Sri Lankan street boys. *Childhood: A Global Journal of Child Research, 3*(2), 247-259.

Errecart, M. T., Walberg, H. J., Ross, J. G., Gold, R. S., Fiedler, J. L., & Kolbe, L. J. (1991). Effectiveness of teenage health teaching modules. *The Journal of School Health*, *61*(1), 26–30. doi:10.1111/j.1746-1561.1991.tb07855.x PMID:2027290

Fernandes, G. T., & Vaughn, M. G. (2008). Brazilian street children: Contextual influences in relation to substance misuse. *International Social Work*, *51*(5), 669–681. doi:10.1177/0020872808093344

Government of India. (2000). *The Juvenile Justice (Care and protection of children) Act, 2000 (Act No. 56 of 2000)*. Retrieved from wcd.nic.in/childprot/jjact2000.pdf

Keriotis, A. A., & Upadhyaya, H. P. (2000). Inhalant dependence and withdrawal symptoms. *Journal of the American Academy of Child and Adolescent Psychiatry*, *39*(6), 679–680. doi:10.1097/00004583-200006000-00004 PMID:10846300

Kilmer, J. R., Cronce, J. M., & Palmer, R. S. (2005). Relapse prevention for abuse of Club Drugs, Hallucinogens, Inhalants, and Steroids. In G. A. Marlatt & D. M. Donovan (Eds.), Relapse prevention: Maintenance strategies in the treatment of addiction behaviors (2nd ed.; pp. 208-247). New York: The Guilford Press.

Kono, J., Miyata, H., Ushijima, S., Yanagita, T., Miyasato, K., Ikawa, G., & Hukui, K. (2001). Nicotine, alcohol, methamphetamine, and inhalant dependence: A comparison with clinical features with the use of a new clinical evaluation form. *Alcohol (Fayetteville, N.Y.)*, *24*(2), 99–106. doi:10.1016/S0741-8329(01)00143-4 PMID:11522430

Kudrati, M., Plummer, M., & Yousif, N. D. E. H. (2008). Children of the sug: A study of the daily lives of street children in Khartoum, Sudan, with intervention recommendations. *Child Abuse & Neglect*, *32*(4), 439–448. doi:10.1016/j.chiabu.2007.07.009 PMID:18457872

Kurtzman, T. L., Otsuka, K. N., & Wahl, R. A. (2001). Inhalant abuse by adolescents. *The Journal of Adolescent Health*, *28*(3), 170–180. doi:10.1016/S1054-139X(00)00159-2 PMID:11226839

Lakshmana, G. (2014). DhanasekaraPandian R., & Prabhat Kumar Chand. (2014). Knowledge on impact of substance use and help seeking behavior among substance using street children. *Indian Journal of Social Psychiatry*, *30*(3-4), 106–114.

Lakshmana, G., Pandian, R. D., Kumar, P. K., & Marimuttu, P. (2013). Street children with substance abuse: Enhancement of motivation and relapse prevention strategies. *The Indian Journal of Social Work*, *74*(1), 131–150.

Lam, D., & Cheng, F. (2008). Chinese policy reaction to the problem of street children: An analysis from the perspective of street children. *Children and Youth Services Review*, *30*(5), 575–584. doi:10.1016/j.childyouth.2007.11.009

Le Roux, J., & Smith, C. S. (1998). Psychological characteristics of South African street children. *Adolescence*, *33*(132), 891–899. PMID:9886016

Malekoff, A. (2007). A flexible organizing framework for group work with adolescents. *Social Work with Groups: A Journal of Community and Clinical Practice, 30*(3), 85-102.

Malhotra, C., Sharma, N., Saxena, R., & Ingle, G. K. (2007). Drug use among juveniles in conflict with the law. *Indian Journal of Pediatrics*, *74*(4), 353–356. doi:10.1007/s12098-007-0059-1 PMID:17476079

Mathur, M. (2009B). Socialization of street children in India: A socio-economic profile. *Psychology and Developing Societies*, *21*(2), 299–325. doi:10.1177/097133360902100207

Merrill, R. M., Njord, L., Njord, R., Read, C., & Pachano, J. D. R. (2010). The effect of family influence on indicators associated with street life among Filipino street children. *Vulnerable Children and Youth Studies*, *5*(2), 142–150. doi:10.1080/17450121003615369

Merriman, B., & Guerin, S. (2007). Exploring the aspirations of Kolkatan (Calcuttan) street children living on an off the streets using drawings. *International Journal of Psychology & Psychological Therapy*, *7*(2), 269–283.

Meyer, A., Madu, S. N., & Mako, M. J. (2002). Self esteem and emotional stability of street children in some townships in South Africa. *The Irish Journal of Psychology*, *23*(1-2), 109–119.

Michale, C. (2001). *A feasibility study on life skills education for street children.* (Unpublished M.Phil Dissertation). National Institute of Mental Health and Neuro Sciences, Bangalore, India.

Moolla, A., Myburgh, C., & Poggenpoel, M. (2008). Street children's experiences of aggression during interaction with police. *Journal of Psychology in Africa*, *18*(4), 597–602.

Nalkur, P. G. (2009a). Achievement orientations and strategies: A cultural comparison of Tanzanian street children, former street children, and school-going children. *Journal of Cross-Cultural Psychology*, *40*(6), 1012–1027. doi:10.1177/0022022109346954

Newbauer, J. F., & Blanks, J. W. (2001). Group work with adolescent sexual offenders. *Journal of Individual Psychology*, *57*(1), 37–50.

Njord, L., Merrill, R. M., Njord, R., Lindsay, R., & Pachano, J. D. R. (2010). Drug use among street children and non-street children in the Philippines. *Asia-Pacific Journal of Public Health*, *22*(2), 203–211. doi:10.1177/1010539510361515 PMID:20457649

Olley, B. O. (2006). Social and health behaviors in youth of the streets of Ibadan, Nigeria. *Child Abuse & Neglect*, *30*(3), 271–282. doi:10.1016/j.chiabu.2005.10.011 PMID:16519940

Patterson, G. T. (2007). Examining missing person police reports to identify the service needs of runaway youth and their families. *Journal of Human Behavior in the Social Environment*, *16*(3), 73–88. doi:10.1300/10911350802107751

Peterson, P. L., Baer, J. S., Wells, E. A., Ginzler, J. A., & Garrett, S. B. (2006). Short-term effects of a brief motivational intervention to reduce alcohol and drug risk among homeless adolescents. *Psychology of Addictive Behaviors*, *20*(3), 254–264. doi:10.1037/0893-164X.20.3.254 PMID:16938063

Pinzón-Rondón, A. M., Hofferth, S., & Briceño, L. (2008). Children working in the streets of Colombian cities: Different pathways to the street lead to different populations. *Children and Youth Services Review*, *30*(12), 1417–1424. doi:10.1016/j.childyouth.2008.04.009

Plummer, M. L., & Mustafa, K. (2007). Beginning street life: Factors contributing to children working and living on the streets of Khartoum, Sudan. *Children and Youth Services Review*, *29*(12), 1520–1536. doi:10.1016/j.childyouth.2007.06.008

Praharaj, S. K., Verma, P., & Arora, M. (2008). Inhalant abuse (typewriter correction fluid) in street children. *Journal of Addiction Medicine*, *2*(4), 175–177. doi:10.1097/ADM.0b013e31817be5bc PMID:21768989

Rakshit, R. (2004). *An intervention study on the coping skills of the street children with substance abuse.* Bangalore: National Institute of Mental Health and Neuro Sciences.

Rhodes, J., & Jason, L. (1988). *Preventing Substance Abuse Among young children and adolescents.* New York: Pergamon Press.

Schimmel, N. (2008). A humanistic approach to caring for street children: The importance of emotionally intimate and supportive relationships for the successful rehabilitation of street children. *Vulnerable Children and Youth Studies*, *3*(3), 214–220. doi:10.1080/17450120802032883

Schurink, E., & Tiba, M. (1993). Street children as a world phenomenon. In Schurink (Ed.), Street children. Pretoria: Human Sciences Research Council.

Seth, R., Kotwal, A., & Ganguly, K. K. (2005). Street and working children of Delhi, India, misusing toluene: An ethnographic exploration. *Substance Use & Misuse*, *40*(11), 1659–1679. doi:10.1080/10826080500222792 PMID:16253933

Sharry, J., & Owens, C. (2000). The rules of engagement': A case study of a group with 'angry' adolescents. *Clinical Child Psychology and Psychiatry*, *5*(1), 53–62. doi:10.1177/1359104500005001006

UNICEF. (1993). *The state of the world's children* (1st ed.). New York: Oxford University.

UNICEF. (1998). *A background paper on street children.* Paper presented at the National Workshop on Street Children.

Veale, A., & Donà, G. (2003). Street children and political violence: A socio-demographic analysis of street children in Rwanda. *Child Abuse & Neglect*, *27*(3), 253–269. doi:10.1016/S0145-2134(03)00005-X PMID:12654324

WHO. (2000). *Working with street children: A training package on substance use, sexual and reproductive health including HIV/AIDS and STDs.* Geneva: WHO- Department of Mental Health and Substance Dependence.

World Health Organization. (1993). *WHO programme on substance abuse, 'one way street': A report on phase I of street children project.* Geneva: WHO.

Xue, Z. (2009). Urban street children in China: A social exclusion perspective. *International Social Work*, *52*(3), 401–408. doi:10.1177/0020872808102072

KEY TERMS AND DEFINITIONS

Intervention: An intervention is defined as an action or activity that helps in the prevention, modification, or treatment of problems related to substance use and other health problems.

Motivation: Motivation refers to one's willingness to change/stop/cut down his undesired behaviour. In substance abuse, Motivation refers to one's willingness to change/stop/cut down his substance use or abuse.

Psychoactive Substance: Refers to a substance that produces a change in mental processes, e.g. altering mood or state of consciousness.

Social Group Work: According to Konopka (1963) Social group work is a method of social work which helps individuals to enhance their social functioning through purposeful group experiences and to cope more effectively with their personal, group and community problems.

Street Children: According to Juvenile Justice (care and protection of children) Government of India (GOI) act 2000, a person who has not completed 18 years, living on the street in the presence of the family or absent of the family is a street child.

Street Life: In the present study, street life refers to children staying on the street with or without parental supervision and engaging with any kind of activities for survival.

Substance: Any product that affects the way people feel, think, see, taste, smell, hear or behave (psychoactive substance). A substance can be a medicine or it can be an industrial product, such as glues, fluids, petroleum products, paint thinner. Some substances are legal, such as approved medicines and cigarettes and others are illegal as with heroin and cocaine.

Chapter 14
Chronic Mental Illness and the Changing Scope of Intervention Strategies, Diagnosis, and Treatment in Child and Adolescent Population

Bhavuk Garg
IHBAS, India

Prerna Khanna
Pushpanjali Crosslay Hospital, India

Amit Khanna
IHBAS, India

ABSTRACT

A significant proportion of the Child and Adolescent population suffer from a psychological or psychiatric disorder. It is estimated that at least 20% of the child and adolescent population is affected mental health problems and largely this is undetected. Some of the mental health problems are severe and disabling and tend to be chronic in nature. Childhood forms an important phase in the development period of life during which one develops physically, emotionally, socially, intellectually and morally. Chronic and severe mental health problems in children impact the overall development of the child thereby leading to significant and lifelong disability. The scope of this chapter has been narrowed to include two important chronic mental illness in children mainly Schizophrenia and Bipolar Mood Disorder. The Authors will discuss the clinical features, course, outcome and treatment strategies. Special issues in children are also discussed in terms of diagnosis and treatment.

DOI: 10.4018/978-1-5225-0519-8.ch014

INTRODUCTION

Although it is sometimes assumed that childhood and adolescence are times of carefree bliss, as many as 20% of children and adolescents have one or more diagnosable mental disorders. Most of these disorders may be viewed as exaggerations or distortions of normal behaviour and emotions. Like adults, children and adolescents vary in temperament. Some are shy and reticent; others are socially exuberant. Some are methodical and cautious; others are impulsive and careless. Whether a child is behaving like a typical child or has a disorder is determined by the presence of impairment and the degree of distress related to the symptoms. For example, a 12-yr-old girl may be frightened by the prospect of delivering a book report in front of her class. This fear would be viewed as social anxiety disorder only if her fears were severe enough to cause significant distress and avoidance. There is much overlap between the symptoms of many disorders and the challenging behaviours and emotions of normal children. Thus, many strategies useful for managing behavioural problems in children can also be used in children who have mental disorders. Furthermore, appropriate management of childhood behavioural problems may decrease the risk of temperamentally vulnerable children developing a full-blown disorder. Also, effective treatment of some disorders (eg, anxiety) during childhood may decrease the risk of mood disorders later in life. The most common mental disorders of childhood and adolescence fall into the following categories:

- Anxiety disorders,
- Mood disorders,
- Disruptive behavioural disorders (e.g., attention-deficit/hyperactivity disorder [ADHD]).

Schizophrenia and related disorders are much less common.

However, more often than not, children and adolescents have symptoms and problems that cut across diagnostic boundaries. For example, > 25% of children with ADHD also has an anxiety disorder, and 25% meet the criteria for a mood disorder.

In this chapter were covered two important chronic mental illnesses in children- Schizophrenia and Bipolar Mood Disorder. This chapter discusses the clinical features, course, outcome and treatment strategies. Special issues in children are also discussed in terms of diagnosis and treatment.

Early Onset of Schizophrenia

Schizophrenia is a chronic, disabling severe mental illness. The incidence of schizophrenia during childhood is rare. The peak age of onset is in early adult life. Most of the cases of childhood schizophrenia diagnosed earlier were actually cases of autism. Currently the same diagnostic criteria are applied for children and adults although as described below there are significant differences between the two.

Classification of Early Onset Schizophrenia

In terms of age of onset,

- Early onset Schizophrenia- onset prior to age 18 years,
- Very early onset schizophrenia- onset prior to age 13.

Epidemiology

There are very few studies about the population prevalence of childhood schizophrenia. There are numerous reasons for this. The challenges in diagnosis make this a difficult disorder to study. Gillberg, Wahlstrom, Forsman, Hellgren, and Gillberg (1986) found that in the age group of 13-18 years, out of all psychosis 41% had schizophrenia. Prevalence of all psychoses at age 13 years was 0.9 in 10,000. The figure increases during adolescence.

Etiology and Risk Factors

Pregnancy and birth complications have been found to be a risk factor for schizophrenia. However it is not clear whether they are a consequence of or cause of abnormal neurodevelopment leading to schizophrenia. Cannabis use has also been proposed to be a risk factor for schizophrenia. However a causal relationship has not been established and a common genetic susceptibility has been proposed. Expressed emotions like critical comments, hostility and over involvement have been found to be associated with relapse of schizophrenia. The role of childhood abuse and neglect in schizophrenia etiology has been found to be inconclusive. Schizophrenia is also heritable many genetic factors have been implicated in the etiology of schizophrenia, however, a direct causal association has not been established.

Diagnostic Criteria and Clinical Features

ICD-10

1. Thought echo, thought insertion or withdrawal, and thought broadcasting;
2. Delusions of control, influence, or passivity, clearly referred to body or limb movements or specific thoughts, actions, or sensations; delusional perception;
3. Hallucinatory voices giving a running commentary on the patient's behaviour, or discussing the patient among themselves, or other types of hallucinatory voices coming from some part of the body;
4. Persistent delusions of other kinds that are culturally inappropriate and completely impossible, such as religious or political identity, or superhuman powers and abilities (e.g. being able to control the weather, or being in communication with aliens from another world);
5. Persistent hallucinations in any modality, when accompanied either by fleeting or half-formed delusions without clear affective content, or by persistent over-valued ideas, or when occurring every day for weeks or months on end;
6. Breaks or interpolations in the train of thought, resulting in incoherence or irrelevant speech, or neologisms;
7. Catatonic behaviour, such as excitement, posturing, or waxy flexibility, negativism, mutism, and stupor;
8. "Negative" symptoms such as marked apathy, paucity of speech, and blunting or incongruity of emotional responses, usually resulting in social withdrawal and lowering of social performance; it must be clear that these are not due to depression or to neuroleptic medication;
9. A significant and consistent change in the overall quality of some aspects of personal behaviour, manifest as loss of interest, aimlessness, idleness, a self-absorbed attitude, and social withdrawal.

The normal requirement for a diagnosis of schizophrenia is that a minimum of one very clear symptom (and usually two or more if less clear-cut) belonging to any one of the groups listed as (1) to (4) above, or symptoms from at least two of the groups referred to as (5) to (8), should have been clearly present for most of the time during a period of 1 month or more.

Schizophrenia is characterized mainly by positive and negative symptoms. Positive symptoms consist of delusions, hallucinations, thought alienation and passivity phenomena. Negative symptoms include poverty of speech, a motivation, anhedonia, restricted affect and attention deficits. Persons may also have cognitive symptoms, symptoms of disorganization and disturbances of affect. In children it may be difficult to elicit and establish the core features of schizophrenia. The onset may be characterized by social withdrawal, decline in school performance, odd behaviours. These symptoms may occur around a year before the onset of clear schizophrenic symptoms. Many children may experience prodromal symptoms which consist of nonspecific symptoms such as bizarre perceptual experiences, odd ideas, eccentric interests and odd behaviours. This may be confused with Schizotypal personality.

Though the diagnostic criteria as per ICD-10 and DSM 5 are similar for children and adults, child and adolescent onset schizophrenia is characterized by hallucinations in different modalities, less systematized and fragmented delusions and more negative symptoms as compared to adults.

Rating Scales

The Schedule for Affective Disorders and Schizophrenia for School-Age Children-Present and Lifetime version (K-SADS-PL) (Kaufman et al., 1997) is a reliable and valid tool to diagnose schizophrenia in children. This tool is used in diagnosis, monitoring of symptoms and also for research purposes. Other than this specific tool in children, other tools like Brief Psychiatric Rating Scale (Overall & Gorham, 1962) and Positive and Negative Symptom Scale (Kay, Flszbein., & Opfer, 1987) are also used.

Course, Outcome, and Prognosis

Child and adolescent onset schizophrenia typically runs a chronic course. The short term outcome is worse as compared to first episode psychoses in adults. Only a minority of cases make full recovery after the first episode. The child usually has an unremitting chronic course and there are long term functional impairments in adulthood. The prognostic factors include premorbid cognitive and social functioning. Premorbid cognitive and social impairment predict a poorer prognosis. Extended duration of untreated psychosis, prolonged first episode and presence of negative symptoms also predict a poor outcome.

Treatment

The treatment strategies are similar to adult schizophrenia. Antipsychotics are the mainstay of treatment. An important point to consider is that the antipsychotic drugs should be started at lowest possible dose and should be optimized gradually. Treatment should be multimodal including pharmacotherapy, illness education, family intervention and taking care of educational and social needs. There has been ongoing work on early detection and intervention in schizophrenia. Studies have aimed at identifying "ultra-high risk" group for this purpose. Pharmacological intervention in this group has been found to delay the onset of psychosis but not necessarily reduce the incidence of schizophrenia. (McGorry et al., 2002). A meta-analysis done in 2013 (Stafford, 2013) did not find the pharmacological intervention using risperidone and olanzapine to be more effective than a psychosocial intervention in preventing the transition to psychosis in the ultra-high risk group. National Institute of Health and Care Excellence [NICE] clinical guideline (NICE, 2013) do not recommend the use of antipsychotics in young people to manage attenuated psychosis symptoms or prevent the transition to psychosis.

Pharmacological Approaches

Studies of antipsychotics in children are limited and most of the literature consists of extrapolation of findings from the adult population. Antipsychotic drugs are broadly classified into two groups- Typical and Atypical antipsychotics. The typical antipsychotics include Haloperidol, Trifluoperazine, Chlorpromazine, and the atypical agents include Risperidone, Olanzapine, Clozapine, Quetiapine and Aripiprazole. Aripiprazole, olanzapine, quetiapine, risperidone, and paliperidone have been FDA approved for treatment of pediatric schizophrenia (ages 13-17 yrs). Haloperidol has been found to be effective in children. In head to head trials, atypical antipsychotics have been found to have similar efficacy as typical antipsychotics (Sikich, Hamer, Bashford, Sheitman., & Lieberman, 2004) but better safety profile in terms of extra pyramidal symptoms. However, atypical antipsychotics have some metabolic side effects which requires regular monitoring. The principle is to start with the lowest possible dose of the agent as children are sensitive to the side effects of these medications. Most of the guidelines recommend starting with a low dose of atypical antipsychotic in first episode patients. Children have been found to have more treatment resistance as compared to adults. Clozapine is useful in such cases. However, cloazpine requires regular monitoring of serious adverse effects like neutropenia.

Psychosocial Approaches

Psychoeducation and family interventions form an integral part of management of schizophrenia. Explaining about the illness to family, identifying and reducing the burden of family and handling expressed emotions are important components of management. The role of Cognitive- Behaviour Therapy in adults is established for treatment resistant positive symptoms but studies about its efficacy in children are lacking. Cognitive remediation may also be a useful approach in managing cognitive dysfunction.

DIAGNOSIS AND TREATMENT OF SCHIZOPHRENIA

The presentation of schizophrenia in children is an atypical presentation with respect to the age of onset. In the beginning, any self-absorbed child would be diagnosed as Schizophrenia. But with progress in the science, newer disorders came to be identified such as Autistic Spectrum Disorder. Many developmental conditions were identified. Many children who were diagnosed with schizophrenia in the 1970s would now be diagnosed with Autism. To diagnose schizophrenia in children, emphasis was put on hallucinations. The criteria given by ICD-10 and DSM-5 are same for children and adults but it is difficult to apply the same criteria directly to diagnose schizophrenia in children. However, the presentation, course and prognosis of Schizophrenia in this age group tend to be different from the adult population. There is a need to follow the course of schizophrenia in children for a longer duration.

Intervention strategies and treatment have also borrowed the broader concepts from studies done in adult population. The studies done in the pediatric age group have mainly focused on establishing the safety of medications. Recently, efficacy studies have also been done. The psychosocial interventions have not been studied systematically in this age group.

BIPOLAR DISORDER

Pediatric bipolar disorder (PBD) has been a diagnostic challenge for the clinicians. The overlap with many disorders, comorbidities and variable course are important aspects of this disorder in this age group.

There are two main phenotypes of pediatric bipolar disorder. The "narrow" phenotype is defined by recurrent episodes of major depression and mania, with manic symptoms including elated/expansive mood and grandiosity. The "broad" phenotype of PBD is characterized by chronic, severe mood dysregulation and hyperarousal. Although the mood states in the broad phenotype may evidence episodic variations, they are unlikely to be of the intensity or duration necessary to meet criteria for bipolar disorder (type I or II), and are categorises as Bipolar Disorder Not Otherwise Specified.

Epidemiology

In a meta-analysis done by Van Meter, Moreira, and Youngstrom (2011) in participants upto 21 years of age, the overall rate of bipolar disorder was 1.8%. The studies have found marked variations in data because of the methodological differences e.g. whether ICD-10 or DSM criterions are used. The majority of youth with BD experience a depressive episode as the first mood episode, and the mean age of onset of this first episode was 11.75 years (Lewinsohn, Klein., & Seeley, 1995). The prevalence increases nearly twofold from the 13–14-years to the 17–18-years age group (Merikangas, He., & Burstein, 2010).

Comorbidity

Comorbidity is high with pediatric BD, particularly with ADHD, anxiety disorders, conduct disorder and ODD, and substance use disorders. It is important to recognize these comorbidities as they influence the course and outcome of pediatric BD. The overlap of the symptoms between pediatric BD and these disorders also needs to be recognized.

Diagnostic Criteria and Clinical Features

As per ICD-10, "This disorder is characterized by repeated (i.e. at least two) episodes in which the patient's mood and activity levels are significantly disturbed, this disturbance consisting on some occasions of an elevation of mood and increased energy and activity (mania or hypomania), and on others of a lowering of mood and decreased energy and activity (depression). Characteristically, recovery is usually complete between episodes, and the incidence in the two sexes is more nearly equal than in other mood disorders. As patients who suffer only from repeated episodes of mania are comparatively rare, and resemble (in their family history, premorbid personality, age of onset, and long-term prognosis) those who also have at least occasional episodes of depression, such patients are classified as bipolar."

As per DSM 5 (American Psychiatric Association, [APA] 2013), for Bipolar Disorder(BD) Type I, person has had at least one manic episode plus any number of hypomanic or depressive episodes. In BD Type II, person has had at least one major depressive episode plus any number of hypomanic episodes, but no manic episode.

Mania/hypomania is defined as a distinct period of "abnormally and persistently elevated, expansive or irritable mood" and increased energy or activity for 1 week/4 or more days, lasting most of the day and changes in three or more of the following:

1. Self-esteem/grandiosity,
2. Need for sleep (decreased),
3. Talkativeness,
4. Racing thoughts,
5. Distractibility,
6. Goal-directedness,
7. Involvement in risky activities.

In a manic episode, individual is noted to have marked impairment in functioning, psychotic features, or the need to be hospitalized to ensure safety. For a hypomanic episode, the disturbance in mood and change in functioning is uncharacteristic and observable by others, but the episode is not severe enough to case marked impairment in functioning or to necessitate hospitalization. An episode of mania or hypomania must not be attributable to the physiological effects of a substance or to a medical condition.

Major Depressive Episode

Five (or more) of the following symptoms have been present during the same 2-week period and represent a change from previous functioning; at least one of the symptoms

1. Depressed mood most of the day, nearly every day. In children and adolescents, can be irritable mood.
2. Markedly diminished interest or pleasure in all, or almost all, activities most of the day, nearly every day.
3. Significant weight loss when not dieting or weight gain (e.g., a change of more than 5% of body weight in a month), or decrease or increase in appetite nearly every day. In children, consider failure to make expected weight gain.
4. Insomnia or hypersomnia nearly every day.
5. Psychomotor agitation or retardation nearly every day.
6. Fatigue or loss of energy nearly every day.
7. Feelings of worthlessness or excessive or inappropriate guilt nearly every day.
8. Diminished ability to think or concentrate, or indecisiveness, nearly every day.
9. Recurrent thoughts of death (not just fear of dying), recurrent suicidal ideation without a specific plan, or a suicide attempt or a specific plan for committing suicide.

The symptoms cause clinically significant distress or impairment in social, occupational, or other important areas of functioning and the episode is not attributable to the physiological effects of a substance or another medical condition.

Diagnostic Challenges

Pediatric bipolar disorder is a difficult condition to diagnose. Children do not present with the typical manic symptoms as seen in adults during a manic episode. Children present with irritability. It is difficult for a child to express euphoria. In children rapid shifts of mood are common further causing difficulty in diagnosing. There is also significant overlap in symptom profile with some major childhood disorders. Attention Deficit Hyperactivity Disorder is difficult to distinguish from a manic episode. Episodic nature and elation may help in diagnosing as Bipolar disorder. Conduct disorder and Oppositional defiant disorder may also resemble manic presentation. Substance use in adolescents also poses challenge towards diagnosis of Bipolar disorder.

Chronic irritability needs to be differentiated from Bipolar disorder. The debate about whether chronic irritability is a developmental form of BD has given rise to the introduction of Disruptive Mood Dysregulation Disorder (DMDD) in DSM-5, intended in part to decrease inaccurate diagnoses of BD.

- **Rating Scales:** K-SADS-PL can be used for affective disorders in children. In addition, for manic episode, Child Mania Rating Scale (Pavuluri, Henry, Devineni, Carbray., & Birmaher, 2006), and the parent version of Young Mania Rating Scale (P-YMRS) (Gracious, Youngstorm., & Findling, 2002) can be used. These scales have items specific to this age group.

Course and Outcome

The COBY study (Birmaher et al., 2009) is a landmark study that has provided great insights into the course of bipolar disorder in youth. Early onset of bipolar disorder predicts a more chronic and fluctuating course. There are more chances of mixed and cycling episodes. Early onset bipolar disorder is also associated with higher comorbidity and suicidality. The episodes tend to be longer. Rapid mood changes and subsyndromal episodes are common in this population.

Treatment

The treatment of bipolar disorder is divided into three phases- Acute, Continuation and Maintenance. The acute phase is concerned with the control of the acute symptoms that the child presents with. Continuation phase consists of continuing the medicines with which the child responded in the acute phase with monitoring of side effects. Maintenance phase aims at long term prophylaxis to prevent relapse.

Pharmacological Treatment

Pharmacological treatment studies in pediatric bipolar disorder have mainly focused on the manic episode and minimally on the depressive episode. There are no FDA-approved medications for the treatment of bipolar depression in children and adolescents. Atypical antipsychotics (risperidone, quetiapine, ziprasidone, and olanzapine) and lithium (ages 12–17years) have been approved for mania or mixed episodes in youth (DeFilippis & Wagner, 2013). Recently Asenapine has also obtained approval for use in Pediatric Bipolar disorder. No agent is approved for children less than 10 years' age. It has been seen that children are often prescribed a combination of many drugs by clinicians in a bid to get response. However, combination treatment does not offer any additional benefit and only adds to the side effects. For a manic episode, starting an atypical antipsychotic is a good option (Hauser & Correll, 2013). Lithium and Valproate are also useful options. Some evidence exists for Carbamazepine. The metabolic side effects of atypical antipsychotics are an important source of concern and need to be monitored regularly. For a bipolar depressive episode, not many trials are available. Studies support use of Lithium, Aripoprazole (Findling, Nyilas., & Forbes, 2009; Correll, & Nyilas, 2013) and Quetiapine (Delbello, Schwiers., & Rosenberg, 2002). An important aspect of management is use of Selective Serotonin Reuptake Inhibitors (SSRIs). SSRIs are frequently prescribed in depressive episodes, but their efficacy in bipolar depression in this age group has not been established. In fact, they may lead to treatment emergent affective switch to a hypomanic/manic episode.

Psychosocial Intervention

Psychosocial treatments are useful adjunct to pharmacological treatment in pediatric bipolar disorder. According to American Academy of Child and Adolescent Psychiatry Practice Parameter for the treatment of PBD (McClellan, Kowatch., & Findling, 2007), "a comprehensive multimodal treatment approach combining psychopharmacology with adjunctive psychosocial therapies is almost always indicated for early-onset BD".

Psychoeducational approaches, Family Focused Therapy (FFT), Inter personal and Social Rhythm Therapy (IPSRT) and Cognitive Behavior Therapy (CBT) are useful approaches in Pediatric Bipolar Disorder. These therapies were mainly developed for adult bipolar disorder but modules have been developed for Pediatric Bipolar Disorder as well and have been subjected to randomized controlled trials.

DIAGNOSIS AND TREATMENT OF PEDIATRIC BIPOLAR DISORDER

The diagnosis and intervention strategies in Pediatric Bipolar disorder have been borrowed heavily from the adult counterparts. Over the years, important differences in the presentation, course and outcome of pediatric bipolar disorders have been identified. The nature of presentation, comorbidities and the chronic course make this a difficult disorder to manage. Studies are focusing on evaluating the long term course of this disorder. More and more studies are also focussing on the management strategies of this disorder. The pharmacological and non-pharmacological intervention strategies need more systematic evaluation in this group especially less than 10 years' age.

CONCLUSION

As researchers support the early intervention affirm, the at risk mental state represents an intermediate state, which begins to be followed up by specialists, and, therefore, no longer summarizes the health state, but does not necessarily implies the development of the disorder, and it is not equivalent to the diagnosis of the disease. If the interventions constructed in the context of the services of early detection, in a first moment, represented the refinement of clinical instruments, especially for patients living the first episode, for risk cases, it is not known what to offer exactly; thus, an intervention that can change the alleged vulnerability of child adolescents remains undefined. In the clinical dimension, the discussion on the early intervention directed to the first break, with special attention to the period of untreated psychosis, may represent the construction of care instruments and strategies useful in the assistance to the psychopathology of child and adolescent population. At the same time, the formalization of the diagnostic category of bipolar disorder and psychosis points more to an intention of applying the risk thinking to the psychiatric field, and of carrying out preventive actions whose efficacy and safety are not known. The questioning about the boundaries between normality and pathology is not only beneficial, but also essential to the construction of care practices that are more sensitive to psychic suffering.

REFERENCES

American Psychiatric Association. (2013). *Diagnostic and statistical manual of mental disorders* (5th ed.). Washington, DC: Author.

Birmaher, B., Axelson, D., Goldstein, B., Strober, M., Gill, M. K., Hunt, J., & Keller, M. et al. (2009). Four-Year Longitudinal Course of Children and Adolescents with Bipolar Spectrum Disorder: The Course and Outcome of Bipolar Youth (COBY) Study. *The American Journal of Psychiatry*, *166*(7), 795–804. doi:10.1176/appi.ajp.2009.08101569 PMID:19448190

DeFilippis, M. S., & Wagner, K. D. (2013). Bipolar depression in children and adolescents. *CNS Spectrums*, *18*(04), 209–213. doi:10.1017/S1092852913000217 PMID:23570693

DelBello, M. P., Schwiers, M. L., Rosenberg, H. L., & Strakowski, S. M. (2002). A double-blind, randomized, placebo-controlled study of quetiapine as adjunctive treatment for adolescent mania. *Journal of the American Academy of Child and Adolescent Psychiatry*, *41*(10), 1216–1223. doi:10.1097/00004583-200210000-00011 PMID:12364843

Findling, R. L., Correll, C. U., Nyilas, M., Forbes, R. A., McQuade, R. D., Jin, N., & Carlson, G. A. et al. (2013). Aripiprazole for the treatment of pediatric bipolar I disorder: A 30-week, randomized, placebo controlled study. *Bipolar Disorders*, *15*(2), 138–149. doi:10.1111/bdi.12042 PMID:23437959

Findling, R. L., Nyilas, M., Forbes, R. A., McQuade, R. D., Jin, N., Iwamoto, T., & Chang, K. et al. (2009). Acute treatment of pediatric bipolar I disorder, manic or mixed episode, with aripiprazole: A randomized, double-blind, placebo-controlled study. *The Journal of Clinical Psychiatry*, *70*(10), 1441–1451. doi:10.4088/JCP.09m05164yel PMID:19906348

Gillberg, C., Wahlstrom, J., Forsman, A., Hellgren, L., & Gillberg, J. C. (1986). Teenage psychoses: Epidemiology, classification and reduced optimality in the pre-, peri- and neonatal periods. *Journal of Child Psychology and Psychiatry, and Allied Disciplines*, *27*(1), 87–98. doi:10.1111/j.1469-7610.1986.tb00624.x PMID:3949910

Gracious, B. L., Youngstorm, E. A., & Findling, R. L. (2002). Discriminative validity of a parent version of the Young Mania rating Scale. *Journal of the American Academy of Child and Adolescent Psychiatry*, *41*(11), 1350–1359. doi:10.1097/00004583-200211000-00017 PMID:12410078

Hauser, M., & Correll, C. U. (2013). The significance of at-risk or prodromal symptoms for bipolar I disorder in children and adolescents. *Canadian Journal of Psychiatry*, *58*, 22–31. PMID:23327753

Kaufman, J., Birmaher, B., Brent, D., Rao, U. M. A., Flynn, C., Moreci, P., & Ryan, N. (1997). Schedule for affective disorders and schizophrenia for school-age children-present and lifetime version (K-SADS-PL): Initial reliability and validity data. *Journal of the American Academy of Child and Adolescent Psychiatry*, *36*(7), 980–988. doi:10.1097/00004583-199707000-00021 PMID:9204677

Kay, S. R., Flszbein, A., & Opfer, L. A. (1987). The positive and negative syndrome scale (PANSS) for schizophrenia. *Schizophrenia Bulletin*, *13*(2), 261–276. doi:10.1093/schbul/13.2.261 PMID:3616518

Lewinsohn, P. M., Klein, D. N., & Seeley, J. R. (1995). Bipolar disorders in a community sample of older adolescents: Prevalence, phenomenology, comorbidity, and course. *Journal of the American Academy of Child and Adolescent Psychiatry*, *34*(4), 454–463. doi:10.1097/00004583-199504000-00012 PMID:7751259

McClellan, J., Kowatch, R., & Findling, R. L. (2007). Practice parameter for the assessment and treatment of children and adolescents with bipolar disorder. *Journal of the American Academy of Child and Adolescent Psychiatry*, *46*(1), 107–125. doi:10.1097/01.chi.0000242240.69678.c4 PMID:17195735

McGorry, P. D., Yung, A. R., Phillips, L. J., Yuen, H. P., Francey, S., Cosgrave, E. M., & Jackson, H. et al. (2002). Randomized controlled trial of interventions designed to reduce the risk of progression to first-episode psychosis in a clinical sample with subthreshold symptoms. *Archives of General Psychiatry*, *59*(10), 921–928. doi:10.1001/archpsyc.59.10.921 PMID:12365879

Merikangas, K. R., He, J. P., Burstein, M., Swanson, S. A., Avenevoli, S., Cui, L., & Swendsen, J. et al. (2010). Lifetime prevalence of mental disorders in U.S. adolescents: Results from the National Comorbidity Survey Replication – Adolescent Supplement (NCS-A). *Journal of the American Academy of Child and Adolescent Psychiatry*, *49*(10), 980–989. doi:10.1016/j.jaac.2010.05.017 PMID:20855043

National Institute of Health and Care Excellence. (2013). *Psychosis and schizophrenia in children and young people*. Retrieved 09 January, 2106, from https://www.nice.org.uk/guidance/indevelopment/gid-cgwave0797

Overall, J. E., & Gorham, D. R. (1962). The brief psychiatric rating scale. *Psychological Reports*, *10*(3), 799–812. doi:10.2466/pr0.1962.10.3.799

Pavuluri, M. N., Henry, D. B., Devineni, B., Carbray, J. A., & Birmaher, B. (2006). Child mania rating scale: Development, reliability, and validity. *Journal of the American Academy of Child and Adolescent Psychiatry*, *45*(5), 550–560. doi:10.1097/01.chi.0000205700.40700.50 PMID:16601399

Sikich, L., Hamer, R. M., Bashford, R. A., Sheitman, B. B., & Lieberman, J. A. (2004). A pilot study of risperidone, olanzapine, and haloperidol in psychotic youth: A double-blind, randomized, 8-week trial. *Neuropsychopharmacology*, *29*(1), 133–145. doi:10.1038/sj.npp.1300327 PMID:14583740

Stafford, M. R., Jackson, H., Mayo-Wilson, E., Morrison, A. P., & Kendall, T. (2013). Early interventions to prevent psychosis: Systematicreviewandmeta-analysis. *British Medical Journal*, *346*(jan18 1), f185. doi:10.1136/bmj.f185 PMID:23335473

Van Meter, A. R., Moreira, A. L., & Youngstrom, E. A. (2011). Meta-analysis of epidemiologic studies of pediatric bipolar disorder. *The Journal of Clinical Psychiatry*, *72*(9), 1250–1256. doi:10.4088/JCP.10m06290 PMID:21672501

World Health Organization. (1992). *The ICD-10 classification of mental and behavioural disorders: clinical descriptions and diagnostic guidelines*. Geneva: World Health Organization.

KEY TERMS AND DEFINITIONS

Childhood Schizophrenia: A type of schizophrenia, present in children. Children's symptoms start before the age of 13 and characterized by hallucinations, delusions, disordered thoughts and negative symptoms. The onset is often insidious with cognitive deterioration.

Depression: A state of low mood and aversion to activity that can affect a person's thoughts, behavior, feelings and sense of well-being. People with depressed mood can feel sad, anxious, empty, hopeless, helpless, worthless, guilty, irritable, ashamed or restless. They may lose interest in activities that were once pleasurable, experience loss of appetite or overeating, have problems concentrating, remembering details or making decisions, and may contemplate, attempt or commit suicide. Insomnia, excessive sleeping, fatigue, aches, pains, digestive problems or reduced energy may also be present.

Early Onset Schizophrenia: A type of schizophrenia, present in children. Children's symptoms start before the age of 13 and characterized by hallucinations, delusions, disordered thoughts and negative symptoms. The onset is often insidious with cognitive deterioration.

Mania: The mood of an abnormally elevated arousal energy level, or "a state of heightened overall activation with enhanced affective expression together with lability of affect. Although mania is often conceived as a "mirror image" to depression, the heightened mood can be either euphoric or irritable; indeed, as the mania worsens, irritability often becomes more pronounced and may eventuate in violence.

Pediatric Bipolar Disorder: Bipolar disorder starts during childhood or the early teen years is called pediatric bipolar disorder. The onset in characterized with mixed-dysphoric, labile and rapid changing presentation; the symptoms are more or less commons.

Section 6

Chronic Mental Illness:
Advanced Treatment Strategies

Chapter 15
Advanced Intervention Strategies for Suicide in Patients with Chronic Mental Illness

Shailesh Jha
IHBAS, India

Amit Khanna
IHBAS, India

Prerna Khanna
Pushpanjali Crosslay Hospital, India

ABSTRACT

Chronic mental illnesses are common to find in routine clinical practice and suicide is one of the dreaded outcomes. The concept under defining chronic mental illness has evolved in few decades as now the critical elements for defining the chronic mental illness are psychiatric diagnosis, functional disability, and illness duration. There are various studies on prevalence of suicide and especially in patients with CMI. There is rising trend of research on suicide in patient with psychiatric illness in last decade and found ever over thousand published article in year 2014. This chapter will include literature based on various aspect of suicide including neurobiological factors like neurotransmitters, neural circuits, genetic and epigenetic factors, response on pharmacotherapy and newer generation novel treatment strategies and various psychosocial factors.

INTRODUCTION

Chronic Mental Illnesses (CMI) are common to find in routine clinical practice. The concept for defining chronic mental illness has evolved in few decades. The three critical elements for defining the chronic mental illness are psychiatric diagnosis, functional disability and illness duration. Based on these elements there will be different understanding regarding outcome of CMI. Among various outcomes based on psychiatric diagnosis and associated disability, the most dreaded one is suicide. The great majority of

DOI: 10.4018/978-1-5225-0519-8.ch015

people who experience a mental illness do not die by suicide. However, of those who die from suicide, more than 90 percent have a diagnosable mental disorder. Suicide has been studied in various populations and attempts were made to understand these above factors mentioned. Based on the projected rising trend of diagnosable psychiatric illness in general population and undoubtedly more indulgence of stressful life, the trend of suicide seems to be reciprocative. This concern has been acknowledged and appreciated by service providers since long back but still seems unmatched with current need. There are various Intervention Strategies brought into practice which are broadly grouped as pharmacological, non-pharmacological and novel techniques but two extreme aspects of spectrum which required specific intervention are early detection of suicide risk and intervention in suicide rescued victims. These have been the area of research not only for mental health professionals but also for other medical disciplines like forensic medicine, internal medicine, emergency and trauma etc. This chapter will detail about suicide in CMI, prevalence, burden, factors related to suicide and different advanced interventional strategies as part of management.

Prevalence

There are various studies on prevalence of suicide and especially in patients with CMI. According to calculations based on data reported to World Health Organization [WHO] (2015), by its Member States, in 1998 suicide represented 1.8% of the global burden of disease and it is expected to increase to 2.4% by the year 2020. Suicide is among the 10 leading causes of death for all ages in most of the countries for which information is available. There may be differences in statistical data among various dependent variables like age, gender, ethnicity and other sociodemographic profile in suicide epidemiology but at same time it is difficult to draw qualitative analogy among the same. In some countries, it is among the top three causes of death for people aged 15-34 years. Suicide does not just occur in high-income countries, but in fact, 75% of global suicides occurred in low and middle income countries in 2012. In the year 2020, approximately 1.53 million people will die from suicide based on current trends and according to WHO estimates. Ten to twenty times more people will attempt suicide worldwide. This represents on average one death every 20 seconds and one attempt every 1-2 seconds. In India (based on National Crime Records Bureau [NCBR] report, 2014), more than one lakh persons commit suicides every year in the country during the decadal period from 2004 to 2014. The number of suicides in the country during the decade (2004–2014) has recorded an increase of 15.8% (1,31,666 in 2014 from 1,13,697 in 2004). The increase in incidence of suicides was reported each year till 2011 thereafter a declining trend was noticed. The population has increased by 14.6% during the decade while the rate of suicides has slightly increased by 1.0% (from 10.5 in 2004 to 10.6 in 2014).

Burden

Mental health conditions are the leading cause of Disability-Adjusted Life Years (DALYs) worldwide and account for 37% of healthy life years lost from Non-Communicable Diseases (NCD). By disease, mental illness will account for the largest share of the economic burden in both 2010 and 2030, just slightly greater than cardiovascular diseases (figure-1). They are followed by cancer, chronic respiratory disease and diabetes.

Among these conditions, unipolar depressive disorder, alcohol use disorders and schizophrenia constitute the greatest global burden in terms of disability (see the Table 1).

Figure 1. Mental health and cardiovascular diseases are top drivers of lost output breakdown of NCD cost by disease type, based on EPIC model

Source: The Global Economic Burden of Non Communicable Diseases. Geneva: World Economic Forum (Bloom et al., 2011)

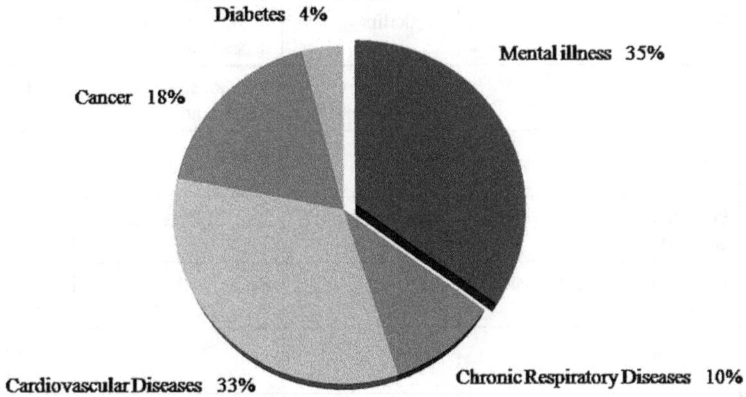

In a study by Greenberg et al. (2015), the economic burden of individuals with chronic psychiatric illness with high suicide rate especially in major depressive disorder has increased by 21.5% from 2005 to 2010. The composition of these costs remained stable, with approximately 45% attributable to direct costs, 5% to suicide-related costs, and 50% to workplace costs. The global cost of mental health conditions in 2010 was estimated at US$ 2.5 trillion, with the cost projected to surge to US$ 6.0 trillion by 2030. The nationwide attempts to curtail health expenditures have resulted in pressure to demonstrate

Table 1. Disability-Adjusted life years associated with mental health conditions

Types of Disorders	DALYs (Millions)	% Mental Health DALYs, World
All Neuropsychiatric disorders	**199**	
Unipolar depressive disorders	65	32.9
Bipolar affective disorder	14	7.2
Schizophrenia	17	8.4
Epilepsy	8	3.9
Alcohol use disorders	24	11.9
Alzheimer and other dementias	11	5.6
Parkinson disease	2	0.9
Multiple sclerosis	2	0.8
Drug use disorders	8	4.2
Post-traumatic stress disorder	3	1.7
Obsessive-compulsive disorder	5	2.6
Panic disorder	7	3.5
Insomnia (primary)	4	1.8
Migraine	8	3.9

Source: The Global Economic Burden of Noncommunicable Diseases. Geneva: World Economic Forum (Bloom et al., 2011).

Table 2. Risk Factors for suicide

Primary Diagnosis	Sociodemographic and Miscellaneous Factors	Personality	Co-Morbidities	Social Factors	Other Factors
Bipolar	Male	Borderline	Substance abuse/ dependence	Divorced	Means available
Schizophrenia	Older age	Narcissistic	Alcohol abuse/ dependence	Widower	abuse
Major Depressive Episode	White race	Antisocial	Anxiety	Lives alone	Few reasons
Dysthymia	Prior depression or Suicide attempts	Conduct Disorder	Axis III Diagnosis	Isolated	To live
Adjustment Disorder with Depression	Family history of Depression/ attempts	Impulsive	Panic	Financial Worries	Adverse events
Delirium or Dementia	Homosexuality			Other losses	Change of grades
Any psychosis	Suicidal Ideation			No religion	Change of friends
Hallucinations/ delusions: especially poverty	Hopeless/Helpless				Giving away possessions
	Agitation/ desperation				Guns in home

Source: Kaplan and Sadock's Comprehensive Textbook of Psychiatry, 9th Ed.

treatment effectiveness in most areas of health. However according to Atkinson, Zibin and Chuang (1997) as psychiatry deal with chronic illness with complex etiology and pervasive psychosocial effects on disorders leading to serious challenges to those who endeavor to assess program effectiveness in terms of economic burden.

FACTORS FOR SUICIDE RISK

Many risk factors and their relationship with underlying mental disorders and suicides have come from "psychological autopsy" studies (Cavanagh, Carson, Sharpe., & Lawrie, 2003). It is detailed investigations rely on interviews with family, close friends, and others who were in close contact with the person who died by suicide, in order to identify factors that likely contributed to the death (Table 2). Such studies have consistently found that the overwhelming majority of people who die by suicide i.e. 90% or more had a mental disorder at the time of their deaths. Often, however, these disorders had not been recognized, diagnosed, or adequately treated. While nearly all mental disorders have the potential to increase the risk for suicide, Bertolote and Fleischmann (2002) have shown that the most common disorders among people who die by suicide are major depression or with other mood disorders, substance use disorders, schizophrenia and personality disorders.

The various risk factors for suicide has been discussed which are as follows.

Previous Suicide Attempt

According to Tidemalm, Langstrom, Lichtenstein, and Runeson (2008) about 20% of people who die by suicide have made a prior suicide attempt and clinical studies have confirmed that such prior attempts increase a person's risk for subsequent suicide death. Suicide risk appears to be especially elevated during the days and weeks following hospitalization for a suicide attempt, especially in people with diagnoses of major depression, bipolar disorder, and schizophrenia.

The majority of people who make a suicide attempt, however, do not ultimately die by suicide. There are studies that have followed suicide attempters identified in hospital emergency rooms have found that just 7–10% died by suicide over the next two decades (Carter, Child, Page, Clover, & Taylor, 2007).

Family History of Suicide

There are systematic reviews by Thelma Beatriz, Isela, Alma, María Lilia, and Carlos Alfonso, (2014) which have shown that the risk for suicide can be inherited. Pandey (2013) has reported that among the most studied genes are the ones that codify tryptophan hydroxylase 1 and 2 (TPH-1 and TPH-2), the serotonin transporter (5-HTT or SLC6A4) and the serotonin receptors (5-HTR1A, 5-HTR1B, 5-HTR2A, 5-HTR2C, etc.). Identical twins, for example, have been found to have stronger concordance for suicide than fraternal twins, even when they are raised separately. Study by de Leo and Heller (2008) on people who were adopted and subsequently died by suicide have found suicide to be more common among these individuals' biological parents than their adopted parents. Exposure to completed and attempted suicide in the family has also been found to increase suicide risk among family members by providing a "social model" of self-harm behavior. While these studies indicate that a family history of suicide can be a risk factor for suicide, they do not suggest that a suicide in the family automatically heightens suicide risk for all family members. Family history is one among many factors that can contribute to a person's vulnerability or resilience. As with other genetically-linked illnesses and conditions, awareness of possible risk and attention to early signs of problems in oneself or a loved one can be protective if it leads those who have lost a relative to suicide to seek timely treatment or intervention.

Relationship between Sociodemographic Factors and Suicide Risk

One of the major challenges of suicide research is determining how mental disorders and sociodemographic factors with certain environmental stressors interact to create a pathway to suicide. Data collected by the Centers for Disease Control and Prevention showed clear differences in the gender and age patterns in those who die by suicide or even suicide attempters. For example, young women are estimated to make 100 or more suicide attempts for every completed suicide, but yet they have a low rate of completed suicide. In contrast, the elderly have a suicide rate that is twice the rate among youth, but make relatively few non-fatal suicide attempts. Greater frailty and increased likelihood of physical illnesses are the factors which contribute to the lethality of suicide attempts in older adults.

Suicide Contagion

That imitative behavior ("contagion") plays a role in suicide has long been observed. Recent studies have concluded that media coverage of suicide is connected to the increase or decrease in subsequent suicides, particularly among adolescents (Sisask &Varnik, 2012). High volume, prominent, repetitive coverage that glorifies, sensationalizes or romanticizes suicide has been found to be associated with an increase in suicides (Bohanna & Wang, 2012). There is also evidence that when coverage includes detailed description of specific means used, the use of that method may increase in the population as a whole (Yip et al., 2012).

In recent years, the internet has become a particular concern because of its reach and potential to communicate information about notorious suicides and those that occur among celebrities. However, when media follows appropriate reporting recommendations, studies show that the risk of suicide contagion can be decreased (Bohanna & Wang, 2012).

Access to Lethal Methods of Suicide

There is strong evidence that the availability and use of different modes of suicide impacts suicide rates among different population and different geographical areas. In the U.S., the most common method of suicide is firearms, used in 51% of all suicides. Currently, firearms are involved in 56% of male suicides and 30% of female suicides. Among U.S. women, the most common suicide method involves poisonous substances, especially overdoses of medications. Poisoning accounts for 37% of female suicides, compared to only 12% of male suicides. Hanging or other means of suffocation are used in about 25% of both male and female suicides. The difference in death rates among the most common suicide methods estimated at 80-90% for firearms and 1.5-4% for overdoses helps to account for the roughly 4: 1 ratio of male-to-female suicides (Yip et al., 2012). The greater availability of firearms in rural parts of the country also contributes to higher suicide rates in the more rural Western states. Studies have shown that many suicide attempts are unplanned and occur during an acute period of ambivalence (Bohanna & Wang, 2012). Therefore, restricting access to lethal methods is a key suicide prevention strategy.

Biological Factors

Postmortem studies of the brains of people who have died by suicide have shown a number of visible differences in the brains of people who died by suicide, compare to those who died from other causes, suicide is a result of a disease of the brain (Mann & Currier, 2012). There is possible strong association with neuroplastic effect due to chronic mental illness and prolonged drug exposure leading to suicidality. The brain systems that have been most frequently studied as factors in suicide are the serotonergic system, adrenergic system and the Hypothalamic-Pituitary Axis (HPA), which relate to mood, thinking and stress response, respectively. This research has also identified neurobiological impairments related to depression and other underlying mental disorders, as well as to acute or prolonged stressors. One of the key challenges of neurobiological studies is to determine the abnormalities in genes, brain structures or brain function that differentiate patients from CMI who died by suicide from who died by other causes.

ADVANCE INTERVENTION STRATEGIES

It can be as a part of preventive strategies, treatment and rehabilitative strategies. There have been several reviews of interventions that may be considered effective in reducing suicides. Under the framework of universal, selective, and indicated interventions (Mrazek & Haggerty, 1994) the general population is targeted by universal interventions (e.g. restricting access to means of suicide) and selective interventions focus on high-risk subgroups (e.g. people with mental disorders), whereas those who have attempted suicide are considered high-risk individuals and are therefore addressed with indicated interventions, which include a range of pharmacotherapy, non-pharmacotherapy like behavioral therapies and approaches such as cognitive therapy (Brown et al., 2005) including mindfulness based cognitive behavior therapy and novel treatment approaches particularly in active suicidal or in rescued cases as a part of rehabilitation. As it is indicated in the first report in WHO Preventing suicide: a global imperative (2014), many universal, selected and indicated strategies have been implemented worldwide to improve the knowledge about suicide, increase the access to health care professionals, train the gatekeepers and therefore lead to an improvement in identification and management of people at risk.

How to Assess Suicidality

The rising trend of suicide in community has other way raised the concern of unidentified underlying psychiatric illness possibly of chronic nature. Over the past several decades our knowledge about suicidal behavior has greatly increased. Research could prove the importance of the interplay between neurobiological, social, psychological, cultural and environmental factors for the development of suicidal behavior. Epidemiological studies have led to more information about risk and protective factors in general population and in patients with psychiatric diseases. Apart from various tools available for suicide risk assessment, there are various recent advances and research in developing easy accessible tools for assessment of suicide. One of the larger initiativeshas been taken by Substance Abuse and Mental Health Services Administration (SAMHSA) and the Health Resources and Services Administration (HRSA). The Center for Integrated Health Solutions (CIHS) promotes the development of integrated primary and behavioral health services to better address the needs of individuals with mental health and substance use conditions, whether seen in specialty behavioral health or primary care provider settings. CIHS is funded jointly by SAMHSA and HRSA and run by the National Council for Behavioral Health.

The various screening tools for suicide assessment are:

- Columbia Classification Algorithm of Suicide Assessment (C-CASA) by Posner, Oquendo and Gould (2007).
- Substance Abuse and Mental Health Services Administration (SAMHSA) Suicide Assessment Five-Step Evaluation and Triage (SAFE-T): Pocket Card for Clinicians which is a Suicide Safe mobile app (based on the SAFE-T is available on the app stores).
- The Columbia-Suicide Severity Rating Scale (C-SSRS) by Posner, Brown and Stanley, (2011), is a questionnaire used for suicide assessment. It is available in 114 country-specific languages.
- PHQ-9 and SBQ-R and other regular screenings by Bluml et al. (2013) in primary care and other healthcare settings enable earlier identification of suicide risk and mental health disorders.
- QPR Institute's risk audit can help in your organization's current operational and training approach to suicidal patient safety.

- Stories of Hope and Recovery, is a video guide for Suicide Attempt Survivors and features inspiring stories from three people who survived an attempted suicide.
- The MacArthur Depression Toolkit assists primary care clinicians with recognizing and managing depression. This toolkit includes user-friendly instruments to assist with recognizing, diagnosing, treating, and monitoring depression (Han, Voils, & Williams, 2011).
- A Discussion Guide for Primary Health Care Providers is an online guide to equip primary health care providers with questions to begin discussions with their patients about alcohol, illicit drug, and mental health problems, as well as co-occurring disorders. This brief guide also includes resources for patients who need an evaluation based on positive screening results.

What Are the Preventive Strategies?

Among indicated interventions, various approaches have been tested to prevent subsequent suicidal behavior by suicide attempters; extensive review articles are available. Usually, the primary outcome measure used for these interventions was repeated suicide attempts. Previously, completed suicides were used as an outcome measure in a study that investigated the maintenance of long-term contact (i.e. a total of 5 years and 24 contacts) with high suicide-risk psychiatric patients refusing further treatment (Motto, 1976; Motto, Heilbron, Juster., & Bostrom, 1981; Motto & Bostrom, 2001). The contact comprised regular short letters expressing concern for the person's well-being and inviting them to respond. This was associated with a significant reduction in suicide rates for at least 2 years after discharge from the in-patient setting.

The Crisis Intervention and Suicide Prevention Centre of BC (Crisis Centre) is a non-profit, volunteer organization committed to helping people help themselves and others deal with crisis. The Crisis Centre has been providing emotional support to youth, adults and seniors in distress since 1969. As a safe place to turn when there seems to be no hope, the Crisis Centre is operated by 450+ frontline volunteers and a small team of professional staff who support and empower individuals to see their own strengths and options, 24 hours a day in 7 days a week. We work at the community level to provide education and training aimed at fostering resiliency and building capacity to respond to crisis and suicide. In 2014, the Crisis Centre impacted more than 127,000 lives across BC through its three core services: 24/7 Distress Phone Services, Online Distress Services (YouthInBC.com, CrisisCentreChat.ca) and Community Education.

In addition, in the elderly who typically have an elevated risk of suicide compared with an age-adjusted number for the general population, a "tele-help/tele-check" service (i.e. an alarm system that can be activated to call for help and a service that contacts a person twice a week for assessment of their needs and to provide emotional support) could significantly reduce the number of suicide deaths (De Leo, Carollo., & DelloBuono, 1995; De Leo, DelloBuono., & Dwyer, 2002).

The multisite intervention study on suicidal behaviours (SUPRE-MISS), launched by WHO in 2000, evaluated an innovative intervention in a large randomized controlled trial, that brought together the elements of information, education, and practical advice from brief interventions with the maintenance of long-term follow-up contact on a regular basis. It used completed suicides as the primary outcome measure because the reduction in suicide mortality is the most convincing evidence for the effectiveness of suicide prevention (Moller, 1989). The multisite randomized controlled trial of different treatment strategies for suicide attempters represented one component of SUPRE-MISS, which, overall, aimed at increasing knowledge about suicidal behaviours and effective interventions for suicide attempters (Bertolote et al., 2005).

The main crucial factor for prevention of suicide is the time of contact. In an analysis of separate 40 postmortem studies found that 45% of those had seen a primary care provider within the month before their death, and 77% had such contact within the past year (Luoma, Martin, & Pearson, 2002). Older adults who died by suicide were even more likely to have had recent contact with a primary care provider. By contrast, only about 30% of all those who died by suicide had received mental health services during the last year of life, and only 19% in the last month. These findings suggest that suicides may be reduced if primary care providers and their staffs were better able to recognize and treat (or refer for specialty care) patients who show signs of the mental disorders that are most commonly associated with suicide. In a recent meta-analysis (Inagaki et al., 2015), the interventions of active contact and follow-up have been recommended to reduce the risk of a repeat suicide attempt.

Substance Abuse and Mental Health Services Administration (SAMHSA) and the Health Resources and Services Administration (HRSA) have come up with general resources for suicide prevention strategies keeping view on recent technological advances like:

- An edition of solutions which focuses on Suicide Prevention in Primary Care, common suicide warning signs, featured resources, etc.
- The Suicide Resource Prevention Center, funded by SAMHSA, provides technical assistance, training, and materials to increase the knowledge of professionals serving people at risk for suicide.
- The 2012 National Strategy for Suicide Prevention: Goals and Objectives for Action is a joint effort by the U.S. Surgeon General and the National Action Alliance for Suicide Prevention.
- Suicide Prevention Toolkit for Rural Primary Care, developed by Western Interstate Commission for Higher Education (WICHE) Mental Health Program, in collaboration with the Suicide Prevention Resource Center, assists rural primary care providers in effectively identifying and intervening with individuals who are suicidal.
- Suicide Prevention: Not Another Life to Lose, the most recent edition of National Council Magazine, provides insights from leaders in the field, extensive community resources, and inspiring, poignant stories of survival, resiliency, and courage.
- Suicide Safe: a suicide prevention, mobile-learning tool to help providers integrate suicide prevention strategies into their practice and reduce suicide risk among their patients. SAMHSA'S free app is available for Android and iOS operating systems.

There are attempts to curtail health expenditures which have resulted in pressure to demonstrate most effective treatment outcome models in practice. However, as psychiatry deal with chronic illness with complex etiology hassled to serious challenges to those who endeavor to assess program effectiveness in terms of economic burden. Such difficulties include: Disease states of a chronic nature, multi determinant treatment outcome indicators and lack clear causal specificity, indicators of effectiveness that involve complex psychosocial systems, and treatment approaches that often focus on the prevention or maintenance of psychosocial function as opposed to circumscribed curative goals. One of the major factors which prevent patients to seek treatment is perceived stigma. This underlies even when such subjects do not have any CMI but are only under severe emotional crises. There are some policies and programs in match with current advancement for its early detection and interventions like online suicide helpline etc.

Table 3. Selected suicide risk factors and interventions: individual, family, and community levels

Risk Factors	Interventions
Individual Level: • Sex/gender • Occupation • History of suicide attempts • Mental disorder (anxiety, mood) • Addictions • Physical illness • Financial stress • Personality disorders/impulsivity/aggression • Legal problems • Lack of religious affiliation	• Timely access to evidence-based interventions in various settings: college,workplace, justice, primary care, organized faith settings, specialty care (S/I) • Postdischarge follow-up contact for patients hospitalized for suicidal behavior (I)
Family Level: • Childhood maltreatment • Intimate partner violence • Addictions, mental disorders, suicide in family members	• Positive parenting programs (U/S) • Family-based interventions (U/S) • Peer support for young mothers (S) • Support for the bereaved (S)
Community Level: • Suicide in peers • Sensational media reporting of suicide • Specific cultural factors (e.g., Native Americans, immigrants, refugees) • Access to lethal means: guns, pesticides	• School-based evidence based programs (U) • Media education of safe reporting (U) • Culturally grounded interventions (U/I/S) • Means restriction (U) • Crisis lines (U)

Source: Promising Strategies for Advancement in Knowledge of Suicide Risk Factors and Prevention (Sareen et al., 2014)

Note: Institute of Medicine [IOM] -defined prevention programs: I, indicated; S, selective; U, universal.

I programs target groups that have already developed the disease and aim to reduce severe problems. S programs target groups at high risk for the outcome or disease.

U programs include all people in a certain community in the intervention.

Table 4. Strengths and limitations of proposed research pathways

Research Pathways	Strengths	Limitations
Analysis of existing epidemiologic samples and clinical trial databases	• Data already collected • Inexpensive to conduct analysis • Large sample size	• Limited by what is already collected in data sets • Observational studies, causal inferences cannot be made
Networks and consortia of researchers	• Multi-site prospective cohorts (history of suicide attempts, family history of suicide) • Sufficient sample sizes to examine biomarkers, genetics, and imaging work to understand biological factors related to suicide • Understand the natural trajectory of suicidal behavior	• Large infrastructure support required • Observational studies • Substantial effort to create the network and develop partnerships
Evaluation of current or new policies and programs	• Creates partnerships between policymakers and researchers in suicide • Bidirectional knowledge exchange leads to rapid uptake of new knowledge in suicide • Prevention • Careful evaluation of large-scale policies leads to an understanding of which suicide policies have an impact on suicide • Multi-site clinical trials with high-risk	• Large-scale policies are heterogeneous and it may be difficult to discern which parts of the policies are associated with reductions in suicide • Quasi-experimental designs preclude causal inferences • Ethical issues of conducting RCTs in high-risk groups samples

Source: Promising Strategies for Advancement in Knowledge of Suicide Risk Factors and Prevention (Sareen et al., 2014).

Note: IOM-defined prevention programs: I, indicated; S, selective; U, universal.

I programs target groups that have already developed the disease and aim to reduce severe problems. S programs target groups at high risk for the outcome or disease.

U programs include all people in a certain community in the intervention (see the Table 3 & 4)

Treatment

Suicidality represents trans-diagnostic issue, so matter of the fact is to make the correct diagnosis. There have not been a large number of programs and practices identified that can be said to be truly "evidence based" in terms of suicide prediction or treatment because first, completed suicide is relatively uncommon and researchers have become ethically constrained. This has led deficit in methodological consideration in studying suicide or suicidality even in general populations (Till, Strauss, Sonneck., & Niederkrotenthaler, 2015; Jha & Kumar, 2015). Treated versus treatment as usual (TAU) rather than randomized, treated versus untreated controls and the utilization of suicide attempt data as a proxy for completed suicides are not entirely satisfactory substitutes. Of the handful of evidence-based programs or practices, the use of clozapine in schizophrenia, lithium in bipolar patients, dialectical behavioral therapy (DBT) in patients with borderline personality disorder, and cognitive behavioral therapy (CBT) in depressed patients stand out as providing strong evidence of their effectiveness in diminishing suicide attempts or completions (Kaplan & Sadock, pp. 2717–2732). Other interventions and programs have lesser degrees of proven efficacy. With advent of newer interventions in terms of pharmacotherapy, psychotherapy and novel treatments like Transcranial Magnetic Stimulation (TMS), transcranial Direct Current Stimulation (tDCS) along with gold standard modified Electro-Convulsive Therapy (ECT), has led path for promising outcome.

Pharmacotherapy

The primary determinant of the pharmacotherapy is the underlying disorder like antidepressants for patients with depressions, mood stabilizers in bipolar patients, atypical antipsychotics for psychotic patients and substance use disorder patients may receive methadone, naltrexone or disulfiram, etc. Based on various researches on biological basis of suicide and its implications in understanding treatments strategies have helped in formulating different pharmacotherapuetic regimes for preventing suicide. The genetic and epigenetic factors, dysfunction of neurotransmitter, neuroendocrine system and stress response system has been determining for neurobiology of suicidality. Therefore, pharmacotherapeutic approach should be focused, not only on prevention and reduction of suicidality, but adjusted for general and diagnosis-specific risk factors.

The serotoninergic drugs have neutral or mildly protective effect on potential suicidal behaviour while noradrenergic drugs may have activating effect or could even worsen suicidal ideation in certain phase of the illness. There is perennial debate regarding the use of antidepressant medications themselves may induce suicidal behavior in youths. But based on research it was reported that there were no completed suicides occurred in children treated with SSRI medications. However, about four percent of those taking SSRI medications experienced suicidal thinking or behavior, including actual suicide attempts-twice the rate of those taking placebo, or sugar pills. In response, the U.S. Food and Drug Administration (FDA) adopted a "black box" label warning indicating that antidepressants may increase the risk of suicidal thinking and behavior in some children and adolescents with major depressive disorder. When given in appropriate dose and the right time, dual or noradrenergic antidepressants, could also have good protective impact on specific patient. There is emergence of four new antidepressants among two are essentially old wines in new bottles i.e. trazodone extended-release and doxepin, one is a reissue of as is ocarboxazid and one is actually a new molecule vilazodone (Rickels et al., 2009). However, their efficacy comparing with existing antidepressant in management of suicide risk is yet to be studied.

Psychotherapy

The psychopathological dynamics in suicidality overcomes actual diagnostic distribution therefore pharmacotherapy has restricted role in overall prevention of suicidal behaviour among mentally ill and is demanding for clinician. Searches for relevant literatures were carried out using electronic databases. Pubmed (including Pubmed Central) and Google Scholar were used to identify published studies. Searches were carried out using Medical Subject Headings (MeSH) terms "psychotherapy" and "Suicide". Additional searches were carried out using related keywords of "suicidal behaviors" and "psychotherapy". There were studies on specific therapies providing evidence of their effectiveness directed towards preventing suicidal behavior or suicide in respective disorders like unguided online self-help to reduce suicidal thoughts, an adjunctive Emotion Regulation Group Therapy (ERGT) for Deliberate Self-Harm among women with BPD, Interpersonal Psychotherapy (IPT) adapted for older depressive patients at risk for suicide, Internet-delivered CBT programs, MIDSHIPS: multi-centre intervention designed for self-harm using interpersonal problem-solving, Mindfulness-based stress reduction, Dialectical Behavioral Therapy (DBT) and DBT Prolonged Exposure in patients with borderline personality disorder and PTSD, and Cognitive Behavioral Therapy (CBT) in depressed patients.

Based on recent systematic review and meta-analysis (Cuijpers et al., 2013), there is insufficient evidence for making assumption that the suicidality in depressed patients can be reduced with psychotherapy. Although psychotherapy of depression may have small positive effects on suicidality, available data suggest that psychotherapy for depression cannot be considered to be a sufficient treatment.

Novel Treatments

Apart from above mentioned therapeutic interventions, there are few novel techniques like Electro-Convulsive Therapy (ECT), Triple Chronotherapy, Transcranial Magnetic Stimulation (TMS), Transcranial Direct Current Stimulation (tDCS) and Vagal Nerve Stimulation (VNS). Among these techniques, ECT has proven its efficacy over the time in improving depressive symptom and subsequently in suicide prevention. The rapid relief of severe depression, mania and psychosis by electroconvulsive therapy (ECT) is accompanied by the rapid reduction in suicide drive. These have led to the consideration of ECT in treatment algorithms to reduce suicide rates. The benefit of ECT in reducing suicide risk is widely acknowledged by National Psychiatric Associations (NPA) in Great Britain and the United States although supporting studies are few (Fink, Kellner, & McCall, 2014). Studies have demonstrated that combined total sleep deprivation (Wake therapy), sleep phase advance, and bright light therapy (Triple Chronotherapy) produce a rapid and sustained antidepressant effect in acutely depressed individuals. The results of this small pilot trial demonstrate that adjunctive Triple Chronotherapy is feasible and tolerable in acutely suicidal and depressed inpatients (Sahlem et al., 2014).

ECT is an intervention for which its role in suicide prevention is not based on any robust, formalized study, but rather relies on a long clinical history of successful use in the treatment of depression associated with suicidal thoughts and behaviors. Despite expert consensus that ECT is effective, it has a limited role in the general prevention of suicide given its cost, limited availability, and procedural logistics with associated stigma. Each treatment requires several hours for administration of anesthesia and recovery in a monitored medical setting, and it is generally given 3 times per week for 2–4 weeks, making it a very involved process for patients, clinicians, and family members. Unlike the pharmacotherapies discussed above, convulsive treatments can work rather quickly to reduce suicidal ideation, but their long-term impact is not as clear, and the potential for cognitive side effects can be limiting.

TMS is a newer neurostimulatory technique that is less invasive than ECT and does not require sedation. It utilizes alternating magnetic fields to induce neuronal firing in targeted brain regions. There are studies on efficacy of perfusional imaging assisted TMS in treatment resistant depression (Jha, Chadda, Kumar, & Bal, 2013) which alleviates risk of suicide. In a clinical trial (Ferrucci et al., 2009) that included some patients with a history of suicide attempt, tDCS was shown to have an effect on depressive symptoms, including suicidal ideation, comparable to that of a 6-week course of standard antidepressant medications. One weakness of the study was it did not take into account the proximity of attempts to the treatment. Direct evaluation of this novel therapy with regard to suicide has not been conducted.

There are studies on suicide rescued patient (Kumar & Jha, 2013) particularly post hanging that soon or later manifest with some neuropsychiatric deficit like amnesia, orbitofrontal syndromes or based on extent and area of brain insult. The brain SPECT assisted TMS has shown some evidence in such rescued patient in overcoming those residual deficits though it requires further research.

SPECIAL TOPICS

Extended Suicide

Extended suicide is a dramatic event in which an individual commits suicide shortly after homicide. In German-speaking countries Nacke first introduced the term “extended suicide”. In extended suicide the person sees the murdered person as an extension of self (Cooke, 2013). Extended suicide is the most tragic associations between depression and criminality. In a study on Austrian females who committed a serious extended suicide attempt, it was found that factor associated were first, chronic severe depression with or without psychotic features, anxious-avoidant personality disorder, committed at least one suicide attempt in the past, long standing overstrain, marital or financial problems. An altruistic, hypernomic motive for killing and psychotic identification with the victim were found to be the basic understanding behind extended suicide (Meszaros & Fischer-Danzinger, 2000).

Suicide Victim

The majority of patients who make a suicide attempt, however, do not ultimately die by suicide. Studies that have followed suicide attempters identified in hospital emergency rooms have found that just 7–10% died by suicide over the next two decades (Jenkins, Hale, Papanastassiou, Crawford, & Tyrer, 2002). In rescued cases of suicide by hanging, there are hypoxic or anoxic changes occur in brain which may later lead to behavioral abnormality and personality change (Kumar & Jha, 2013). Single-Photon Emission Computed Tomography (SPECT) is a valuable tool to investigate regional cerebral blood flow (rCBF) deficits in such patients especially correlating the stable neuropsychiatric deficits. The perfusion studies have shown diffusely scattered area of hypoperfusion involving various cortical and subcortical structures. These neuropsychiatric deficits do add up to the existing burden of chronic psychiatric illness and subsequently requires intensive interventions (Kumar & Jha, 2013) with rehabilitation plan.

WHO Response

WHO is recognized suicide as a priority in public health perspective. The first WHO World Suicide Report "Preventing suicide: a global imperative" published in 2014. It was aimed to increase the awareness of the public health significance of suicide and suicide attempts and to make suicide prevention a high priority on the global public health agenda. It also aimed to encourage and support countries to develop or strengthen comprehensive suicide prevention strategies in a multisectoral public health approach. Suicide is one of the priority conditions in the WHO Mental Health Gap Action Programme (mhGAP) launched in 2008, which provides evidence-based technical guidance to scale up service provision and care in countries for mental, neurological and substance use disorders. In the WHO Mental Health Action Plan 2013-2020, WHO Member States have committed themselves to working towards the global target of reducing the suicide rate in countries by 10% by 2020.

Indian Scenario

The suicide rate in India is comparable to that of developed countries and the increasing rate during recent decades is consistent with the global trend. More than one lakh lives are lost every year due to suicide in India. There had been a gradual increasing trend of suicide rate in the past decades (from 1975 to 2005), the suicide rate increased by 43%. The rates were approximately the same in 1975 and 1985; from 1985 to 1995 there was an increase of 35% and from 1995 to 2005, the increase was 5%. In the NCRB report the rate in 2010 rose to 11.4 per 100,000 population; an increase of 5.9% in the number of suicides (Radhakrishnan & Andrade, 2012). Based on NCRB report, 2014 the number of Suicides in 2013 was 1,34,799 i.e. 11.0 per one lakh persons and in 2014 was 1,31,666 i.e. 10.6 per one lakh persons. The problem is however a difficult one as expressed by Gajalakshmi and Peto (2007) as "a complex array of factors such as poverty, low literacy level, unemployment, family violence, breakdown of the joint family system, unfulfilled romantic ideals, inter-generational conflicts, loss of job or loved one, failure of crops, growing costs of cultivation, huge debt burden, unhappy marriages, harassment by in-laws and husbands, dowry disputes, depression, chronic physical illness, alcoholism/drug addiction, and easy access to means of suicide."47 the prevention is being the main intervention and based on same there are various crisis intervention centers came into existence. There had been research on suicide which are categorized under (1) Incidence and prevalence studies (2) Profiling and identification of risk factors (3) Suicide and suicidal behavior in specific communities (4)Studies on Non-Fatal Deliberate Self Harm (DSH) (5) Suicide prevention strategies.

Nandi, Banarjee and Boral, (1978) and Hegde, (1980) studied incidence rates in Bengal and patterns of suicide in a rural community in northern Karnataka respectively using data available in the public domain across a hundred-year period (1872-1972) and reported increasing incidence of suicide rate with male preponderance along with the most common method identified was poisoning. Regarding clinical profile and factors associated, Rao, (1965) in his hospital based study on suicide attempts reported a male preponderance and vulnerable age group as being from 15 to 25 years. 20% of the attempters had a family history of mental illness/suicidal attempts. He also recommended that education of general physicians, limiting access to availability of antidepressants, paracetemol and pesticides would lower the rates of suicide (Rao, 1999).

Vijayakumar, (2007) in an editorial expresses the urgent need for suicide prevention in India and stresses that suicide is a multifaceted problem and hence suicide prevention programs should also be multidimensional. Collaboration, coordination, cooperation and commitment are needed to develop and implement a national plan, which is cost-effective, appropriate and relevant to the needs of the community. For the suicide risk assessment, Gupta, Anand, and Trivedi (1983) published an article on the development of a 10 item suicidal intent questionnaire. The article established that the questionnaire was fairly valid but stated that further work was necessary to establish its statistical validity and reliability.

Based on the research evidences (Vijayakumar, 2010), a social and public health approach acknowledged that suicide is preventable, and initiated a framework to be made in integrated system of interventions across multiple levels within society including the individual, the family, the community and the health care system. A key step in such an approach involves modifying attitudes toward suicide via educational efforts and legal levers (e.g. decriminalizing suicide).

Moving ahead on policy level, the landmark initiative had been taken by the government of India indecriminalizing the "attempt to suicide" by deleting Section 309 of the Indian Penal Code (IPC) from the statute book after 18 states and 4 Union territories backed the recommendation of the Law Commission of India in this regard.

Further in an attempt to make crisis intervention accessible to every people in crisis, the initiatives taken by SAMHSA and manyonline crisis intervention sites like IMAlive: An Online Crisis Network, Crisis Chat, National Suicide Prevention Lifeline and others. Similarly, in India such center is "AASRA". It is a crisis intervention center for the lonely, distressed and suicidal. Aasra functions as a unit of Befrienders Worldwide/Samaritans and is a non-religious, non-political and non-sectarian organization, registered as a Public Charity under the Bombay Charity Act, 1960. There are many such reforms required even at the level of policy making for some population specific crisis or suicide like farmers' suicide in India.

Few Facts about NCRB Report, 2014:

- 15 Suicides take place every one hour in the year 2014.
- Like previous years, more than one lakh persons (1,31,666) in the country lost their lives by committing suicide during the year 2014.
- Maximum suicides were reported in Maharashtra (16,307) followed by Tamil Nadu (16,122) and West Bengal (14,310) accounting for 12.4%, 12.2% and 10.9% respectively of total suicides reported in the country during 2014. Puducherry reported the highest rate of suicides (40.4) followed by Sikkim (38.4) during 2014.
- Like previous year, 'Hanging' (41.8%), Consuming 'Poison' (26.0%), 'Self-Immolation' (6.9%) and 'Drowning' (5.6%) were the prominent means of committing suicides during 2014.
- 1 suicide out of every 6 suicides was committed by a 'homemaker'; nearly 67.0% of the male victims were married while 63.6% of female victims were married.
- 69.7% of victims having income of less than 1 lakh have committed suicides during 2014. 26.9% of suicides victims belong to income group of 1 lakh and above to less than 5 lakh. 20.2% of the suicide victims were educated up to middle level, 19.0% of the suicide victims were educated up to primary level and 14.3% of victims of suicide were illiterate.
- Family problem (other than marriage related issues) was the major cause of suicide in cities in 2014 which accounted for 25.0% (5,157 out of 20,621) of total suicides followed by 'Illness' which accounted for 19.0% (3,920 victim out of 20,621 victim)

- Out of total 20,621 suicides in cities during 2014, 23.6% were educated up to matriculate/secondary level (4,867) The highest number of mass/family suicide deaths were reported from Uttar Pradesh (66) followed by Karnataka (52), Andhra Pradesh (33), Maharashtra (23), Kerala and Telangana (22 each) out of 275 deaths during the year 2014.

CONCLUSION

Suicide is major public health issue. Mental illness is a risk factor for suicide and uniformly studied all across the globe. With such rising trend, it requires specific attention in all domains among public service providers along with specific targeted population of patients suffering from psychiatric illness. A social and public health response to suicide is crucial and should complement a mental health response. However, additional risk factors are prominent in India. These tend to relate to societal structures and specific stressors. Among people who die by suicide, identifiable psychiatric diagnosis either independent or comorbid are common. Therefore, efforts to educate primary care providers about the diagnosis and treatment of such condition including referral to specialized center are especially important. However, the enormity of the problem has led to several major public health initiatives and a growth in research funding for suicide prevention and specific interventions. The national strategy should focus on promoting awareness that suicide is public health problem and it is preventable, to develop support for suicide prevention, implement strategies to reduce the stigma, implement suicide prevention programs, efforts to reduce access to lethal means and methods, implement training for recognition of at-risk behavior and delivery of effective treatment, improve access to and community linkages with mental health and substance abuse services, promote and support research on suicide and suicide prevention, improve and expand surveillance systems. Twenty-eight countries have established national suicide prevention programs dedicated to suicide research and prevention. However, there is still a need to expand suicide prevention research and anti-suicidal strategies. With vigorousness in research methodology and in era of technological advancement, there have been various treatment alternatives now available which has emerged and hold great promises in future prospect. But due to limited resources especially in under-develop or developing nation, the accessibility to all is still a concern by service providers. Besides all the commitment perceived at all sections including community, professional bodies and policy makers, it is yet not impossible to provide helping hand to the person in crisis.

REFERENCES

Atkinson, M., Zibin, S., & Chuang, H. (1997). Characterizing Quality of Life Among Patients With Chronic Mental Illness: A Critical Examination of the Self-Report Methodology. *The American Journal of Psychiatry*, *154*(1), 99–105. doi:10.1176/ajp.154.1.99 PMID:8988966

Bertolote, J. M., & Fleischmann, A. (2002). Suicide and psychiatric diagnosis: A worldwide pe4rspective. *World Psychiatry; Official Journal of the World Psychiatric Association (WPA)*, *1*(3), 181–185. PMID:16946849

Bertolote, J. M., Fleischmann, A., De Leo, D., Bolhari, J., Botega, N., De Silva, D., & Wasserman, D. et al. (2005). Suicide attempts, plans, and ideation in culturally diverse sites: The WHO SUPRE-MISS community survey. *Psychological Medicine*, *35*(10), 1457–1465. doi:10.1017/S0033291705005404 PMID:16164769

Bloom, D. E., Cafiero, E. T., Jané-Llopis, E., Abrahams-Gessel, S., Bloom, L. R., Fathima, S., Weinstein, C. (2011). *The Global Economic Burden of Noncommunicable Diseases*. Geneva: World Economic Forum.

Bluml, V., Kapusta, N. D., Doering, S., Brahler, E., Wagner, B., & Kersting, A. (2013). Personality Factors and Suicide Risk in a Representative Sample of the German General Population. *PLoS ONE*, *8*(10), e76646. doi:10.1371/journal.pone.0076646 PMID:24124582

Bohanna, I., & Wang, X. (2012). Media guidelines for the responsible reporting of suicide: A review of effectiveness. Crisis. *Journal of Crisis Intervention & Suicide*, *33*(4), 190–198. doi:10.1027/0227-5910/a000137 PMID:22713977

Brown, G. K., Ten Have, T., Henriques, G. R., Xie, S. X., Hollander, J. E., & Beck, A. T. (2005). Cognitive therapy for the prevention of suicide attempts: A randomized controlled trial. *Journal of the American Medical Association*, *294*(5), 563–570. doi:10.1001/jama.294.5.563 PMID:16077050

Carter, G. L., Child, C., Page, A., Clover, K., & Taylor, R. (2007). Modifiable risk factors for attempted suicide in Australian clinical and community samples. *Suicide & Life-Threatening Behavior*, *37*(6), 671–680. doi:10.1521/suli.2007.37.6.671 PMID:18275373

Cavanagh, J. T., Carson, A. J., Sharpe, M., & Lawrie, S. M. (2003). Psychological autopsy studies of suicide: A systematic review. *Psychological Medicine*, *33*(3), 395–405. doi:10.1017/S0033291702006943 PMID:12701661

Cooke, B. K. (2013). Extended Suicide With a Pet. *The Journal of the American Academy of Psychiatry and the Law*, *41*, 437–443. PMID:24051598

Cuijpers, P., de Beurs, D. P., van Spijker, B. A., Berking, M., Andersson, G., & Kerkhof, A. J. (2013). The effects of psychotherapy for adult depression on suicidality and hopelessness: A systematic review and meta-analysis. *Journal of Affective Disorders*, *144*(3), 183–190. doi:10.1016/j.jad.2012.06.025 PMID:22832172

De Leo, D. (2002). Suicide among the elderly: The long-term impact of a telephone support and assessment intervention in northern Italy. *The British Journal of Psychiatry*, *181*(3), 226–229. doi:10.1192/bjp.181.3.226 PMID:12204927

De Leo, D., Carollo, G., & DelloBuono, M. (1995). Lower suicide rates associated with a tele-help/tele-check service for the elderly at home. *The American Journal of Psychiatry*, *152*(4), 632–634. doi:10.1176/ajp.152.4.632 PMID:7694919

de Leo, D., & Heller, T. (2008). Social modeling in the transmission of suicidality. Crisis. *Journal of Crisis Intervention & Suicide*, *29*(1), 11–19. doi:10.1027/0227-5910.29.1.11

Ferrucci, R., Bortolomasi, M., Vergari, M., Tadini, L., Salvoro, B., Giacopuzzi, M., & Priori, A. (2009). Transcranial direct current stimulation in severe, drug-resistant major depression. *Journal of Affective Disorders*, *118*(1-3), 215–219. doi:10.1016/j.jad.2009.02.015 PMID:19286265

Fink, M., Kellner, C. H., & McCall, W. V. (2014). The role of ECT in suicide prevention. *Journal of Electric Convulsive Therapy*, *30*(1), 5–9. PMID:24091903

Gajalakshmi, V., & Peto, R. (2007). Suicide rates in rural Tamil Nadu, south India: Verbal autopsy of 39 000 deaths in 1997-98. *International Journal of Epidemiology*, *36*(1), 203–207. doi:10.1093/ije/dyl308 PMID:17301103

Greenberg, P. E., Fournier, A. A., Sisitsky, T., Pike, C. T., & Kessler, R. C. (2015). The Economic Burden of Adults With Major Depressive Disorder in the United States (2005 and 2010). *The Journal of Clinical Psychiatry*, *76*(2), 155–162. doi:10.4088/JCP.14m09298 PMID:25742202

Gupta, S. C., Anand, R., & Trivedi, J. K. (1983). Development of a suicidal intent questionnaire. *Indian Journal of Psychiatry*, *25*, 57–62. PMID:21847253

Han, C., Voils, C. I., & Williams, J. W. (2011). Uptake of Web-Based Clinical Resources from the MacArthur Initiative on Depression and Primary Care. *Community Mental Health Journal*, 1. PMID:22038376

Hegde, R. S. (1980). Suicide in rural community. *Indian Journal of Psychiatry*, *22*, 368–370. PMID:22058501

Inagaki, M., Kawashima, Y., Kawanishi, C., Yonemoto, N., Sugimoto, T., Furuno, T., & Yamada, M. (2015). Interventions to prevent repeat suicidal behavior in patients admitted to an emergency department for a suicide attempt: A meta-analysis. *Journal of Affective Disorders*, *175*, 66–78. doi:10.1016/j.jad.2014.12.048 PMID:25594513

Jenkins, G. R., Hale, R., Papanastassiou, M., Crawford, M. J., & Tyrer, P. (2002). Suicide rate 22 years after parasuicide: Cohort study. *British Medical Journal*, *325*(7373), 1155. doi:10.1136/bmj.325.7373.1155 PMID:12433767

Jha, S., Chadda, R. K., Kumar, N., & Bal, C. S. (2016). Brain SPECT guided repetitive transcranial magnetic stimulation (rTMS) in treatment resistant major depressive disorder. *Asian Journal of Psychiatry*, *21*, 1–6. doi:10.1016/j.ajp.2016.02.003

Jha, S., & Kumar, R. (2015). Methodological considerations in determining the effects of films with suicidal content. *The British Journal of Psychiatry*, *207*(6), 562. doi:10.1192/bjp.207.6.562

Kaplan & Sadock. (2010). *Comprehensive Textbook of Psychiatry* (9th ed.; Vol. 2). Philadelphia: Lippincott Williams and Wilkins.

Kumar, N., & Jha, S. (2013). Repetitive Transcranial Magnetic Stimulation (RTMS) in organic personality and behavioral disorder, secondary to suicide attempt by hanging. *Clinical Neurophysiology*, *124*(10), 165–166.

Luoma, J. B., Martin, C. E., & Pearson, J. L. (2002). Contact with mental health and primary care providers before suicide: A review of the evidence. *The American Journal of Psychiatry*, *159*(6), 909–916. doi:10.1176/appi.ajp.159.6.909 PMID:12042175

Mann, J. J., & Currier, D. (2012). Neurobiology of Suicidal Behavior. In R.I. Simon & R.E. Hales (Eds.), The American Psychiatric Publishing Textbook of Suicide Assessment and Management (pp. 481–500). Academic Press.

Meszaros, K., & Fischer-Danzinger, D. (2000). Extended suicide attempt: Psychopathology, personality and risk factors. *Psychopathology*, *33*(1), 5–10. doi:10.1159/000029111 PMID:10601820

Moller, H. J. (1989). Efficacy of different strategies of after-care for patients who have attempted suicide. *Journal of the Royal Society of Medicine*, *82*, 643–648. PMID:2556579

Motto, J. A. (1976). Suicide prevention for high-risk persons who refuse treatment. *Suicide & Life-Threatening Behavior*, *6*, 223–230. PMID:1023455

Motto, J. A., & Bostrom, A. G. (2001). A randomized controlled trial of postcrisis suicide prevention. *Psychiatric Services (Washington, D.C.)*, *52*(6), 828–833. doi:10.1176/appi.ps.52.6.828 PMID:11376235

Motto, J. A., Heilbron, D. C., Juster, R. P., & Bostrom, A. G. (1981). Communication as a suicide prevention program. In J. P. Soubrier & J. Vedrienne (Eds.), *Depression and suicide* (pp. 143–166). Paris: Pergamon.

Mrazek, P. J., & Haggerty, R. J. (1994). *Reducing risks for mental disorders: frontiers for preventive intervention research*. Washington, DC: National Academy Press.

Nandi, D. N., Banarjee, G., & Boral, G. C. (1978). Suicide in West Bengal - A century apart. *Indian Journal of Psychiatry*, *20*, 155–160.

National Crime Records Bureau. (2014). Retrieved from India.ncrb.gov.in/ADSI2014/adsi-2014%20 full%20report.pdf

Pandey, G. N. (2013). Biological basis of suicide and suicidal behavior. *Bipolar Disorders*, *15*(5), 524–541. doi:10.1111/bdi.12089 PMID:23773657

Posner, K., Brown, G. K., Stanley, B., Brent, D. A., Yershova, K. V., Oquendo, M. A., & Mann, J. J. et al. (2011). The Columbia–Suicide Severity Rating Scale: Initial Validity and Internal Consistency Findings From Three Multisite Studies With Adolescents and Adults. *The American Journal of Psychiatry*, *168*(12), 1266–1277. doi:10.1176/appi.ajp.2011.10111704 PMID:22193671

Posner, K., Oquendo, M. A., Gould, M., Stanley, B., & Davies, M. (2007). Columbia Classification Algorithm of Suicide Assessment (C-CASA): Classification of Suicidal Events in the FDA's Pediatric Suicidal Risk Analysis of Antidepressants. *The American Journal of Psychiatry*, *164*(7), 1035–1043. doi:10.1176/ajp.2007.164.7.1035 PMID:17606655

Radhakrishnan, R., & Andrade, C. (2012). Suicide: An Indian perspective. *Indian Journal of Psychiatry*, *54*(4), 304–319. doi:10.4103/0019-5545.104793 PMID:23372232

Rao, V. A. (1965). Attempted suicide. *Indian Journal of Psychiatry*, *7*, 253–264.

Rao, V. A. (1999). Toward suicide prevention. *Indian Journal of Psychiatry*, *41*, 280–288. PMID:21430799

Rickels, K., Athanasiou, M., Robinson, D. S., Gibertini, M., Whalen, H., & Reed, C. R. (2009). Evidence for efficacy and tolerability of vilazodone in the treatment of major depressive disorder: A randomized, double-blind, placebo-controlled trial. *The Journal of Clinical Psychiatry*, *70*(3), 326–333. doi:10.4088/JCP.08m04637 PMID:19284933

Sahlem, G. L., Kalivas, B., Fox, J. B., Lamb, K., Roper, A., Williams, E. N., & Short, E. B. et al. (2014). Adjunctive triple chronotherapy (combined total sleep deprivation, sleep phase advance, and bright light therapy) rapidly improves mood and suicidality in suicidal depressed inpatients: An open label pilot study. *Journal of Psychiatric Research*, *59*, 101–107. doi:10.1016/j.jpsychires.2014.08.015 PMID:25231629

Sareen, J., Isaak, C., Katz, L.Y., Bolton, J., Enns, M.W, & Steinet M. B. (2014). Promising Strategies for Advancement in Knowledge of Suicide Risk Factors and Prevention. *American Journal of Preventive Medicine*, *47*(3S2), S257–S263.

Sisask, M., & Varnik, A. (2012). Media roles in suicide prevention: A systematic review. *International Journal of Environmental Research and Public Health*, *9*(1), 123–138. doi:10.3390/ijerph9010123 PMID:22470283

Substance Abuse and Mental Health Services Administration (SAMHSA). (n.d.). Retrieved from http://www.integration.samhsa.gov/clinical-practice/suicide-prevention

Thelma Beatriz, G.-C., Isela, J.-R., Alma, G., María Lilia, L.-N., & Carlos Alfonso, T.-Z. (2014). Association between HTR2C gene variants and suicidal behaviour: A protocol for the systematic review and meta-analysis of genetic studies. *BMJ Open*, *4*(9), e005423. doi:10.1136/bmjopen-2014-005423 PMID:25190618

Tidemalm, D., Langstrom, N., Lichtenstein, P., & Runeson, B. (2008). Risk of suicide after suicide attempt according to coexisting psychiatric disorder: Swedish cohort study with long term follow-up. *British Medical Journal*, *337*(nov18 3), a2205. doi:10.1136/bmj.a2205 PMID:19018040

Till, B., Strauss, M., Sonneck, G., & Niederkrotenthaler, T. (2015). Determining the effects of films with suicidal content: A laboratory experiment. *The British Journal of Psychiatry*, *207*(1), 72–78. doi:10.1192/bjp.bp.114.152827 PMID:25906792

Vijayakumar, L. (2007). Suicide and its prevention: The urgent need in India. *Indian Journal of Psychiatry*, *49*(2), 81–84. doi:10.4103/0019-5545.33252 PMID:20711387

Vijayakumar, L. (2010). Indian research on suicide. *Indian Journal of Psychiatry*, *52*(7ll), S291–S296. doi:10.4103/0019-5545.69255 PMID:21836697

World Health Organization. (2015). *Preventing suicide: a global imperative*. World Health Organization. Retrieved from http://www.who.int/mental_health/suicide-prevention/world_report_2014/en/

Yip, P. S., Caine, E., Yousuf, S., Chang, S. S., Wu, K. C., & Chen, Y. Y. (2012). Means restriction for suicide prevention. *Lancet*, *379*(9834), 2393–2399. doi:10.1016/S0140-6736(12)60521-2 PMID:22726520

KEY TERMS AND DEFINITIONS

Novel Treatments in Suicide: There are few novel techniques, what we call as an advance treatment modalities like Electro-Convulsive Therapy (ECT), Triple Chronotherapy, Transcranial Magnetic Stimulation (TMS), Transcranial Direct Current Stimulation (tDCS) and Vagal Nerve Stimulation (VNS). Among these techniques, ECT has proven its efficacy over the time in improving depressive symptom and subsequently in suicide prevention.

Suicide: The act of intentionally causing one's own death. Suicide is often carried out as a result of despair, the cause of which is frequently attributed to a mental disorder such as depression, bipolar disorder, schizophrenia, borderline personality disorder, alcoholism, or drug abuse, as well as stress factors such as financial difficulties, troubles with interpersonal relationships, and bullying.

Suicide in Depression: A morbidity associated with depression is difficult to quantify, but the lethality of depression takes the measurable form of completed suicide.

Suicide in Schizophrenia: A chronic disabling mental illness, characterized by a wide range of symptoms including abnormal thinking, loss of contact with the reality and hallucinations. It is strongly linked to an increased risk of suicideattempts and completed suicides.

Suicide in Bipolar Disorder: Bipolar disorder (manic-depressive illness) is a neurobiological disorder that severely affects patients with depression. Individuals diagnosed with this disease have mood swings that alternate from periods of severe highs (mania) to extreme lows (depression). Suicide is the number one cause of premature death among people with bipolar disorder.

Chapter 16
Cognitive Remediation Therapy in Chronic Schizophrenia

Susmita Halder
Amity University, India

Akash Mahato
Amity University, India

ABSTRACT

Cognitive impairments are now recognized as one of the most ubiquitous features of schizophrenia. Cognitive deficits appear to play a large role in how patients with schizophrenia function in their everyday lives. The role of cognitive deficits in schizophrenia may be gauged by the fact that even when patients with schizophrenia are relatively free of psychotic symptoms, many still have extraordinary difficulty with communication, motivation, self-care, and establishing and maintaining relationships with others. Patients with schizophrenia are often additionally treated with supportive psychotherapy, behavioral management, or social skills training as required. However, the efficacy of these adjunct therapies could be limited in presence of marked cognitive deficits. Thus it becomes crucial to have specific intervention for the underlying cognitive deficits that appear detrimental to improvement of functioning of patients with schizophrenia. The present chapter focuses on cognitive training based intervention program for schizophrenia patients and its efficacy.

INTRODUCTION

Schizophrenia is a major psychiatric disorder characterized by a disruption in affective, cognitive and social domains, which results in compromised ability to adapt to a changing environment and to function adequately in the community. It is a hypothetical construct that clinicians and scientists have developed in an attempt to capture a complex reality (Morey, 1991). As a diagnostic construct, it is inferred from behaviour of a client or the symptoms reported by him. The complexity of the illness is such that even psychiatric experts concede on hypothetical construct nature of the diagnostic categories in schizophrenia (Wong, 2014).

DOI: 10.4018/978-1-5225-0519-8.ch016

The deterioration in cognitive and behavioural functions has been implicit in initial conceptualization of the illness to an extent that Kraeplin (1919) described the illness as an irreversible and deteriorating condition like dementia (Goldman, Axlerod, & Taylor, 1996). Cognitive impairments are now recognized as one of the most ubiquitous features of schizophrenia. It is suggested that these impairments are very apparent and detectable before the onset of symptoms that meet diagnostic criteria for schizophrenia. The severity of these impairments may vary from moderate to severe even at the time of the first break of the symptoms and they tend to persist throughout the course of the illness (Bowie & Harvey, 2005). Meta-analytical studies provide substantial evidences that these cognitive impairments are present significantly at early stage of the illness even in drug naive patients; thus they are not resulting from other symptoms or antipsychotic treatment (Bergman, Cervenka, Flyckt, Edman, & Farde, 2014). The recognition that cognitive dysfunction is a central feature of schizophrenia has elevated its importance for both research and treatment. One of the main incentives for understanding the signature of cognitive impairment in schizophrenia is the strong relationship between cognitive performance and functional skills and functional outcome.

Despite the widespread prevalence of cognitive impairment in schizophrenia, there is considerable controversy as to whether the deficits reflect a generalized and a global neuropsychological impairment. The presence of diffuse cognitive impairment has been documented in patients with schizophrenia across a range of cognitive measures (Hoff et al. 1999; Mohamed, Paulsen, O'Leary, Arndt, & Andreasen,1999; Saykin et al., 1994). Although there appears to be a group of patients who are impaired only minimally, most patients are characterized as having at least some impairment across a number of domains.

SPECIFIC NEUROPSYCHOLOGICAL DEFICITS IN SCHIZOPHRENIA

Several studies identify selective impairments of a greater magnitude against a background of global impairment. Specifically, the cognitive deficits appear to be larger in areas of attention, memory and executive function.

- **Attention:** Schizophrenia is characterized by deficits in attention (Bleuler, 1911; Kraepelin, 1919; Shakow, 1962) and it has been claimed that these attention deficits are related to dysfunctional brain systems that underlie the pathophysiology of the disease (Robbins, 1990; Norman et al., 1997). Attention skills are disrupted by a wide variety of causes and attention is a critical underlying component of many cognitive functions. Without intact attention skills; many other skills, including learning, communication, and problem-solving become difficult or impossible. Furthermore, attention deficits can be mistaken for memory deficits when memory functions are in fact intact.
- **Memory:** Memory impairment is one of the most common cognitive problems in schizophrenia patients (Gourovitch & Goldberg, 1996). This type of impairment is usually long- term, debilitating and difficult to treat (Chen& McKenna, 1996). In last many years, an increasing amount of research has investigated memory deficits in schizophrenia. Schizophrenia patients have been found to be impaired on their ability to recall, recognize, and learn both visual and verbal materials (Gold, Carpenter, Randolph, Goldberg, & Weinberger, 1997; Tamlyn et al., 1992; Paulsen et al., 1995). These findings have been postulated to result from neuropathological abnormalities in the temporal- hippocampal area (Goldman et al., 1996). Consistent with learning theory, three

phases of learning are implemented in memory training: acquisition, application, and adaptation. Each phase imposes different demands on the learner and requires adjustment in instructional strategies.

- **Executive Function:** Executive functions include the capacity to formulate goals, plan and organize goal- directed behavior, carry out goal directed behavior fully and effectively, and monitor and self- correct one's behavior needed. Disturbances in executive functions have been structurally related to the prefrontal lobes, neuropsychological to defective performance in tests of problem- solving abilities, and functionally to disability in maintaining a complex behavior sequence without help. Schizophrenics have varying grades of impairment of executive processes, which result in difficulties during extended and multifaceted interpersonal interactions. Carter and Barch (2000) relate the neural basis of executive functions to the dorsolateral prefrontal cortex and anterior cingulated cortex, and show that functional imaging studies identified disturbances in other areas as well, particularly the temporolimbic region. Disturbances in higher cognitive functions may have an engaging relationship to the functional hypofrontality observed among these patients during positron emission tomography (PET) and functional MRI studies. Luria (1973) have referred to the loss of meaningful, directed behaviour resulting from frontal lobe lesions, in the absence of marked disturbances in motor activity or sensitivity, agnosis or praxis as a construct in rehabilitation.

EFFECT ON REAL-WORLD FUNCTIONING

Cognitive deficits appear to play a large role in how patients with schizophrenia function in their everyday lives. Impaired cognition can harm patient compliance to treatment regimens and reduce motivation to engage in a therapeutic alliance (Olfson et al., 2000). Cognitive deficits may be the most vital factor in predicting real-world functioning in patients with schizophrenia, such as availing public transport and doing financial transactions in shops or bank. In a study, geriatric patients who were able to live in the community in comparison to institutionalized patients were found not differing from them on most measures, including the severity of their positive symptoms; however, their cognitive functioning was dramatically better than the institutionalized patients, suggesting that a patient's level of cognitive functioning might be the most important determinant of real-world outcomes (Harvey & Keefe, 1997). Similarly, Green (1996) tried to determine which, if any, neurocognitive deficits restrict the functioning of schizophrenic patients in the outside world. He reviewed studies that have evaluated neurocognitive measures as predictors and correlates of functional outcome for schizophrenic patients. The review included seventeen studies that evaluated specific neurocognitive correlates of community functioning, social problem solving, and psychosocial skill acquisition. Results suggested that despite wide variation among studies in the selection of neurocognitive measures, some consistencies emerged. The most consistent finding was that verbal memory was associated with all types of functional outcome. Vigilance was related to social problem solving and skill acquisition. Negative symptoms were associated with social problem solving but not skill acquisition. Notably, psychotic symptoms were not significantly associated with outcome measures in any of the studies reviewed. Verbal memory and vigilance appear to be necessary for adequate functional outcome. Deficiencies in these areas may prevent patients from attaining optimal adaptation and hence act as neurocognitive rate-limiting factors.

Addington and Addington (2000) examined the relationships between neurocognitive and social functioning in 80 schizophrenia outpatients. They found social functioning as assessed by the Social Functioning Scale was unrelated to neurocognitive functioning. However, poor cognitive flexibility was associated with low scores on the Quality of Life Scale and the Assessment of Interpersonal Problem-Solving Skills (AIPSS). Verbal ability and verbal memory were also significantly associated with the AIPSS. Visual-spatial ability and vigilance were associated with the sending skills subscale of the AIPSS. In this study, which used a wide range of neurocognitive tests and measures of community functioning and social problem solving, results support earlier research that suggests an association between certain aspects of neurocognitive functioning and social functioning. Perhaps one of the most challenging aspects of treating patients with schizophrenia is coping with the severe cognitive deficits that accompany the disease. These deficits are evident in nearly all individuals diagnosed with schizophrenia (Keefe & Harvey, 2012) and their impact on the employment, social relationships and living status of patients is devastating. Cognitive deficits impair motivation and insight about one's illness and treatment as well as negatively affecting the therapeutic alliance.

Diminished attention disrupts the ability of a patient to follow a conversation, comply with medication instructions, complete a course of therapy and hold a job. Poor memory has many consequences harming social functioning, employment and quality of life. Patients with schizophrenia also tend to have greater trouble with tasks that require executive functions in that they have impaired ability to shift from one set of rules to another. This difficulty, also known as a perseveration, makes the process of adapting to change very difficult. It is evident that each of these cognitive deficits may pose a problem during non-pharmacological form of therapy. For example, patients with poor verbal memory will find it difficult to benefit from cognitive-behavioral therapy techniques if they cannot easily remember them. A physician's awareness of these deficiencies will help patients receive the best possible treatment.

COGNITIVE REMEDIATION THERAPY

While Cognitive Remediation Therapy and Cognitive Rehabilitation Therapy sound very similar, there are certain differences. Cognitive rehabilitation is a form of intervention in which a series of procedures are applied by a trained practitioner to retain or alleviate problems due to deficits in underlying cognitive functions (Sohlberg & Mateer, 1989). While, cognitive remediation is a teaching process that targets areas of neuropsychological functioning involved in learning and basic day-to-day functioning. It itself is a behavioural training based rehabilitative exercise aiming to improve attention, memory, language, executive functions and social cognition. It is an art and science of restoring these mental processes and teaching compensatory strategies. Overall, any cognitive rehabilitation procedure must be based on solid, scientific knowledge of brain- behaviour relationships and designed to meet specifically defined treatment goals.

TYPES OF COGNITIVE REHABILITATION THERAPY (CRT)

- **Stimulation Therapy:** It is based on the assumption that cognitive functions will improve by stimulating the cognitive system. The therapy usually includes paper-and-pencil exercises or computer training that stimulates one or more mental skills. Presumably, by using these skills, a person's cognition will improve and the improvement will transfer to his or her activities of daily living.

- **Process Training:** Process training is similar to stimulation training, but process training focuses on specific areas of cognition. For example, Bracy's (1986) process approach to CRT emphasizes assessment and treatment of specific cognitive defects, such as poor visual scanning or visual neglect.
- **Attention-Concentration Training:** It is designed to improve a person's ability to focus attention, to maintain vigilance, to resist distraction, and to perform mental manipulations quickly and efficiently. It is one of the most widely researched areas of CRT and the researcher has produced commercially available training programs with proven efficacy (Sohlberg & Mateer, 1987).
- **Strategy Training:** As the name suggests, strategy training imparts specific strategies to a deal with situations which a person finds difficult to handle, e.g. remembering information, or skill to continue on a particular task like conversation. These kinds of trainings have been used on patients with traumatic brain injury (Richardson, 1992).
- **Nutrient and Drug Treatment:** It operates on the premise that various substances can affect cognition by correcting chemical imbalance. For example, memory deficits secondary to long term alcohol abuse can often be arrested with thiamine treatments (Elovic, 2000). This type of CRT is relatively new although the results are promising.
- **Prosthetic-Orthotic Devices:** External aids are sometimes referred to as prosthetic-orthotic devices. Their purpose is to obviate a cognitive problem rather than to retrain a defective process. Using an external aid is often the most efficient and expedient way to treat certain cognitive deficits. For example, training a person with a poor memory to use a tape recorder can improve his or her functional memory immediately but it may not have any effect on the underlying physiological cause of the deficit. Although the prosthetic devices do not rectify a person's memory deficit, the devices are especially effective and efficacious methods of treatment.
- **Domain-Specific Training:** These techniques emphasize training a person with simulated life experiences or within a specific functional domain. For example, Schacter and Glisky (1986) described the use of computer simulation to train a person to perform data entry.
- **Indirect Training:** This is based on the idea that although CRT methods like those previously discussed may be the most direct ways to improve cognitive problems, other indirect methods may also be effective (Herrmann & Parente, 1994; Yesavage, Rose, & Spiegel, 1982). For example, teaching a person to adhere to better sleeping and eating habits can improve cognitive function. Training a person to use a variety of external aids can result in a productive and satisfying daily routine (Herrmann & Petro, 1991; Naugle, Prevy, Naugle, & Delaney, 1988). Even the teaching of certain social skills can give some people more control over their everyday living situations so that they can make better use of their reduced cognitive functioning (Best, 1992; McEvoy, 1992).

In recent times, researchers introduce a model of cognition that provides a theoretical backdrop for an eclectic approach to cognitive rehabilitation. This approach is rooted in the theoretical assumption that cognition and the rehabilitation of cognitive functions are influenced by many different factors including a person's physiological state, perceptual skills, emotional status, motivation, and social skills. Changing these factors can improve the person's cognitive functioning as much as any learned compensatory strategies. A combination of environmental changes and cognitive rehabilitation produces the greatest improvement in a person's cognitive functioning (Ben- Yishay & Diller, 1981; Gianutos, 1980). Moreover, this multimodal model provides a blueprint for a holistic approach to cognitive rehabilitation that is grounded in basic and clinical research (Herrmann, Plude, Yoder, & Mullin, 1999; McEvoy & Moon, 1988).

- **Cognitive Remediation:** A behavioural intervention designed to improve cognition in people who have suffered a decline in neuropsychological functioning. The application of cognitive remediation for people with schizophrenia has become increasingly popular. Over the past several years, two models of cognitive rehabilitation are in practice, viz. Cognitive remediation and Cognitive adaptation:
    - **Cognitive Remediation:** In this model cognitive deficits are treated directly through repeated practice and acquisition of compensatory strategies on cognitive exercises designed to engage under functioning brain systems.
    - **Cognitive Adaptation:** In this adaptive model, neurocognitive deficits are addressed through modification of patient's environment to allow patients to bypass their deficits (Kurtz, 2003).

Cognitive remediation packages are usually customized as per the cognitive deficits of the patient. Cognitive training studies in schizophrenia have followed two approaches:

1. In laboratory setting improving individual test; and
2. In clinical setting: paper pencil task along with variety tasks.

NEUROPSYCHOLOGICAL MEASURES IN COGNITIVE REMEDIATION

It could be a big question that which cognitive domains to be included in remediation training programme. Cognitive remediation programmes are more specific and conventionally have targeted on attention, memory, language and executive functions. This is in line with the evident literature on cognitive impairment in schizophrenia, making it a characteristics feature of the illness. Impairments of attention, learning, memory, and executive function have been reliably identified in the context of preserved verbal knowledge (Gold et al., 1997; Heinrichs & Zakzanis, 1998; Saykin, Gur, Gur, & Mozley, 1991). Decline in attention, memory are the common manifestation of cognitive impairment in schizophrenia, which is increasingly recognized as a core symptom of the disorder. It is evident in almost all people who carry the diagnosis. Deficits in the following areas have been consistently highlighted against a background of diffuse impairment: *Attention processes*: slowed cognitive speed. *Memory:* immediate and delayed recall, learning and verbal memory. *Executive functioning*: sequencing, organisation, planning, and flexibility. On the contrary, language, motor and visuo-spatial functions are less consistently impaired. As neuropsychological assessments are integral part of cognitive remediation programmes; the following guidelines for maximally valid neuropsychological assessment has been hypothesized while dealing with clients with severe disabilities like in schizophrenia.

1. Neuropsychological assessment should occur in real world settings.
2. Assessments should be made repeatedly over time.
3. Neuropsychological assessment measures should include the following:
    a. Supervisor ratings of patient's performance and attitudes.
    b. Objective ratings of the work environment.

THE COGNITIVE REMEDIATION PACKAGE

We discuss a remediation package (Halder, 2011) in detail that was done in clinical setting customized for and used on five chronic schizophrenia patients showing evidence of impaired attention, memory and executive functions. It was conducted in a tertiary care psychiatric hospital setting, rather than in laboratory set up, so several external distractions were there, but on the other hand it acted as real life simulation. The programme was structured combining psychoeducation without disturbing other daily schedule of the subjects.

Before selecting any test for administration, it was ensured that:*(a) the test could be easily administered on chronic schizophrenia patients,(b) even patient with impaired cognitive functioning could show some measurable performance on the tests and (c) practice on these tests in diverse set-up should be possible.*

Considering evidence based literature as discussed before, the researcher focussed on intervening on attention, memory and executive functions only.

- **Target for Intervention:** The package was designed so as to:
    - Improve attention, memory and executive function of the patients.
    - Modify the clinical symptoms of the patients.
    - Improve overall daily functioning of the patients.

The package was developed keeping in view, easy availability of the materials used, ease of method, so that it could be easily conducted by trained person in diverse setups and with patients of different background even with minimal educational background. The remediation therapy package basically investigated the efficacy of cognitive remediation program of neuropsychological deficits, in terms of attention, memory, and executive functioning of hospitalized, chronic schizophrenic patients. The overall effects from baseline to the 3-month follow-up were investigated.

- **Therapeutic Package:** The package broadly consisted of:
    - Psychoeducation.
    - **Cognitive Training:** Attention module, Memory module, Executive functions.

Psychoeducation

Psychoeducation refers to the dissemination of information about psychosis and skills of self-management. It has generally been targeted either at neuroleptic medication compliance and/or improving understanding and insights into psychotic illness itself (Goldman & Quinn, 1988). Early studies on psychoeducation on schizophrenia demonstrate that patients can acquire information and skills, but they still beg the question as to whether such information and skills internalize such that these are seen as relevant to the individual and his or her own situations. Keeping this view in mind, the intervention program started with a brief session of psychoeducation to both the groups. It specially helps to prepare the patient for actual therapy. It basically aimed to:

1. Provide information to patients regarding signs and symptoms of schizophrenia;
2. Knowledge and importance of medication and its side effects; and
3. Inform the patients about the cognitive difficulties in simple language that were going to be dealt with the aim to improve that functioning.

The patients were explained briefly about the cognitive problems in schizophrenia. The idea was to improve compliance and effort on part of the patients. Patients were explained how deficits in cognitive functions led to gross deficit in their daily activities, like attending things, remembering (dates, events, work), or organizing. Along with Psychoeducation, the group was continued with group meeting which included

- **Social Interaction:** Interacting with other patients and staff nurses.
- **Recreation:** Participation in activities like singing, games.
- **Involvement in Pre-Vocational Work Assignment:** Engagement in light work like helping the ward staff, carrying water and food from the mess, cleaning etc.

Cognitive Training Programme

The cognitive training program consisted of 30 hours (average) individual training divided into 20 minute sessions. The sessions were done six days a week and lasted for three months. The program consisted of three modules: Attention, Memory, and Executive function apart from psychoeducation.

Training Programme Flow Chart

Brief Education about the cognitive training
↓
Introduce a new task and establish a rationale for the task
↓
Discuss Steps of the task
↓
Demonstration of the task
↓
Practicing the task
↓
Giving feedback and correct mistakes if any
↓
Assignment of Homework
↓
Review of work from previous session.
↓
Assessment

Introducing a new task:

- The cognitive training program consisted of a series of exercises that were hierarchically ordered according to increasing cognitive complexity.
- The program progressed from training the sample on basic and simple stimuli to training on more complex stimuli.

Table 1. The attention, memory and executive functions training module

Intervention Area	Specific Target Area	Task
Attention	• Sustained Attention • Selective Attention • Scanning Ability	• Joining Beads • Grouping of cards • Letter Cancellation • Joining dots • Reading newspaper
Memory	• Verbal Learning • Immediate Memory • Delayed Memory • Recall • Recognition	• Remembering Objects • Picture Recognition • Learning Word list • Story Telling
Executive Function		• Category Matching • Correcting the order • Daily Schedule and 'to do list' • Planning Daily Routine • Problem solving • Extensive training on WCST

- The training programme encompassed training on reasoning skills, training on attention, memory and executive functioning, which were deemed as basic skills for intervention.
- The training exercises were always presented in the same predetermined order, though tailored according to the need of the patient.
- Considering the educational and Sociodemographic background of the subjects, remediation training tasks were formulated as such that they were simple yet effective and feasible to follow at home under supervision. The tasks as per intervention areas are detailed in Table 1.
- **Sessions:** Given that treatment intensity appears to be a salient factor in any cognitive remediation programme, every effort should be made both to provide treatment regularly and to ensure that clients go to sessions. And that was the reason why patient were intervened for three months.
- **No. of Sessions:** The subjects attended at least 10 but typically more than 25 sessions, which involved doing the packaged exercises designed to improve cognitive skills.
- A reminder was given to subjects in each session:
    - To attend each and every session – the more you attend and participate, the more skills you learn.
    - Bring your notebook and do the task what you are asked to do in free time after the session.
    - In event of any problem or difficulty, consult.

Procedure

- Detail and structured interview of the patient, and information from the ward staff were collected in the process of selecting and screening the patients.
- Semi-structured Performa was prepared for collecting data related to socio-demographic detail, clinical variables, and their social functioning.
- Standardized tools were also used for rating patient's psychopathology, handedness, and overall functioning.

- Direct behavioural observation method was also emphasized for the patient in actual or simulated interpersonal situation. Direct observation was done while patient interacted with the therapist, other patients, ward staffs, and other people.
- In addition, two raters (Clinical Psychologists) were engaged, who were unaware about the nature of the study. So the raters could do their rating impartially and in this way, tried to maintain objectivity and prevent rater biasness.

As patients differ widely in pre-morbid cognitive abilities, duration of illness, symptoms and pattern of neuropsychological deficits, the effects of individual differences on sensitivity to remediation procedure could be immense. For this, patient ideally should be screened for significant neurocognitive impairment prior to treatment with these remediation procedures. Thus, the clinical status, psychopathology level, disability and neuropsychological measures of the subjects were assessed thrice; once at the baseline, next post intervention, and lastly at follow up. Before introducing any new task, subjects were explained in simple words the rationale behind it and the impairment of the skills (in daily life) to motivate the patient to involve in that task.

- **Drop Out of Patients:** Out of the total sample two subjects dropped out of the intervention program, as one patient was discharged from the hospital before completion of the study, while one was dropped for increased severity of symptoms.

Treatment Factors Involved

There was no attempt to control the type of medications subjects were getting in the previous study. This was kept in unison to most of the similar treatment efficacy studies done earlier, which did not control this variable, although post hoc analysis of tracked data about medication use suggests that patients taking atypical anti psychotics were more likely to improve in cognitive remediation than those on conventional anti psychotics. In fact, only few remediation studies e.g. Wykes et al. (2007) have reported the type of medication during these training procedures. However, all psychotic medications administered to patients during the study were noted down. Type and doses of antipsychotic medications were determined at the initial assessment. Usually cognitive exercises targeted at specific neurocognitive deficits provide incremental benefit for specific aspects of neurocognition. The intervention program along with psychoeducation improve overall clinical and psychosocial functioning. In the study (Halder, 2011) patients assigned to cognitive remediation demonstrated significantly greater improvements in overall cognitive performance. There are also non-specific effects of participation in the cognitive remediation program, such as improved motivation or sense of self-confidence, which are another potential contributor to improved work outcomes. A greater understanding of the relationship between improved cognitive functioning and better psychosocial functioning in areas such as work is needed to identify appropriate cognitive targets for treatment. This in turn may reinforce motivation and improve a sense of self-mastery, which in itself could contribute to better cognitive performance. Apart from control interventions that systematically teach skills; simply engaging the patient in some active manner may also improve cognitive functioning in patients with schizophrenia. However, more work is needed to evaluate the effects of different types of control groups on cognitive performance in schizophrenia and to identify the common and unique features of active control programs and cognitive remediation programs, based on theories of how each program works.

IMPLICATIONS

One potential implication of these findings is that while neurocognitive deficits and negative symptoms of schizophrenia place large restrictions on patients social and daily work life; any type of sustained, goal-directed cognitive activity in the presence of supportive clinicians, regardless of its content, has the potential to improve neuropsychological function significantly in this patient population. Consistent with this viewpoint, a small but growing number of studies suggest that structured behavioural rehabilitation improves neurocognitive skills in patients with schizophrenia in the absence of any specific cognitive training (Spaulding et al., 1999; Spaulding, Reed, Sullivan, Richardson, & Weiler, 1999; Silverstein & Wilkness, 2004). This possibility also emphasizes the significance of reports showing an advantage of cognitive remediation for a variety of outcome measures, even when cognitive remediation interventions are compared with control interventions that involve considerable non-specific stimulation such as work therapy or supported employment programs (Bell, Bryson, Greig, Corcoran, & Wexler, 2001; McGurk, Mueser, & Pascaris, 2005).

GENERALIZATION

An important issue is the generalizability of the improvement. Literature suggests that performance on the training task can often be improved (Green, Satz, Ganzell, & Vaclav, 1992) but it is doubtful whether these effects generalize meaningfully (Bellack, Blanchard, Murphy, & Podell, 1996). Findings of the previous study discussed (Halder, 2011) suggests that improvement in cognitive function also has effects on social, and daily functions, but overall improvement is not maintained. It also indicates that longer duration of intervention program may lead to more sustained and generalized effect.

Among few methodologically adequate studies, like Wykes, Reeder, Corner, Williams and Everitt (1999); Medalia, Revheim, and Casey (2000; 2001) have investigated the effects of an intensive cognitive rehabilitation programme. The intervention was targeted at deficits of executive functions, based on procedural learning and the principles of errorless learning, targeted reinforcement and massed practice. It consisted of individual daily sessions of 1 hour for up to 3 months. The control therapy was occupational therapy, matched for length of treatment and therapist contact. Seventeen patients received the cognitive treatment and 16 received occupational therapy. Some improvement in cognition followed both therapies, but the cognitive intervention was superior to the occupational therapy with regard to tests of cognitive flexibility and memory. There were no systematic changes in symptoms or social functioning in either group, with one exception: patients in the cognitive treatment showed a significant increase in self-esteem. The study by Medalia et al. (2000, 2001) applied computer-aided training programmes to remediate memory and problem-solving deficits. The subjects failed to apply the mnemonic strategies that they learned successfully within training tasks to other general measures of memory and learning. In contrast, the problem-solving group showed a significant improvement on the outcome measure that assessed problem-solving skills required for independent living, an effect that was not present in the other two groups. The authors concluded that patients with schizophrenia are responsive to problem-solving training techniques.

Reviewing the available set of studies, it is clear that some measures of executive function, attention, and memory can be remediated with extra instructions, repeated practice, or reinforcement or both, but not conclusive about social, daily functions and other areas of disability. Recent researches are targeting those areas of neuropsychological deficit that are particularly responsible for the profound social dysfunction evident in schizophrenia. Different neuropsychological deficits may not contribute to social dysfunction equally. There has been increasing attention to the relationship between specific neuropsychological dysfunction and community outcomes, social problem solving and social skills acquisition over the past several years (Green, 1996).

CONCLUSION

Patients with chronic schizophrenia are impaired in a range of neurocognitive domain, and this is evident in terms of both statistical and clinical significance. The neurocognitive deficits can be improved by continuous cognitive training, along with psychoeducation. There is also strong relation between cognitive functioning and clinical symptoms and social outcome, and that too improve with cognitive intervention program. There is a need of proper standard cognitive remediation package, which should be rich in methods but may not be computerized. Focus on functional deficits is a much neglected area in which further research is urgently needed and cognitive remediation in schizophrenia should be aimed at improving not just specific cognitive deficits, but also the functional deficits that arise from them.

The overall impression of this chapter confirm the notion and suggests that individuals with schizophrenia have cognitive deficit and can learn and perform the skills with proper intervention. The skills taught in remediation programme can be retained without substantial degradation over a considerable period of time, showing the effectiveness of the comprehensive cognitive remediation program along with psychoeducation. The intervention programme also indicated in improvement of clinical symptoms and social functioning of chronic schizophrenia patients. The cognitive remediation programme discussed in the chapter included only three major areas: *attention, memory and executive functions.* Future remediation programmes may be drafted targeting the overall neuropsychological functioning in a comprehensive way. Along with neuropsychological functions, more stress may be put on social and vocational functioning and a combined rehabilitation package should be made in future. A proper, detail manual of cognitive remediation program can be made. The package for cognitive remediation can be standardized in different population and the duration of the remediation programme can be increased.

REFERENCES

Addington, J., & Addington, D. (2000). Neurocognitive and social functioning in schizophrenia: A 2.5 year follow-up study. *Schizophrenia Research*, *44*(1), 47–56. doi:10.1016/S0920-9964(99)00160-7 PMID:10867311

Bell, M., Bryson, G., Greig, T., Corcoran, C., & Wexler, B. E. (2001). Neurocognitive enhancement therapy with work therapy: Effects on neuropsychological test performance. *Archives of General Psychiatry*, *58*(8), 763–768. doi:10.1001/archpsyc.58.8.763 PMID:11483142

Bellack, A. S., Blanchard, J. J., Murphy, P., & Podell, K. (1996). Generalization effects of training on the Wisconsin Card Sorting Test for schizophrenia patients. *Schizophrenia Research*, *19*(2-3), 189–194. doi:10.1016/0920-9964(95)00067-4 PMID:8789917

Ben-Yishay, U., & Diller, L. (1981). Cognitive deficits. In M. Rosenthal (Ed.), *Rehabilitation of the Head Injured Adult*. Philadelphia: F.A. Davis.

Bergman, H. F., Cervenka, S., Flyckt, L., Edman, G., & Farde, L. (2014). Meta-analysis of cognitive performance in drug-naïve patients with schizophrenia. *Schizophrenia Research*, *158*(1-3), 156–162. doi:10.1016/j.schres.2014.06.034 PMID:25086658

Best, D. (1992). The role of social interaction in memory improvement. In D. Herrmann, H. Weingartner, A. Searleman, & C. McEvoy (Eds.), *Memory improvement: Implications for memory theory*. New York: Springer-Verlag. doi:10.1007/978-1-4612-2760-1_8

Bleuler, E. (1950). *Dementia Praecox or The Group of Schizophrenias (Tranl. by Zinkin)*. New York, NY: International Universities Press. (Original work published 1911)

Bowie, C. R., & Harvey, P. D. (2005). Cognition in Schizophrenia: Impairments, Determinants, and Functional Importance. *The Psychiatric Clinics of North America*, *28*(3), 613–633. doi:10.1016/j.psc.2005.05.004 PMID:16122570

Bracy, O. L. (1986). Cognitive rehabilitation: A process approach. *Cognitive Rehabilitation*, *4*, 10–17.

Carter, C. S., & Barch, D. M. (2000). Attention, memory and language disturbances in schizophrenia: Characteristics and implications. In Advances in psychiatry (pp. 45–72). Oxford University Press.

Chen, E. Y. H., & McKenna, P. J. (1996) Memory dysfunction in schizophrenia. In Schizophrenia: A Neuropsychological Perspective (pp. 107-124). New York, NY: John Wiley and Sons.

Elovic, E. (2000). Use of Provigil for under arousal following TBI. *The Journal of Head Trauma Rehabilitation*, *15*(4), 1068–1071. doi:10.1097/00001199-200008000-00009 PMID:10876176

Gianutsos, R. (1980). What is cognitive rehabilitation? *Journal of Rehabilitation*, 36-40.

Gold, J. M., Carpenter, C., Randolph, C., Goldberg, T. E., & Weinberger, D. R. (1997). Auditory working memory and Wisconsin Card Sorting Test performance in schizophrenia. *Archives of General Psychiatry*, *54*(2), 159–165. doi:10.1001/archpsyc.1997.01830140071013 PMID:9040284

Goldman, C. R., & Quinn, F. L. (1988). Effects of a patient education programme in the treatment of schizophrenia. *Hospital & Community Psychiatry*, *39*, 282–286. PMID:3356434

Goldman, R. S., Axelrod, B. N., & Taylor, S. F. (1996). Neuropsychological aspects of schizophrenia. In I. Grant & K. M. Adams (Eds.), *Neuropsychological assessment of neuropsychiatric disorders*. New York: Oxford University press.

Gourovitch, M. L., & Goldberg, T. E. (1996). Cognitive deficits in schizophrenia: Attention, executive functions, memory and language processing. In Schizophrenia: A Neuropsychological Perspective (pp. 72-86). New York, NY: John Wiley and Sons.

Green, M. F. (1996). What are the functional consequences of neurocognitive deficits in schizophrenia? *The American Journal of Psychiatry*, *153*(3), 321–330. doi:10.1176/ajp.153.3.321 PMID:8610818

Green, M. F., Satz, P., Ganzell, S., & Vaclav, J. F. (1992). Wisconsin Card Sorting Test performance in schizophrenia: Remediation of a stubborn deficit. *The American Journal of Psychiatry*, *149*(1), 62–67. doi:10.1176/ajp.149.1.62 PMID:1728187

Halder, S. (2011). *Efficacy of Cognitive Remediation of Neuropsychological Deficits in Patients with Chronic Schizophrenia*. (Unpublished Doctoral thesis). Ranchi Institute of Neuropsychiatry & Allied Sciences, Ranchi University, Ranchi, India.

Harvey, P. D., & Keefe, R. S. E. (1997). Cognitive impairment in schizophrenia and implications of atypical neuroleptic treatment. *CNS Spectrums*, *2*, 1–11.

Heinrichs, R. W., & Zakzanis, K. K. (1998). Neurocognitive deficit in schizophrenia: A quantitative review of the evidence. *Neuropsychology*, *12*(3), 426–445. doi:10.1037/0894-4105.12.3.426 PMID:9673998

Herrmann, D., & Parente, R. (1994). The multi-modal approach to cognitive rehabilitation. *NeuroRehabilitation*, *4*, 133–142. PMID:24525361

Herrmann, D., & Petro, S. (1991). Commercial memory aids. *Applied Cognitive Psychology*, *4*(6), 439–450. doi:10.1002/acp.2350040603

Herrmann, D., Plude, D., Yoder, C., & Mullin, P. (1999). Cognitive processing and extrinsic psychological systems: A holistic model of cognition. *Zeitschrift fur Psychologie mit Zeitschrift fur Angewandte Psychologie*, *207*, 123–147.

Hoff, A. L., Sakuma, M., Wieneke, M., Horon, R., Kushner, M., & DeLisi, L. E. (1999). Longitudinal neuropsychological follow-up study of patients with first-episode schizophrenia. *The American Journal of Psychiatry*, *156*, 1336–1341. PMID:10484942

Keefe, R. S. E., & Harvey, P. D. (2012). Cognitive Impairment in Schizophrenia. In N. A. Treatments (Ed.), Handbook of Experimental Pharmacology: Vol. 213. Springer-Verlag Berlin Heidelberg.

Kraepelin, E. (1919/1971). Dementia Praecox and Paraphrenia. R.E. Krieger.

Kurtz, M. M. (2003). Neurocognitive rehabilitation for schizophrenia. *Current Psychiatry Reports*, *5*(4), 303–310. doi:10.1007/s11920-003-0060-y PMID:12857534

Luria, A. R. (1973). *The Working Brain*. New York: Basic Books.

McEvoy, C. (1992). Memory improvement in context: Implications for the development of memory improvement theory. In Memory improvement: Implications for memory theory (pp. 210-230). New York: Springer-Verlag.

McEvoy, C. L., & Moon, J. R. (1988). Assessment and treatment of everyday memory problems in the elderly. In Practical aspects of memory: Current research and issues. Vol 2: Clinical and educational implications. (pp. 155-160). Chichester, UK: Wiley

McGurk, S. R., Mueser, K. T., & Pascaris, A. (2005). Cognitive training and supported employment for persons with severe mental illness: One-year results from a randomized controlled trial. *Schizophrenia Bulletin*, *31*(4), 898–909. doi:10.1093/schbul/sbi037 PMID:16079391

Medalia, A., Revheim, N., & Casey, M. (2000). Remediation of memory disorders in schizophrenia. *Psychological Medicine*, *30*(6), 1451–1459. doi:10.1017/S0033291799002913 PMID:11097085

Medalia, A., Revheim, N., & Casey, M. (2001). The remediation of problem-solving skills in schizophrenia. *Schizophrenia Bulletin*, *27*(2), 259–267. doi:10.1093/oxfordjournals.schbul.a006872 PMID:11354593

Mohamed, S., Paulsen, J. S., O'Leary, D., Arndt, S., & Andreasen, N. (1999). Generalized cognitive deficits in schizophrenia: A study of firstepisode patients. *Archives of General Psychiatry*, *56*(8), 749–754. doi:10.1001/archpsyc.56.8.749 PMID:10435610

Morey, L. C. (1991). Classification of mental disorder as a collection of hypothetical constructs. *Journal of Abnormal Psychology*, *100*(3), 289–293. doi:10.1037/0021-843X.100.3.289 PMID:1918606

Naugle, R., Prevy, M., Naugle, C., & Delaney, R. (1988). The new digital watch as a compensatory device for memory dysfunction. *Cognitive Rehabilitation*, *6*, 22–23.

Norman, R. M., Malla, A. K., Morrison, S. S. L., Helmes, E., Williamson, P. C., Thomas, J., & Cortese, L. (1997). Neuropsychological correlates of syndromes in schizophrenia. *The British Journal of Psychiatry*, *170*(2), 134–139. doi:10.1192/bjp.170.2.134 PMID:9093501

Olfson, M., Mechanic, D., Hansell, S., Boyer, C. A., Walkup, J., & Weiden, P. J. (2000). Predicting medication noncompliance after hospital discharge among patients with schizophrenia. *Psychiatric Services (Washington, D.C.)*, *51*(2), 216–222. doi:10.1176/appi.ps.51.2.216 PMID:10655006

Paulsen, J. S., Heaton, R. K., Sadek, J. R., Perry, W., Delis, D. C., Braff, D., & Jeste, D. V. et al. (1995). The nature of learning and memory impairments in schizophrenia. *Journal of the International Neuropsychological Society*, *1*(01), 88–99. doi:10.1017/S135561770000014X PMID:9375213

Richardson, J. T. E. (1992). Imagery, mnemonics, and memory remediation. *Neurology*, *42*(2), 283–286. doi:10.1212/WNL.42.2.283 PMID:1736154

Robbins, T. W. (1990). The case for frontostriatal dysfunction in schizophrenia. *Schizophrenia Bulletin*, *16*(3), 391–402. doi:10.1093/schbul/16.3.391 PMID:2287930

Saykin, A. J., Gur, R. E., Gur, R. C., & Mozley, P. D. (1991). Neuropsychological function in schizophrenia: Selective impairment in memory and learning. *Archives of General Psychiatry*, *48*(7), 618–622. doi:10.1001/archpsyc.1991.01810310036007 PMID:2069492

Saykin, A. J., Shtasel, D. L., Gur, R. E., Kester, D. B., Mozley, L. H., Stafiniak, P., & Gur, R. C. (1994). Neuropsychological deficits in neuroleptic naïve patients with first- episode schizophrenia. *Archives of General Psychiatry*, *51*(2), 124–131. doi:10.1001/archpsyc.1994.03950020048005 PMID:7905258

Schacter, D. L., & Glisky, E. L. (1986). Memory remediation: Restoration, alleviation, and the acquisition of domain-specific knowledge. In B. Uzzell & Y. Gross (Eds.), Clinical neuropsychology of intervention (pp. 257-282). Boston: Martinus Nijhoff.

Shakow, D. (1962). Segmental set: A theory of the formal psychological deficit in schizophrenia. *Archives of General Psychiatry*, *6*(1), 1–17. doi:10.1001/archpsyc.1962.01710190003001 PMID:13911157

Silverstein, S. M., & Wilkniss, S. M. (2004). At issue: The future of cognitive rehabilitation of schizophrenia. *Schizophrenia Bulletin*, *30*(4), 679–692. doi:10.1093/oxfordjournals.schbul.a007122 PMID:15954183

Sohlberg, M. M., & Mateer, C. A. (1987). Effectiveness of an attention-training program. *Journal of Clinical and Experimental Neuropsychology*, *9*(2), 117–130. doi:10.1080/01688638708405352 PMID:3558744

Spaulding, W. D., Fleming, S. K., Reed, D., Sullivan, M., Storzbach, D., & Lam, M. (1999). Cognitive functioning in schizophrenia: Implications for psychiatric rehabilitation. *Schizophrenia Bulletin*, *25*(2), 275–289. doi:10.1093/oxfordjournals.schbul.a033378 PMID:10416731

Spaulding, W. D., Reed, D., Sullivan, M., Richardson, C., & Weiler, M. (1999). Effects of cognitive treatment in psychiatric rehabilitation. *Schizophrenia Bulletin*, *25*(4), 657–676. doi:10.1093/oxfordjournals.schbul.a033409 PMID:10667738

Tamlyn, D., McKenna, P. J., Mortimer, A. M., Lund, C. E., Hammond, S., & Baddeley, A. D. (1992). Memory impairment in schizophrenia: Its extent, affiliations, and neuropsychological character. *Psychological Medicine*, *22*(01), 101–115. doi:10.1017/S0033291700032773 PMID:1349439

Wong, S. E. (2014). A Critique of the Diagnostic Construct Schizophrenia. *Research on Social Work Practice*, *24*(1), 132–141. doi:10.1177/1049731513505152

Wykes, T., Reeder, C., Corner, J., Williams, C., & Everitt, B. (1999). The effects of neurocognitive remediation on executive processing in patients with schizophrenia. *Schizophrenia Bulletin*, *25*(2), 291–307. doi:10.1093/oxfordjournals.schbul.a033379 PMID:10416732

Wykes, T., Reeder, C., Landau, S., Everitt, B., Knapp, M., Patel, A., & Romeo, R. (2007). Cognitive remediation therapy in schizophrenia Randomised controlled trial. *The British Journal of Psychiatry*, *190*(5), 421–427. doi:10.1192/bjp.bp.106.026575 PMID:17470957

Yesavage, J. A., Rose, T. L., & Spiegel, D. (1982). Relaxation training and memory improvement in elderly normals: Correlations of anxiety rating and recall improvement. *Experimental Aging Research*, *8*(4), 1982. doi:10.1080/03610738208260365 PMID:6762966

KEY TERMS AND DEFINITIONS

Cognitive Remediation: A behavioural training based rehabilitation treatment, focussing to improve attention, memory, language and executive functions in persons having these impairments.

Neurocognitive Impairment: The impairment of cognitive functions of a person following a neurological illness, mental illness, drug use or brain injury. Most common cognitive domains are attention, memory and executive functions.

Schizophrenia: Schizophrenia is a psychiatric illness characterized by abnormalities in thought, perception, language and speech. The symptoms are manifested variably in combination of hallucinations, delusions, impaired reality contact and abnormal behaviour.

Chapter 17
Efficacy of Art Therapy in Treating Patients with Paranoid Schizophrenia

Deepali Bedi
Sukoon Psychotherapy Center, India

ABSTRACT

Paranoid Schizophrenia chronic mental illnesses according to DSM-IVTR characterized by the presence of delusion of persecution, suspicious, distrusting, guarded, reserved, tensed, and also sometimes hostile or aggressive. Patients also perceive exaggerated warmth and friendship by the professionals as attempt at bribery, manipulation or exploitation. But therapeutic relationship between patient and the professional is integral to the recovery process and the outcome. Good communication on the part of health care professionals is an essential element in developing the strong practitioner-patient relationship necessary in the treatment of schizophrenia. Professionals are usually at a look out for tools to build a working alliance best used in such cases. Usually behavioural therapy, supportive therapy and family therapy are used for such patients. But sometimes with chronic and resistant client will get stuck at the initial rapport itself. At this stage probably art therapy as an advance intervention strategy to work with patient as an advanced intervention strategies and treatment.

INTRODUCTION

Art therapy is based on the idea that the creative process of art making is healing and life enhancing and is a form of nonverbal communication of thoughts and feelings (Malchiodi, 1996). Like other forms of psychotherapy and counselling, it is used to encourage personal growth, increase self-understanding, and assists in emotional reparation and has been employed in a wide variety of settings with children, adults, families, and groups. It is a modality that can help individuals of all ages create meaning and achieve insight, find relief from overwhelming emotions or trauma, resolve conflicts and problems enrich daily life, and achieve an increased sense of well-being (Malchiodi, 1998). Art therapy supports the belief that all individuals have the capacity to express themselves creatively and that the product is less important

DOI: 10.4018/978-1-5225-0519-8.ch017

than the therapeutic process involved. The therapist's focus is not specifically on the aesthetic merits of art making but on the therapeutic needs of the person to express. With the advent of brief forms of therapy and the increasing pressures to complete treatment in a limited number of sessions, therapists are finding that art activities help individuals to communicate relevant issues and problems quickly, thus expediting assessment and intervention. Even the simplest drawing task offers unique possibilities for expression that complements and, in many cases, helps a child or adult to communicate what words cannot.

APPROACHES TO ART THERAPY

Rubin in his book, Approaches *to Art Therapy* (Rubin, 1987/2001), discussed the diversity of theoretical positions within the field of Art therapy.

Psychodynamic Approaches

The ideas of Freud and his followers have been part of art therapy since the earliest days, although contemporary writers are more likely to apply terms such as "transference" and "the defense mechanisms" to articulate a position rather than employ classic psychoanalytic techniques with any degree of orthodoxy. Kramer, Rubin, Ulman, and Wilson (all cited in Rubin, 1987/2001) and Levick (1983) all use psychoanalytic language and concepts. Interpretations of the newer developments in psychoanalysis such as the theories of Klein (Weir, 1987), self-psychology (Lachman-Chapin) and object relations theory (Robbins) can also be found in the art therapy literature (both cited in Rubin, 1987/2001). With his emphasis on images from the unconscious, it was natural for Jung's concepts of analytical and archetypal psychology to cross over into art. Work by Edwards and Wallace (both cited in Rubin, 1987/ 2001), Mcconeghey (1986), and Schaverian (1992) all reflect this emphasis.

Humanistic Approaches

Elkins and Stovall (2000) suggest that only a small number of art therapists operate from a humanistic position (among humanistic, Gestalt, existential, and client centered; the highest response was to the first category with 2.9%). Yet if these approaches can be defined as sharing "an optimistic view of human nature and of the human condition, seeing people in a process of growth and development, with the potential to take responsibility for their fate" (Rubin, 1987/2001), these figures belie a sentiment held by many art therapists. Garai (cited in Rubin, 1987/2001) has written from a general humanistic position, Rogers (1993) and Silverstone (1997) use a person-centered model, and Dreikurs (1986) and Garlock (cited in Rubin, 1987) have adapted ideas first articulated by Alfred Adler. Other models that fall under the humanistic heading include existential (Moon, 1990/1995), phenomenological (Betensky, 1995), and gestalt (Rhyne, 1973/1995) approaches.

Learning and Developmental Approaches

Perhaps because they are perceived to be mechanistic, those psychological theories that emphasize learning tend to be less popular with art therapists. In the Elkins and Stovall (2000) survey, cognitive-behavioural, cognitive, developmental, and behavioural received an endorsement of over 2%. Yet there are art therapy authors whose work has been informed by these theories.

Silver (2000) has written extensively on assessment using a cognitive approach, and the work of Lusebrink (1990) and Nucho (1987) is based in general systems theory. Art therapists working with children with emotional and developmental disabilities have also adapted concepts from developmental (Roth, cited in Rubin, 1987/2001).

Family Therapy and Other Approaches

A number of writers (Landgarten, 1987; Linesch, 1993; Riley & Malchiodi, 1994; Sobol, 1982) have built on Kwiatkowska's early family work, particularly in California where art therapists become licensed as marriage and family therapists. Riley (1999) also incorporates concepts from narrative therapy into her work. Relational (Dalley, Rifkind, & Terry, 1993) and feminist (Hogan, 1997) approaches question the hierarchy in the client/therapist relationship and empowering the client and have also shaped contemporary art therapy practice. Publications by Horovitz-Darby (1994), Farrelly-Hansen (2001), and Mcniff (1992) reflect an emphasis on spiritual and philosophical concepts over psychological theory. Franklin, Farrelly-Hansen, Marek, Swan-Foster, and Wallingford (2000) describe a transpersonal approach to art therapy. Allen (1992) called for a reversal of the perceived trend in overemphasizing the clinical orientation and encouraged art therapists to refocus on their artist identity. Writings by Lachman-Chapin (1983) and Knill (1995), who espouses an expressive arts therapies approach (Moon, 2002) reflect this studio approach to theory and practice.

Clinical Implication of Art Therapy

Art expression has been extensively used in therapy with children for several reasons. It is a natural language for most children and can be a valuable modality in enhancing expression of trauma, distress, or loss (Malchiodi, 1997, 1998). Also, children do not have the verbal capacity to articulate crisis and for those who have been violated or abused, art is a way to communicate feelings and experiences without words. Gross and Haynes (1998) hypothesized that there may be several reasons why art expressions are helpful adjuncts in child therapy:

1. They may reduce anxiety and help children feel more comfortable with the therapist.
2. They may increase memory retrieval.
3. They may help children organize their narratives.
4. They may prompt children to tell more than they would during a solely verbal interview.

Mental health workers may refrain from using art in counselling adults because many adults feel inadequate about their skills or embarrassed over expressing themselves artistically (Gladding, 1998). Nevertheless, there are many documented benefits of employing art as a part of a treatment plan with adult clients including:

1. Taps the unconscious and helps individuals express covert conflicts, bringing into awareness thoughts and feelings that were previously hidden (Liebmann, 1990).
2. Acts as a metaphor for the conflicts, emotions, and situations experienced by clients (Ulak & Cummings, 1997).

3. Assists people in picturing themselves or their situations in a concrete, objectified manner (Rubin, 2001).
4. Acts as a bridge between the counsellor and the client, especially when the subject matter is too embarrassing or difficult to talk about, such as family violence, illicit relationship and abuse (Brooke, 1995; Liebmann, 1990; Trowbridge, 1995).
5. Creates a visible trail, provides a tangible record, and allows clients and counsellors to review a series of past sessions and note development and change (Ganim, 2000; Liebmann, 1990).
6. Inspires and helps people become more connected with the transcendent and growth sides of their personalities (Mills & Crowley, 1986).
7. Provides a process that is energy enhancing (Kahn, 1999); art gets clients "doing" rather than thinking and therefore can be more activating than verbal counselling (France & Allen, 1997).
8. Can easily be combined with other expressive arts such as music, movement, creative writing, and imagery (McNiff, 1997).
9. The case mentioned here very well illustrates most of the benefits of using Art therapy with the client.

Psychoanalytic theories postulated that various symptoms of Schizophrenia have symbolic meaning for individual patient (Sadock & Sadock, 2003). Freud (1920) said that the symptom carries a meaning and is connected with the experience of the patient. According to Jones (1916), 'only what is repressed is symbolised; only what is repressed needs to be symbolised'. Grunbaum (1986) reminded that 'symptoms, as compromise formations, have traditionally been viewed as "symbols", but they are "symbols" in the no semantic sense of being substitutive formations affording replacement satisfactions or outlets, not linguistic representatives of their hypothesized unconscious causes'

The following case of a client who is married and denies her actually identity is because of her unconscious desire to be the wife of the boy she ones loved. In the reality her desire is unacceptable and illicit so her illness gives expression to her illicit desire.

In her art work she drew hearts and flowers on a same stem depicted her conflict. She wants to be a wife of the boy she loved but current a mother of beautiful children who she also loves. There was a huge social taboo to her desire but she could express this much easily with minimum anxiety through art work.

A house without an entry metaphorically depicted her delusive world which no one could entry. It was also about her anger of being unable to meet her loved ones in her ward.

Drawing of umbrella depicted the metaphor of longing for the love and protection of her father.

Thus clinically Art therapy is a very useful modality even with adults specially where the client if not able to verbally express their conflicts due to various reasons.

Art Therapy with Client Having Paranoid Schizophrenia

A patient with paranoid schizophrenia is mainly characterized by the presence of delusion of persecution i.e. a false, firm and fixed believe or a suspicion that people would harm him or her. The said patients are suspicious, distrusting, guarded, reserved, tensed, and also sometimes hostile or aggressive (Sadock & Sadock, 2003). The patient is likely to perceive exaggerated warmth and friendship by the professionals as attempt at bribery, manipulation or exploitation. On the other hand, we know therapeutic relationship between patient and the professional is integral to the recovery process and the outcome of the illness (Ivezic, Ljubimir, & Urlic, 2001) which is also true for treating patients with Schizophrenia (Burns et al., 1999; Eisen, Dickey, & Sederer, 2000). This challenge of building a strong therapeutic alliance with the patient without it being perceived as manipulation or exploitation makes the situation tricky. So there is a constant need for multiple tools which can help a professional in communicating with the patient without making them hostile or defensive.

In the cases presented below, the team of mental health professionals had a similar challenge with the patient diagnosed with Paranoid Schizophrenia. The Psychiatrist tried various combinations of antipsychotics drugs with no change in the symptoms of the patient. During this phase she refused any interaction with any other professional and also denied attending any group activity sessions as she felt she was normal and unnecessarily forced to stay away from her family and the boy she loved. In reality she was talking of her parental family and the boy was actually a relative whom she liked before her marriage. She had denied recognizing her husband, children or any one from his family. At this stage where every other method of communicating with the patient seemed fruitless, a new clinical psychologist was assigned who got a break though with the patient using art therapy.

CASE STUDY

Mrs. H who is a 34 years old house wife, was brought to the clinic by her husband and family. The husband chief complaint was that she talks irrelevant about his illicit relationship with others including his sister. Since six months she is very irritable and use abusive language. There had been frequent incidents of unprovoked aggression. But the situation got worse just six days before this visit, when she left her home and was found wandering near the railway tracks in the absence of her husband. She was brought back home from there. Thereafter she stopped recognizing her husband and children and said she was not married.

To understand the current situation better let's know our Patient, Mrs. H right from her birth. She was born to a low middle class family in a small town in the north. She was the youngest of the five siblings. She had three sisters and one brother. As a child she was very emotional and had limited friends. Like many other girls of her age in her town, she used to be actively involved in house hold chores after returning from school or college. She lost her father in a rail accident when she was 14 years and in the 9th standard. The patient was very attached to her father, thus the event was a traumatic experience for her. Soon she lost companionship of her sister with the latter's love marriage after two years. This marriage led to her first episode of the illness. She would be irritable and would talk of illicit relationships of various people. This had to be treated. She was given electro convulsive therapy (ECT) and medication for the same which lead to remission.

In 1997, she completed her graduation and soon after that, she got married. The marriage was performed against her will as she was interested in a boy known to the family, whom she would have seen at her sister's marriage. Within few days of marriage she had a psychotic breakdown. She again was observed as irritable, used to physically hit people, throw things, smile while she was sitting alone and would eat excessively. She would also blame her husband of illicit affairs. Due to such behavior with in the short duration of her marriage, she was brought back to her parental home and psychiatric treatment was sought. During the same duration, she started calling herself as "Laxmi," who is in love with another boy and is waiting to get married to him. With medication and ECT, her condition improved and there was partial remission after one and a half year of illness. She started helping her brother actively in his shop. However, during her phase of partial remission, symptoms like having doubts on her husband's intentions and having frequent fights with him subsequently continued which led to her divorce in 2007. In the same year she got re-married to a man who was 10 years elder to her and had a son aged 17 from his previous marriage. Since the very initial days of marriage, her husband noticed that she would not trust him and would doubt his intentions and would also blame him for being involved with any female who was around him. In 2008, she gave birth to a baby girl. In April 2012, she aborted her second pregnancy as the fetus was a girl child. After which she started talking irrelevantly about her husband's affair with his sister and would get irritable blaming him of the same. She would also use abusive language. Most of the time, she was observed sitting alone with reduction in her interaction with people. Around, she held the neck of the servant and slapped her without any provocation. Thereafter, six days back, she left home and was found by the police walking on the railway track when her husband was not at home. She could not recall how and when she reached there but gave details of her husband and family to inform them about her wellbeing. Since last four days, she claimed that she is "Laxmi" who has never been married. She is also denying recognizing her parents as her own and identifying her cousin brother as her real brother. During this period she also stopped taking care of her daughter and her step son.

Case Formulation by Using Psychodynamic Approach

Based on the attachment theory client's psychosis can be understood to be triggered by the loss of secured base with the death of the father which made the client insecure. The other boy she saw at her sister's marriage came as a loved object but under family pressure got married to another man this making her ambivalent towards the husband. To understand it further let's understands the attachment theory.

Attachment theory (Bowlby, 1969) has been used as a theoretical base for psychotherapy for many years but has more recently become a major focus of neuroscience and renewed interest among therapists. Siegel (1999) explains attachment as follows: "Attachment is an inborn system in the brain that evolves in ways that influence and organize motivational, emotional, and memory processes with respect to significant care giving figures" (p. 67). Schore (1994) offers a neurological model for the importance of infant attachment throughout life. He notes that soon after birth the caretaker and infant develop interactions that are important to the process of affect regulation. Face-to-face contact and soothing touch are examples of ways the infant learns to respond to stimulation from people and experiences. Perry, Pollard, Blakley, Baker, and Vigilante (1995) propose that successful attachment is critical to optimal development of specific parts of the brain. He believes that a healthy attachment between infant and caretaker sets the stage for the individual to develop the capacity to "self-regulate" stimulating experiences. Early childhood bonding is imprinted on the brain, laying a foundation for relationship patterns later in life; when trauma is present; brain imprinting is changed, but may be corrected with appropriate intervention.

Research in neuroscience is demonstrating that infancy is not the only chance a person has for healthy attachment and there seem to be ways to reshape and repair some early experiences. Art therapy is one way being explored to re-establish healthy attachments, both through therapist and client, and through encouraging healthy interactions between parent and child. Riley (2001) cites how art activities are being used in early childhood attachment programs and how simple drawing exercises can be used to resolve relational problems and strengthen parent–child bonds. She explains that the nonverbal dimensions of art activities tap early relational states before words are dominant, possibly allowing the brain to establish new, and more productive patterns.

Siegel (1999) and Schore (1994) believe that interactions between baby and caretaker are right-brain mediated because during infancy the right cortex is developing more quickly than the left. Siegel also observes that just as the left hemisphere requires exposure to language to grow, the right hemisphere requires emotional stimulation to develop properly. He goes on to say that the output of the right brain is expressed in "non-word-based ways" such as drawing a picture or using a picture to describe feelings or events. According to this idea, art therapy may be an important modality in working with attachment issues, among other emotionally related disorders or experiences).

TREATMENT AND THERAPY

She was given a diagnosis of episodic paranoid schizophrenia with marital discord and she was put on anti-psychotic drugs. She was also admitted in the psychiatric setup for close monitoring of drugs and intervention. There she denied participate in any group activity organized for the patients. Any intervention of any sort was not acceptable and she would keep sleeping in her room with minimal required communication with the staff. She only wanted to go back to her house, her parental house. As every other tool had failed to build a strong therapeutic alliance with the patient, a therapist was given this case, hoped that some innovation and creativity by her might work miracle with the patient.

The new assigned clinical psychologist wanted to use 'Art therapy' because she believed that being a non-directive method it will subtly allow the patient to symbolically reveal the inner conflicts without the fear of disclosure. As Susan Hogan and Annette M. Coulter (2014) said- 'Being revealed can be both cathartic and empowering for the patient.' Indeed, it is believed that even without direct interpretation of art in therapy it can be of great use with a patient with paranoid schizophrenia. Art therapy allows exploration of the patient's inner world in a non-threatening way through a therapeutic relationship and the use of art materials. Indeed, if we look at the history of Art therapy for treatment of schizophrenia has developed its initial stages within Pennsylvania's Western Psychiatric Institute and Clinic with the utmost of success. It was developed in adult psychiatric inpatient units and was designed for use with people for whom verbal psychotherapy would be impossible. Helping people communicate what they are unable to think and feel on a normal level is the ultimate goal of art therapy. Robyn Cruz, director of creative and expressive arts therapies has talked about the success of art therapy program for outpatients with schizophrenia. The reason that art therapy for treatment of schizophrenia is successful is because art therapy is a safe and effective tool to use with people who cannot share their thoughts and feelings adequately through the tried-and-true traditional methods of "talk therapy" conversation. Through art therapy, those with schizophrenia can develop ways to achieve self-expression while simultaneously being able to utilize social skills, new hobbies and personal interests through their creativity. Alison Cobb from the mental health charity mind said, "Art therapy is non-threatening and accessible therapies that can help people express their feelings without the need to talk them over." Thus art therapy with family therapy can be used successfully with eclectic components of other therapeutic approach also.

Being sure about the success of art therapy with such resistant patients of Schizophrenia she was allowed to work with the patient.

The first session with her was in her personal ward in the Psychiatric setup as she denied coming out for any activity or therapy. But this too started only with rejection from her. As she was drowsy with medicine she said she wants to sleep and turned towards the wall ignoring the psychologist's presence and went to sleep. She was found to be unkempt, disoriented and guarded.

Not losing any hope the psychologist went to her room the next day too. On being asked how she was, she again displayed the frustration of being held up in the hospital setup for no visible reason. Even that day too she was feeling drowsy with medicine. Thus, even on the day two nothing could be done with her but then psychologist plan to stay in her room in silence for the complete one hour.

On the visit by the psychologist on day three, she looked better and little receptive of the psychologist. She did complain about being refrained in the hospital with none of the family members with her. She added that her brother (actually her cousin brother who she identifies as her own bother) was not even informed that she is in hospital. MMSE was done on her, which proved she had started reciprocating to the medicine and thus was oriented to time and the place, her recent memory was intact but there was difficulty in recall. The insight into the illness was at Grade 1. She was not ready for any further intervention for the day.

Day four was very similar to day 3 where she was again complaining about being refrained in the hospital with none of the family members, including her brother around. Her insight was still at Grade 1 level.

For facilitating further intervention her family was called to visit her. Her brother knew much about the illness but the husband was ignorant so he psycho-educated about the illness. Besides his initial ignorance, he was very cooperative, and this made things easier. They were allowed to meet the patient with clear instructions not to challenge her delusions till we work through them therapeutically. The husband due to his business could not stay back to actively be part of the therapeutic process any further.

In the next session with the patient, as per the protocol of the clinical institution Sentence Completion Test (SCT) was done on the patient but the patient was not forced to fill all the columns. Expecting early discharge from the hospital she was trying to be very cooperative with the testing. Although she left lot of column unfilled saying she has nothing more to say.

On the analysis of the SCT, the principal conflict areas identified were her relationship with her father, interpersonal relationships with others and fear of her treatment and being alone. The index patient fear loss of her father whom she had already lost in 1993. She feels that people can betray her so she should not trust them. She also expressed her fear of being alone at home and fear of being treated with ECT.

Next day she was encouraged to do Rorschach, she was again very cooperative. The results indicated coping perceptual thinking problems. Further, it indicated that the patient has high vulnerability to loss of control and becoming stressed. There were indications which indicated possibility of chronic vulnerability to become disorganized by natural every day stresses of life. The protocol indicated possible history of numerous events of faulty judgment, emotional disruption and behavioral ineffectiveness.

For adequate functionality, she needs to be in an environment which is highly structured, over which she has some sense of control. She seemed to be overwhelmed or flooded by emotions. This flooding of emotions could have impacted on thinking. There is a possibility of her experiencing seemingly random, disconnecting patterns of thinking due to her ungratified needs.

Relationships with others are likely superficial and thus regarded by others as distant, inept and helpless. She generally prefers passive role in a relationship and avoid the responsibility of decision making.

Now after completing the testing as per the protocol of the institute, we next started with free drawing so that she would easily express her inner conflicts in an indirect manner. She was introduced to the idea of drawing and coloring and expressing about her drawing. She drew Drawing No. 1, which has a house and fruits on 1 side and reddish, peacock, fish, flower, grapes and water on the other side. These drawings on both side of the paper could be pictographically representing the two separate worlds which

Figure 1. Depicted by patients eight of her drawings

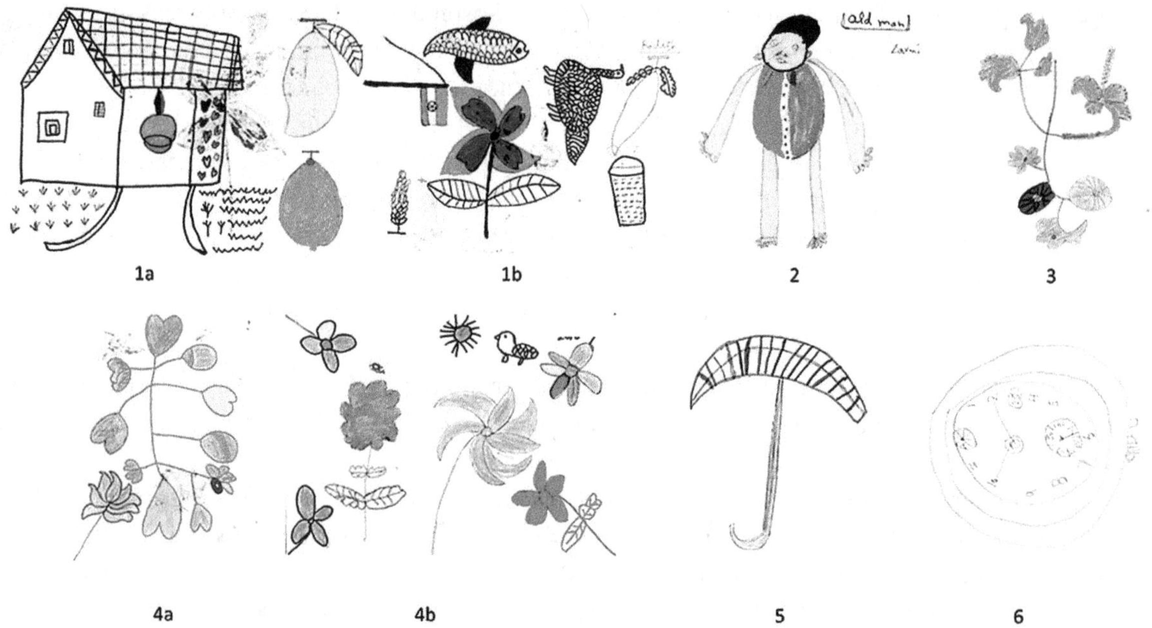

she is experiencing in the in-house setup (see Figure 1). One is the world of her delusion, and other is the world of reality with basic necessary aspects of life. In her delusive world, she is closed in a house with no door to it. With the help of our understanding of drawing of a person with house tree, the analysis of her house showed that she feels she is in a restricted environment and has high sexual fantasy needs which could be the cause of psychotic breakdown.

The receptivity by the therapist about her psychotic delusions and absence of any refutation by the psychologist of her thoughts started bridging the therapeutic alliance between the psychologist and the patient which was visible in the next session. She was in a good mood and she drew a flower stem (Drawing No. 3) and for the first time she wrote her real name on the drawing which was an indication of a big break through. This flower can be interpreted as thanks to the psychologist for welcoming her emotions which would otherwise be seen as illicit and wrong. After her drawing she started talking about her liking for a boy before her marriage and how seeing her love at a common relatives' marriage resurfaced her love for him. She realized about her delusion as part of her illness. She with no hitch expressed her fantasy to have this boy whom she loved as her husband.

Next day was a Sunday, so there was no therapy session as the psychologist was on a holiday.

The following day her drawing had flowers as expression of her various emotions, hearts for the man he loved, ball for her daughter and her desire to connect emotionally to all what her bunch of life has for her. She wanted to connect with her current environment and seek sunshine here. She talked about her fantasy to get married to the young man known to her and thus a conflict of being with an elderly man.

Her mourning couldn't be completed without talking about her loss of her father at that early age. She was intensively attached to her father and he would give her whatever she demanded till his death. She also had a fantasy that had her father been alive he would have married the man of her choice. The next day's drawing was thus an umbrella and she talked elaborately about her father's love, care and protection for her.

On the next day's visit by the psychologist she was asymptomatic of any active symptom. She seemingly didn't want to talk further about her fantasies and past as the realities of the day were very different and she realized the importance of her adjustment to her current situation. She also understood her family condition and lack of funds to work further extensively in therapy. She knew immediate discharge was important which was only possible if she adapts to the current reality and thus that day she drew watch in the newspaper kept in her room.

Being asymptomatic of any active symptom, her family that evening took her back home and the therapy had to be ended there. Although the end of the therapy seemed abrupt as no formal ending was defined but the therapist and the patient both at one level communicated the end in the form of need to live in today.

CONCLUSION

The author says that art therapy even without any formal interpretation during the therapy session communicated a lot of material in the therapy sessions which help the flow of therapy process leading to a successful result. This case is another feather in the hat of an art therapist for its accomplishment with a patient resistant paranoid schizophrenia. This case reassures us that art therapy is a safe, effective and successful tool for the management of schizophrenia with medication and family therapy for a complete biopsychosocial intervention. For sure art therapy is a tool to use with people who cannot share their thoughts and feelings adequately through the tried-and-true traditional methods of "talk therapy" conversation.

REFERENCES

Allen, P. B. (1992). Artist- in –residence: An alternative to "clinification" for art therapist. *Art Therapy: Journal of the American Art Therapy Association*, *9*(1), 22–29. doi:10.1080/07421656.1992.10758933

American Art Therapy Association. (1996). Mission statement. New York: McGraw Hill-NTC.

Betensky, M. G. (1995). *What do you see? Phenomenology of therapeutic art expression*. London: Jessica Kingsley.

Bowlby, J. (1969). *Attachment*. New York: Basic Books.

Brooke, S. L. (1995). Art therapy: An approach to working with sexual abuse survivors. *The Arts in Psychotherapy*, *22*(5), 447–466. doi:10.1016/0197-4556(95)00036-4

Burns, T., Baldwin, D., Emsley, R., Kerwin, R., Steinberg, J., & Van Os, J. (1999). Treatment challenges in schizophrenia. *Primary Care Psychiatry*, *5*(3), 117–123.

Dalley, Rifkind, & Terry. (1993). *Three voices of art therapy: image, client therapist*. London: Routledge.

Dreikurs, S. E. (1986). *Cows can be purple: My life & art therapy*. Chicago: Adler School of Professional Psychology. Dunn, M.B.

Eisen, S. V., Dickey, B., & Sederer, L. I. (2000). A self-report symptom and problem rating scale to increase inpatients' involvement in treatment. *Psychiatric Services (Washington, D.C.)*, *51*(3), 349–353. doi:10.1176/appi.ps.51.3.349 PMID:10686242

Elkins, D. E., & Stovall, K. (2000). American Art Therapy Association, Inc.: 1998–1999 Membership survey report. *Art Therapy: Journal of the American Art Therapy Association*, *17*(1), 41–46. doi:10.1080/07421656.2000.10129431

Farrelly-Hansen, M. (2001). *Spirituality and art therapy: Living the connection*. London: Jessica Kingsley.

France, M. H., & Allen, E. G. (1997). Using art: A gestalt counselling strategy for working with disruptive clients. *Guidance and Counselling*, *12*(4), 24–26.

Franklin, Farrelly-Hansen, & Marek, Swan-Foster, & Wallingford. (2000). Transpersonal art therapy education. *Art Therapy: Journal of the American Art Therapy Association*, 17.

Freud, S. (1920). A General Introduction to Psychoanalysis. New York: Boni and Liveright.

Ganim, B. (2000). *Art and healing: Using expressive art to heal your body, mind, and spirit*. Three Rivers, MI: Three Rivers Press.

Gladding, S. T. (1998). *Counseling as an art: The creative arts in counseling* (2nd ed.). Alexandria, VA: American Counseling Association.

Gross, J., & Haynes, H. (1998). Drawing facilitates children's verbal reports of emotionally laden events. *Journal of Experimental Psychology*, *4*, 163–179.

Grunbaum. (1986). Précis of The Foundations of Psychoanalysis: A Philosophical Critique. *Behavioral and Brain Sciences, 9*(2).

Hogan, S. (1997). *Feminist approach to art therapy*. London: Routledge.

Hogan, S., & Coulter, A. M. (2014). *The Introductory Guide to Art Therapy*. Routledge.

Horovitz-Darby, E. G. (1994). Spiritual art therapy. Springfield, IL: Charlie C. Thomas

Ivezic, S., Ljubimir, V., & Urlic, I. (2001). Therapist-patient relations in treatment of chronic schizophrenic patients. *Medicinski Arhiv*, *55*(1), 39–46. PMID:11795193

Jones, E. (1916). The theory of symbolism. *British Journal of Psychology*, *9*(2), 181–229.

Kahn, B. B. (1999). Art therapy with adolescents: Making it work for school counselors. *Professional School Counseling*, *2*(4), 291–298.

Knill, P. J. (1995). The place of beauty in therapy and the Arts. *The Arts in Psychotherapy*, 22.

Lachman-Chapin, M. (1983). The artist as clinician: An interactive technique in art therapy. *American Journal of Art Therapy*, 23.

Landgarten, H. B. (1987). *Family Art therapy*. New York: Brunner Mazel.

Levick, M. F. (1983). *They could not talk and so they drew: Children's styles of coping and thinking*. Springfield, IL: Charlie C. Thomas.

Liebmann, M. (1990). "It just happened": Looking at crime events. In M. Liebmann (Ed.), *Arttherapy in practice* (pp. 133–155). Bristol, PA: Jessica Kingsley.

Linesch, D. (1993). *Art therapy with families with crisis*. New York: Brunner Mazel.

Lusebrink, V. B. (1990). *Imagery and visual expression in therapy*. New York: Plenum press. doi:10.1007/978-1-4757-0444-0

Malchiodi, C. A. (1996). '*Art therapists* in cyberspace.' *Art Therapy. Journal of the American An Therapy Association*, *13*(4), 150–151.

Malchiodi, C. A. (1997). *Breaking the silence: Art therapy with children from violent homes*. Philadelphia: Brunner/Mazel.

Malchiodi, C. A. (1998). *The Art therapy sourcebook*. Los Angeles, CA: Lowell House.

Malchiodi, C. A. (1998). *Understanding children's drawings*. New York: Guilford Press.

McConeghey, H. (1986). Archetypal art therapy in cross cultural art therapy. *Art Therapy: Journal of the American Art Therapy Association*, 3.

McNiff, S. (1992). *Art as medicine: Creating a therapy of imagination*. Boston: Shambhala.

McNiff, S. (1997). Art therapy: A spectrum of partnerships. *The Arts in Psychotherapy*, *24*(1), 37–44. doi:10.1016/S0197-4556(97)00001-4

Mills, J. C., & Crowley, R. J. (1986). *Therapeutic metaphors for children and the child within*. New York: Brunner/Mazel.

Moon, B. L. (1995). *Existential Art Therapy: The Canvas Mirror*. Springfield, IL: Charlie C. Thomas.

Moon, C. H. (2002). *Studio art therapy: Cultivating the artist identity in the art therapist*. London: Jessica Kingsley.

Nucho, A. O. (1987). The Psychocybernetic model of art therapy. Springfield, IL: Charlie C. Thomas.

Perry, B. D., Pollard, R. A., Blakley, T. L., Baker, W. L., & Vigilante, D. (1995). Childhood trauma, the neurobiology of adaptation and use-dependent development of the brain: How states become traits. *Infant Mental Health Journal*, *16*(4), 271–291. doi:10.1002/1097-0355(199524)16:4<271::AID-IMHJ2280160404>3.0.CO;2-B

Rhyne, J. (1973/1995). *The Gestalt art experience*. Chicago: Magnolia Street.

Riley, S. (1999). *Contemporary art therapy with adolescents*. London: Jessica Kingsley.

Riley, S. (2001). *Group process made visible*. New York: Brunner-Routledge.

Riley, S., & Malchiodi, C. A. (1994). *Integrative approach to family art therapy*. Chicago: Magnolia Street.

Rogers, N. (1993). *The Creative Connection*. Expressive Arts as Healing.

Rubin, J. A. (1987/2001). *Approaches for art therapy* (J. A. Rubin, Ed.). Philadelphia: Brunner- Routledge.

Rubin, J. A. (2001). *Approaches to Art Therapy: Theory and techniques*. New York: Brunner Routledge.

Sadock, B. J., & Sadock, V. (2003). *Kaplan and Sadock's Synopsis of Psychiatry* (9th ed.). Philadelphia: Lippincott Williams and Wilkins.

Schaverian, J. (1992). *The Revealing Image: Analytical Art Psychotherapy in Theory and Practice*. Jessica Kingsley Publishers.

Schore, A. (1994). *Affect regulation and the origin of the self.* Hillsdale, NJ: Erlbaum.

Siegel, D. J. (1999). *The developing mind: Towards a neurobiology of interpersonal experience*. New York: Guilford Press.

Siegel, D. J. (1999). *The developing mind: Towards a neurobiology of interpersonal experience*. New York: Guilford Press.

Silver, R. A. (2000). *Studies in art therapy (1962-2000)*. Sarasota, FL: Ablin Press.

Silverstone, L. (1997). *Art Therapy - The Person-Centred Way: Art and the Development of the Person*. Jessica Kingsley Pub.

Sobol, B. (1982). Art therapy and strategic family therapy. *American Journal of Art Therapy*, 2.

Trowbridge, M. M. (1995). Graphic indicators of sexual abuse in children's drawings: A review of the literature. *The Arts in Psychotherapy*, *22*(5), 485–494. doi:10.1016/0197-4556(95)00052-6

Ulak, B. J., & Cummings, A. L. (1997). Using clients' artistic expressions as metaphor in counselling: A pilot study. *Canadian Journal of Counselling*, *31*(4), 305–316.

Weir, F. (1987). The role of symbolic expression in its relation to art therapy: A Kleinian approach. In Images of art therapys. London: Routledge.

KEY TERMS AND DEFINITIONS

Art Therapy: Art therapy is non directive method that subtly allows the patient to symbolically reveal the inner conflicts without the fear of disclosure by the means of art.

Biopsychosocial Intervention: Approach stating that biological, psychological (which entails thoughts, emotions, and behaviors), and social (socio-economical, socio-environmental, and cultural) factors, all play a significant role in human functioning in the context of disease.

Paranoid Schizophrenia: Paranoid Schizophrenia is one of the chronic mental illnesses according to DSM-IVTR mainly characterized by the presence of delusion of persecution, suspicious, distrusting, guarded, reserved, tensed, and also sometimes hostile or aggressive.

Phases of Sessions: The progress of case of seen in phases like initial rapport building phase, middle phase and ending phase.

Therapeutic Techniques: Skills used in the treatment or management of the illness.

Chapter 18
Psychotherapeutic Interventions in Emotional and Behavioural Problems with Adolescents

Mahesh A. Tripathi
Sweekaar Rehabilitation Institute for Handicapped, India

Godishala Sridevi
Osmania University, India

ABSTRACT

Children undergo a variety of interrelated changes in their adolescence and at times most children exhibits difficult behaviours. The problem becomes more severe in adopted children because such status of adoption affects various aspects of the developing personality. Feeling of rejection in early childhood generates a tendency of insecurity and fear in these children and to overcome from these beliefs they adopt aggressive behaviour. Psychotherapy with adolescents is different in a number of substantive ways from adults, because an adolescent is a person who is no longer a child but is not yet an adult. They are special population for whom psychotherapeutic intervention needs to be customized considering the emotional and behavioural exigencies. Identification and changing unhealthy thoughts and behaviours is the central idea of CBT and is becoming the treatment of choice for children and adolescents. The chapter deals with application of CBT in adolescent.

INTRODUCTION

The origin of the term psychotherapy dates back to 1891, and first appeared in the paper entitled '*Hypnotism, suggestion, psychotherapy*' by Hippolyte Bernheim. Then it was discussed in psychoanalytical approach as a talking cure. In 20th century psychotherapy grew manifold and various form of psychotherapy emerged. Across time, many professionals and writers have defined psychotherapy in their own words. However, the most accepted definition of psychotherapy was given by Wolberg, (1995) who defined psychotherapy "a psychological treatment of emotional problems in which a trained person deliberately establishes a professional relationship with the patient in order to: (a) remove or modify or

DOI: 10.4018/978-1-5225-0519-8.ch018

retard existing symptoms; (b) mediate disturbed patterns of behavior; (c) promote positive personality growth and development". In simple term we can say that psychotherapy is a meet between a clinician and an individual taking place in a trustful environment, and clinician talks through the patient's concerns with the goal of bringing about changes in his thoughts, feelings, and behaviours. It is essential to clarify what not qualifies as psychotherapy. The interventions that use biological means of producing change, such as medication, diet, exercise, and psychosurgery are not psychotherapy. Other intervention such as tuitions and counselling aiming to enhance academic performance and achievement are also excluded. Engagement in leisure time activities such as chatting with friends and relatives, sports activities, or other individual or group activities like dancing, singing; and merely spending time with one's spouse or significant other are also omitted from the standard definitions of psychotherapy, though each of these can be a part of intervention for therapeutic benefit in improving.

TYPES OF THERAPIES

Wolberg, (1995) in his book "The techniques of psychotherapy" discussed psychotherapies in three major categories: Supportive Psychotherapies, Re-educative Psychotherapies and Reconstructive psychotherapies. According to him all psychoanalytical and psychodynamic therapies comes under re-constructive therapy and all time framed, short form, aiming on symptomatology comes under re-educative psychotherapies. While, techniques that are sympathetic in nature and provide hope, and sympathy and are basically uses as an adjunctive therapy are supportive therapies.

Every schools of psychology have different view toward mental illness and their management. Theoretical development of each school was based on particular target group and specific problems. Hence each school have their own understanding for casual and maintaining factors of all type of psychological problems. Therefore, founders and developers of different schools have generated and adopted a little unique way of management. Therapies developed on the theories of these schools are different in nature and we can divide them as follows.

1. Psychoanalysis and Psychodynamic psychotherapies,
2. Humanistic psychotherapy,
3. Gestalt psychotherapy,
4. Existential psychotherapy,
5. Cognitive behaviour therapy,
6. Transactional therapy,
7. Family therapy,
8. Reality therapy.

APPROACHES OF THERAPIES

Psychotherapeutic need of every client differs from another client and Therapists too employ different approaches as per the need. Approaches differ from anything between a few sessions to a number of years of intensive contact between client and therapist. Professionals select a type of psychotherapy for a variety of reasons, including its empirical effectiveness. There are three broad categorical approaches toward all type of psychotherapies. In this, the oldest psychodynamic psychotherapy tends towards a pessimistic view of the human condition whereas a humanistic and integrative approach is essentially optimistic in nature and procedures. Psychodynamic model of psychotherapy give more emphasis on conflict and attempts to resolve it.

Humanistic and integrative psychotherapy includes many different schools of psychotherapy in which there is not one accepted theoretical approach. Most of these have a unique theoretical and methodological approach to psychotherapy. There are some general principles that can be found to lie in all schools related to this group or form of approach. The basic idea of this form of psychotherapy is as being intrinsically involved in facilitating the client's development of their potential. A recent development in this form of psychotherapy is the emergence of integrative psychotherapy. Safran and Messer (1997) have identified three most popular forms currently in practice.

1. **Technical Eclecticism:** Approach in which the therapist selects some core ingredients from different therapies that share common features, with aim to develop more efficacious treatment. (Norcross & Grencavage, 1989).
2. **Common Principles:** In this approach some common factors are identified from variety of psychotherapeutic approaches and are brought together. (Nuttall, 2002) argues that one such 'common principle' is the primacy of the therapeutic relationship as a factor for change. Therefore, an integrative interventionist utilizing this approach is giving more attention to develop the therapeutic relationship.
3. **Theoretical Integration:** Integration is described as "two or more therapies are integrated in the hope that the result will be better than the constituent therapies alone" (Norcross, 2005). In this approach therapist constructs his own theory of psychotherapy that draws on other approaches.

The third major approach was identified as Cognitive and behavioral therapy (CBT). Identification and changing unhealthy thoughts and behaviors is the central idea of CBT. Mainly used in a one-to-one setting, CBT is symptom-based, and in a collaborative effort client and therapist both decide the outcome from the therapy and measures its success as therapy progress. Homework and willingness to engage in activities between sessions is the main ingredient of CBT approach.

PSYCHOTHERAPIES FOR ADOLESCENTS WITH EMOTIONAL BEHAVIOURAL PROBLEMS

Psychotherapy with adolescents is different in a number of substantive ways from adults, because an adolescent is a person who is no longer a child but is not yet an adult. Children undergo variety of interrelated changes in these years. The physical changes are associated with puberty, cognitive changes are likely to be intellectual, social changes appear in increased peer-focused orientation, and educational move from elementary to secondary education (Moshman, 2005). In this period of development, most children are prone to exhibit difficult behaviour such as temper tantrums or occasional aggressive outbursts, but this behaviour becomes problematic when it is persistent. The problem could become more severe in special cases like adopted children, who spent their early childhood in and orphanages. The child who is placed with adoptive parents at or soon after birth misses the mutual and deeply satisfying mother and child relationship (Clothier, 1943). The belief of "I'm no good: because my parents gave me away, because I was no good and I am going to prove them right" is common in adoptive children (Schechter, 1960). There are various emotional and psychodynamic issues behind this recurrent behavioural and personality pattern that are specifically linked to adoption. Studies support that extreme provocative, aggressive, antisocial, and delinquent conducts are much more consistently among adoptees than their non-adopted counterparts (Kirshner, & Nagel, 1988). Large percentage of adopted children eventually comes to psychiatric or other professional attention because of emotional, educational or social problems (Toussieng, 1962). The most common behavior problems among these adopted children are externalized behavior problems indicative of children diagnosed as having "conduct disorders," who are acting out anti-socially in response to a number of internal negative feelings such as anger, powerlessness, low self-esteem, fear, and anxiety (Smith & Howard, 1991). Rejected children are more physically aggressive and more disruptive and used more verbal threats than other children (Coie, 1990; Newcomb, Bukowski., & Pattee, 1993) when confronted with social problems, conduct disordered children generate fewer solutions than children who do not have conduct disorder. There are also long term consequences for such children as they grow into adulthood, as about 80% of youths who demonstrate severe acting-out are likely to meet criteria for some type of psychiatric disorder in the future (Kazdin, 2004). It is also reported that girls significantly have more number of problems and lower self-esteem then boys (Harper & Marshall, 1991). Moreover, fathers play a much important role in the life of girls, who feels rejected by their fathers often have more adjustment and personality problems (Fish & Biller, 1993). Cognitive behaviour therapy (CBT) usually targets the attitudes and beliefs underlying such type of behaviours. Behavioural problems in children may be affected by both family and child factors, and problems may occur during interactions with parents. Individual intervention strategies are more desirable and effective in adolescent groups. There is some evidence that CBT interventions for adolescents administered in groups may make conduct problems worse (Fonagy et al., 2002). A meta-analysis based on 50 studies incorporating 1640 subject reveals that CBT recipient was better than 76% of untreated subjects in term of anger reduction (Beck & Fernandez, 1998). Cognitive behaviour and skills based approaches are the most widely studied and empirically validated treatments for anger and aggression in youth. Commonly used therapeutic techniques include affective education, relaxation training, and cognitive restructuring, problem solving skills, social skill training, and conflict resolution. These techniques tailored to the individual child and or families need and can foster the development of more adaptive and pro-social behaviour (Blake & Hamrin, 2007). A study revealed that CBT has improved the self-confidence and self-esteem of adolescent and effectively worked in adolescents with depressive and anxiety features (Tripathi & Sridevi, 2014).

It is important to note that anger outburst, aggression difficulties in regulating negative emotions are significant psychological problems of adolescent. Anger and aggression can be understood as a part of other psychological disorder such as conduct disorder, anxiety disorder or as an independent problem maintained by contingencies in the environment. They facilitate negative emotions and impact in interpersonal relationships. Therefore, it is necessary to adapt a little different psychotherapeutic approach in order to assist adolescents in managing such changes. It is also important to adopt a contextual and developmental perspective for describing, understanding, and treating adolescents. Usually, a difficulty in relating with other people and circumstances brings adolescents to psychotherapy, irrespective of the etiological factors of their problems. When specific type of treatment or intervention, especially meant for the adolescents uses psychological constructs and mechanisms it is known as 'adolescent psychotherapy'. Different therapists have developed their own strategies to work with children and adolescents. Like, Kazdin, (2002) described self-instructional program including cognitive problem-solving skills to help adolescents in building competencies to deal with anger and aggression. Social skill training (SST) proposed by Bandura (1977) is another approach to deal with adolescents' problems. This include behavioral and social skills training, which involves accurate interpretation of social cues from others, self-instruction/self-regulation training. Other strategies involve the use of self-talk, self-reinforcement in response to appropriate social behaviors, social problem-solving skills. SST also includes the reduction of inappropriate, inhibiting or competing social behaviors that interfere with appropriate social interactions. SST is an essential component of therapeutic program designed for emotional and behavior disorders.

CBT FOR ADOLESCENT

CBTs include a variety of cognitive and behavioural techniques that target on symptom reduction and changes through identification and modification of dysfunctional thoughts, cognitive errors and interpersonal skill building. It is derived from learning theories and gradually moved on to incorporating the mediational role of cognitions in the perpetuation of emotional disorders. All CBTs have some common features consists a comprehensive cognitive and behavioural assessment of thoughts, emotions and behaviours. The core ingredients of cognitive therapies are negative automatic thoughts, cognitive errors or distortions and schema and CB therapist works on these components simultaneously. However, CBT in its conventional form for adults may or may not be indicative for adolescents. There is a need to adopt evidence-based therapies in order to make interventions scientific and effective. Evidence-based interventions are practices that are based on empirical research studies and interventions have been demonstrated to be superior to no treatment or alternative interventions for people with specific diagnoses (Sudhir, 2015).

An integrative approach to psychotherapy may often be a necessity due to the unique demands of working with children and adolescents (Coonerty, 1993). Through integration of different perspectives, both in conceptualizing and responding to child or adolescent difficulties, therapists may ensure a better fit between the interventions and the individual's specific needs. Child and adolescent cognitive styles and self-concepts are still developing, so interventions must be tailored to match these emerging abilities. Furthermore, because children are more contextually dependent than adults (Fitz Patrick, 1993), effective treatments often focus on creating a developmentally appropriate environment and modifying patterns of reinforcement, in addition to improving self-regulatory skills. For example, clinicians could respond to a child's problem behaviours by helping parents implement appropriate sleep routines to address inadequate sleep, as well as helping the child learn to better modulate his or her feelings. Integrative approaches allow clinicians to address interpersonal challenges while also addressing external realities. CBT is becoming the treatment of choice for children and adolescents because it is flexible and includes a variety of behavioural and cognitive strategies that the therapist can choose and apply during the progress of therapy.

STRUCTURE OF CBT SESSIONS

- Review of mood state and recent events,
- Setting agenda,
- Review of homework,

- Working on targets, like defining problems, identifying & challenging negative thoughts,
- Establishment of home practice (Homework) based on work during the session,
- Feedback and planning for the next appointment.

Literature

CBT is a well-established therapeutic approach for adult as well young people and there are various studies to support the effectiveness in adolescent's behavior and emotional problems. In a meta-analysis of all psychological treatments for depression in child and adolescence CBT was found to be more effective (Weisz et al., 2006). The treatment effects were described as modest compared with outcomes for other disorders, such as anxiety. Watanabe et al., (2007) conducted a further meta-analysis of psychotherapies used a different methodology, including intention-to-treat analyses, and took a clinical perspective on outcomes and found that psychotherapies, especially CBT, which had the largest body of evidence, and interpersonal therapy (IPT) were more effective than no treatment, waiting list or attention placebo at post-treatment in youths. Effectiveness was greatest for 12–18-year-olds. A meta-analysis of child and adolescent psychotherapy outcome research indicates positive and highly significant effect. These effects were more positive for behavioural than for non-behavioural treatments, and samples of adolescent girls showed better outcomes than other Age and Gender groups. Results supported the specificity of treatment effects: Outcomes were stronger for the particular problems targeted in treatment than for problems not targeted (Weisz, Weiss, Han, Granger., & Morton, 1995). Though there is a strong empirical support for CBT in dealing with various disorders of all age groups. Most of the studies has been conducted on adolescent are targeting on externalizing behaviour, especially substance abuse, risk sex behaviour, and aggression but most of the studies are carried out in orphanage or institutions. Only few studies are available on adopted adolescents emotional and behaviour problem whose early life was belonged to an orphanage. There is no such study available in Indian context where cultural attributes are very prominent and adaptation is still not so popular, accepted and children or families both are facing different type of difficulties after adaptation. Therefore, there is strong need to find out some effective treatment strategy to address the issues related to anger and interpersonal conflict. Our aim is to find out a better comprehensive intervention plan to deal with such problems.

Case Study of CBT in an Adopted Adolescent

The authors worked with a case of an adopted adolescent, on whom CBT was employed. Miss "A", 14 yrs old girl, studying in IXth grade, belongs to nuclear family, from Hyderabad, India. She was adopted from a Government Orphanage home at the age of 2 yrs 6 months. She was dropped at orphanage when she was 15 days old. Initially she used to sit alone and remained aloof but gradually, she started interacting with family members. She was short tempered and impulsive since her childhood and she used to break her toys and her belongings whenever she became angry or frustrated. She was admitted in the play school at the age of 2 and ½ years and she loved to go to school and used to participate in all activities. She was an average student since her childhood and no disciplinary complaints from school about her. She maintained a good and healthy relationship with classmates and teachers and had good number of friends in school from both genders. She was a Gymnastic player at national level and practised till 8th standard but discontinued as her father did not want to continue it. She participated in a science exhibition during current academic session and was appreciated by the school. According to school authorities she was a well-disciplined, regular, obedient student and always respected the teachers and staffs. She was very much kind towards poor people and beggars since her childhood as she used to bring extra pencils, erasers and sharpeners to donate among needy children. She also used to give her pocket money to beggars and poor children.

As per history, patient A's mother' nature was calm, quiet and sensitive while father had very low emotional tolerance and he used to become aggressive for simple reasons and used abusive language at that time. However, he was a responsible person to his family and always fulfilled the demands as far as possible. But he used to scold 'A' whenever she did any mistake and mentioned that she was an orphan child. While both parents were suffering from some health conditions, Miss A was sympathetic towards mother only as whenever mother felt sick she used to take care of her and always seems worry. She made three attempts to harm her mother in past 8 months, first time she bought acid bottle, second time pushed her, and last time she mixed excessive sleeping pills in her food. After each attempt she felt guilt and accepted her fault (all attempts were on planning phase and before execution of act she was caught by family). She gave the explanation to her mother for such behaviours that she wanted to throw her out from home and send her to other people as she is an orphan child.

Child was diagnosed as "Other mixed disorder of conduct and emotion" as per ICD-10 classification and CBT techniques were used in intervention program. Pre- post research design was used to study the efficacy of Cognitive Behaviour Therapy. She was assessed using Human Figure Drawing Test (HFDT) (Mitchel, Rechard., & Roland,1993). Bender-Gestalt Test (BGT-II) (Brannigan, & Decker, 2003), Malin's Intelligence Scale for Indian Children (MISIC), (Malin,1971). Rorschach's Test, Strength and Difficulties Questionnaire (SDQ-Self report) (Goodman, 1997) and Beck Depression Inventory (BDI-II) (Beck, Ward, Mendelson, Mock., & Erbaugh, 1961). BDI-II and SDQ was administered for pre-post assessment of the intervention.

INTERVENTION

Procedure and Therapeutic Process

Therapist targeted emotional and behaviour problems with integrated therapeutic approach. Intervention was done in two sessions in a week, each session for 55 minutes and total 24 sessions within 12 weeks were planned. Component of intervention comprised with psycho-education, relaxation therapy, anger management, cognitive restructuring, activity scheduling, role playing, social skill training, positive self -statement, and yoga.

Therapeutic Formulation

Miss "A" showed affective, cognitive, and behavioural features consistent with a diagnosis of other mixed disorder of conduct and emotion, increased since last 3 years. In addition, she shows a variety of emotional problems with fluctuation since early childhood. Predisposing factors for her emotional disorder included orphan and institutionalized in infant age. Perpetuating factors were father's aggressive nature and mother's over-concern on her studies. She has deep feeling of inferiority and father's critical approach toward her provoking to negative thoughts. Her anxious and irritable state was maintained by her self- criticizing style of thought, and the fact that she and her parents have developed a style of interacting that is either critical or over involved. These maintaining factors occurred within a family situation. There were a number of important protective factors in this case which suggested that could be a positive outcome. These included her average overall level of academic ability and problem solving skills; ability to make and maintain friendships and effective behaviour with relatives; at times she cared for both parents.

Initial Sessions

In the initial session informal conversation including sharing of likes, dislikes, interests and hobbies were carried out to develop rapport with the client. After successfully establishing rapport she was psycho-educated about the nature, course, prognosis and management program. Psycho-education was also given to the mother to gain her support in psychotherapeutic process as psycho-education to the family members improves social functioning and adolescent-parent relationships and it provides great satisfaction with treatment (Stanford et al., 2006). She was educated about the functions of anger and about her personal anger patterns.

Initially clinical interview technique was used for assessing cognition, emotion and behaviour in which client was asked to describe the thoughts, feelings and actions. It has been argued that much important cognition is not accessible to self-monitoring and that individual's reports concerning their own cognitions are often no more accurate (Nisbett & Wilson, 1977). She was asked to maintain a self-monitoring record (thought sheet) and demonstration was given to her by hypothetical examples. It was a three column DTR chart in which she has to write stimulus situation, emotional response, and cognition that helps as a database for discussion of therapeutic principles and goals (Freeman et al., 1990). Through interview, thought sheet (dairy), and with the help of Socratic questioning, following triggering events were identified-

- Mother's excessive concern towards study.
- Father's shouting and criticizing attitude.

Middle Sessions

These sessions were purely cognitive in which underlying cognitive errors or beliefs were indentified with the help of thought challenging and Socratic questioning. She has belief that, her parents do not love her as she is not their biological child and they leave her. Initially thought challenging was used by examining the evidence such as she was asked to explain that how she came to know that her parents do not love her? She described some incidents where she felt that father was humiliating her and mother also support him. She was also elaborated the situations which made her to feel the same. The logical disputing was also used to change her irrational belief with some examples such as biological parents are more demanding and authoritarian. It was also noticed that her mother and maternal family has accepted her very well and she remained happy with them but father and few members of paternal family were used to criticize her. Initially she tried a lot to defend her beliefs but when other meanings of interactions were introduced, she started to accept that, maybe I was wrong. After convincing the patient that her underlying beliefs were maladaptive by providing lot of examples and she was suggested to write sentences which consisting positive and motivating words, for (e.g., My parents and friends likes me, as they take care of me, "I am also the part of society and there are so many children like me, I am in better place than other orphan children" and 'I have to take care of my parents).

The next target was to make her understand about the determents of the anger and distinguish anger from aggression. She was explained regarding expectation and appraisals which are linked with anger arousal. Particular attention was paid to inordinately high expectations of others behaviours and to the appraisal of the events as personal affronts or ego threats. This was done to increase her cognitive flexibility. Therefore, started intervening for skill acquisition in which first target was to create ability to "not take things personally", and the behavioural strategies were introduced such as self- instructions in the form of coping and self-statements were designed for specific provocative events (Bellack & Hersen, 1989). E.g (translated) – "when angry, my father can say anything, but my father cares for me, and that's why he scolds me". After setting set of instructions she was asked to start repeating the self-instructions out loud. With practice she learned to use the instructions and eventually instruction become automatic. Behaviour change can be brought about by changing the instructions that Patient give themselves, away from maladaptive and upsetting thoughts to more adaptive self-talk (Meichenbaum, 1977).

Two sessions were planned with parents to involve them in therapy process mainly the father because he did not believe in psychotherapy but after seeing some improvement he willingly came for the session. Initially his point of view was listened carefully. Therefore, He was psycho-educated about the maintaining factors. Therapist explained him the procedure of therapy and he was happy with the progress. Finally, he asked that in what way he can support in the therapy and he was advised to avoid criticizing or comparing with others and to spend quality of time with her. Mother was very much co-operative and ready to follow each and every instruction she was instructed to appreciate and appraise her, whenever she controls her temper. She was also advised to hug the child to make her calm whenever she becomes frustrated. Relationship between the adolescents and their fathers is particularly important for therapy prognosis and one has to consider the respective relations with both parents for therapy prognosis. Interest and readiness of parents (mothers as well as fathers) for a close cooperation are higher than generally expected (Mattejat & Remschmidt, 1997).

In these sessions relaxation technique was introduced and rationale behind this technique was discussed in detail. She was taught to relax muscles (e g, arms, face, jaw, tongue, neck, shoulders, trunk, and lower limbs) one by one. In first session all the procedure regarding relaxation was taught by demonstration. She was instructed to sit on the chair comfortably, close eyes and try to concentrate on breathing and asked to follow the instructions. (Ex- Clench the right fist, feeling tension in the fist and forearm, clinch the left fist, feeling the tension in the fist and forearm, bend the elbows and tensed the biceps keeping the hands relaxed, straighten the arm and tensed the triceps leaving the lower arms supported by the chair with the hands relaxed and so on). Initially she was not able to concentrate and used to open her eyes in between but later she started doing well and immediate after each session her subjective feeling was recorded on 10-point scale. After third session she rated 6 on 10-point scale. She was advised to follow the procedure by her own and also asked to practice it two to three time at home and she went fluent in next few sessions.

Meanwhile, she was targeted on communication skills as it was found through interview and thought dairy that she had a problem in interaction with parents. The role play technique was introduced and initially, she was asked to play her father's role and demonstrated how to control and divert the situation. Some communication strategies were taught to handle her mother that starts the conversation with mother after reaching home before she asks. Role playing is a very common strategy to assess and train clients in social skills training (Bellack & Hersen, 1989).

To improve her mental well-being and positive attitude toward self, she was introduced to yoga techniques in which five Asna's including Padmasna, Sarvangasna, Pashchimottasna, Bhujang asna and "Om chanting. Yoga was introduced for arousal reduction as it is personally suited program (Bellack & Hersen, 1989). In fact, later mother was also advised to join the client in yoga session.

Terminal Sessions

In these sessions homework dairy was checked and self-rating and evaluation of therapy was obtained. Activity scheduling was done to bring her in more active and worthy life which was done on the basis of her previous routine such as early morning yoga, spend time with parents, fix time for homework and other studies, playing outdoor game (Badminton), weekly visit to grandparents or outing, etc. All scheduling was done with her concern which helps in reducing an apparently overwhelming mass of tasks (Hawton, 1989). Post therapeutic assessment was carried out with BDI-II, and SDQ. In the terminal session she was encouraged to maintain the improvements and advised to follow up once in a month for three months and reported the progress. Parents reported that her behaviour was significantly improving and she was doing well in academics as well as at home. She has started to maintain herself calm at home and used to help her mother and prepares favourite food for her father on holidays. She is developed to be clam when her father shouts on her. She practiced yoga regularly with her mother. Overall an integrated approach had good prognostic effect on the client.

IMPLICATIONS FOR CBT OUTCOME RESEARCH

Parental Involvement in therapeutic process with adolescents becomes an important for many of the behavioral and emotional problems. Research evidence suggests that parent involvement is likely to improve treatment outcome in anxious children and adolescents (Albano & Kendall, 2002; Barrett, Dadds., & Rapee,1996). Parents can be involved as a co- therapist, as collaborators or as a consultant who provide important assistance during therapeutic process. Parents are also instructed to provide positive reinforcements during the course of therapy and their active involvement in the therapeutic plan will vary depending upon degree of impairment, co-morbidity, age, and gender. Conflict resolution skills and handling negative self talk affect regulation skills such as learning to relax or use social problem-solving skills that are used in the management of problems related to anger (Novaco, 1979).

CONCLUSION

Integrated psychotherapeutic approach will improve the self-confidence, feeling of security and improving self-esteem, self-respect, confidence and emotional well –being of an adopted adolescent with emotional and behavioural problems. Yoga could be effective in improving emotional well- being and anger management techniques helps to control the emotions in adolescents. Parental involvement in therapy with adolescents is much needed. Findings of the case study mentioned in the chapter are difficult to generalize, however, the case was unique in nature and finding a group for such type of problems is a difficult task. CBT techniques with yoga can be applied with techniques such as stress inoculation and anger management in adolescents.

FUTURE RESEARCH DIRECTION

The assumption that a single form of therapy can be generically applied to a broad range of adolescent problems has been laid to rest. Similarly, the assumption that all forms of therapy are equally effective has not been supported. A range of adolescent disorders and a number of widely practiced forms of therapy have not been adequately evaluated. Although anxiety, depressive, and conduct disorders make up the bulk of adolescent referrals, there are a number of clinical problems in adolescents that need to be evaluated and evidence based managements for them.

REFERENCES

Albano, A. M., & Kendall, P. C. (2002). Cognitive behavioural therapy for children and adolescents with anxiety disorders: Clinical research advances. *International Review of Psychiatry (Abingdon, England), 14*(2), 129–134. doi:10.1080/09540260220132644

Bandura, A. (1977). *Social Learning Theory*. Englewood Cliffs, NJ: Prentice-Hall.

Barrett, P. M., Dadds, M. R., & Rapee, R. M. (1996). Family treatment of childhood anxiety: A controlled trial. *Journal of Consulting and Clinical Psychology, 64*(2), 333–342. doi:10.1037/0022-006X.64.2.333 PMID:8871418

Beck, R., & Fernandez, E. (1998). Cognitive Behaviour Therapy in the treatment of anger: A meta analysis. *Cognitive Therapy and Research, 22*(1), 63–74. doi:10.1023/A:1018763902991

Bellack, A. S., & Hersen, M. (1989). Dictionary of behaviour therapy techniques. Pregamon Press.

Blake, C.S., & Hamrin, V. (2007). Current approaches to the assessment and management of anger and aggression in youth: A review. *Journal of Child and Adolescent Psychiatric Nursing, 20*(4), 209-221.

Brannigan, G. G., & Decker, S. L. (2003). *Bender Visual-Motor Gestalt Test* (2nd Ed). Itasca, IL: Riverside Publishing. Retrieved from www.riversidepublishing.com

Clothier, F. (1943). The Psychology of the Adopted Child. The National Committee for Mental Hygiene. *Mental Hygiene*, 27.

Coie, J. D. (1990). Toward a theory of peer rejection. In S. R. Asher, & J. D. Coie (Eds.), Peer rejection in childhood (pp. 365–401). New York: Cambridge University Press.

Coonerty, S. (1993). Integrative child therapy. In G. Stricker & J. R. Gold (Eds.), *Comprehensive handbook of psychotherapy integration*. New York, NY: Plenum Press; doi:10.1007/978-1-4757-9782-4_28

Fish, C., & Biller, S. (1993). Advances in Clinical Child Psychology. In T. H. Ollendick & R. J. Prinz (Eds.), *Plenum Press*. New York.

FitzPatrick, M. (1993). Adolescents. In G. Stricker & J. R. Gold (Eds.), *Comprehensive handbook of psychotherapy integration*. New York, NY: Plenum Press; doi:10.1007/978-1-4757-9782-4_29

Fonagy, P., Target, M., Cottrell, D., Phillips, J., & Kurtz, Z. (2002). *What works for whom? A critical review of treatments for children and adolescents*. Guildford Press.

Freeman, A., Pretzer, J., Fleming, B., & Simon, K. M. (1990). *Clinical Application of Cognitive Therapy*. New York: Plenum Press. doi:10.1007/978-1-4684-0007-6

Goodman, R. (1997). The Strength and Difficulties Questionnaire: A research note. *Journal of Child Psychology and Psychiatry, and Allied Disciplines*, *38*(5), 581–586. doi:10.1111/j.1469-7610.1997.tb01545.x PMID:9255702

Harper, J. F., & Marshall, E. (1991). Adolescents problems and their relationship to self esteem. *Adolscence*, *26*, 799–808. PMID:1789167

Hawton, K., Salkvskis, P., Kirk, J., & Clark, D. M. (1989). Cognitive behaviour therapy for psychiatric problems: A practical guide. Oxford University Press. doi:doi:10.1093/med:psych/9780192615879.001.0001 doi:10.1093/med:psych/9780192615879.001.0001

Kazdin, A. E. (2002). Psychosocial treatments for conduct disorder in children and adolescent. In P. E. Nathan & J. M. Gorman (Eds.), *Guides to treatments that work* (2nd ed.). New York: Oxford University Press.

Kazdin, W. E. (2004). Psychotherapy with children. In M. J. Lambert (Ed.), *Bergin and Garfield's handbook of psychotherapy and behavior change* (5th ed.). New York: Wiley.

Malin, A. J. (1971). *Manual Malin's intelligence scale for Indian children (Indian Adaptation of W.I.S.I.C.)*. Lucknow: Indian Psychological Corpoation.

Mattejat, F., & Remschmidt, H. (1997). Significance of family relations for coping with psychological disorders--results of an empirical study of therapy prognosis of children and adolescents with psychological disorders. *Praxis der Kinderpsychologie und Kinderpsychiatrie*, *46*(5), 371–392. PMID:9273537

Meichenbaum, D. (1977). *Cognitive- behaviour modification: An integrative approach*. New York: Plenum Press. doi:10.1007/978-1-4757-9739-8

Moshman, D. (2005). Adolescent Psychological Development Rationality, Morality and Identity (2nd Ed.) Lawrence Erlbaum Associates, Inc.

Nisbett, R. E., & Wilson, T. D. (1977). Telling more than we can know: Verbal reports on mental processes. *Psychological Review*, *84*(3), 231–259. doi:10.1037/0033-295X.84.3.231

Norcross, J. C. (2005). A primer on psychotherapy integration. In J. C. Norcross & M. R. Goldfried (Eds.), Handbook of psychotherapy integration (2nd ed.). New York: Oxford. doi:doi:10.1093/med:psych/9780195165791.003.0001 doi:10.1093/med:psych/9780195165791.003.0001

Norcross, J. C., & Grencavage, L. M. (1989). Eclecticism and integration in psychotherapy: Major themes and obstacles. *British Journal of Guidance & Counselling*, *19*, 227–247.

Novaco, R. W. (1979). *Therapist manual for stress inoculation training. Therapeutic interventions for anger problems*. Irvine, CA: University of California.

Nuttall, J. (2002). Modes of therapeutic relationship in brief dynamic psychotherapy: A case study. *Psychodynamic Practice*, *8*(4), 505–523. doi:10.1080/1353333021000038854

Safran, J. D., & Messer, S. B. (1997). Psychotherapy integration: A postmodern critique. *Clinical Psychology: Science and Practice*, *4*(2), 140–192. doi:10.1111/j.1468-2850.1997.tb00106.x

Sanford, M., Boyle, M., Mccleary, Z., Miller, J., Steele, M., Duku, E., & Offord, D. (2006). A Pilot Study. *Mental Hygiene*, 27. PMID:16601642

Schechter, M. D. (1960). *Fantasies and behaviour of the adopted child*. Beverly Hills, CA; Academic Press.

Smith, S. L., & Howard, J. A. (1991). A comparative study of successful and disrupted adoptions. *The Social Service Review*, *65*(2), 248–261. doi:10.1086/603836

Sudhir, P. M. (2015). A practical Approach to cognitive behaviour therapy for adolescent. Springer.

Toussieng, W. P. (1962). Disabilities in adopted children and adoptive parents, The National Committee for Mental Hygiene. *Mental Hygiene*, 27.

Tripathi, M. A., & Sridevi, G. (2014). CBT and remedial training in adolescent with writing difficulty and emotional problem: A case study, *Proceedings of International Conference on Developmental Disability*.

Watanabe, N., Hunot, V., Omori, I. M., Churchill, R., & Furukawa, T. A. (2007). Psychotherapy for depression among children and adolescents: A systematic review. *Acta Psychiatrica Scandinavica*, *116*(2), 84–95. doi:10.1111/j.1600-0447.2007.01018.x PMID:17650269

Weisz, J. R., McCarty, C. A., & Valeri, S. M. (2006). Effects of psychotherapy for depression in children and adolescents a meta-analysis. *Psychological Bulletin*, *132*(1), 132–149. doi:10.1037/0033-2909.132.1.132 PMID:16435960

Weisz, J. R., Weiss, B., Han, S. S., Granger, D. A., & Morton, T. (1995). Effects of psychotherapy with children and adolescents revisited: A meta-analysis of treatment outcome studies. *Psychological Bulletin*, *117*(3), 450–468. doi:10.1037/0033-2909.117.3.450 PMID:7777649

Wolberg, L. R. (1995). *The techniques of psychotherapy* (4th ed.). Jason Aronson Inc.

KEY TERMS AND DEFINITIONS

Adolescent: In the process of developing from a child to an adult.

Adoption: The action or fact of adopting or being adopted.

Aggression: Feelings of anger or antipathy resulting in hostile or violent behaviour; readiness to attack or confront.

Cognitive Behaviour Therapy: A type of psychotherapy in which negative patterns of thought about the self and the others or world are challenged in order to alter unwanted behaviour patterns or mood.

Integrated Psychotherapy: An openness for various ways of integrating diverse theories and techniques.

Intervention: The action or process of intervening.

Sessions: A fixed time for therapy.

Compilation of References

Aaron, R., Joseph, A., & Abraham, S. (2004). Suicides in young people in rural southern India. *Lancet, 363*(9415), 1117-8.

Abraham, K. (1911). Notes on the psychoanalytic investigation and treatment of manic-depressive insanity and allied conditions. In *Selected papers on psychoanalysis.* Hogarth Press and the Institute of Psychoanalysis.

Addington, J., & Addington, D. (2000). Neurocognitive and social functioning in schizophrenia: A 2.5 year follow-up study. *Schizophrenia Research, 44*(1), 47–56. doi:10.1016/S0920-9964(99)00160-7 PMID:10867311

Addington, J., Cadenhead, K. S., Cannon, T. D., Cornblatt, B., McGlashan, T. H., Perkins, D. O., & Heinssen, R. et al. (2007). North American prodrome longitudinal study: A collaborative multisite approach to prodromal schizophrenia research. *Schizophrenia Bulletin, 33*(3), 665–672. doi:10.1093/schbul/sbl075 PMID:17255119

Addington, J., Coldham, E. L., Jones, T., & Addington, K. D. (2003). The first episode of psychosis: The experience of relatives. *Acta Psychiatrica Scandinavica, 108*(4), 285–289. doi:10.1034/j.1600-0447.2003.00153.x PMID:12956829

Agarwal, N., & Jhingan, H. P. (2002). Life events and depression in elderly. *Indian Journal of Psychiatry, 44*, 34–40. PMID:21206879

Agbahowe, S. A., Ohaeri, J. U., Ogunlesi, A. O., & Osahon, R. (1998). Prevalence of psychiatric morbidity among convicted inmates in a Nigerian prison community. *East African Medical Journal, 75*(1), 19–26. PMID:9604530

Agnelli, S. (1986). *Street Children: A growing urban tragedy* (1st ed.). London: George Weiden Field & Nicholson.

Agosti, V., Nunes, E., & Levin, F. (2002). Rates of psychiatric comorbidity among U.S. residents with lifetime cannabis dependence. *The American Journal of Drug and Alcohol Abuse, 28*(4), 643–652. doi:10.1081/ADA-120015873 PMID:12492261

Aguilar, M. C., Gurpegui, M., Diaz, F. J., & de Leon, J. (2005). Nicotine dependence and symptoms in schizophrenia: Naturalistic study of complex interactions. *The British Journal of Psychiatry, 186*(3), 215–221. doi:10.1192/bjp.186.3.215 PMID:15738502

Ahmadkhaniha, H. R., Shariat, S. V., Torkaman-nejad, S., & Moghadam, M. M. H. (2007). The frequency of sexual abuse and depression in a sample of street children of one of deprived districts of Tehran. *Journal of Child Sexual Abuse, 16*(4), 23–35. doi:10.1300/J070v16n04_02 PMID:18032244

Aidan, M. (1997). Stress and coping strategies among street children in Lusaka. *Journal of Psychology in Africa, 2*(1), 24–33.

Albano, A. M., & Kendall, P. C. (2002). Cognitive behavioural therapy for children and adolescents with anxiety disorders: Clinical research advances. *International Review of Psychiatry (Abingdon, England), 14*(2), 129–134. doi:10.1080/09540260220132644

Albee, G. W., Bond, L. A., Monsey, T., & Cook, V. (Eds.). (1992). Improving children's lives: Global perspectives on prevention. In *Primary Prevention of Psychopathology* (vol. 14, pp. 279-295). Thousand Oaks, CA: Sage Publications, Inc.

Allen, P. B. (1992). Artist- in –residence: An alternative to "clinification" for art therapist. *Art Therapy: Journal of the American Art Therapy Association, 9*(1), 22–29. doi:10.1080/07421656.1992.10758933

Alonso, J., Codony, M., & Kovess, V. (2007). Population level of unmet need for mental healthcare in Europe. The British Journal of Psychiatry, 190(4), 299–306. PubMed PMID:17401035

Altanis, P., & Goddard, J. (2004). Street children in contemporary Greece. *Children & Society, 18*(4), 299–311. doi:10.1002/chi.797

Alvarez-Jimenez, M., Priede, A., Hetrick, S. E., Bendall, S., Killackey, E., Parker, A. G., & Gleeson, J. F. et al. (2012). Risk factors for relapse following treatment for first episode psychosis: A systematic review and meta-analysis of longitudinal studies. *Schizophrenia Research, 139*(1-3), 116–128. doi:10.1016/j.schres.2012.05.007 PMID:22658527

American Art Therapy Association. (1996). Mission statement. New York: McGraw Hill-NTC.

American Psychiatric Association. (1994). *Diagnostic and statistical manual of mental disorders* (4th ed.). Washington, DC: Author.

American Psychiatric Association. (2000). Diagnostic and statistical manual of the mental disorders (4 TR ed.). Washington, DC: Author.

American Psychiatric Association. (2000). *Task Force on DSM-IV: Diagnostic and statistical manual of mental disorders.* Author.

American Psychiatric Association. (2013). Diagnostic and Statistical Manual of mental Disorders (5th ed.). Washington, DC: American Psychiatric Association.

Ames, D. (1990). Depression among elderly residents of local authority residential homes.It's nature and efficacy of intervention. *The British Journal of Psychiatry, 156*(5), 667–675. doi:10.1192/bjp.156.5.667 PMID:2095943

Amminger, G. P., Leicester, S., Yung, A. R., Phillips, L. J., Berger, G. E., Francey, S. M., & McGorry, P. D. et al. (2006). Early onset of symptoms predicts conversion to non-affective psychosis in ultra-high risk individuals. *Schizophrenia Research, 84*(1), 67–76. doi:10.1016/j.schres.2006.02.018 PMID:16677803

Amore, K., Baker, M., & Chapman, P. H. (2011). The ETHOS Definition and Classification of Homelessness: An Analysis. *European Journal of Homelessness, 5*(2), 19–37.

Andersen, H. S. (2004). Mental health in prison populations. A review – With special emphasis on a study of Danish prisoners on remand. *Acta Psychiatrica Scandinavica, 424*(s424), 5–59. doi:10.1111/j.1600-0447.2004.00436_2.x PMID:15447785

Anderson, C. M., Reiss, D. J., & Hogarty, G. E. (1986). *Schizophrenia in the Family: A Practitioner's Guide to Psychoeducation and Management.* New York: Guilford Press.

Anderson, H. S., Sestoft, D., Lillebaek, T., Gabrielsen, G., Hemmingsen, R., & Kramp, P. (2000). A longitudinal study of prisoners on remand: Psychiatric prevalence, incidence and psychopathology in solitary vs non-solitary confinement. *Acta Psychiatrica Scandinavica, 102*(1), 19–25. doi:10.1034/j.1600-0447.2000.102001019.x PMID:10892605

Anderson, I., Baptista, I., Wolf, J., Edgar, B., Benjaminsen, L., & Sapounakis, A. (2006). *The changing role of service provision: barriers of access of health services for homeless people. European Federation of National Organizations Working with Homeless (FEANTSA).* European Observatory on Homelessness.

Andlin-Sobocki, P., Jonsson, B., Wittchen, H. U., & Olesen, J. (2005). Cost of disorders of the brain in Europe. European Journal of Neurology, 12(1), 1–27. doi:10.1111/j.1468-1331.2005.01202.x PubMed doi:10.1111/j.1468-1331.2005.01202.x PMID:15877774

Andreasen, N. C., & Black, D. W. (2006). Introductory Textbook of Psychiatry (4th ed.). Washington, DC: American Psychiatric Publishing.

Andreasen, N. C. (1999). A unitary model of schizophrenia: Bleuler's "fragmented phrene" as schizencephaly. *Archives of General Psychiatry*, *56*(9), 781–787. doi:10.1001/archpsyc.56.9.781 PMID:12884883

Andréasson, S., Allebeck, P., Engström, A., & Rydberg, U. (1987). Cannabis and schizophrenia. A longitudinal study of Swedish conscripts. *Lancet*, *2*(8574), 1483–1486. doi:10.1016/S0140-6736(87)92620-1 PMID:2892048

Andrew, M. (2007). A flexible organizing framework for group work with adolescents. Social Work with Groups. *A Journal of Community and Clinical Practice, 30*(3), 85-102.

Andrews, G., Stewart, G., Morris-Yates, A., Holt, P., & Henderson, S. (1990). Evidence for a general neurotic syndrome. *The British Journal of Psychiatry*, *157*(1), 6–12. doi:10.1192/bjp.157.1.6 PMID:2397364

Angermeyer, M. C., Kilian, R., Wilms, H. U., & Wittmund, B. (2006). Quality of life of spouses of mentally ill people. *The International Journal of Social Psychiatry*, *52*(3), 278–285. doi:10.1177/0020764006067186 PMID:16875199

Anish, K. R. (2013). An evaluation of psychosocial rehabilitation facilities for homeless mentally ill in India. *Arthraties Journal of Social Sciences*, *12*(2), 1–19.

Anthony, W., Cohen, M., & Farkas, M. (1991). *Psychiatric Rehabilitation.* Boston, MA: Boston University, Centre for Psychiatric Rehabilitation.

Appelbaum, K. L., Manning, T. D., & Noonan, J. D. (2002). A university-state-corporation partnership for providing correctional mental health services. *Psychiatric Services (Washington, D.C.)*, *53*(2), 185–189. doi:10.1176/appi.ps.53.2.185 PMID:11821549

Arias, F., Szerman, N., Vega, P., Mesias, B., Basurte, I., Morant, C., & Babin, F. (2013). Abuse or dependence on cannabis and other psychiatric disorders. Madrid study on dual pathology prevalence. *Actas Españolas de Psiquiatría*, *41*(2), 122–129. PMID:23592072

Arieti, S. (1959). Manic-Depressive Psychosis. American Handbook of Psychiatry, (1), 419-454.

Arseneault, L., Cannon, M., Poulton, R., Murray, R., Caspi, A., & Moffitt, T. E. (2002). Cannabis use in adolescence and risk for adult psychosis: Longitudinal prospective study. *BMJ (Clinical Research Ed.)*, *325*(7374), 1212–1213. doi:10.1136/bmj.325.7374.1212 PMID:12446537

Aschbrenner, A.K., Greenberg, J.S., & Seltzer, M. M. (2008). The long- term impact of parenting and adult child with bipolar disorder. *Research that Matters,* 17-20.

Assadi, S. M., Noroozian, M., Pakravannejad, M., Yahyazadeh, O., Aghayan, S., Shariat, S. V., & Fazel, S. (2006). Psychiatric morbidity among sentenced prisoners: Prevalence study in Iran. *The British Journal of Psychiatry*, *188*(2), 159–164. doi:10.1192/bjp.188.2.159 PMID:16449704

Atkinson, M., Zibin, S., & Chuang, H. (1997). Characterizing Quality of Life Among Patients With Chronic Mental Illness: A Critical Examination of the Self-Report Methodology. *The American Journal of Psychiatry*, *154*(1), 99–105. doi:10.1176/ajp.154.1.99 PMID:8988966

Awadalla, W. A., Ohaeri, J. U., Salih, A. A., & Tawfiq, A. M. (2005). Subjective quality of life of family caregivers of community living Sudanese psychiatric patients. *Social Psychiatry Epidemiology*, *40*(9), 755–763. doi:10.1007/s00127-005-0947-x PMID:16151598

Awad, G., & Voruganti, L. (2008). The Burden of Schizophrenia on Caregivers. *PharmacoEconomics*, *26*(2), 149–162. doi:10.2165/00019053-200826020-00005 PMID:18198934

Bachrach, L. L. (1988). Defining chronic mental illness: A concept pape. Hospital and Community, 398, 383–288.

Baer, J. S., Beadnell, B., Garrett, S. B., Hartzler, B., Wells, E. A., & Peterson, P. L. (2008). Adolescent change language within a brief motivational intervention and substance use outcomes. *Psychology of Addictive Behaviors*, *22*(4), 570–575. doi:10.1037/a0013022 PMID:19071983

Baer, J. S., Garrett, S. B., Beadnell, B., Wells, E. A., & Peterson, P. L. (2007). Brief Motivational Intervention With Homeless Adolescents: Evaluating Effects on Substance Use and Service Utilization. *Psychology of Addictive Behaviors*, *21*(4), 582–586. doi:10.1037/0893-164X.21.4.582 PMID:18072842

Baillargeon, J., Binswanger, I. A., Penn, J. V., Williams, B. A., & Murray, O. J. (2009). Psychiatric disorders and repeat incarcerations: The revolving prison door. *The American Journal of Psychiatry*, *166*(1), 103–109. doi:10.1176/appi.ajp.2008.08030416 PMID:19047321

Baker, A., Bucci, S., Lewin, T. J., Kay-Lambkin, F., Constable, P. M., & Carr, V. J. (2006). Cognitive-behavioural therapy for substance use disorders in people with psychotic disorders: Randomised controlled trial. *The British Journal of Psychiatry*, *188*(5), 439–448. doi:10.1192/bjp.188.5.439 PMID:16648530

Bal, B., Mitra, R., Mallick, A. H., Chakraborti, S., & Sarkar, K. (2010). Nontobacco substance use, sexual abuse, HIV, and sexually transmitted infection among street children in Kolkata, India. *Substance Use & Misuse*, *45*(10), 1668–1682. doi:10.3109/10826081003674856 PMID:20590379

Balmer, N., Pleasence, P., Buck, A., & Walker, H. (2006). Worried sick: The experience of debt problems and their relationship with health, illness and disability. *Social Policy and Society*, *5*(1), 39–51. doi:10.1017/S147474640500271X

Baltes, P. B., & Smith, J. (1999). Multilevel and systemic analyses of old age: theoretical and empirical evidence for a fourth age. In Handbook of Theories of Aging. Springer.

Baltes, P. B., & Baltes, M. M. (Eds.). (1990). *Successful Aging: Perspectives from the Behavioural Sciences*. New York: Cambridge University Press. doi:10.1017/CBO9780511665684

Balye, F.J., Krebs, M.O., Epelbaum, C., Levy, D., & Hardy, P. (2001). Clinical Features of panic attacks in schizophrenia. *European Psychiatry: The Journal of the Association of European Psychiatrist*, (6), 349-353.

Bandura, A. (1977). *Social Learning Theory*. Englewood Cliffs, NJ: Prentice-Hall.

Barch, D. M., & Sheffield, J. M. (2014). Cognitive impairments in psychotic disorders: Common mechanisms and measurement. *World Psychiatry; Official Journal of the World Psychiatric Association (WPA)*, *13*(3), 224–232. doi:10.1002/wps.20145 PMID:25273286

Barrett, P. M., Dadds, M. R., & Rapee, R. M. (1996). Family treatment of childhood anxiety: A controlled trial. *Journal of Consulting and Clinical Psychology*, *64*(2), 333–342. doi:10.1037/0022-006X.64.2.333 PMID:8871418

Bathla, M., Chandan, S., Bathla, J., & Kaloiya, G. S. (2015). Faith healers in morden psychiatric practice: Result of a four year study. *Delhi Psychiatric Journal*, 18(10).

Beach, S. R., Schulz, R., Yee, J. L., & Jackson, S. (2000). Negative and positive health effects of caring for a disabled spouse: Longitudinal findings from the caregiver health effects study. *Psychology and Aging*, *15*(2), 259–271. doi:10.1037/0882-7974.15.2.259 PMID:10879581

Bechdolf, A., Maier, S., Knost, B., & Wagner, M. (2003). A psychological early intervention program for the prepsychotic prodromal state. A case report. *Der Nervenarzt*, *74*, 436–439. doi:10.1007/s00115-002-1322-3 PMID:12966818

Beck, A. T. (1976). Cognitive therapy and the emotional disorders. International University Press.

Beck, R., & Fernandez, E. (1998). Cognitive Behaviour Therapy in the treatment of anger: A meta analysis. *Cognitive Therapy and Research*, *22*(1), 63–74. doi:10.1023/A:1018763902991

Bellack, A. S., & Hersen, M. (1989). Dictionary of behaviour therapy techniques. Pregamon Press.

Bellack, A. S., Blanchard, J. J., Murphy, P., & Podell, K. (1996). Generalization effects of training on the Wisconsin Card Sorting Test for schizophrenia patients. *Schizophrenia Research*, *19*(2-3), 189–194. doi:10.1016/0920-9964(95)00067-4 PMID:8789917

Bellack, A. S., Mueser, K. T., Gingerich, S., & Agresta, J. (2004). *Social skills training for schizophrenia: A step-by-step guide* (2nd ed.). New York: Guilford Press.

Bell, M., Bryson, G., Greig, T., Corcoran, C., & Wexler, B. E. (2001). Neurocognitive enhancement therapy with work therapy: Effects on neuropsychological test performance. *Archives of General Psychiatry*, *58*(8), 763–768. doi:10.1001/archpsyc.58.8.763 PMID:11483142

Benegal, V., Bhushan, K., Seshadri, S. P., & Karott, M. (1999). *Drug Abuse Among Street Children in Bangalore*. Unpublished manuscript, Bangalore.

Benegal, V., Sheshadri, S. P., Chand, P. K., Pandian, D., Lakshmana, G., & Subodh, B. N. (2010).Inhalant use among street children in Bangalore (Project report). Bangalore: NIMHANS (Unpublished Document).

Bengston, M. (2013). Types of Schizophrenia. *Psych Central*. Retrieved on February 4, 2016, from http://psychcentral.com/lib/types-of-schizophrenia

Ben-Yishay, U., & Diller, L. (1981). Cognitive deficits. In M. Rosenthal (Ed.), *Rehabilitation of the Head Injured Adult*. Philadelphia: F.A. Davis.

Bergman, H. F., Cervenka, S., Flyckt, L., Edman, G., & Farde, L. (2014). Meta-analysis of cognitive performance in drug-naïve patients with schizophrenia. *Schizophrenia Research*, *158*(1-3), 156–162. doi:10.1016/j.schres.2014.06.034 PMID:25086658

Bermu´dez, C.E., Romero Mendoza, M.P., Rodrı´guez Ruiz, E.M., Durand-Smith, A.L., & Saldı´var Herna´ndez, G.J. (2007). *Female depression and substance dependence in the Mexico City penitentiary system*. Academic Press.

Bertolote, J. M., & Fleischmann, A. (2002). Suicide and psychiatric diagnosis: A worldwide pe4rspective. *World Psychiatry; Official Journal of the World Psychiatric Association (WPA)*, *1*(3), 181–185. PMID:16946849

Bertolote, J. M., Fleischmann, A., De Leo, D., Bolhari, J., Botega, N., De Silva, D., & Wasserman, D. et al. (2005). Suicide attempts, plans, and ideation in culturally diverse sites: The WHO SUPRE-MISS community survey. *Psychological Medicine*, *35*(10), 1457–1465. doi:10.1017/S0033291705005404 PMID:16164769

Best, D. (1992). The role of social interaction in memory improvement. In D. Herrmann, H. Weingartner, A. Searleman, & C. McEvoy (Eds.), *Memory improvement: Implications for memory theory*. New York: Springer-Verlag. doi:10.1007/978-1-4612-2760-1_8

Betensky, M. G. (1995). *What do you see? Phenomenology of therapeutic art expression.* London: Jessica Kingsley.

Bhagwagar, Z. (2007). Bipolar disorder and its comorbidities. *Medscape Psychiatry.* Retrieved from http://www.medscape.org/viewarticle/558733

Bhattacharyya, S., Prasanna, C. L. N., Khanna, S., Janardhan Reddy, Y. C., & Sheshadri, S. (2005). A family Genetic study of clinical subtypes of obsessive-compulsive disorder. *Psychiatric Genetics, 15*(3), 175–180. doi:10.1097/00041444-200509000-00007 PMID:16094251

Bhushan, V., & Sachdeva, D. R. (2002). *An Introduction to Sociology* (34th ed.). Allahabad, India: Kitab Mahal.

Bianco, C., & Wells, S. M. (Eds.). (2001). *Overcoming Barriers to Community Integration for People with Mental Illnesses. Center for Mental Health Services Substance Abuse and Mental Health Services Administration (SAMHSA).* U.S. Department of Health and Human Services.

Bibring, E. (1953). The Mechanism of Depression. In P. Greenacre (Eds.), Affective disorders. New York: The University Press.

BienBOSCO. (1998). *In partnership for children.* Bangalore: Adithya.

Bines, W. (1994). *The health of single homeless people.* York, UK: Centre for Housing Policy, University of York.

Binswanger, I. A., Stern, M. F., & Deo, R. A. (2007). Release from prison: A high risk of death for former inmates. *Cross Ref Medline, 356*, 157–165. PMID:17215533

Birmaher, B., Axelson, D., Goldstein, B., Strober, M., Gill, M. K., Hunt, J., & Keller, M. et al. (2009). Four-Year Longitudinal Course of Children and Adolescents with Bipolar Spectrum Disorder: The Course and Outcome of Bipolar Youth (COBY) Study. *The American Journal of Psychiatry, 166*(7), 795–804. doi:10.1176/appi.ajp.2009.08101569 PMID:19448190

Birmaher, B., Brent, D. A., Kolko, D., Baugher, M., Bridge, J., Holder, D., & Ulloa, R. E. et al. (2000). Clinical outcome after short term psychotherapy for adolescents with major depressive disorder. *Archives of General Psychiatry, 57*(1), 29–86. doi:10.1001/archpsyc.57.1.29 PMID:10632230

Birmingham, L., Mason, D., & Grubin, D. (1996). Prevalence of mental disorder in remand prisoners: Consecutive case study. *British Medical Journal, 313*(7071), 1521-4.

Bjorgvinsson, T., Wetterneck, C. T., Powell, D. M., Chasson, G. S., Webb, S. A., Hart, J., & Stanley, M. A. et al. (2008). Treatment outcome for adolescent obsessive-compulsive disorder in a specialized hospital setting. *Journal of Psychiatric Practice, 14*(3), 137–145. doi:10.1097/01.pra.0000320112.36648.3e PMID:18520782

Black, D. W., & Blum, N. S. (1992). Obsessive-compulsive disorder support groups: The Iowa model. *Comprehensive Psychiatry, 33*(1), 65–71. doi:10.1016/0010-440X(92)90082-2 PMID:1555412

Blake, C.S., & Hamrin, V. (2007). Current approaches to the assessment and management of anger and aggression in youth: A review. *Journal of Child and Adolescent Psychiatric Nursing, 20*(4), 209-221.

Bleuler, E. (1950). *Dementia Praecox or The Group of Schizophrenias (Tranl. by Zinkin).* New York, NY: International Universities Press. (Original work published 1911)

Bloom, D. E., Cafiero, E. T., Jané-Llopis, E., Abrahams-Gessel, S., Bloom, L. R., Fathima, S., … Weinstein, C. (2011). *The Global Economic Burden of Noncommunicable Diseases.* Geneva: World Economic Forum.

Blow, F. C., Brockmann, L. M., & Barry, K. L. (2004). Role of alcohol in late-life suicide. *Alcoholism, Clinical and Experimental Research, 28*(5Suppl), 48S–56S. doi:10.1111/j.1530-0277.2004.tb03603.x PMID:15166636

Bluml, V., Kapusta, N. D., Doering, S., Brahler, E., Wagner, B., & Kersting, A. (2013). Personality Factors and Suicide Risk in a Representative Sample of the German General Population. *PLoS ONE*, *8*(10), e76646. doi:10.1371/journal.pone.0076646 PMID:24124582

Bobes, J., Gonzalez, M. P., Bascaran, M. T., Arango, C., Saiz, P. A., & Bousono, M. (2001). Quality of life and disability in patient with obsessive-compulsive disorder. *European Psychiatry*, *16*(4), 239–245. doi:10.1016/S0924-9338(01)00571-5 PMID:11418275

Boeding, S. E., Paprocki, C. M., Baucom, D. H., Abramowitz, J. S., Wheaton, M. G., Fabricant, L. E., & Fischer, M. S. (2013). Let me check that for you: Symptom accommodation in romantic partners of adults with obsessive–compulsive disorder. *Behaviour Research and Therapy*, *51*(6), 316–322. doi:10.1016/j.brat.2013.03.002 PMID:23567474

Bohanna, I., & Wang, X. (2012). Media guidelines for the responsible reporting of suicide: A review of effectiveness. Crisis. *Journal of Crisis Intervention & Suicide*, *33*(4), 190–198. doi:10.1027/0227-5910/a000137 PMID:22713977

Bombay prevention of begging Act (1959) Complete Act- Bare Act.

Bora, E., Yucel, M., & Pantelis, C. (2009). Cognitive functioning in schizophrenia, schizoaffective disorder and affective psychoses: Meta-analytic study. *The British Journal of Psychiatry*, *195*(6), 475–482. doi:10.1192/bjp.bp.108.055731 PMID:19949193

Botvin, G. J., Baker, E., Botvin, E. M., Filazzola, A. D., & Millman, R. B. (1984). Alcohol abuse prevention through the development of personal and social competence: A pilot study. *Journal of Studies on Alcohol*, *45*, 550–554. doi:10.15288/jsa.1984.45.550 PMID:6521482

Boundless. (2015). Continuity Theory. *Boundless Sociology*. Retrieved 20 Dec. 2015 from https://www.boundless.com/sociology/textbooks/boundless-sociology-textbook/aging-18/the-functionalist-perspective-on-aging-128/continuity-theory-723-3593/

Bowie, C. R., & Harvey, P. D. (2005). Cognition in Schizophrenia: Impairments, Determinants, and Functional Importance. *The Psychiatric Clinics of North America*, *28*(3), 613–633. doi:10.1016/j.psc.2005.05.004 PMID:16122570

Bowie, C. R., Leung, W. W., Reichenberg, A., McClure, M. M., Patterson, T. L., Heaton, R. K., & Harvey, P. D. (2008). Predicting schizophrenia patients' real-world behavior with specific neuropsychological and functional capacity measures. *Biological Psychiatry*, *63*(5), 505–511. doi:10.1016/j.biopsych.2007.05.022 PMID:17662256

Bowie, C. R., Reichenberg, A., Patterson, T. L., Heaton, R. K., & Harvey, P. D. (2006). Determinants of real-world functional performance in schizophrenia subjects: Correlations with cognition, functional capacity, and symptoms. *The American Journal of Psychiatry*, *163*(3), 418–425. doi:10.1176/appi.ajp.163.3.418 PMID:16513862

Bowlby, J. (1969). *Attachment*. New York: Basic Books.

Bracy, O. L. (1986). Cognitive rehabilitation: A process approach. *Cognitive Rehabilitation*, *4*, 10–17.

Brady, K. T., & Verduin, M. L. (2005). Pharmacotherapy of comorbid mood, anxiety, and substance use disorders. *Substance Use & Misuse*, *40*(13-14), 2021–2041, 2043–2048. doi:10.1080/10826080500294924 PMID:16282091

Branch, L. G., Wetle, T. T., Scherr, P. A., Cook, N. R., Evans, D. A., Hebert, L. E., & Taylor, J. O. et al. (1988). A prospective study of incident comprehensive medical home care use among the elderly. *American Journal of Public Health*, *78*(3), 255–259. doi:10.2105/AJPH.78.3.255 PMID:3124639

Brands, B., Leslie, K., Catz-Biro, L., & Li, S. (2005). Heroin use and barriers to treatment in street-involved youth. *Addiction Research and Theory*, *13*(5), 477–487. doi:10.1080/16066350500150624

Brannigan, G. G., & Decker, S. L. (2003). *Bender Visual-Motor Gestalt Test* (2nd Ed). Itasca, IL: Riverside Publishing. Retrieved from www.riversidepublishing.com

Brenes, G. A., Guralnik, J. M., Williamson, J. D., Fried, L. P., Simpson, C., Simonsick, E. M., & Penninx, B. W. J. H. (2005). The influence of anxiety on the progression of disability. *Journal of the American Geriatrics Society*, *53*(1), 34–39. doi:10.1111/j.1532-5415.2005.53007.x PMID:15667373

Brenes, G. A., Kritchevsky, S. B., & Mehta, K. M. (2007). Scared to death: Results from the Health, Aging, and Body Composition study. *The American Journal of Geriatric Psychiatry*, *15*, 262–265. PMID:17322138

Brinded, P. M., Simpson, A. I. F., Laidlaw, T. M., Fairley, N., & Malcolm, F. (2001). Prevalence of psychiatric disorders in New Zealand prisons: A national study. *The Australian and New Zealand Journal of Psychiatry*, *35*(2), 166–173. doi:10.1046/j.1440-1614.2001.00885.x PMID:11284897

Brissos, S., Balanzá-Martinez, V., Dias, V. V., Carita, A. I., & Figueira, M. L. (2011). Is personal and social functioning associated with subjective quality of life in schizophrenia patients living in the community? *European Archives of Psychiatry and Clinical Neuroscience*, *261*(7), 509–517. doi:10.1007/s00406-011-0200-z PMID:21384166

Brissos, S., Molodynski, A., Vasco Videira Dias, V. V., & Figueira, M. L. (2011). The importance of measuring psychosocial functioning in schizophrenia. *Annals of General Psychiatry*, *10*(1), 18. doi:10.1186/1744-859X-10-18 PMID:21702932

Brooke, S. L. (1995). Art therapy: An approach to working with sexual abuse survivors. *The Arts in Psychotherapy*, *22*(5), 447–466. doi:10.1016/0197-4556(95)00036-4

Brown, G.K., & Gibbs, J. (1996). *Community Mental Health Centers and Homeless Persons: A report from the office of the Inspector General of HHS*. Washington, DC: U.S. Department of Health and Human Services.

Browne, G. M., Morick, E., Carstairs, G., & Wing, J. (1962). Influence of family life on the course of Schizophrenia illness. *British Journal of Preventive & Social Medicine*, *16*, 55–68.

Browne, K., & Falshaw, L. (1998). Street children and crime in the UK: A case of abuse and neglect. *Child Abuse Review*, *7*(4), 241–253. doi:10.1002/(SICI)1099-0852(199807/08)7:4<241::AID-CAR501>3.0.CO;2-0

Brownell, B. (2014). *Crime and Justice, Health Care, Human Rights, Prisons, op Stories, There Are 10 Times More Mentally Ill People Behind Bars Than in State Hospitals*. Academic Press.

Browne, S., Clarke, M., & Gervin, M. (2000). Determinants of quality of life at first presentation with schizophrenia. *The British Journal of Psychiatry*, *176*(2), 173–176. doi:10.1192/bjp.176.2.173 PMID:10755056

Brown, G. K., Ten Have, T., Henriques, G. R., Xie, S. X., Hollander, J. E., & Beck, A. T. (2005). Cognitive therapy for the prevention of suicide attempts: A randomized controlled trial. *Journal of the American Medical Association*, *294*(5), 563–570. doi:10.1001/jama.294.5.563 PMID:16077050

Brugha, T., Singleton, N., Meltzer, H., Bebbington, P., Farrell, M., Jenkins, R., & Lewis, G. et al. (2005). Psychosis in the community and in prisons: A report from the British National Survey of psychiatric morbidity. *The American Journal of Psychiatry*, *162*(4), 774–780. doi:10.1176/appi.ajp.162.4.774 PMID:15800152

Brunet, G. E., & Decety, J. (2006). Social brain dysfunctions in schizophrenia: A review of neuroimaging studies. *Psychiatry Research*, *148*(2-3), 75–92. doi:10.1016/j.pscychresns.2006.05.001 PMID:17088049

Bryson, G. J., Silverstein, M. L., Nathan, A., & Stephen, L. (1993). Differential rate of neuropsychological dysfunction in psychiatric disorders: Comparison between the Halstead-Reitan and Luria-Nebraska batteries. *Perceptual and Motor Skills*, *76*, 305–306. PMID:8451141

Burlingame, G. M., Fuhriman, A., & Johnson, J. E. (2001). Cohesion in group psychotherapy. *Psychotherapy (Chicago, Ill.), 38*(4), 373–379. doi:10.1037/0033-3204.38.4.373

Burnam, M. A., & Watkins, K. E. (2006). Substance abuse with mental disorders: Specialized public systems and integrated care. *Health Affairs (Project Hope), 25*(3), 648–658. doi:10.1377/hlthaff.25.3.648 PMID:16684728

Burns, T., Baldwin, D., Emsley, R., Kerwin, R., Steinberg, J., & Van Os, J. (1999). Treatment challenges in schizophrenia. *Primary Care Psychiatry, 5*(3), 117–123.

Burt, M. R. (2001). *Helping America's homeless.* Washington, DC: Urban InstitutePress.

Busch-Geertsema, V., Edgar, W., O'Sullivan, E., & Pleace, N. (2010). *Homelessness and Homeless policies in Europe: lessons from research.* In FEANTSA: A report prepared for the European Consensus Conference on Homelessness.

Butler, T. K., Males, J. J., Robinson, L. P., Wechsler, A. W., Sutton, G. L., Cheng, J., & McClellan, K. et al. (1997). Six-year review of Acanthamoeba keratitis in New South Wales, Australia: 1997-2002. *Clinical & Experimental Ophthalmology, 33*(1), 41–46. doi:10.1111/j.1442-9071.2004.00911.x PMID:15670077

Butler, T., & Allnutt, S. (2003). *Mental Illness among New South Wales Prisoners.* NSW Correction Health Service.

Calabrese, J. R., Hirschfeld, R. M., Reed, M., Davies, M. A., Frye, M. A., Keck, P. E. Jr, & Wagner, K. D. et al. (2003). Impact of bipolar disorder on a U.S. community sample. *The Journal of Clinical Psychiatry, 64*(4), 425–432. doi:10.4088/JCP.v64n0412 PMID:12716245

California Department of Corrections and Rehabilitation Report. (2014). *Unless otherwise noted, all data in this report were provided by the For purposes of this report, "mental illness" is defined as a condition that qualifies for placement in the prison's Mental Health Delivery System within the last year.* Academic Press.

Callahan, A. M., & Bauer, M. S. (1999). Psychosocial interventions for bipolar disorder. *The Psychiatric Clinics of North America, 22*(3), 675–688. doi:10.1016/S0193-953X(05)70102-7 PMID:10550862

Calvocoressi, L., Mazure, C. M., Kasl, S. V., Skolnick, J., Fisk, D., Vegso, S. J., & Price, L. H. et al. (1999). Family accommodation of obsessive-compulsive symptoms: Instrument development and assessment of family behavior. *The Journal of Nervous and Mental Disease, 187*(10), 636–642. doi:10.1097/00005053-199910000-00008 PMID:10535658

Canavan, R., Barry, M. M., Matanov, A., Barros, H., Gabor, E., Greacen, T., & Priebe, S. et al. (2012). Service provision and barriers to care for homeless people with mental health problems across 14 European capital cities. *BMC Health Services Research, 12*(1), 222. doi:10.1186/1472-6963-12-222 PMID:22838503

Canaway, R., & Merkes, M. (2010). Barriers to comorbidity service delivery: the complexities of dual diagnosis and the need to agree on terminology and conceptual frameworks. *Australian Health Review: A Publication of the Australian Hospital Association, 34*(3), 262–268.

Cannon, M., & Jones, P. (1996). Schizophrenia. *Journal of Neurology, Neurosurgery and Psychiatry,* (60), 604-613.

Caplan, C. (1964). Principles of Preventive Psychiatry. New York: Basic Books, Inc.

Carey, K. B. (1996). Substance use reduction in the context of outpatient psychiatric treatment: A collaborative, motivational, harm reduction approach. *Community Mental Health Journal, 32*(3), 291–306, discussion 307–310. doi:10.1007/BF02249430 PMID:8790970

Caron, J., Mercier, C., Diaz, P., & Martin, A. (2005). Socio-demographic and clinical predictors of quality of life in patients with schizophrenia or schizo-affective disorder. *Psychiatry Research, 137*(3), 203–213. doi:10.1016/j.psychres.2005.07.002 PMID:16298428

Carpentier, N., Lesage, A., & Goulet, J. (1992). Burden of care of families not living with young Schizophrenia relatives. *Hospital & Community Psychiatry*, *43*, 38–43. PMID:1544645

Carson, V. B., & Saunders, W. B. (2000). *Mental health nursing: the nurse-patient journey*. Schizophrenia.

Carter, C. S., & Barch, D. M. (2000). Attention, memory and language disturbances in schizophrenia: Characteristics and implications. In Advances in psychiatry (pp. 45–72). Oxford University Press.

Carter, G. L., Child, C., Page, A., Clover, K., & Taylor, R. (2007). Modifiable risk factors for attempted suicide in Australian clinical and community samples. *Suicide & Life-Threatening Behavior*, *37*(6), 671–680. doi:10.1521/suli.2007.37.6.671 PMID:18275373

Caspi, A., Moffitt, T. E., Cannon, M., McClay, J., Murray, R., Harrington, H., & Craig, I. W. (2005). Moderation of the effect of adolescent-onset cannabis use on adult psychosis by a functional polymorphism in the catechol-O-methyltransferase gene: Longitudinal evidence of a gene X environment interaction. *Biological Psychiatry*, *57*(10), 1117–1127. doi:10.1016/j.biopsych.2005.01.026 PMID:15866551

Caspi, A., Reichenberg, A., Weiser, M., Rabinowitz, J., Kaplan, Z., Knobler, H., & Davidson, M. et al. (2003). Cognitive performance in schizophrenia patients assessed before and following the first psychotic episode. *Schizophrenia Research*, *65*(2-3), 87–94. doi:10.1016/S0920-9964(03)00056-2 PMID:14630301

Cavanagh, J. T., Carson, A. J., Sharpe, M., & Lawrie, S. M. (2003). Psychological autopsy studies of suicide: A systematic review. Psychological Medicine, 33(3), 395–405. doi:10.1017/S0033291702006943 PubMed doi:10.1017/S0033291702006943 PMID:12701661

Census of India report, homeless population. (2001). Office of registrar general & census commissioner, India.

Centers for Disease Control and Prevention. (2010). Attitudes toward Mental Illness-35 States, District of Columbia, and Puerto Rico, 2007. *Morbidity and Mortality Weekly Report*, *59*(20), 619–625. Available from http://www.cdc.gov/mmwr/preview/mmwrhtml/mm5920a3.htm

Centre for Mental Health. (2010). Economic and social costs of mental health problems in 2009/10. London: Author.

Chadda, R. K. (2014). Caring for the family caregivers of persons with mental illness. *Indian Journal of Psychiatry*, *56*(3), 221–227. doi:10.4103/0019-5545.140616 PMID:25316932

Chadda, R. K., Singh, T. B., & Ganguly, K. K. (2007). Caregiver burden and coping: A prospective study of relationship between burden and coping in caregivers of patients with schizophrenia and bipolar affective disorder. *Social Psychiatry and Psychiatric Epidemiology*, *42*(11), 923–930. doi:10.1007/s00127-007-0242-8 PMID:17700975

Chakraborty, S., Kulahara, P., & Verma, S. K. (1992). Extent and determinants of burden among families of patients with affective disorders. *Acta Psychiatrica Scandinavica*, *86*(3), 247–252. doi:10.1111/j.1600-0447.1992.tb03261.x PMID:1414422

Chalise, H. N. (2014). *Depression among elderly living in Briddashram (OAH). Advances in Aging Research*. AAR. doi:10.4236/aar.31002

Chamberlain, C., & Johnson, G. (2002). The development of Prevention and early intervention services for homeless youth: Intervening successfully (Position Paper). Melbourne: Australian Urban Housing Research Institute (AUHRI).

Chamberlain, C., & MacKenzie, D. (2008). Youth Homelessness. *Youth Studies*, (27), 17-25.

Chamberlain, C. (1999). *Counting the homeless: Implications for policy development*. Canberra: Australian Bureau of Statistics.

Chamberlain, C., & MacKenzie, D. (1992). Understanding Contemporary Homelessness: Issues of Definition and Meaning. *The Australian Journal of Social Issues*, *27*(4), 274–297.

Chambers, R. A., Krystal, J. H., & Self, D. W. (2001). A neurobiological basis for substance abuse comorbidity in schizophrenia. *Biological Psychiatry*, *50*(2), 71–83. doi:10.1016/S0006-3223(01)01134-9 PMID:11526998

Chambless, D., & Steketee, G. (1999). Expressed emotion and behavior therapy outcome: A prospective study with obsessive-compulsive and agoraphobic outpatients. *Journal of Consulting and Clinical Psychology*, *67*(5), 658–665. doi:10.1037/0022-006X.67.5.658 PMID:10535232

Chandrashekar, H., Prashanth, N.R., Kasthuri, P., & Madhusudan, S. (2010). Psychiatric Rehabilitation. *Indian Journal of Psychiatry, 52*(1), 278-280.

Chapman, D. P., Perry, G. S., & Strine, T. W. (2005). The vital link between chronic disease and depressive disorders. *Preventing Chronic Disease*, *2*(1). Available from http://www.cdc.gov/pcd/issues/2005/jan/04_0066.htm PMID:15670467

Chaudhury, P. K., Deka, K., & Chetia, D. (2006). Disability associated with mental disorders. Indian Journal of Psychiatry, 48(2), 95–101. doi:10.4103/0019-5545.31597 PubMed doi:10.4103/0019-5545.31597 PMID:20703393

Chen, E. Y. H., & McKenna, P. J. (1996) Memory dysfunction in schizophrenia. In Schizophrenia: A Neuropsychological Perspective (pp. 107-124). New York, NY: John Wiley and Sons.

Chien, W. T., Chan, S. W., & Morrissey, J. (2007). The perceived burden among Chinese family caregivers of people with schizophrenia. *Journal of Clinical Nursing*, *16*(6), 1151–1161. doi:10.1111/j.1365-2702.2007.01501.x PMID:17518890

Christopher, J.L., & Murray, M.D. (2013). *UK health performance: findings of the Global Burden of Disease Study 2010*. Academic Press.

Cisneros. (1997). Searching for Home: Mentally Ill Homeless People in America. *Cityscape (Washington, D.C.)*, 155–172.

Clothier, F. (1943). The Psychology of the Adopted Child. The National Committee for Mental Hygiene. *Mental Hygiene*, 27.

Code of Civil Procedure. (1908). *Bare Act; Bare Act*. Lucknow: Eastern Book Company.

Code of Criminal Procedure Amendment Act. (2010). Bare Act; Eastern Book Company, Lucknow.

Cohen, C. I., Magai, C., Yaffee, R., & Walcott-Brown, L. (2006). The prevalence of anxiety and associated factors in a multiracial sample of older adults. *Psychiatric Services (Washington, D.C.)*, *57*(12), 1719–1725. doi:10.1176/ps.2006.57.12.1719 PMID:17158485

Cohen, S. (1984). The Hallucinogens and the inhalants. *The Psychiatric Clinics of North America*, *7*, 681–688. PMID:6097885

Coid, J. (1984). How many psychiatric patients in prison? *The British Journal of Psychiatry*, *145*(1), 78–86. doi:10.1192/bjp.145.1.78 PMID:6743949

Coie, J. D. (1990). Toward a theory of peer rejection. In S. R. Asher, & J. D. Coie (Eds.), Peer rejection in childhood (pp. 365–401). New York: Cambridge University Press.

Coldham, E.L., Addington, J., & Addington, D. (2002). *Medication adherence of individuals with a first episode of psychosis*. Academic Press.

Cole, J. D., & Kazarian, S. S. (1993). Predictive validity of the Level of Expressed Emotion (LEE) Scale: Readmission follow-up data for 1, 2, and 5-year periods. *Journal of Clinical Psychology*, *49*(2), 216–218. doi:10.1002/1097-4679(199303)49:2<216::AID-JCLP2270490214>3.0.CO;2-G PMID:8098049

Colton, C. W., & Manderscheid, R. W. (2006). Congruencies in increased mortality rates, years of potential life lost, and causes of death among public mental health clients in eight states. *Preventing Chronic Disease*, *3*(2). Available from http://www.cdc.gov/pcd/issues/2006/apr/05_0180.htm PMID:16539783

Commission for Architecture and the Built Environment .(2009). Independent living by design CABE London

Conrod, P. J., Castellanos-Ryan, N., & Strang, J. (2010). Brief, Personality-Targeted Coping Skills Interventions and Survival as a Non–Drug User Over a 2-Year Period During Adolescence. *Archives of General Psychiatry*, *67*(1), 85–93. doi:10.1001/archgenpsychiatry.2009.173 PMID:20048226

Consortium For Street Children. (2011). *Street Children Statistics*. Retrieved on 5 July 2011 from http://www.streetchildren.org.uk/reports/State%20of%20he%20World's%20Street%20Children-Violence.pdf

Convention on Rights of Person with Disability. (n.d.). Available online on website http://www.un.org/disabilities/countries.asp?id=166htm

Conway, K. P., Compton, W., Stinson, F. S., & Grant, B. F. (2006). Lifetime comorbidity of DSM-IV mood and anxiety disorders and specific drug use disorders: Results from the National Epidemiologic Survey on Alcohol and Related Conditions. *The Journal of Clinical Psychiatry*, *67*(2), 247–257. doi:10.4088/JCP.v67n0211 PMID:16566620

Cooke, B. K. (2013). Extended Suicide With a Pet. *The Journal of the American Academy of Psychiatry and the Law*, *41*, 437–443. PMID:24051598

Coonerty, S. (1993). Integrative child therapy. In G. Stricker & J. R. Gold (Eds.), *Comprehensive handbook of psychotherapy integration*. New York, NY: Plenum Press; doi:10.1007/978-1-4757-9782-4_28

Cooper, M. (1996). Obsessive-compulsive disorder: Effects on family members. *TheAmerican Journal of Orthopsychiatry*, *66*(2), 296–304. doi:10.1037/h0080180 PMID:8860758

Cornelius, J. R., Bukstein, O., Salloum, I., & Clark, D. (2003). Alcohol and psychiatric comorbidity. Recent Developments in Alcoholism: An Official Publication of the American Medical Society on Alcoholism, the Research Society on Alcoholism, and the National Council on Alcoholism, 16, 361–374.

Cornish, J. W., Metzger, D., Woody, G. E., Wilson, D., McLellan, A. T., Vandergrift, B., & O'Brien, C. P. (1997). Naltrexone pharmacotherapy for opioid dependent federal probationers. *Journal of Substance Abuse Treatment*, *14*(6), 529–534. doi:10.1016/S0740-5472(97)00020-2 PMID:9437624

Corrigan, P. W., Markowitz, F. E., & Watson, A. C. (2004). Structural levels of mental illness: Stigma and discrimination. *Schizophrenia Bulletin*, *20*(3), 481–491. doi:10.1093/oxfordjournals.schbul.a007096 PMID:15631241

Coumarelos, C., Wei, Z., & Zhou, A. (2006). *Justice made to measure: NSW Legal Needs Survey in disadvantaged areas*. Sydney: Law and Justice Foundation of NSW.

Council of Europe. (1998). *Recommendation NO R (98) 11 on the organisation of health care services for the chronically ill (Adopted by the Committee of Ministers at the 641st meeting of the Ministers' Deputies)*. Author.

Cowen, R. (1968). A new type of delthyrial cover in the Devonian brachiopod Mucrospirifer. Palaeontology, 11, 317–327.

Coyle, J. (2006). The Neurochemistry of Schizophrenia. In *Basic Neurochemistry: Molecular, Cellular and Medical Aspects* (7th ed.; p. 876). Burlington, MA: Elsevier Academic Press.

Crane, M. (1998). The associations between mental illness and homelessness among older people: An exploratory study. *Aging & Mental Health*, *2*(3), 171–180. doi:10.1080/13607869856641

Creado, D. A., Parkar, S. R., & Kamath, R. M. (2006). A comparison of the level of functioning in chronic schizophrenia with coping and burden in caregivers. *Indian Journal of Psychiatry*, *48*(1), 27–33. doi:10.4103/0019-5545.31615 PMID:20703411

Crowther, R., Marshall, M., Bond, G., & Huxley, P. (2001). Vocational Rehabilitation for people with severe mental illness. *Cochrane Database of Systematic Reviews*, *2*, CD00380. doi:10.1002/14651858.CD003080 PMID:11406069

Cuffel, B. J., Heithoff, K. A., & Lawson, W. (1993). Correlates of patterns of substance abuse among patients with schizophrenia. *Hospital & Community Psychiatry*, *44*, 247–251. PMID:8444435

Cuijpers, P., de Beurs, D. P., van Spijker, B. A., Berking, M., Andersson, G., & Kerkhof, A. J. (2013). The effects of psychotherapy for adult depression on suicidality and hopelessness: A systematic review and meta-analysis. *Journal of Affective Disorders*, *144*(3), 183–190. doi:10.1016/j.jad.2012.06.025 PMID:22832172

Cullen, K. R., Kumra. S., & Regan, J. (2008). Atypical Antipsychotics for Treatment of Schizophrenia Spectrum Disorders. *Psychiatric Times*, *25*(3).

Current Statistics on the Prevalence and Characteristics of People Experiencing Homelessness in the United States. (2011). SAMHSA.

Currie, A. (2007). Civil justice problems and the disability and health status of Canadians. In P. Pleasence, A. Buck, & N. Balmer (Eds.), *Transforming lives: law and social process*. London: The Stationary Office.

D'ambrosio, V., Albert, U., Bogetto, F., & Maina, G. (2010). Obsessive-compulsive disorder and cyclothymic temperament: An exploration of clinical features. *Journal of Affective Disorders*, *127*(1-3), 295–299. doi:10.1016/j.jad.2010.06.007 PMID:20591494

da Silva Gdel, G., Jansen, K., Barbosa, L. P., Branco Jda, C., Pinheiro, R. T., Magalhães, P. V., & da Silva, R. A. et al. (2013). Burden and related factors in caregivers of young adults presenting bipolar and unipolar mood disorder. *TheInternational Journal of Social Psychiatry*, *60*(4), 396–402. doi:10.1177/0020764013491740 PMID:23828767

Dalack, G. W., Healy, D. J., & Meador-Woodruff, J. H. (1998). Nicotine dependence in schizophrenia: Clinical phenomena and laboratory findings. *The American Journal of Psychiatry*, *155*(11), 1490–1501. doi:10.1176/ajp.155.11.1490 PMID:9812108

Dale, D. M. (2000). The state of access to justice in Oregon, part 1: assessment of legal needs. Portland, OR: Oregon State Bar. Retrieved from http://www.nlada.org/DMS/Documents/1028902493.69/ LegalNeedsreport.pdf

Dalley, Rifkind, & Terry. (1993). *Three voices of art therapy: image, client therapist*. London: Routledge.

Daniel, A. E. (2006). Preventing suicide in prison: A collaborative responsibility of administrative, custodial, and clinical staff. *The Journal of the American Academy of Psychiatry and the Law*, *34*(2), 165–175. PMID:16844795

Daniels, J., D'Andrea, M., Omizo, M., & Pier, P. (1999). Group work with homeless youngsters and their mothers. *Journal for Specialists in Group Work*, *24*(2), 164–185. doi:10.1080/01933929908411428

Davenport, L. (2008). Patient depression predicts bipolar disorder caregiver burden. *Acta Psychiatrica Scandinavica*, *118*, 49–56. doi:10.1111/j.1600-0447.2008.01201.x PMID:18582347

Davenport, L. (2008). Quality of life reduced in euphoric bipolar disorder. *Perspectives in Psychiatric Care*, *44*, 275–284. PMID:18826466

Davies, R. D., Gabbert, S. L., & Riggs, P. D. (2001). Anxiety disorders in neurologic illness. *Current Treatment Options in Neurology*, *3*(3), 333–346. doi:10.1007/s11940-001-0038-1 PMID:11389804

De geus, F., Denys, D. A., Sitskoorn, M.M., & Westenberg, H.G. (2007). Attention and cognition in patients with obsessive-compulsive disorder. *Psychiatry and Clinical Neuroscience, 61*(1), 45-53.

De Leo, D. (2002). Suicide among the elderly: The long-term impact of a telephone support and assessment intervention in northern Italy. *The British Journal of Psychiatry, 181*(3), 226–229. doi:10.1192/bjp.181.3.226 PMID:12204927

De Leo, D., Carollo, G., & DelloBuono, M. (1995). Lower suicide rates associated with a tele-help/tele-check service for the elderly at home. *The American Journal of Psychiatry, 152*(4), 632–634. doi:10.1176/ajp.152.4.632 PMID:7694919

de Leo, D., & Heller, T. (2008). Social modeling in the transmission of suicidality. Crisis. *Journal of Crisis Intervention & Suicide, 29*(1), 11–19. doi:10.1027/0227-5910.29.1.11

de Mathis, M. A., do Rosario, M. C., Diniz, J. B., Torres, A. R., Shavitt, R. G., Ferrao, Y. A., & Miguel, E. C. et al. (2008). Obsessive-compulsive disorder: Influence of age at onset on comorbidity patterns. *European Psychiatry, 23*(3), 187–194. doi:10.1016/j.eurpsy.2008.01.002 PMID:18329252

Dean, B., Sundram, S., Bradbury, R., Scarr, E., & Copolov, D. (2001). Studies on [3H]CP-55940 binding in the human central nervous system: Regional specific changes in density of cannabinoid-1 receptors associated with schizophrenia and cannabis use. *Neuroscience, 103*(1), 9–15. doi:10.1016/S0306-4522(00)00552-2 PMID:11311783

DeFilippis, M. S., & Wagner, K. D. (2013). Bipolar depression in children and adolescents. *CNS Spectrums, 18*(04), 209–213. doi:10.1017/S1092852913000217 PMID:23570693

DelBello, M. P., Schwiers, M. L., Rosenberg, H. L., & Strakowski, S. M. (2002). A double-blind, randomized, placebo-controlled study of quetiapine as adjunctive treatment for adolescent mania. *Journal of the American Academy of Child and Adolescent Psychiatry, 41*(10), 1216–1223. doi:10.1097/00004583-200210000-00011 PMID:12364843

Demyttenaere, K., Bruffaerts, R., & Posada, V. J. (2004). Prevalence, Severity, and Unmet Need for Treatment of Mental Disorders in the World Health Organization World Mental Health Surveys. *JAMA, 291*(21), 2581-90.

Demyttenaere, K., Bruffaerts, R., Posada-Villa, J., Gasquet, I., Kovess, V., & Lepine, J. P. (2004). World Health Organization (WHO) World Mental Health Survey Consortium. Prevalence, severity, and unmet need for treatment of mental disorders in the WHO, World Mental Health Surveys. *Journal of the American Medical Association, 291*, 2581–2590. doi:10.1001/jama.291.21.2581 PMID:15173149

Denys, D., Tenney, N., vanMegen, H. J., de Geus, F., & Westenberg, H. G. (2004). Axis I and II comorbidity in a large sample of patients with obsessive-compulsive disorder. *Journal of Affective Disorders, 80*(2-3), 155–162. doi:10.1016/S0165-0327(03)00056-9 PMID:15207928

Desai, N. G., & Gupta, D. K. (1999). Substance use disorders. In *Textbook of post graduate Psychiatry* (2nd ed., pp. 76–89). New Delhi: Jaypee Publishers.

Dhanda, A. (2000). *Legal order and mental disorder*. New Delhi: Sage Publications.

Dhawan, A., Chopra, A., Ambekar, A., & Ray, R. (2015). Treatment seeking behavior of Inhalant using street children: Are we prepared to meet their treatment needs. *Indian Journal of Psychological Medicine, 37*(3), 282–287. doi:10.4103/0253-7176.162918 PMID:26664076

Diagnostic and Statistical Manual of Mental Disorders. (1994). Washington, DC: American psychiatric association.

Dickey, B., & Azeni, H. (1996). Persons with dual diagnoses of substance abuse and major mental illness: Their excess costs of psychiatric care. *American Journal of Public Health, 86*(7), 973–977. doi:10.2105/AJPH.86.7.973 PMID:8669521

Directorate of Welfare of Disabled and Senior Citizens, Government of Karnataka. (2008).

Disability-adjusted life year (DALY). (2016). From *Wikipedia, the free encyclopedia*. Retrieved from https://en.wikipedia.org/wiki/Disability-adjusted_life_year

Donald, B. (1963). *Skid Row in American Cities*. Chicago: Community and Family Studies Centre, University of Chicago.

Dore, G., & Romans, S. E. (2001). Impact of bipolar affective disorder on family and partners. *Journal of Affective Disorders*, *67*(1-3), 147–158. doi:10.1016/S0165-0327(01)00450-5 PMID:11869762

Doris, J. J., & Lauren, E. G. (2006). *Mental Health Problems of Prison and Jail Inmates*. Bureau of Justice Statistics.

Dowling, S., Manthorpe, J., Cowley, S., King, S., Raymond, V., & Perez, W. (2006). *Person-centred planning in social care: A scoping review*. Joseph Rowntree Foundation, King's College London.

Drake, R. E., Goldman, H. H., Leff, H. S., Lehman, A. F., Dixon, L., Mueser, K. T., & Torrey, W. C. (2001). Implementing evidence-based practices in routine mental health service settings. *Psychiatric Services (Washington, D.C.)*, *52*(2), 179–182. doi:10.1176/appi.ps.52.2.179 PMID:11157115

Drake, R. E., Mercer-McFadden, C., Mueser, K. T., McHugo, G. J., & Bond, G. R. (1998). Review of integrated mental health and substance abuse treatment for patients with dual disorders. *Schizophrenia Bulletin*, *24*(4), 589–608. doi:10.1093/oxfordjournals.schbul.a033351 PMID:9853791

Drake, R. E., Mueser, K. T., Brunette, M. F., & McHugo, G. J. (2004). A review of treatments for people with severe mental illnesses and co-occurring substance use disorders. *Psychiatric Rehabilitation Journal*, *27*(4), 360–374. doi:10.2975/27.2004.360.374 PMID:15222148

Drake, R. E., Mueser, K. T., Clark, R. E., & Wallach, M. A. (1996). The course, treatment, and outcome of substance disorder in persons with severe mental illness. *The American Journal of Orthopsychiatry*, *66*(1), 42–51. doi:10.1037/h0080153 PMID:8720640

Drake, R. E., & Wallach, M. A. (2000). Dual diagnosis: 15 years of progress. *Psychiatric Services (Washington, D.C.)*, *51*(9), 1126–1129. doi:10.1176/appi.ps.51.9.1126 PMID:10970914

Drake, R. J., & Lewis, S. W. (2005). Early detection of schizophrenia. *Current Opinion in Psychiatry*, *144*, 718–726. PMID:16639167

Dreikurs, S. E. (1986). *Cows can be purple: My life & art therapy*. Chicago: Adler School of Professional Psychology. Dunn, M.B.

Drew, A. E., Derbez, A. E., & Werling, L. L. (2000). Nicotinic receptor-mediated regulation of dopamine transporter activity in rat prefrontal cortex. *Synapse (New York, N.Y.)*, *38*(1), 10–16. doi:10.1002/1098-2396(200010)38:1<10::AID-SYN2>3.0.CO;2-T PMID:10941136

Dubey, A., Bhasin, S., Gupta, N., & Sharma, N. (2011). A Study of elderly livingin old age home and with infamily set-up in Jammu. *Studies on Home and Community Science*, *5*(2), 93–98.

Duffy, D., Linehan, S., & Kennedy, H.G. (2006). *Psychiatric morbidity in the male sentenced Irish prisons population*. Academic Press.

Dybicz, P. (2005). Interventions for street children: An analysis of current best practices. *International Social Work*, *48*(6), 763–771. doi:10.1177/0020872805057083

Dyck, D. G., Short, R., & Vitaliano, P. P. (1999). Predictors of burden and infectious illness in schizophrenia caregivers. *Psychosomatic Medicine*, *61*(4), 411–419. doi:10.1097/00006842-199907000-00001 PMID:10443748

Edgar, B. (2009). *European Review of Statistics on Homelessness*. Brussels: FEANTSA.

Edgar, W., Doherty, J., & Meert, H. (2003). *Second Review of Statistics on Homelessness in Europe*. Brussels: FEANTSA.

Einar, H. (1996). Finding care on the street: Processes in the careers of Sri Lankan street boys. *Childhood: A Global Journal of Child Research, 3*(2), 247-259.

Eisen, S. V., Dickey, B., & Sederer, L. I. (2000). A self-report symptom and problem rating scale to increase inpatients' involvement in treatment. *Psychiatric Services (Washington, D.C.), 51*(3), 349–353. doi:10.1176/appi.ps.51.3.349 PMID:10686242

El-Gabalawy, R., Cox, B., Clara, I., & Mackenzie, C. (2010). Assessing the validity of social anxiety disorder subtypes using a nationally representative sample. *Journal of Anxiety Disorders, 24*(2), 244–249. doi:10.1016/j.janxdis.2009.11.003 PMID:19963338

Elkins, D. E., & Stovall, K. (2000). American Art Therapy Association, Inc.: 1998–1999 Membership survey report. *Art Therapy: Journal of the American Art Therapy Association, 17*(1), 41–46. doi:10.1080/07421656.2000.10129431

Elovic, E. (2000). Use of Provigil for under arousal following TBI. *The Journal of Head Trauma Rehabilitation, 15*(4), 1068–1071. doi:10.1097/00001199-200008000-00009 PMID:10876176

Elvevag, B., & Goldberg, T. E. (2000). Cognitive impairment in schizophrenia is the core of the disorder. *Critical Reviews in Neurobiology, 14*(1), 1–21. doi:10.1615/CritRevNeurobiol.v14.i1.10 PMID:11253953

Errecart, M. T., Walberg, H. J., Ross, J. G., Gold, R. S., Fiedler, J. L., & Kolbe, L. J. (1991). Effectiveness of teenage health teaching modules. *The Journal of School Health, 61*(1), 26–30. doi:10.1111/j.1746-1561.1991.tb07855.x PMID:2027290

European Monitoring Centre for Drugs and Drug Addiction (EMCDDA). (2008). *Substance use among older adults: a neglected problem.* Available at http://www.emcdda.europa.eu/html.cfm/ index50563EN.html

Fadden, G., Bebbington, P., & Kuipers, L. (1987). The burden of care: The impact of functional psychiatric illness on the patient's family. *The British Journal of Psychiatry, 150*(3), 285–292. doi:10.1192/bjp.150.3.285 PMID:3311267

Falloon, I. R. H., Boyd, J. L., & McGill, C. W. (1985). Family management in the prevention of morbidity of schizophrenia: I. Clinical outcome of a two-year longitudinal study. *Archives of General Psychiatry, 42*(9), 887–896. doi:10.1001/archpsyc.1985.01790320059008 PMID:2864032

Falloon, I. R., Boyd, J. L., & McGill, C. W. (1984). *Family Care of Schizophrenia.* New York: Guilford Press.

Faraone, S. V., Sergeant, J., Gillberg, C., & Biederman, J. (2003). The worldwide prevalence of ADHD: Is it an American condition? *World Psychiatry; Official Journal of the World Psychiatric Association (WPA), 2*, 104–113. PMID:16946911

Farrelly-Hansen, M. (2001). *Spirituality and art therapy: Living the connection.* London: Jessica Kingsley.

Fatséas, M., Denis, C., Lavie, E., & Auriacombe, M. (2010). Relationship between anxiety disorders and opiate dependence--a systematic review of the literature: Implications for diagnosis and treatment. *Journal of Substance Abuse Treatment, 38*(3), 220–230. doi:10.1016/j.jsat.2009.12.003 PMID:20116963

Fazel, S., Cartwright, J., Norman-Nott, A., & Hawton, K. (2008). Suicide in prisoners: A systematic review of risk factors. *The Journal of Clinical Psychiatry, 69*(11), 1721–1731. doi:10.4088/JCP.v69n1107 PMID:19026254

Fazel, S., & Danesh, J. (2002). Serious mental disorder in 23 000 prisoners: a systematic review of 62 surveys. Severe mental illness in 33 588 prisoners worldwide: systematic review and meta regression analysis. *Lancet, 359*(9306), 545–550. doi:10.1016/S0140-6736(02)07740-1 PMID:11867106

Fazel, S., & Seewald, K. (2012). Severe mental illness in 33,588 prisoners worldwide: Systematic review and meta-regression analysis. *The British Journal of Psychiatry, 200*(5), 364–373. doi:10.1192/bjp.bp.111.096370 PMID:22550330

Fazel, S., & Yu, R. (2011). Psychotic disorders and repeat offending: Systematic review and meta-analysis. *Schizophrenia Bulletin, 37*(4), 800–810. doi:10.1093/schbul/sbp135 PMID:19959703

FEANTSA & Mental Health Europe. (2009). *Joint statement in homelessness and mental health*. Mental Health Europe. Retrieved September 12, 2014, from http:/www.mhesme.org/assets/files/Common%20statement%20FEANTSA%20 MHE%20.pdf)

FEANTSA European typology on homelessness and housing exclusion (ETHOS). (2005). Brussels: FEANTSA. Retrieved September 12, 2014, fromhttp://www.feantsa.org/files/ freshstart/Toolkits/ Ethos / Leaflet/EN.pdf

FEANTSA Proposal, . (2007). *A Retrospective Module on Homelessness for Household Surveys*. Brussels: FEANTSA.

FEANTSA. (2006). *The right to health is a human right: ensuring access to health for people who are homeless*. In Feantsa Annual European Report.

Feinstein, A.R. (1970). The pre-therapeutic classification of co-morbidity in chronic disease. *Journal of Chronic Disease,* (23), 455-468.

Fellner, J. (2006). A Corrections Quandary. *Harvard Civil Rights-Civil Liberties Law, 29*, 773–789.

Fennell, M. J. V. (1998). Depression. In Cognitive behaviour therapy for psychiatric problems a practical guide. Oxford University Press.

Fernandes, G. T., & Vaughn, M. G. (2008). Brazilian street children: Contextual influences in relation to substance misuse. *International Social Work, 51*(5), 669–681. doi:10.1177/0020872808093344

Ferrucci, R., Bortolomasi, M., Vergari, M., Tadini, L., Salvoro, B., Giacopuzzi, M., & Priori, A. et al. (2009). Transcranial direct current stimulation in severe, drug-resistant major depression. *Journal of Affective Disorders, 118*(1-3), 215–219. doi:10.1016/j.jad.2009.02.015 PMID:19286265

Findling, R. L., Correll, C. U., Nyilas, M., Forbes, R. A., McQuade, R. D., Jin, N., & Carlson, G. A. et al. (2013). Aripiprazole for the treatment of pediatric bipolar I disorder: A 30-week, randomized, placebo controlled study. *Bipolar Disorders, 15*(2), 138–149. doi:10.1111/bdi.12042 PMID:23437959

Findling, R. L., Nyilas, M., Forbes, R. A., McQuade, R. D., Jin, N., Iwamoto, T., & Chang, K. et al. (2009). Acute treatment of pediatric bipolar I disorder, manic or mixed episode, with aripiprazole: A randomized, double-blind, placebo-controlled study. *The Journal of Clinical Psychiatry, 70*(10), 1441–1451. doi:10.4088/JCP.09m05164yel PMID:19906348

Fink, M., Kellner, C. H., & McCall, W. V. (2014). The role of ECT in suicide prevention. *Journal of Electric Convulsive Therapy, 30*(1), 5–9. PMID:24091903

First, M. B. (2005). Mutually Exclusive versus co-occurring Diagnostic Categories: The challenge of diagnostic comorbidity. *Psychopathology, 38*(4), 206–210. doi:10.1159/000086093 PMID:16145276

Fischer, P. J. (1990). *Alcohol and drug abuse and mental health problems among homeless persons: A review of the literature, 1980-1990*. Rockville, MD: National Institute of Alcohol Abuse and Alcoholism and National Institute of Mental Health.

Fischer, P. J., & Breakey, W. R. (1991). The epidemiology of alcohol, drug and mental disorders among homeless persons. *The American Psychologist, 46*(11), 1115–1128. doi:10.1037/0003-066X.46.11.1115 PMID:1772149

Fish, F. (1967). Clinical psychopathology: Sign and symptoms in psychiatry. Bristol, UK: John Wright & Sons.

Fish, C., & Biller, S. (1993). Advances in Clinical Child Psychology. In T. H. Ollendick & R. J. Prinz (Eds.), *Plenum Press*. New York.

FitzPatrick, M. (1993). Adolescents. In G. Stricker & J. R. Gold (Eds.), *Comprehensive handbook of psychotherapy integration*. New York, NY: Plenum Press; doi:10.1007/978-1-4757-9782-4_29

Foldemo, A., Gullberg, M., Ek, A. C., & Bogren, L. (2005). Quality of life and burden in parents of outpatients with schizophrenia. *Social Psychiatry and Psychiatric Epidemiology*, *40*(2), 133–138. doi:10.1007/s00127-005-0853-x PMID:15685405

Folsom, D. P., Hawthorne, W., Lindamer, L., Gilmer, T., Bailey, A., Golshan, S., & Jeste, D. V. et al. (2005). Prevalence and risk factors for homelessness and utilization of mental health services among 10,340 patients with serious mental illness in a large public mental health system. *The American Journal of Psychiatry*, *162*(2), 370–376. doi:10.1176/appi.ajp.162.2.370 PMID:15677603

Folsom, D., & Jeste, D. (2002). Schizophrenia in homeless persons: A systematic review of the literature. *Acta Psychiatrica Scandinavica*, *104*, 1–10. PMID:12059843

Fonagy, P., Target, M., Cottrell, D., Phillips, J., & Kurtz, Z. (2002). *What works for whom? A critical review of treatments for children and adolescents*. Guildford Press.

Ford, D. E., & Erlinger, T. P. (2004). Depression and C-reactive protein in US adults: Data from the third National Health and Nutrition Survey. Archieves of International Medicine, 168, 284–290. PubMed PMID:15136311

France, M. H., & Allen, E. G. (1997). Using art: A gestalt counselling strategy for working with disruptive clients. *Guidance and Counselling*, *12*(4), 24–26.

Frank, E. (2005). *Treating Bipolar Disorder: A clinician's guide to Interpersonal and social rhythm therapy*. New York: Guilford.

Franklin, Farrelly-Hansen, & Marek, Swan-Foster, & Wallingford. (2000). Transpersonal art therapy education. *Art Therapy: Journal of the American Art Therapy Association*, 17.

Freeman, A., Pretzer, J., Fleming, B., & Simon, K. M. (1990). *Clinical Application of Cognitive Therapy*. New York: Plenum Press. doi:10.1007/978-1-4684-0007-6

Freeman, D., Dunn, G., Startup, H., Pugh, K., Cordwell, J., Mander, H., & Kingdon, D. et al. (2015). Effects of cognitive behavior therapy for worry on persecutory delusions in patients with psychosis (WIT): A parallel, single-blind, randomized controlled trial with a mediation analysis. *The Lancet Psychiatry*, *2*(4), 305–313. doi:10.1016/S2215-0366(15)00039-5 PMID:26360083

Frei, A., & Rehm, J. (2002). The prevalence of psychiatric co-morbidity among opioid addicts. *Psychiatrische Praxis*, *29*(5), 258–262. doi:10.1055/s-2002-32713 PMID:12101492

Freud, S. (1920). A General Introduction to Psychoanalysis. New York: Boni and Liveright.

Frost, R. O., Krause, M. S., & Steketee, G. (1996). The hoarding and obsessive-compulsive symptoms. *Behavior Modification*, *20*(1), 116–132. doi:10.1177/01454455960201006 PMID:8561769

Gajalakshmi, V., & Peto, R. (2007). Suicide rates in rural Tamil Nadu, south India: Verbal autopsy of 39 000 deaths in 1997-98. *International Journal of Epidemiology*, *36*(1), 203–207. doi:10.1093/ije/dyl308 PMID:17301103

Gallagher, S. K., & Mechanic, D. (1996). Living with the mentally ill: Effects on the health and functioning of other members. *Social Science & Medicine*, *42*(12), 1691–1701. doi:10.1016/0277-9536(95)00296-0 PMID:8783431

Ganesan, V., Kumar, R., & Khanna, S. (2001). Obsessive compulsive disorder and psychosis. *Canadian Journal of Psychiatry*, (46): 750–754. PMID:11692979

Gangadhar, B. N., Thirthali, J., Venkatesh, B. K., Naveen, M. N., & Arunchala, U. (2007). Co-morbid substance use disorder in Schizophrenia: Results from a community survey. *Indian Journal of Psychiatry*, *49*, S30.

Ganim, B. (2000). *Art and healing: Using expressive art to heal your body, mind, and spirit*. Three Rivers, MI: Three Rivers Press.

Gautam, S., Jain, S., Batra, L., Sharma, R., & Munshi, D. (2009). Human rights and privileges of mentally ill persons. In S. Gautam & A. Avasthi (Eds.), *Forensic Psychiatry, Clinical Practice Guidelines for Psychiatrists in India* (pp. 82–112). New Delhi: Indian Psychiatric Society.

Geller, D. A., Biederman, J., Faraone, S., Agranat, A., Cradock, K., Hagermoser, L., & Coffey, B. J. et al. (2001). Developmental aspects of obsessive-compulsive disorder: Findings in children, adolescents and adults. *The Journal of Nervous and Mental Disease*, *189*(7), 471–477. doi:10.1097/00005053-200107000-00009 PMID:11504325

Genn, H. (1999). *Paths to justice: what people do and think about going to law*. Portland, OR: Hart Publishing.

George, & Lakshmi. (2007). The burden of schizophrenia on caregivers: A review. *PharmacoEconomics*, *26*, 149–162. PMID:18198934

Ghosh, A. B. (2006). Psychiatry in India: Need to focus on geriatric Psychiatry. *Indian Journal of Psychiatry*, *48*(1), 4–9. doi:10.4103/0019-5545.31612 PMID:20703408

Gianutsos, R. (1980). What is cognitive rehabilitation? *Journal of Rehabilitation*, 36-40.

Giel, R., de Arango, M. V., Hafeiz Babikir, A., Bonifacio, M., Climent, C. E., Harding, T. W., & Wig, N. N. et al. (1983). The burden of mental illness on the family. Results of observations in four developing countries. A report from the WHO collaborative study on strategies for extending mental healthcare. *Acta Psychiatrica Scandinavica*, *68*(3), 186–201. doi:10.1111/j.1600-0447.1983.tb06998.x PMID:6637556

Gillberg, C., Wahlstrom, J., Forsman, A., Hellgren, L., & Gillberg, J. C. (1986). Teenage psychoses: Epidemiology, classification and reduced optimality in the pre-, peri- and neonatal periods. *Journal of Child Psychology and Psychiatry, and Allied Disciplines*, *27*(1), 87–98. doi:10.1111/j.1469-7610.1986.tb00624.x PMID:3949910

Gill, P., & de Wildt, G. (Eds.). (2003). *Housing and Health: The Role of Primary Care*. Oxford, UK: Radcliffe Medical.

Girimaji, S.R., Biju, S.T., Srinath, S., & Seshadri, S.P. (2005). Co-morbid psychiatric disorders in pervasive developmental disorders. *Journal of Indian Association for Child and Adolescent Mental Health, 1*(2), 7.

Giuffrida, A., Leweke, F. M., Gerth, C. W., Schreiber, D., Koethe, D., Faulhaber, J., & Piomelli, D. (2004). Cerebrospinal anandamide levels are elevated in acute schizophrenia and are inversely correlated with psychotic symptoms. *Neuropsychopharmacology: Official Publication of the American College of Neuropsychopharmacology*, *29*(11), 2108–2114. doi:10.1038/sj.npp.1300558 PMID:15354183

Gladding, S. T. (1998). *Counseling as an art: The creative arts in counseling* (2nd ed.). Alexandria, VA: American Counseling Association.

Goeree, R., Farahati, F., Burke, N., Blackhouse, G., O'Reilly, D., Pyne, J., & Tarride, J. E. (2005). The economic burden of schizophrenia in Canada in 2004. Current Medical Research and Opinion, 21(12), 2017–2028. doi:10.1185/030079905X75087 PubMed doi:10.1185/030079905X75087 PMID:16368053

Goerke, D., & Kumra, S. (2013). Substance abuse and psychosis. *Child and Adolescent Psychiatric Clinics of North America*, *22*(4), 643–654. doi:10.1016/j.chc.2013.06.001 PMID:24012078

Gold, J. M., Carpenter, C., Randolph, C., Goldberg, T. E., & Weinberger, D. R. (1997). Auditory working memory and Wisconsin Card Sorting Test performance in schizophrenia. *Archives of General Psychiatry*, *54*(2), 159–165. doi:10.1001/archpsyc.1997.01830140071013 PMID:9040284

Goldman, C. R. (1998). *Handout*. Retrieved 04 January, 2016. Available at www.karunadu.gov.in/welfareofdisabled/Documents/RTI.pdf

Goldman, C. R., & Quinn, F. L. (1988). Effects of a patient education programme in the treatment of schizophrenia. *Hospital & Community Psychiatry*, *39*, 282–286. PMID:3356434

Goldman, R. S., Axelrod, B. N., & Taylor, S. F. (1996). Neuropsychological aspects of schizophrenia. In I. Grant & K. M. Adams (Eds.), *Neuropsychological assessment of neuropsychiatric disorders*. New York: Oxford University press.

Goldstein, M. (1985). Family factors that antedate the onset of schizophrenia and related disorders: The results of a fifteen year prospective longitudinal study. *Acta Psychiatrica Scandinavica*, *71*(319), 7–18. doi:10.1111/j.1600-0447.1985.tb08520.x PMID:3863461

Goldstein, M. J., Rea, M., & Miklowitz, D. J. (1996). Family factors related to the course and outcome of bipolar disorder. In M. J. Mundt, K. Goldstein, & K. Hahlweg et al. (Eds.), *Interpersonal Factors in the Origin and Courses of Affective Disorder*. Washington, DC: American Psychiatric Press.

Gómez-de-Regil, L., Kwapil, T. R., & Barrantes-Vidal, N. (2014). Predictors of expressed emotion, burden and quality of life in relatives of Mexican patients with psychosis. *Journal of Psychiatric and Mental Health Nursing*, *21*(2), 170–179. doi:10.1111/jpm.12071 PMID:23551489

Goodman, R. (1997). The Strength and Difficulties Questionnaire: A research note. *Journal of Child Psychology and Psychiatry, and Allied Disciplines*, *38*(5), 581–586. doi:10.1111/j.1469-7610.1997.tb01545.x PMID:9255702

Goodwin, R. D., & Roy Byrne, P. (2006). Panic and suicidal ideation and suicidal attempts: Results from the National Comorbidity Survey. *Depression and Anxiety*, *23*(3), 124–132. doi:10.1002/da.20151 PMID:16502406

Goreishizadeh, M. A., Mohagheghi, A., Farhang, S., & Alizadeh, L. (2012). Psychosocial Disabilities in Patients with Schizophrenia. *Iranian Journal of Public Health*, *41*(5), 116–121. PMID:23113186

Gorman, M. (1999). Development and the rights of older people. In J. Randel et al. (Eds.), *The aging and development report: poverty, independence and the world's older people* (pp. 3–21). London: Earthscan Publications Ltd.

Gourovitch, M. L., & Goldberg, T. E. (1996). Cognitive deficits in schizophrenia: Attention, executive functions, memory and language processing. In Schizophrenia: A Neuropsychological Perspective (pp. 72-86). New York, NY: John Wiley and Sons.

Government of India. (2000). *The Juvenile Justice (Care and protection of children) Act, 2000 (Act No. 56 of 2000)*. Retrieved from wcd.nic.in/childprot/jjact2000.pdf

Govt. of India. (2012). *Draft Mental Health Care Bill*. Retrieved from http://mohfw.nic.in/WriteReadData/l892s/6420662643DRAFT%20THE%20MENTAL%20HEALTH%20CARE%20BILL.pdf

Gowri, G. B. (2003). Attitudes towards old age and aging as shown by humor. *The Gerontologist*, *17*(2), 220–226.

Gracious, B. L., Youngstorm, E. A., & Findling, R. L. (2002). Discriminative validity of a parent version of the Young Mania rating Scale. *Journal of the American Academy of Child and Adolescent Psychiatry*, *41*(11), 1350–1359. doi:10.1097/00004583-200211000-00017 PMID:12410078

Grad, J., & Sainsbusy, P. (1963). Mental illness and the family. *Lancet*, *281*(7280), 544–549. doi:10.1016/S0140-6736(63)91339-4 PMID:13949711

Grady, C. L., & Craik, F. I. M. (2000). Changes in memory processing with age. *Current Opinion in Neurobiology*, *10*(2), 224–231. doi:10.1016/S0959-4388(00)00073-8 PMID:10753795

Grandon, P., Jenaro, C., & Lemos, S. (2008). Primary caregivers of schizophrenia outpatients: Burden and predictor variables. *Psychiatry Research*, *158*(3), 335–343. doi:10.1016/j.psychres.2006.12.013 PMID:18280584

Grant, B. F., Stinson, F. S., Dawson, D. A., Chou, S. P., Dufour, M. C., Compton, W., & Kaplan, K. (2004). Prevalence and co-occurrence of substance use disorders and independent mood and anxiety disorders: Results from the National Epidemiologic Survey on Alcohol and Related Conditions. *Archives of General Psychiatry*, *61*(8), 807–816. doi:10.1001/archpsyc.61.8.807 PMID:15289279

Green, H., McGinnity, A., Meltzer, H., Ford, T., & Goodman, R. (2005). *Mental health of children and young people in Great Britain 2004*. Academic Press.

Greenberg, P. E., Sisitsky, T., Kessler, R. C., Finkelstein, S. N., Berndt, E. R., Davidson, J. R., . . . Fyer, A. J. (1999). The economic burden of anxiety disorders in the 1990s. The Journal of Clinical Psychiatry, 60(7), 427–435. doi:10.4088/JCP.v60n0702 PubMed doi:10.4088/JCP.v60n0702 PMID:10453795

Greenberg, P. E., Fournier, A. A., Sisitsky, T., Pike, C. T., & Kessler, R. C. (2015). The Economic Burden of Adults With Major Depressive Disorder in the United States (2005 and 2010). *The Journal of Clinical Psychiatry*, *76*(2), 155–162. doi:10.4088/JCP.14m09298 PMID:25742202

Greenberg, P., Stiglin, L., Finkelstain, S., & Berndt, E. (1993). Depression: A neglected major illness. *The Journal of Clinical Psychiatry*, *54*, 419.

Greene-Shortridge, T. M., Britt, T. W., & Castro, C. A. (2007). The stigma of mental health problems in the military. *Military Medicine*, *172*(2), 157–161. doi:10.7205/MILMED.172.2.157 PMID:17357770

Greene, V. L., & Ondrich, J. I. (1990). Risk factors for nursing home admissions and exits: A discrete-time hazard function approach. *Journal of Gerontology Social Science*, *45*(6), 275–276. PMID:2229951

Green, M. F. (1996). What are the functional consequences of neurocognitive deficits in schizophrenia? *The American Journal of Psychiatry*, *153*(3), 321–330. doi:10.1176/ajp.153.3.321 PMID:8610818

Green, M. F., Kern, R. S., Braff, D. L., & Mintz, J. (2000). Neurocognitive deficits and functional outcome in schizophrenia: Are we measuring the "right stuff"? *Schizophrenia Bulletin*, *26*(1), 119–136. doi:10.1093/oxfordjournals.schbul.a033430 PMID:10755673

Green, M. F., Satz, P., Ganzell, S., & Vaclav, J. F. (1992). Wisconsin Card Sorting Test performance in schizophrenia: Remediation of a stubborn deficit. *The American Journal of Psychiatry*, *149*(1), 62–67. doi:10.1176/ajp.149.1.62 PMID:1728187

Gregg, L., Barrowclough, C., & Haddock, G. (2007). Reasons for increased substance use in psychosis. *Clinical Psychology Review*, *27*(4), 494–510. doi:10.1016/j.cpr.2006.09.004 PMID:17240501

Gregory, B.S., Andrew, I.S., Ryan, L.D., & Stephanie, D. M. (1993). *The International Journal of Psychosocial Rehabilitation*. The Role of Psychologists in the Treatment, Management, and Prevention of Chronic Mental Illness.

Griffiths, C. T., Dandurand, Y. V., & Murdoch, D. (2007). *The Social Reintegration of Offenders and Crime Prevention-The International Centre for Criminal Law Reform and Criminal Justice Policy*. ICCLR.

Griffiths, S. (2002). *Addressing the health needs of rough sleepers. Homelessness Directorate*. London: Office of the Deputy Prime Minister.

Grimier, H. (2012). Are elderly people living in old age home, less depressed than those of community? Findings from a comparative study. *Journal of Chitwan Medical College*, *1*(2), 2–8.

Gros, D. F., Milanak, M. E., Brady, K. T., & Back, S. E. (2013). Frequency and severity of comorbid mood and anxiety disorders in prescription opioid dependence. *The American Journal on Addictions / American Academy of Psychiatrists in Alcoholism and Addictions, 22*(3), 261–265.

Gross, J., & Haynes, H. (1998). Drawing facilitates children's verbal reports of emotionally laden events. *Journal of Experimental Psychology*, *4*, 163–179.

Grover, S., & Dutt, A. (2011). Perceived burden and quality of life of caregivers in obsessive–compulsive disorder. *Psychiatry and Clinical Neurosciences*, *65*(5), 416–422. doi:10.1111/j.1440-1819.2011.02240.x PMID:21851450

Grunbaum. (1986). Précis of The Foundations of Psychoanalysis: A Philosophical Critique. *Behavioral and Brain Sciences, 9*(2).

Gupta & Sharma. (1992). The oldest old and the use of institutional long term care from an international perspective. New York: Oxford University Press.

Gupta, A., Mohan, U., Tiwari, S. C., Singh, S. K., Manar, M. K., & Singh, V. K. (2014). Home away from Home: Quality of Life, Assessment of Facilities and Reason for Settlement in OAH of Lucknow, India. *Indian Journal of Community Health*, *26*(2), 165–169.

Gupta, R., Nehra, D. K., Kumar, V., Sharma, P., & Kumar, P. (2013). Psychiatric illnesses in homeless (runaway or throwaway) girl inmates: A preliminary study. *Dysphrenia*, *4*(1), 31–35.

Gupta, S. C., Anand, R., & Trivedi, J. K. (1983). Development of a suicidal intent questionnaire. *Indian Journal of Psychiatry*, *25*, 57–62. PMID:21847253

Gutierrez-Maldonado, J., Caqueo-Urizar, A., & Kavanagh, D. J. (2005). Burden of care and general health in families of patients with schizophrenia. *Social Psychiatry and Psychiatric Epidemiology*, *40*(11), 899–904. doi:10.1007/s00127-005-0963-5 PMID:16245190

Halder, S. (2011). *Efficacy of Cognitive Remediation of Neuropsychological Deficits in Patients with Chronic Schizophrenia*. (Unpublished Doctoral thesis). Ranchi Institute of Neuropsychiatry & Allied Sciences, Ranchi University, Ranchi, India.

Halder, S., Mahato, A., & Jahan, M. (2015). Cognitive profile of paranoid schizophrenia on LNNB. *The international. Journal of Indian Psychology*, *2*(3), 174–181.

Halikas, A. J., Crosby, D. R., Pearson, L. V., Nugent, M. S., & Carlson, A. G. (1994). Psychiatric comorbidity in treatment-seeking cocaine abusers. *The American Journal on Addictions*, *3*(1), 25–35. doi:10.1111/j.1521-0391.1994.tb00223.x

Han, C., Voils, C. I., & Williams, J. W. (2011). Uptake of Web-Based Clinical Resources from the MacArthur Initiative on Depression and Primary Care. *Community Mental Health Journal*, 1. PMID:22038376

Han, O., Lee, H. B., Ahn, J., Park, J., Cho, M., Hong, J., & Kim, C.-Y. et al. (2003). Lifetime and current prevalence of mental disorders among homeless men in Korea. *The Journal of Nervous and Mental Disease*, *191*(4), 272–275. doi:10.1097/01.NMD.0000061151.19363.82 PMID:12695742

Hantouche, E. G., Angst, J., Demonfaucon, C., Perugi, G., Lancrenon, S., & Akiskal, H. S. (2003). Cyclothymic OCD:a distinct form? *Journal of Affective Disorders*, *75*(1), 1–10. doi:10.1016/S0165-0327(02)00461-5 PMID:12781344

Hanzawa, S., Tanaka, G., Inadomi, H., Urata, M., & Ohta, Y. (2008). Burden and doping strategies in mothers of patients with schizophrenia in Japan. *Psychiatry Journal of Clinical Neurosciences*, *62*(3), 256–263. doi:10.1111/j.1440-1819.2008.01791.x PMID:18588584

Harbishettar, V., Kumar, P., Janardhan Reddy, Y. C., & Thennarasu, K. (2005). Is there a relationship between Parkinson's disease and obsessive-compulsive disorder? *Parkinsonism & Related Disorders*, *11*(11), 85–88. doi:10.1016/j.parkreldis.2004.07.006 PMID:15734665

Harding, T. W., De Arango, V., Baltazar, J., Climent, C. E., Ibrahim, H. H. A., Ladrido-Ignacio, L., & Wig, N. N. (1980). Mental disorders in primary health care: A study of their frequency and diagnosis in four developing countries. *Psychological Medicine*, *10*(02), 231–241. doi:10.1017/S0033291700043993 PMID:7384326

Harper, J. F., & Marshall, E. (1991). Adolescents problems and their relationship to self esteem. *Adolscence*, *26*, 799–808. PMID:1789167

Hartwell, S. W., & Orr, K. (1999, September). The massachusetts forensic transition program for mentally ill offenders reentering the community. *Psychiatric Services (Washington, D.C.)*, *50*(9), 1220–1222. doi:10.1176/ps.50.9.1220 PMID:10478911

Harvey, P. D. (2009). When Does Cognitive Decline Occur in the Period Prior to the First Episode of Schizophrenia? *Psychiatry*, *6*(7), 12–14. PMID:19724764

Harvey, P. D. (2011). Mood Symptoms, Cognition, and Everyday Functioning in Major Depression, Bipolar Disorder, and Schizophrenia. *Innovations in Clinical Neuroscience*, *8*(10), 14–18. PMID:22132366

Harvey, P. D., & Keefe, R. S. E. (1997). Cognitive impairment in schizophrenia and implications of atypical neuroleptic treatment. *CNS Spectrums*, *2*, 1–11.

Hasson-Ohayon, I., Kravetz, S., Roe, D., David, A. S., & Weiser, M. (2006). Insight into psychosis and quality of life. *Comprehensive Psychiatry*, *47*(4), 265–269. doi:10.1016/j.comppsych.2005.08.006 PMID:16769300

Hauser, M., & Correll, C. U. (2013). The significance of at-risk or prodromal symptoms for bipolar I disorder in children and adolescents. *Canadian Journal of Psychiatry*, *58*, 22–31. PMID:23327753

Havens, J. R., & Strathdee, S. A. (2005). Antisocial Personality Disorder and Opioid Treatment Outcomes: A Review. *Addictive Disorders & Their Treatment*, *4*(3), 85–97. doi:10.1097/01.adt.0000155725.14375.6e

Hawton, K., Salkvskis, P., Kirk, J., & Clark, D. M. (1989). Cognitive behaviour therapy for psychiatric problems: A practical guide. Oxford University Press. doi:10.1093/med:psych/9780192615879.001.0001

Hayes, R., & McGrath, J. (2000). *Cognitive rehabilitation for people with schizophrenia and related conditions (Cochrane Review)*. Oxford, UK: Update Software.

Heffner, J. L., Anthenelli, R. M., Adler, C. M., Strakowski, S. M., Beavers, J., & DelBello, M. P. (2013). Prevalence and correlates of heavy smoking and nicotine dependence in adolescents with bipolar and cannabis use disorders. *Psychiatry Research*, *210*(3), 857–862. doi:10.1016/j.psychres.2013.04.010 PMID:23684537

Hegde, R. S. (1980). Suicide in rural community. *Indian Journal of Psychiatry*, *22*, 368–370. PMID:22058501

Heinrichs, R. W., & Zakzanis, K. K. (1998). Neurocognitive deficit in schizophrenia: A quantitative review of the evidence. *Neuropsychology*, *12*(3), 426–445. doi:10.1037/0894-4105.12.3.426 PMID:9673998

Heinssen, R. K., Liberman, R. P., & Kopelowicz, A. (2000). Psychosocial skills training for schizophrenia: Lessons from the laboratory. *Schizophrenia Bulletin*, *26*, 21–46.

Hennessy, K. D., Green-Hennessy, S., & Marshall, C. (2012). Datapoints: Receipt of reported mental health specialty care in the 2010 Health Styles Survey. *Psychiatric Services (Washington, D.C.)*, *63*(4), 306. doi:10.1176/appi.ps.20120p306 PMID:22476296

Henquet, C., Krabbendam, L., de Graaf, R., ten Have, M., & van Os, J. (2006). Cannabis use and expression of mania in the general population. *Journal of Affective Disorders*, *95*(1-3), 103–110. doi:10.1016/j.jad.2006.05.002 PMID:16793142

Herrmann, D., & Parente, R. (1994). The multi-modal approach to cognitive rehabilitation. *NeuroRehabilitation*, *4*, 133–142. PMID:24525361

Herrmann, D., & Petro, S. (1991). Commercial memory aids. *Applied Cognitive Psychology*, *4*(6), 439–450. doi:10.1002/acp.2350040603

Herrmann, D., Plude, D., Yoder, C., & Mullin, P. (1999). Cognitive processing and extrinsic psychological systems: A holistic model of cognition. *Zeitschrift fur Psychologie mit Zeitschrift fur Angewandte Psychologie*, *207*, 123–147.

Heru, A. M., & Ryan, C. E. (2008). Burden, reward and family functioning of caregivers for relatives with mood disorders: 1 year follow-up. *Journal of Affective Disorders*, *83*, 221–225. doi:10.1016/j.jad.2004.04.013 PMID:15555717

Hindu Adoption and Maintenance Act. (1956). Bare Act; Eastern Book Company, Lucknow.

Hirschfeld, R., Lewis, L., & Vornik, L. A. (2003). Perception and Impact of bipolar disorders how far have we really come? Results of the National Depressive and Manic-Depressive association 2000 survey of Individuals with bipolar disorder. *The Journal of Clinical Psychiatry*, *64*, 161–174. doi:10.4088/JCP.v64n0209 PMID:12633125

Hoeing, J., & Hamilton, M. (1969). *The Degeneration of Mentally Ill*. London: Routledge and Kegan Paul.

Hofer, A., Baumgartner, S., Bodner, T., Edlinger, M., Hummer, M., Kemmler, G., & Fleischhacker, W. W. et al. (2005). Patient outcomes in schizophrenia II: The impact of cognition. *European Psychiatry*, *20*(5-6), 395–402. doi:10.1016/j.eurpsy.2005.02.006 PMID:16171654

Hoff, A. L., Sakuma, M., Wieneke, M., Horon, R., Kushner, M., & DeLisi, L. E. (1999). Longitudinal neuropsychological follow-up study of patients with first-episode schizophrenia. *The American Journal of Psychiatry*, *156*, 1336–1341. PMID:10484942

Hogan, S. (1997). *Feminist approach to art therapy*. London: Routledge.

Hogan, S., & Coulter, A. M. (2014). *The Introductory Guide to Art Therapy*. Routledge.

Holley, H. L., Arboleda, F. J., & Love, E. (1995). Lifetime prevalence of prior suicide attempts in a remanded population and relationship to current mental illness. *International Journal of Offender Therapy and Comparative Criminology*, *10*(2), 239–256.

Homelessness – Provision of Mental Health and Substance Abuse Services. (2003). *Substance Abuse and Mental Health Services Administration (SAMHSA), Center for Mental Health Services*. Retrieved September12, 2014, from http://mentalhealth.samhsa.gov

Hooley, J. M. (1986). An introduction to expressed emotion measurement and research. In M. J. Goldstein, I. Hand, & K. Hahlweg (Eds.), *Treatment of schizophrenia: family assessment and intervention* (pp. 25–34). Berlin: Springer- Verlag. doi:10.1007/978-3-642-95496-2_3

Hooley, J. M., & Hiller, J. B. (2000). Personality and expressed emotion. *Journal of Abnormal Psychology*, *109*(1), 40–44. doi:10.1037/0021-843X.109.1.40 PMID:10740934

Hooley, J. M., & Teasdale, J. D. (1989). Predictors of relapse in unipolar depressives: Expressed emotion, marital distress, and perceived criticism. *Journal of Abnormal Psychiatry*, *98*(3), 229–235. doi:10.1037/0021-843X.98.3.229 PMID:2768657

Horovitz-Darby, E. G. (1994). Spiritual art therapy. Springfield, IL: Charlie C. Thomas

Horowitz, M. (2013). *The burden of disease due to chronic illnesses, especially mental health illnesses is rising in the UK*. Academic Press.

Houet, S. Y., Ke, C. L., Su, Y. C., Lung, F. W., & Huang, C. J. (2008). Exploring the burden of the primary family caregivers of schizophrenia patients in Taiwan. *Psychiatry and Clinical Neurosciences*, *62*(5), 508–514. doi:10.1111/j.1440-1819.2008.01843.x PMID:18950369

Howes, O. D., & Kapur, S. (2009). The dopamine hypothesis of schizophrenia:version III- the final common pathway. *Schizophrenia Bulletin*, *3*(3), 549–562. doi:10.1093/schbul/sbp006 PMID:19325164

Hsieh, H. F., & Shannon, S. E. (2005). Three Approaches to Qualitative Content Analysis. *QHR*, *15*, 1277–1288. PMID:16204405

Hughes, J. F. (2000). Evidence for and against the self-medication hypothesis for smoking. *Journal of Neuropsychopharmacology*, *3*, S58–S59.

Hughes, R. (1994). In IAPSRS Publications Committee (1994). An Introduction to Psychiatric Rehabilitation. Columbia, MD: IAPSRS individuals with a first episode of psychosis. *Acta Psychiatrica Scandinavica*, *106*, 286–290.

Hunter, R., & Barry, S. (2012). Negative symptoms and psychosocial functioning in schizophrenia: Neglected but important targets for treatment. *European Psychiatry*, *27*(6), 432–436. doi:10.1016/j.eurpsy.2011.02.015 PMID:21602034

Hwang, M.Y., & Hollander, E. (1993). Schizo-obsessive disorders. *Psychiatric Annals, 23*(7), 396-401.

Idstad, M., Ask, H., & Tambs, K. (2010). Mental disorder and caregiver burden in spouses: The Nord-Trøndelag health study. *Bio Med Central Public Health*, *26*, 34–51. PMID:20796279

IHME. (2010). *Global Burden of Disease Study: Data Downloads*. Retrieved from http://ghdx.healthmetricsandevaluation.org/global-burden-diseasestudy-2010-gbd-2010-data-downloads

Inagaki, M., Kawashima, Y., Kawanishi, C., Yonemoto, N., Sugimoto, T., Furuno, T., & Yamada, M. et al. (2015). Interventions to prevent repeat suicidal behavior in patients admitted to an emergency department for a suicide attempt: A meta-analysis. *Journal of Affective Disorders*, *175*, 66–78. doi:10.1016/j.jad.2014.12.048 PMID:25594513

Indian Contract Act. (1872). *Bare Act*. Lucknow: Eastern Book Company.

Indian Council of Medical Research. (2005). *Mental health research in India*. Author.

Indian Psychiatric Society. (2002). *IDEAS (Indian Disability Evaluation and Assessment Scale) - A scale for measuring and quantifying disability in mental disorders*. Retrieved from http://www.indianjpsychiatry.org/cpg/cpg2009/article3.pdf

Inskip, H. M., Harris, E. C., & Barraclough, B. (1998). Lifetime risk of suicide for affective disorder, alcoholism and schizophrenia. *The British Journal of Psychiatry*, *172*(1), 35–37. doi:10.1192/bjp.172.1.35 PMID:9534829

Institute of Medicine (IOM). (2012). *Living well with chronic illness: A call for public health action*. Washington, DC: The National Academies Press.

Ivarsson, A. B., Sidenvall, B., & Carlsson, M. (2004). The factor structure of the Burden Assessment Scale and the perceived burden of caregivers for individuals with severe mental disorders. *Scandinavian Journal of Caring Sciences*, *18*(4), 396–401. doi:10.1111/j.1471-6712.2004.00298.x PMID:15598247

Ivezic, S., Ljubimir, V., & Urlic, I. (2001). Therapist-patient relations in treatment of chronic schizophrenic patients. *Medicinski Arhiv*, *55*(1), 39–46. PMID:11795193

Jablensky, A. (2011). *People living with psychotic illness 2010, Australian national survey*. Retrieved from https://www.health.gov.au/internet/main/publishing.nsf/.../psych10.pdf

Jablensky, A., Sartorious, N., Ernberg, G., Anker, M., Korten, A., Cooper, J. E., …Bertelsen, A. (1992). Schizophrenia: Manifestations, incidence and course in different cultures: A world Health Organization ten-country study. Cambridge, UK: Cambridge University Press.

Jacobsen, L. K., Southwick, S. M., & Kosten, T. R. (2001). Substance use disorders in patients with posttraumatic stress disorder: A review of the literature. *The American Journal of Psychiatry*, *158*(8), 1184–1190. doi:10.1176/appi.ajp.158.8.1184 PMID:11481147

Jaisoorya, T. S., Janardhan Reddy, Y. C., & Srinath, S. (2003). Is Juvenile obsessive-compulsive disorder a developmental subtype of the disorder. Findings from an Indian study? *European Child & Adolescent Psychiatry*, *12*(12), 290–297. doi:10.1007/s00787-003-0342-2 PMID:14689261

James, D.J., & Glaze, L.E. (2006). *Mental health problems of prison and jails inmates*. U.S. Dept. of Justice: Office of Justice Programs.

Jané-Llopis, E., & Gabilondo, A. (Eds.). (2008). Mental Health in Older People. Consensus Paper. Luxembourg: European Communities.

Janet, P. (1903). Les obsessions et la psychasthenie (vol. 2). Felix Alcan.

Jeffrey, M., & Dvoskin, J. (2006). An overview of correctional psychiatry. *The Psychiatric Clinics of North America*, *29*, 773–789. PMID:16904511

Jenkins, G. R., Hale, R., Papanastassiou, M., Crawford, M. J., & Tyrer, P. (2002). Suicide rate 22 years after parasuicide: Cohort study. *British Medical Journal*, *325*(7373), 1155. doi:10.1136/bmj.325.7373.1155 PMID:12433767

Jha, S., Chadda, R. K., Kumar, N., & Bal, C. S. (2013). *Brain SPECT Assisted Repetitive Transcranial Magnetic Stimulation (rTMS) in Treatment Resistant Major Depressive Disorder*. (Unpublished master's thesis). All India Institute of Medical Sciences, New Delhi, India.

Jha, B. K. (1968). A study of the nature of criminal offences of mental patients. *Indian Journal of Psychiatry*, *10*(1), 166–176.

Jha, S., & Kumar, R. (2015). Methodological considerations in determining the effects of films with suicidal content. eLetter "Till B, Strauss M, Sonneck G, Niederkrotenthaler T. Determining the effects of films with suicidal content: A laboratory experiment". *The British Journal of Psychiatry*, *207*(1), 72–78. Retrieved from http://bjp.rcpsych.org/content/early/2015/04/14/bjp.bp.114.152827.e-letters PMID:25906792

Joe, V. (2015). *Theories ofAging (Part 3) - Sociological Theories*. Retrieved 20 Dec. 2015 from http://allnurses-breakroom.com/geriatrics-aging-elderly/theories-of-aging-412760.html

Jolly, C. D. (1996). *Stress taking charge: All about stress*. Retrieved April 30, 2003, from Iowa State University Extension, Department of Human Development and Family Studies Web site: http://www.extension.iastate.edu/Publications/PM1660A.pdf

Jones, E. (1916). The theory of symbolism. *British Journal of Psychology*, *9*(2), 181–229.

Jungbauer, J., Wittmund, B., Dietrich, S., & Angermeyer, M. C. (2004). The disregarded caregivers: Subjective burden in spouses of schizophrenia patients. *Schizophrenia Bulletin*, *30*(3), 665–675. doi:10.1093/oxfordjournals.schbul.a007114 PMID:15631259

Junginger, J., Phelan, E., Cherry, K., & Levy, J. (1993). Prevalence of psychopathology in elderly persons in nursing homes and in the community. *Hospital & Community Psychiatry*, *44*, 381–383. PMID:8462948

Justice, J. (Care and protection of children) Amendment Act, 2006 (Act No. 33 of 2006), Ministry of Law and Justice, India.

Kadri, N., & Sartorius, N. (2005). The global fight against the stigma of schizophrenia. *PLoS Medicine*, *2*(7), 597–599. doi:10.1371/journal.pmed.0020136 PMID:16033301

Kahn, B. B. (1999). Art therapy with adolescents: Making it work for school counselors. *Professional School Counseling*, *2*(4), 291–298.

Kalra, H., Kamath, P., Trivedi, J. K., & Janca, A. (2008). Caregiver burden in anxiety disorders. *Current Opinion in Psychiatry*, *21*(1), 70–73. doi:10.1097/YCO.0b013e3282f2dfca PMID:18281843

Kane, J. M. (2007). Treatment strategies to prevent relapse and encourage remission. *The Journal of Clinical Psychiatry*, *68*(14), 27–30. PMID:18284275

Kanter, J., Lamb, R., & Loeper, C. (1987). Expressed emotion in families: A critical review. *Hospital & Community Psychiatry*, *338*, 374–380. PMID:3552930

Kaplan & Sadock. (2010). *Comprehensive Textbook of Psychiatry* (9th ed.; Vol. 2). Philadelphia: Lippincott Williams and Wilkins.

Kaplan, P. W. (2010). Epilepsy and Obsessive-compulsive disorder. *Dialogues in Clinical Neuroscience*, (12), 241–248. PMID:20623928

Kariminia, A., Law, M., Butler, T., Corben, S. P., Levy, M. H., Kaldor, J. M., & Grant, L. (2007). Factors associated with mortality in a cohort of Australian prisoners. *European Journal of Epidemiology*, *22*(7), 417–428. doi:10.1007/s10654-007-9134-1 PMID:17668280

Karnataka State Mental Health Rules. (2007). Retrieved from karhfw.gov.in/Karnataka_state_mental_health_authority.pdf

Karras, M., McCarron, E., Gray, A., & Ardasinski, S. (2006). *On the edge of justice: the legal needs of people with a mental illness in NSW*. Sydney: Law and Justice Foundation of NSW.

Kate, N., Grover, S., Kulhara, P., & Nehra, R. (2013). Caregiving appraisal in schizophrenia: A study from India. *Social Science & Medicine*, *98*, 135–140. doi:10.1016/j.socscimed.2013.09.005 PMID:24331891

Kaufman, J., Birmaher, B., Brent, D., Rao, U. M. A., Flynn, C., Moreci, P., & Ryan, N. (1997). Schedule for affective disorders and schizophrenia for school-age children-present and lifetime version (K-SADS-PL): Initial reliability and validity data. *Journal of the American Academy of Child and Adolescent Psychiatry*, *36*(7), 980–988. doi:10.1097/00004583-199707000-00021 PMID:9204677

Kay, S. R., Flszbein, A., & Opfer, L. A. (1987). The positive and negative syndrome scale (PANSS) for schizophrenia. *Schizophrenia Bulletin*, *13*(2), 261–276. doi:10.1093/schbul/13.2.261 PMID:3616518

Kazarian, S. S., Malla, A. K., Cole, J. D., & Baker, B. (1990). Comparisons of two expressed emotion scales with the Camberwell Family Interview. *Journal of Clinical Psychology*, *46*(3), 306–309. doi:10.1002/1097-4679(199005)46:3<306::AID-JCLP2270460310>3.0.CO;2-2 PMID:2347936

Kazdin, A. E. (2002). Psychosocial treatments for conduct disorder in children and adolescent. In P. E. Nathan & J. M. Gorman (Eds.), *Guides to treatments that work* (2nd ed.). New York: Oxford University Press.

Kazdin, W. E. (2004). Psychotherapy with children. In M. J. Lambert (Ed.), *Bergin and Garfield's handbook of psychotherapy and behavior change* (5th ed.). New York: Wiley.

Keefe, R. S. E., & Fenton, W. S. (2007). How Should DSM-V Criteria for Schizophrenia Include Cognitive Impairment? *Schizophrenia Bulletin*. Retrieved from schizophreniabulletin.oxfordjournals.org/content/early/2007/06/13/schbul.sbm046. full.pdf

Keefe, R. S. E. (2008). Should cognitive impairment be included in the diagnostic criteria for schizophrenia? *World Psychiatry; Official Journal of the World Psychiatric Association (WPA)*, *7*(1), 22–28. doi:10.1002/j.2051-5545.2008.tb00142.x PMID:18458774

Keefe, R. S. E. (2014). The Longitudinal course of cognitive impairment in schizophrenia: An examination of data from premorbid through post treatment phases of illness. *The Journal of Clinical Psychiatry*, *75*(2suppl 2), 8–13. doi:10.4088/JCP.13065su1.02 PMID:24919165

Keefe, R. S. E., & Harvey, P. D. (2012). Cognitive Impairment in Schizophrenia. In M. A. Geyer & G. Gross (Eds.), Handbook of Experimental Pharmacology: Vol. 213. *Novel Antischizophrenia Treatments* (pp. 11–37). Springer-Verlag Berlin Heidelberg. doi:10.1007/978-3-642-25758-2_2

Keefe, R. S. E., & Harvey, P. D. (2012). Cognitive Impairment in Schizophrenia. In N. A. Treatments (Ed.), Handbook of Experimental Pharmacology: Vol. 213. Springer-Verlag Berlin Heidelberg.

Kelly, T. M., Daley, D. C., & Douaihy, A. B. (2012). Treatment of substance abusing patients with comorbid psychiatric disorders. *Addictive Behaviors*, *37*(1), 11–24. doi:10.1016/j.addbeh.2011.09.010 PMID:21981788

Kensinger, E. A. (2004). *Remembering emotional information: Effects of aging and Alzheimer's disease. In Progress in Alzheimer's Disease Research*. Nova.

Keriotis, A. A., & Upadhyaya, H. P. (2000). Inhalant dependence and withdrawal symptoms. *Journal of the American Academy of Child and Adolescent Psychiatry*, *39*(6), 679–680. doi:10.1097/00004583-200006000-00004 PMID:10846300

Kessler, R. C., & Ustun, T. B. (2004). The World Mental Health (WMH) Survey Initiative version of the World Health Organization (WHO) Composite International Diagnostic Interview (CIDI). [Pubmed Abstract Full Text]. International Journal of Methods in Psychiatric Research, 13(2), 93–121. doi:10.1002/mpr.168 PubMed doi:10.1002/mpr.168 PMID:15297906

Kessler, R.C., Aguilar-Gaxiola, S., Alonso, J., Chatterji, S., Lee, S., Johan Ormel, T.J., … Philip, S. W. (2009). *The global burden of mental disorders: An update from the WHO World Mental Health (WMH) Surveys*. Academic Press.

Kessler, R. C., Aguilar-Gaxiola, S., Andrade, L., Bijl, R., Borges, G., & Caraveo-Anduaga, J. J. et al.. (2001). Mental-substance comorbidities in the ICPE surveys. *Psychiatria Fennica*, *32*, 62–80.

Kessler, R. C., Barker, P. R., Colpe, L. J., Epstein, J. F., Gfroerer, J. C., Hiripi, E., & Zaslavsky, A. M. et al. (2003). Screening for serious mental illness in the general population. *Archives of General Psychiatry*, *60*(2), 184–189. doi:10.1001/archpsyc.60.2.184 PMID:12578436

Kessler, R. C., Chiu, W. T., Demler, O., & Walters, E. E. (2005). Prevalence, severity, and comorbidity of 12-month DSM-IV disorders in the National Comorbidity Survey Replication. *Archives of General Psychiatry*, *62*(6), 617–627. doi:10.1001/archpsyc.62.6.617 PMID:15939839

Kessler, R. C., Crum, R. M., Warner, L. A., Nelson, C. B., Schulenberg, J., & Anthony, J. C. (1997). Lifetime co-occurrence of DSM-III-R alcohol abuse and dependence with other psychiatric disorders in the National Comorbidity Survey. *Archives of General Psychiatry*, *54*(4), 313–321. doi:10.1001/archpsyc.1997.01830160031005 PMID:9107147

Kessler, R. C., Nelson, C. B., McGonagle, K. A., Liu, J., Swartz, M., & Blazer, D. G. (1996). Comorbidity of DSM-III-R major depressive disorder in the general population: Results from the US National Comorbidity Survey. *The British Journal of Psychiatry. Supplement*, (30): 17–30. PMID:8864145

Khess, C.R., Dutta, I., Chakrabarty, I., & Bhattacharya, P., Das, J., & Kothari, S. (1998). Comorbidity in children with mental retardation. *Indian Journal of Psychiatry*, (40), 289–294. PMID:21494486

Kilmer, J. R., Cronce, J. M., & Palmer, R. S. (2005). Relapse prevention for abuse of Club Drugs, Hallucinogens, Inhalants, and Steroids. In G. A. Marlatt & D. M. Donovan (Eds.), Relapse prevention: Maintenance strategies in the treatment of addiction behaviors (2nd ed.; pp. 208-247). New York: The Guilford Press.

Kim, E.Y., & Miklowitz., & D.J. (2004). Expressed emotion as a predictor of outcome among bipolar patients undergoing family therapy. *Journal of Affective Disorders*, *82*, 343–352. PMID:15555685

Kimmett, E., & Dora, R. (2009). *An independent review of unmet mental health need in prison*. Prison Reform Trust.

King, C., Feldman, J., Waithaka, Y., Aban, I., Hu, J., Zhang, S., & Bachmann, L. H. et al. (2008). Sexual risk behaviors and sexually transmitted infection prevalence in an outpatient Psychiatry Clinic. *Sexually Transmitted Diseases*, *35*(10), 877–882. doi:10.1097/OLQ.0b013e31817bbc89 PMID:18607313

Kinsella & Phillips. (2005). Global Aging: The Challenge of Success. Population Bulletin, 60(1).

Knapp, M., Mangalore, R., & Simon, J., (2004). The Global Costs of Schizophrenia. *Schizophrenia Bulletin,* (30), 279-293.

Kneisl, C., & Trigoboff, E. (2009). Contemporary Psychiatric- Mental Health Nursing (2nd ed.), London.

Knill, P. J. (1995). The place of beauty in therapy and the Arts. *The Arts in Psychotherapy*, 22.

Koegel, P., Sullivan, G., Burnam, A., Morton, S. C., & Wenzel, S. (1999). Utilization of mental health and substance abuse services among homeless adults in Los Angeles. *Medical Care*, *37*(3), 306–317. doi:10.1097/00005650-199903000-00010 PMID:10098574

Kohn, R., Saxena, S., Levav, I., & Saraceno, B. (2004). The treatment gap in mental health. Bulletin of the World Health Organization. PubMed PMID:15640922

Kono, J., Miyata, H., Ushijima, S., Yanagita, T., Miyasato, K., Ikawa, G., & Hukui, K. (2001). Nicotine, alcohol, methamphetamine, and inhalant dependence: A comparison with clinical features with the use of a new clinical evaluation form. *Alcohol (Fayetteville, N.Y.)*, *24*(2), 99–106. doi:10.1016/S0741-8329(01)00143-4 PMID:11522430

Konrad, N., Daigle, M. S., & Daniel, A. E. (2007). *Preventing suicide in jails and prisons*. Geneva: World Health Organization.

Koujalgi, S. R., Nayak, R. B., Patil, N. M., & Chate, S. S. (2014). Expressed emotions in patients with obsessive compulsive disorder: A case control study. *Indian Journal of Psychological Medicene*, *36*(2), 138–141. doi:10.4103/0253-7176.130972 PMID:24860213

Kovasznay, B., Fleischer, J., Tanenberg-Karant, M., Jandorf, L., Miller, A. D., & Bromet, E. (1997). Substance use disorder and the early course of illness in schizophrenia and affective psychosis. *Schizophrenia Bulletin*, *23*(2), 195–201. doi:10.1093/schbul/23.2.195 PMID:9165630

Kozaric-Kovacic, D., Folnegovic-Smalc, V., Folnegovic, Z., & Maruic, A. (1995). Influence of alcoholism on the prognosis of schizophrenic patients. *Journal of Studies on Alcohol*, *56*(6), 622–627. doi:10.15288/jsa.1995.56.622 PMID:8558893

Kraepelin, E. (1919/1971). Dementia Praecox and Paraphrenia. R.E. Krieger.

Krishnadas, R., Moore, B. P., Nayak, A., & Patel, R. R. (2007). Relationship of cognitive function in patients with schizophrenia in remission to disability: A cross-sectional study in an Indian sample. *Annals of General Psychiatry*, *6*(1), 19. http://www.annals-general-psychiatry.com/content/6/1/19 doi:10.1186/1744-859X-6-19 PMID:17663763

Kudrati, M., Plummer, M., & Yousif, N. D. E. H. (2008). Children of the sug: A study of the daily lives of street children in Khartoum, Sudan, with intervention recommendations. *Child Abuse & Neglect*, *32*(4), 439–448. doi:10.1016/j.chiabu.2007.07.009 PMID:18457872

Kuipers, L., Leff, J., & Lam, D. (1992). *Family Work for Schizophrenia: A Practical Guide*. London: Gaskell.

Kumar, N., & Jha, S. (2013). *Repetitive Transcranial Magnetic Stimulation (RTMS) in organic personality and behavioral disorder, secondary to suicide attempt by hanging*. Academic Press.

Kumar, S.P.N. (1998). Impact of substance abuse comorbidity on psychopathology and pattern of remission in mania. *Indian Journal of Psychiatry, 40*(4), 357-363.

Kumar, M., Bansal, R. K., & Bansal, M. (2008). Need to Support Old-age Home Residents. *Indian Journal of Community Medicine*, *33*(2), 131. doi:10.4103/0970-0218.40887 PMID:19967043

Kumar, V., & Daria, U. (2013). Psychiatric morbidity in prisoners. *Indian Journal of Psychiatry*, *55*(4), 366–370. doi:10.4103/0019-5545.120562 PMID:24459308

Kunikata, H., Mino, Y., & Nakajima, K. (2005). Quality of life of Schizophrenia patients living in the community: The relationships with personal characteristics, objective indicators and self-esteem. *Psychiatry and Clinical Neurosciences*, *59*(2), 163–169. doi:10.1111/j.1440-1819.2005.01352.x PMID:15823162

Kurtz, M. M. (2003). Neurocognitive rehabilitation for schizophrenia. *Current Psychiatry Reports*, *5*(4), 303–310. doi:10.1007/s11920-003-0060-y PMID:12857534

Kurtzman, T. L., Otsuka, K. N., & Wahl, R. A. (2001). Inhalant abuse by adolescents. *The Journal of Adolescent Health*, *28*(3), 170–180. doi:10.1016/S1054-139X(00)00159-2 PMID:11226839

Labbate, L. A., Young, P. C., & Arana, G. W. (1999). Panic disorder in schizophrenia. *Canadian Journal of Psychiatry*, (44), 488–490. PMID:10389611

Lachman-Chapin, M. (1983). The artist as clinician: An interactive technique in art therapy. *American Journal of Art Therapy*, 23.

Lakshmana, G. (2014). DhanasekaraPandian R., & Prabhat Kumar Chand. (2014). Knowledge on impact of substance use and help seeking behavior among substance using street children. *Indian Journal of Social Psychiatry*, *30*(3-4), 106–114.

Lakshmana, G., Pandian, R. D., Kumar, P. K., & Marimuttu, P. (2013). Street children with substance abuse: Enhancement of motivation and relapse prevention strategies. *The Indian Journal of Social Work*, *74*(1), 131–150.

Lamb, H., Weinberger, L., & Gross, B. (2004). Mentally Ill Persons in the Criminal Justice System: Some Perspectives. *The Psychiatric Quarterly*, *75*(2), 107–126. doi:10.1023/B:PSAQ.0000019753.63627.2c PMID:15168834

Lam, D., & Cheng, F. (2008). Chinese policy reaction to the problem of street children: An analysis from the perspective of street children. *Children and Youth Services Review*, *30*(5), 575–584. doi:10.1016/j.childyouth.2007.11.009

Lam, J., & Rosencheck, R. (1999). Street outreach for homeless persons with serious mental illness: Is it effective? *Medical Care*, *37*(9), 894–907. doi:10.1097/00005650-199909000-00006 PMID:10493468

Landgarten, H. B. (1987). *Family Art therapy*. New York: Brunner Mazel.

Lautenschlager, N. T., Kurz, A. F., Loi, S., & Cramer, B. (2013). Personality of mental health caregivers. *Current Opinion in Psychiatry*, *26*(1), 97–101. doi:10.1097/YCO.0b013e32835997b3 PMID:23041793

Laxman, K. E., Lovibond, K. S., & Hassan, M. K. (2008). Impact of bipolar disorder in employed populations. The American Journal of Managed Care, 14(11), 757–764. PubMed PMID:18999910

Le Roux, J., & Smith, C. S. (1998). Psychological characteristics of South African street children. *Adolescence*, *33*(132), 891–899. PMID:9886016

Lebowitz, E. R., Woolston, J., Bar-Haim, Y., Calvocoressi, L., Dauser, C., Warnick, E., & Leckman, J. F. et al. (2012). Family accommodation in pediatric anxiety disorders. *Depression and Anxiety*, *30*(1), 47–54. doi:10.1002/da.21998 PMID:22965863

Lee, T., Yang, Y., Chen, P., Hung, N., Lin, S., Chang, F., & Cheng, S. (2006). Different dimensions of social support for caregivers for patient with schizophrenia: Main effect and stress-buffering models. *Psychiatric Journal of Clinical Neurosciences*, *60*(5), 546–550. doi:10.1111/j.1440-1819.2006.01556.x PMID:16958936

Leff, J. P., & Vaughn, C. (1985). *Expressed emotion in families*. New York: Guildford Press.

Leff, J., Berkowitz, R., Shavit, N., Strachan, A., Glass, I., & Vaughn, C. (1990). A trial of family therapy versus a relatives' group for schizophrenia.Two year follow-up.Comparative study journal article. *The British Journal of Psychiatry*, *157*(4), 571–577. doi:10.1192/bjp.157.4.571 PMID:2131140

Lehman, A. F., Dixon, L. B., Kernan, E., DeForge, B. R., & Postrado, L. T. (1997). A randomized trial of assertive community treatment for homeless persons with severe mental illness. *Archives of General Psychiatry*, *54*(11), 1038–1043. doi:10.1001/archpsyc.1997.01830230076011 PMID:9366661

Lehman, A. F., Myers, C. P., Thompson, J. W., & Corty, E. (1993). Implications of mental and substance use disorders: A comparison of single and dual diagnosis patients. *The Journal of Nervous and Mental Disease*, *181*(6), 365–370. doi:10.1097/00005053-199306000-00005 PMID:8388914

Leifker, F. R., Bowie, C. R., & Harvey, P. D. (2009). Determinants of everyday outcomes in schizophrenia: The influences of cognitive impairment, functional capacity, and symptoms. *Schizophrenia Research*, *115*(1), 82–87. doi:10.1016/j.schres.2009.09.004 PMID:19775869

Lejoyeux, M., & Marinescu, M. (2006). Alcohol dependence and abuse and psychiatric disorders. *La Revue du Praticien*, *56*(10), 1081-1085. Retrieved from http://www.ncbi.nlm.nih.gov/pubmed/16836203.oyeux

Lenze, E. J., Karp, J. F., & Mulsant, B. H. (2005). Somatic symptoms in late-life anxiety: Treatment issues. *Journal of Geriatric Psychiatry and Neurology*, *18*(2), 89–96. doi:10.1177/0891988705276251 PMID:15911937

Lepage, M., Bodnar, M., & Bowie, C. R. (2014). Neurocognition: Clinical and Functional Outcomes in Schizophrenia. *Canadian Journal of Psychiatry*, *59*(1), 5–12. PMID:24444318

Leroy, S., Griffon, N., Bourdel, M. C., Olie, J. P., Poirier, M. F., & Krebs, M. O. (2001). Schizophrenia and the cannabinoid receptor type 1 (CB1): Association study using a single-base polymorphism in coding exon 1. *American Journal of Medical Genetics*, *105*(8), 749–752. doi:10.1002/ajmg.10038 PMID:11803524

Lester, H., & Bradley, C. P. (2001). Barriers to primary healthcare for the homeless: The general practitioner's perspective. *The European Journal of General Practice*, *7*(1), 6–12. doi:10.3109/13814780109048777

Levick, M. F. (1983). *They could not talk and so they drew: Children's styles of coping and thinking*. Springfield, IL: Charlie C. Thomas.

Levin, F. R., & Hennessy, G. (2004). Bipolar disorder and substance abuse. *Biological Psychiatry*, *56*(10), 738–748. doi:10.1016/j.biopsych.2004.05.008 PMID:15556118

Lewin, B. D. (1950). *The Psychoanalysis of elation*. New York: W.W.Norton.

Lewinsohn, P. M., Klein, D. N., & Seeley, J. R. (1995). Bipolar disorders in a community sample of older adolescents: Prevalence, phenomenology, comorbidity, and course. *Journal of the American Academy of Child and Adolescent Psychiatry*, *34*(4), 454–463. doi:10.1097/00004583-199504000-00012 PMID:7751259

Lewis, R. (2014). *US prisons home to 10 times as many mentally ill as in state hospitals: New report slams lack of treatment for seriously ill inmates as 'inhumane,' calls for reforms*. Extracted from http://america.aljazeera.com/articles/2014/4/8/mental-illness-prison.html

Lieberman, J. A., Alvir, J. M., Koreen, A., Geisler, S., Chakos, M., & Sheitman, B. (1996). Psychobiologic correlates of treatment response in schizophrenia. *Neuropsychopharmacology*, *14*(3), 13S–21S. doi:10.1016/0893-133X(95)00200-W PMID:8866739

Liebmann, M. (1990). "It just happened": Looking at crime events. In M. Liebmann (Ed.), *Arttherapy in practice* (pp. 133–155). Bristol, PA: Jessica Kingsley.

Lin, C. H., Huang, C. L., Chang, Y. C., Chen, P. W., Lin, C. Y., Tsai, G. E., & Lane, H. Y. (2013). Clinical symptoms, mainly negative symptoms, mediate the influence of neurocognition and social cognition on functional outcome of schizophrenia. *Schizophrenia Research*, *146*(1-3), 231–237. doi:10.1016/j.schres.2013.02.009 PMID:23478155

Lincoln Police Department. (2004). Emergency Protective Custody Issues for the Police. Mimeo.

Lindenmayer, J. P., Khan, A., Iskander, A., Abad, M. T., & Parker, B. (2007). A randomized controlled trial of olanzapine versus haloperidol in the treatment of primary negative symptoms and neurocognitive deficits in schizophrenia. *The Journal of Clinical Psychiatry*, *68*(3), 368–379. doi:10.4088/JCP.v68n0303 PMID:17388705

Linesch, D. (1993). *Art therapy with families with crisis*. New York: Brunner Mazel.

Link, B. G., & Phelan, J. C. (2001). Conceptualizing stigma. *Annual Review of Sociology*, *27*(1), 363–385. doi:10.1146/annurev.soc.27.1.363

LLerena, A., de la Rubia, A., Peñas-Lledó, E. M., Diaz, F. J., & de Leon, J.LLerena. (2003). Schizophrenia and tobacco smoking in a Spanish psychiatric hospital. *Schizophrenia Research*, *60*(2-3), 313–317. doi:10.1016/S0920-9964(02)00508-X PMID:12591592

Los Angeles Times. (2010). Sheriff says proposed mental health cuts would burden L.A. jails. *Los Angeles Times*.

Lovell, D. (2008). Patterns of disturbed behavior in a supermax prison. *Criminal Justice and Behavior*, *35*(8), 985–1004. doi:10.1177/0093854808318584

Luoma, J. B., Martin, C. E., & Pearson, J. L. (2002). Contact with mental health and primary care providers before suicide: A review of the evidence. *The American Journal of Psychiatry*, *159*(6), 909–916. doi:10.1176/appi.ajp.159.6.909 PMID:12042175

Luria, A. R. (1973). *The Working Brain*. New York: Basic Books.

Lusebrink, V. B. (1990). *Imagery and visual expression in therapy*. New York: Plenum press. doi:10.1007/978-1-4757-0444-0

Maden, A., Swinton, M., & Gunn, J. (1992). A survey of pre-arrest drug use in sentenced prisoners. *British Journal of the Addictions, 87*, 27-33.

Magan˜a, A. B., Goldstein, J. M., Karno, M., Miklowitz, D. J., Jenkins, J., & Falloon, I. R. (1986). A brief method for assessing expressed emotion in relatives of psychiatric patients. *Psychiatry Research, 17*(3), 203–212.

Magliano, L., Fadden, G., Madianos, M., De Almeida, J. M., Held, T., Guarneri, M., & Maj, M. et al. (1998). Burden on the families of patients with schizophrenia: Results of the BIOMED I study. *Social Psychiatry and Psychiatric Epidemiology*, *33*(9), 405–412. doi:10.1007/s001270050073 PMID:9766166

Magliano, L., Fiorillo, A., De Rosa, C., Malangone, C., & Maj, M. (2005). Family burden in long-term diseases: A comparative study in schizophrenia vs. physical disorders. *Social Science & Medicine*, *61*(2), 313–322. doi:10.1016/j.socscimed.2004.11.064 PMID:15893048

Magliano, L., Marasco, C., Fiorillo, A., Malangone, C., Guarneri, M., & Maj, M. (2003). The impact of professional and social network support on the burden of families of patients with schizophrenia in Italy. *Acta Psychiatrica Scandinavica*, *106*(4), 291–298. doi:10.1034/j.1600-0447.2002.02223.x PMID:12225496

Mahajan, A., & Ray. (2013). *Hindu scriptures*. Retrieved from www.hindubooks.org/scriptures/manusmriti/ch2/ch2_121_130.html

Mahato, A. (2011). *A correlational study of neurocognitive factors and psychosocial functioning in schizophrenic patients*. (Unpublished Doctoral dissertation). RINPAS, Ranchi University, Ranchi, India.

Making a Difference: Interim Status Report of the McKinney Research Demonstration Program for Homeless Mentally Ill Adults. (1995). Retrieved December 18, 2015, from https://aspe.hhs.gov/report/performance-improvement-1995/making-difference-interim-status-report-mckinney-research-demonstration-program-homeless-mentally-ill-adults

Malchiodi, C. A. (1996). '*Art therapists* in cyberspace.' *Art Therapy. Journal of the American An Therapy Association*, *13*(4), 150–151.

Malchiodi, C. A. (1997). *Breaking the silence: Art therapy with children from violent homes*. Philadelphia: Brunner/Mazel.

Malchiodi, C. A. (1998). *The Art therapy sourcebook*. Los Angeles, CA: Lowell House.

Malchiodi, C. A. (1998). *Understanding children's drawings*. New York: Guilford Press.

Malekoff, A. (2007). A flexible organizing framework for group work with adolescents. *Social Work with Groups: A Journal of Community and Clinical Practice, 30*(3), 85-102.

Malhotra, C., Sharma, N., Saxena, R., & Ingle, G. K. (2007). Drug use among juveniles in conflict with the law. *Indian Journal of Pediatrics*, *74*(4), 353–356. doi:10.1007/s12098-007-0059-1 PMID:17476079

Malin, A. J. (1971). *Manual Malin's intelligence scale for Indian children (Indian Adaptation of W.I.S.I.C.)*. Lucknow: Indian Psychological Corpoation.

Maniglio, R. (2009). The impact of child sexual abuse on health: A systematic review of reviews. *Clinical Psychology Review*, *29*(7), 647–657. doi:10.1016/j.cpr.2009.08.003 PMID:19733950

Mann, J. J., & Currier, D. (2012). Neurobiology of Suicidal Behavior. In R.I. Simon & R.E. Hales (Eds.), The American Psychiatric Publishing Textbook of Suicide Assessment and Management (pp. 481–500). Academic Press.

Mann, A. H., Graham, N., & Ashby, D. (1984). Psychiatric illness in residential homes for the elderly: A survey in one London borough. *Age and Aging*, *13*(5), 257–265. doi:10.1093/ageing/13.5.257 PMID:6496236

Mann, A. H., Schneider, J., Mozley, C. G., Levin, E., Blizard, R., Netten, A., & Todd, C. et al. (2000). Depression and the response of residential homes to physical health needs. *International Journal of Geriatric Psychiatry*, *15*(12), 1105–1012. doi:10.1002/1099-1166(200012)15:12<1105::AID-GPS252>3.0.CO;2-W PMID:11180466

March, J. S., Franklin, M. E., Leonard, H., Garcia, A., Moore, P., Freeman, J., & Foa, E. (2007). Tics moderate treatment outcome with sertraline but not cognitive-behaviour therapy in pediatric obsessive-compulsive disorder. *Biological Psychiatry*, *61*(3), 344–347. doi:10.1016/j.biopsych.2006.09.035 PMID:17241830

Maremmani, A. G. I., Rovai, L., Bacciardi, S., Rugani, F., Pacini, M., Pani, P. P., & Maremmani, I. (2013). The long-term outcomes of heroin dependent-treatment-resistant patients with bipolar 1 comorbidity after admission to enhanced methadone maintenance. *Journal of Affective Disorders*, *151*(2), 582–589. doi:10.1016/j.jad.2013.06.054 PMID:23931828

Markowitz, J. C., & Weissman, M. M. (2010). Interpersonal Psychotherapy: Past, Present and Future. *Clinical Psychology & Psychotherapy*, *19*(2), 99–105. doi:10.1002/cpp.1774 PMID:22331561

Martens, L., & Addington, J. (2001). The psychological well-being of family members of individuals with schizophrenia. *Social Psychiatry and Psychiatric Epidemiology*, *36*(3), 128–133. doi:10.1007/s001270050301 PMID:11465784

Martha, L., Gail, J., Patrick, J., Ellen, L., Barnett, S., & Denis, J. (2002). Major depression in elderly home health care patients. *The American Journal of Psychiatry*, *159*(8), 1367–1374. doi:10.1176/appi.ajp.159.8.1367 PMID:12153830

Mason, D., Birmingham, L., & Grubin, D. (1997). Substance use in remand prisoners: A consecutive case study. *British Medical Journal*, *315*(7099), 8–21. doi:10.1136/bmj.315.7099.18 PMID:9233320

Massachusetts Biotechnology Council. (2004). *White paper executive summary on prescription drug cost, access and affordability*. Cambridge, MA: Author.

Mathers, C.D., & Loncar, D. (2006). *Projections of global mortality and burden of disease from 2002 to 2030*. doi: 10.1371/journal.pmed.00304424.

Mathur, M. (2009B). Socialization of street children in India: A socio-economic profile. *Psychology and Developing Societies*, *21*(2), 299–325. doi:10.1177/097133360902100207

Mattejat, F., & Remschmidt, H. (1997). Significance of family relations for coping with psychological disorders--results of an empirical study of therapy prognosis of children and adolescents with psychological disorders. *Praxis der Kinderpsychologie und Kinderpsychiatrie*, *46*(5), 371–392. PMID:9273537

Maulik, S., & Dasgupta, A. (2012). Depression and Determinents in rural elderly of west Bengal-a cross sectional study. *International Journal Biological Medicine Research*, *3*(1), 1299–1302.

Maureen, L. (2007). Offenders with mental illness in the correctional system. *Journal of Offender Rehabilitation*, *45*(1-2), 81–104. doi:10.1300/J076v45n01_08

Maurice, J. K. (1970). group therapy in schizophrenia. *The International Journal of Social Psychiatry*, *16*(4), 266–274. doi:10.1177/002076407001600402

McCauley, E., Myers, K., Mitchell, J., Calderon, R., Schloredt, K., & Treder, R. (1993). Depression in young people; initial presentation and clinical course. *Journal of the American Academy of Child and Adolescent Psychiatry*, *32*(4), 714–722. doi:10.1097/00004583-199307000-00003 PMID:8340290

McClellan, J., Kowatch, R., & Findling, R. L. (2007). Practice parameter for the assessment and treatment of children and adolescents with bipolar disorder. *Journal of the American Academy of Child and Adolescent Psychiatry*, *46*(1), 107–125. doi:10.1097/01.chi.0000242240.69678.c4 PMID:17195735

McClure, M. M., Bowie, C. R., Patterson, T. L., Heaton, R. K., Weaver, C., Anderson, H., & Harvey, P. D. (2007). Correlations of functional capacity and neuropsychological performance in older patients with schizophrenia: Evidence for specificity of relationships? *Schizophrenia Research*, *89*(1-3), 330–338. doi:10.1016/j.schres.2006.07.024 PMID:16982175

McConeghey, H. (1986). Archetypal art therapy in cross cultural art therapy. *Art Therapy: Journal of the American Art Therapy Association*, 3.

McCreadie, R. G.Scottish Comorbidity Study Group. (2002). Use of drugs, alcohol and tobacco by people with schizophrenia: Case-control study. *The British Journal of Psychiatry*, *181*(4), 321–325. doi:10.1192/bjp.181.4.321 PMID:12356659

McEvoy, C. (1992). Memory improvement in context: Implications for the development of memory improvement theory. In Memory improvement: Implications for memory theory (pp. 210-230). New York: Springer-Verlag.

McEvoy, C. L., & Moon, J. R. (1988). Assessment and treatment of everyday memory problems in the elderly. In Practical aspects of memory: Current research and issues. Vol 2: Clinical and educational implications. (pp. 155-160). Chichester, UK: Wiley

Mcglashan, T.H., & Carpenter, W.T. (1976). Post psychotic depression in schizophrenia. *Archives of General Psychiatry*, (33), 231-239.

McGlashan, T. H. (1994). Psychosocial treatments of schizophrenia: The potential of relationships. In N. C. Andreasen (Ed.), *Schizophrenia: From mind to molecule*. Washington, DC: American Psychiatric Press.

McGlashan, T. H. (2009). Psychosis as a disorder of reduced cathectic capacity: Freud's analysis of the schreber case Revisited. *Schizophrenia Bulletin*, *35*(3), 476–481. doi:10.1093/schbul/sbp019 PMID:19357240

McGorry, P. D., Yung, A. F., Phillips, L. J., Yuen, H. P., Francey, S., Cosgrave, E. M., & Jackson, H. et al. (2002). Randomized controlled trial of interventions designed to reduce the risk of progression to first-episode psychosis in a clinical sample with subthreshold symptoms. *Archives of General Psychiatry*, *59*(10), 921–928. doi:10.1001/archpsyc.59.10.921 PMID:12365879

McGurk, S. R., Mueser, K. T., & Pascaris, A. (2005). Cognitive training and supported employment for persons with severe mental illness: One-year results from a randomized controlled trial. *Schizophrenia Bulletin*, *31*(4), 898–909. doi:10.1093/schbul/sbi037 PMID:16079391

McHugo, G. J., Drake, R. E., Burton, H. L., & Ackerson, T. H. (1995). A scale for assessing the stage of substance abuse treatment in persons with severe mental illness. *The Journal of Nervous and Mental Disease*, *183*(12), 762–767. doi:10.1097/00005053-199512000-00006 PMID:8522938

McLean, C. P., Asnaani, A., Litz, B. T., & Hofmann, S. G. (2011). Gender differences in anxiety disorders: Prevalence, course of illness, comorbidity and burden of illness. Journal of Psychiatric Research, 45(8), 1027–1035. doi:10.1016/j.jpsychires.2011.03.006 PubMed doi:10.1016/j.jpsychires.2011.03.006 PMID:21439576

McNiff, S. (1992). *Art as medicine: Creating a therapy of imagination*. Boston: Shambhala.

McNiff, S. (1997). Art therapy: A spectrum of partnerships. *The Arts in Psychotherapy*, *24*(1), 37–44. doi:10.1016/S0197-4556(97)00001-4

Medalia, A., Revheim, N., & Casey, M. (2000). Remediation of memory disorders in schizophrenia. *Psychological Medicine*, *30*(6), 1451–1459. doi:10.1017/S0033291799002913 PMID:11097085

Medalia, A., Revheim, N., & Casey, M. (2001). The remediation of problem-solving skills in schizophrenia. *Schizophrenia Bulletin, 27*(2), 259–267. doi:10.1093/oxfordjournals.schbul.a006872 PMID:11354593

Meichenbaum, D. (1977). *Cognitive- behaviour modification: An integrative approach.* New York: Plenum Press. doi:10.1007/978-1-4757-9739-8

Mencimer, S. (2014). *Crime and Justice, Health Care, Human Rights, Prisons, Top Stories. There Are 10 Times More Mentally Ill People Behind Bars Than in State Hospitals*. Academic Press.

Mental health foundation. (2006). Retrieved September12, 2014, fromwww.mentalhealth.org.uk

Mental Health Promotion Unit (MHPU) of the Public Health Agency of Canada. (2003). *Mental Health Promotion: Frequently Asked Questions*. Retrieved February 22, 2007 from http://www.phac-aspc.gc.ca/mh- sm/mhp-psm/faq_e.html

Mental Illness, Human Right, and US Prisons. (2009). *Human Rights Watch Statement for the Record to the Senate Judiciary Committee Subcommittee on Human Rights and the Law*. Author.

Mercer-McFadden, C., Drake, R. E., Brown, N. B., & Fox, R. S. (1997). The community support program demonstrations of services for young adults with severe mental illness and substance use disorders, 1987–1991. *Psychiatric Rehabilitation Journal, 20*(3), 13–24. doi:10.1037/h0095368

Merikangas, K. R., He, J. P., Burstein, M., Swanson, S. A., Avenevoli, S., Cui, L., & Swendsen, J. et al. (2010). Lifetime prevalence of mental disorders in U.S. adolescents: Results from the National Comorbidity Survey Replication – Adolescent Supplement (NCS-A). *Journal of the American Academy of Child and Adolescent Psychiatry, 49*(10), 980–989. doi:10.1016/j.jaac.2010.05.017 PMID:20855043

Merrill, R. M., Njord, L., Njord, R., Read, C., & Pachano, J. D. R. (2010). The effect of family influence on indicators associated with street life among Filipino street children. *Vulnerable Children and Youth Studies, 5*(2), 142–150. doi:10.1080/17450121003615369

Merriman, B., & Guerin, S. (2007). Exploring the aspirations of Kolkatan (Calcuttan) street children living on an off the streets using drawings. *International Journal of Psychology & Psychological Therapy, 7*(2), 269–283.

Meszaros, K., & Fischer-Danzinger, D. (2000). Extended suicide attempt: Psychopathology, personality and risk factors. *Psychopathology, 33*(1), 5–10. doi:10.1159/000029111 PMID:10601820

Meyer, A., Madu, S. N., & Mako, M. J. (2002). Self esteem and emotional stability of street children in some townships in South Africa. *The Irish Journal of Psychology, 23*(1-2), 109–119.

Michalak, E. E., Yatham, L. N., & Lam, R. W. (2004). The role of psychoeducation in the treatment of bipolar disorder: A clinical perspective. *Clinical Approaches in Bipolar Disorder, 3*, 5–11.

Michale, C. (2001). *A feasibility study on life skills education for street children.* (Unpublished M.Phil Dissertation). National Institute of Mental Health and Neuro Sciences, Bangalore, India.

Miguel, E. C., Rauch, S. L., & Jenike, M. A. (1997). Obsessive Compulsive Disorder. *The Psychiatric Clinics of North America, 20*(4), 863–883. doi:10.1016/S0193-953X(05)70349-X PMID:9443354

Miklowitz, D., Goldstein, M. J., Nuechterlein, K. H., & Synder, K. S. (1998). Family factors and the course of BPAD. *Archives of General Psychiatry, 45*, 225–231. doi:10.1001/archpsyc.1988.01800270033004 PMID:3341878

Miller, B. J., Bodenheimer, C., & Crittenden, K. (2011). Second-Generation Antipsychotic discontinuation in first episode psychosis: An updated review. *Cliincal Psychopharmacological Neuroscience, 9*(2), 45–53. doi:10.9758/cpn.2011.9.2.45 PMID:23429653

Miller, W., & Rollnick, S. (1991). *Motivational Interviewing: Preparing People to Change Addictive Behavior*. New York: Guilford.

Mills, J. C., & Crowley, R. J. (1986). *Therapeutic metaphors for children and the child within*. New York: Brunner/Mazel.

Mills, K. L., Teesson, M., Ross, J., & Peters, L. (2006). Trauma, PTSD, and substance use disorders: Findings from the Australian National Survey of Mental Health and Well-Being. *The American Journal of Psychiatry*, *163*(4), 652–658. doi:10.1176/ajp.2006.163.4.652 PMID:16585440

Ministerial Round Tables. (2011). *54th World Health Assembly Mental Health, A call for Action by World Health Ministers*. Author.

Ministry of Health and Family Welfare (2013). *Annual report 2012-13*. Author.

Ministry of housing & urban poverty alleviation annual report. (2012-13). Government of India.

Ministry of Social Justice and Empowerment (Disabilities Division). Government of India. (2007). Retrieved, 23 February, 2016 from http://socialjustice.nic.in/incentdd.php

Ministry of Social Justice and Empowerment. Government of India. (2009). *Annual report*. Retrieved 4 January, 2016, from http://socialjustice.nic.in/annualreports.php

Minkoff, K. (1989). An integrated treatment model for dual diagnosis of psychosis and addiction. *Hospital & Community Psychiatry*, *40*(10), 1031–1036. PMID:2807203

Mishra, M., Trivedi, J.K., & Sinha, P.K. (2005). Burden of care of key relatives of chronic depressives. *SAARC Psychiatric Foundation Souvenir, 56*.

Mohamed, S., Paulsen, J. S., O'Leary, D., Arndt, S., & Andreasen, N. (1999). Generalized cognitive deficits in schizophrenia: A study of firstepisode patients. *Archives of General Psychiatry*, *56*(8), 749–754. doi:10.1001/archpsyc.56.8.749 PMID:10435610

Mohammadi, M. R., Ghanizadeh, A., Rahgozar, M., Noorbala, A. A., Davidian, H., Afzali, H. M., & Tehranidoost, M. et al. (2004). Prevalence of obsessive-compulsive disorder in Iran. *BMC Psychiatry*, *4*(2). PMID:15018627

Mohan, C., & Dhar, V. (2001). Study of psychiatric status of Central Jail under trials at psychiatric hospitals, Government Medical College, Jammu. *Indian Journal of Psychiatry*, *43*, 59.

Mohan, I., Tandon, R., Kalra, H., & Trivedi, J. K. (2005). Disability assessment in mental illnesses using Indian Disability Evaluation Assessment Scale (IDEAS). *The Indian Journal of Medical Research*, *121*, 759–763. PMID:16037620

Moller, H. J. (1989). Efficacy of different strategies of after-care for patients who have attempted suicide. *Journal of the Royal Society of Medicine*, *82*, 643–648. PMID:2556579

Möller-Leimkühler, A. M., & Obermeier, M. (2008). Predicting caregiver burden in first admission psychiatric patients: 2 year follow up results. *European Archives of Psychiatry and Clinical Neuroscience*, *258*(7), 406–413. doi:10.1007/s00406-008-0818-7 PMID:18574613

Montross, L. P., Barrio, C., Yamada, A., Lindamer, L., Golshan, S., & Garcia, P. et al.. (2005). Tri-ethnic variations of co-morbid substance and alcohol use disorders in schizophrenia. *Schizophrenia Research*, *79*, 297–A305. PMID:15978782

Moodie, R. & Jenkins, R. (2005). I'm from the government and you want me to invest in mental health promotion. Well why should I? *Promotion and Education: The evidence of mental health promotion effectiveness: Strategies for action*, 37-41.

Moolla, A., Myburgh, C., & Poggenpoel, M. (2008). Street children's experiences of aggression during interaction with police. *Journal of Psychology in Africa, 18*(4), 597–602.

Moon, B. L. (1995). *Existential Art Therapy: The Canvas Mirror*. Springfield, IL: Charlie C. Thomas.

Moon, C. H. (2002). *Studio art therapy: Cultivating the artist identity in the art therapist*. London: Jessica Kingsley.

Morey, L. C. (1991). Classification of mental disorder as a collection of hypothetical constructs. *Journal of Abnormal Psychology, 100*(3), 289–293. doi:10.1037/0021-843X.100.3.289 PMID:1918606

Morgan, C. J. A., & Curran, H. V. (2008). Effects of cannabidiol on schizophrenia-like symptoms in people who use cannabis. *The British Journal of Psychiatry, 192*(4), 306–307. doi:10.1192/bjp.bp.107.046649 PMID:18378995

Morse, G. A., Calsyn, R. J., Allen, G., Tempelhoff, B., & Smith, R. (1992). Experimental comparison of the effects of three treatment programs for homeless mentally ill people. *Hospital & Community Psychiatry, 43*, 1005–1010. PMID:1398563

Morse, G. A., Calsyn, R. J., & Klinkenberg, W. D. (1997). An experimental comparison of three types of case management for homeless mentally ill persons. *Psychiatric Services (Washington, D.C.), 48*(4), 497–503. doi:10.1176/ps.48.4.497 PMID:9090733

Moshman, D. (2005). Adolescent Psychological Development Rationality, Morality and Identity (2nd Ed.) Lawrence Erlbaum Associates, Inc.

Motto, J. A. (1976). Suicide prevention for high-risk persons who refuse treatment. *Suicide & Life-Threatening Behavior, 6*, 223–230. PMID:1023455

Motto, J. A., & Bostrom, A. G. (2001). A randomized controlled trial of postcrisis suicide prevention. *Psychiatric Services (Washington, D.C.), 52*(6), 828–833. doi:10.1176/appi.ps.52.6.828 PMID:11376235

Motto, J. A., Heilbron, D. C., Juster, R. P., & Bostrom, A. G. (1981). Communication as a suicide prevention program. In J. P. Soubrier & J. Vedrienne (Eds.), *Depression and suicide* (pp. 143–166). Paris: Pergamon.

Mowrer, O. H. (1969). Psychoneurotic defenses (including deception) as punishment avoidance strategies. In Punishment and aversive behavior. New York: Crofts-Crofts.

Mrazek, P. J., & Haggerty, R. J. (1994). *Reducing risks for mental disorders: frontiers for preventive intervention research*. Washington, DC: National Academy Press.

Mroziewicz, M., & Tyndale, R. F. (2010). Pharmacogenetics: A tool for identifying genetic factors in drug dependence and response to treatment. *Addiction Science & Clinical Practice, 5*(2), 17–29. PMID:22002450

Mueller, T. I., Lavori, P. W., Keller, M. B., Swartz, A., Warshaw, M., Hasin, D., & Akiskal, H. (1994). Prognostic effect of the variable course of alcoholism on the 10-year course of depression. *The American Journal of Psychiatry, 151*(5), 701–706. doi:10.1176/ajp.151.5.701 PMID:8166311

Mueser, K. T., Deavers, F., Penn, D. L., & Cassisi, J. (2013). Psychosocial treatments for schizophrenia. *Annual Review of Clinical Psychology, 9*(1), 465–497. doi:10.1146/annurev-clinpsy-050212-185620 PMID:23330939

Mueser, L. (2005). Psychosocial interventions for adult with severe mental illness and co-occurring substance use conditions: A review of specific interventions. *Journal of Dual Diagnosis, 1*, 57. doi:10.1300/J374v01n02_05

Murray, C. J. L., & Lopez, A. D. (1996). The Global Burden of Disease: A Comprehensive Assessment of Mortality and Disability From Diseases, Injuries and Risk Factors in 1990 and Projected to 2020. Boston: Harvard School of Public Health, World Health Organization, World Bank.

Murray, C. J. L., & Lopez, A. D. (1999). Global burden of disease. Geneva: World Health Organisation.

Murray, C. J. L., & Lopez, A. D. (1996). *The Global Burden of Diseases: A Comprehensive Assessment of Mortality and Disability from Diseases, Injuries and Risk Factors in 1990 and Projected to 2020*. Boston: Harvard School of Public Health, World Health Organization and World Bank.

Murthy, P., & Chand, P. (2012). Treatment of dual diagnosis disorders. *Current Opinion in Psychiatry*, *25*(3), 194–200. doi:10.1097/YCO.0b013e328351a3e0 PMID:22395768

Nadeem, E., Lange, J. M., Edge, D., Fongwa, M., Belin, T., & Miranda, J. (2007). Does stigma keep poor young immigrant and U.S. born black and Latina women from seeking mental health care? *Psychiatric Services (Washington, D.C.)*, *58*(12), 1547–1554. doi:10.1176/ps.2007.58.12.1547 PMID:18048555

Naidoo, S., & Mkize, D.L. (2012). Prevalence of mental disorders in a prison population in Durban, South Africa. *African Journal of Psychiatry*, *15*(1).

Nalkur, P. G. (2009a). Achievement orientations and strategies: A cultural comparison of Tanzanian street children, former street children, and school-going children. *Journal of Cross-Cultural Psychology*, *40*(6), 1012–1027. doi:10.1177/0022022109346954

Nambi, S. (2014). Forensic Psychiatry (Psychiatry & Law). Jaypee Brothers Medical Publishers.

Nambi, S. (2005). Marriage, mental health and the Indian legislation. *Indian Journal of Psychiatry*, *47*(1), 3–14. doi:10.4103/0019-5545.46067

Nambi, S. (2008). *Legal aspects in Psychiatry – Indian Perspective*. Manashanthi Mental Health Care Publications.

Nandi, D. N., Banarjee, G., & Boral, G. C. (1978). Suicide in West Bengal - A century apart. *Indian Journal of Psychiatry*, *20*, 155–160.

Nandi, P. S., Banerjee, G., & Mukherjee, S. P. (1997). A study of psychiatric morbidity of elderly population of a rural community in West Bengal. *Indian Journal of Psychiatry*, *39*, 122–129. PMID:21584058

Narasipuram, S., & Kasimahanti, S. (2012). Quality of life and perception of burden among caregivers of persons with mental illness. *Applied Journal of Psychological Medicine*, *13*, 99–103.

Narayanaswamy, J. C., Viswanath, B., Cherian, A. V., Bada Math, S., Kandavel, T., & Janardhan Reddy, Y. C. (2012). Impact of age of onset of illness on clinical phenotype in OCD. *Psychiatry Research*, *200*(2-3), 554–559. doi:10.1016/j.psychres.2012.03.037 PMID:22503329

Narendra, K. S., Bhattacharjee, D., Nishant, G., Sanjay, K. M., & Nizamie, S. H. (2011). Perceived burden and social support of caregivers in early onset psychosis and epilepsy: A comparative study. *Malaysian Journal of Psychiatry*, *20*, 2.

National Crime Records Bureau. (2014). Retrieved from India.ncrb.gov.in/ADSI2014/adsi-2014%20full%20report.pdf

National electronic Library for Mental Health (NeLMH). (2004). *Defining mental health promotion: risk and protective factors*. Retrieved March 27, 2007 from http://www.nelmh.net/page_view.asp?c=22&did=2358&fc=004002

National Human Rights Commission. NHRC, (2015). Extracted from http://nhrc.nic.in/disparchive.asp?fno=13716

National Institute for Clinical Excellence. (2009). *Schizophrenia (update) Clinical Guidelines CG82*. NICE. Available from: http://www.guidance.nice.org.uk/CG82

National Institute of Health and Care Excellence. (2013). *Psychosis and schizophrenia in children and young people*. Retrieved 09 January, 2106, from https://www.nice.org.uk/guidance/indevelopment/gid-cgwave0797

National Policy for Persons with Disabilities. (1993). Government of India. Handbook on Disability Rehabilitation. New Delhi: National Information Centre on Disability Rehabilitation, Ministry of Social Justice and Empowerment.

Naugle, R., Prevy, M., Naugle, C., & Delaney, R. (1988). The new digital watch as a compensatory device for memory dysfunction. *Cognitive Rehabilitation*, *6*, 22–23.

NDTV. (2014). *Harsh conditions found in Indian mental health facilities for women*. Extracted from http://www.ndtv.com/india-news/harsh-conditions-found-in-indian-mental-health-facilities-for-women-708087

Neale, J., & Kennedy, C. (2002). Good practice towards homeless drug users: Research evidence from Scotland. *Health & Social Care in the Community*, *10*(3), 196–205. doi:10.1046/j.1365-2524.2002.00357.x PMID:12121256

Newbauer, J. F., & Blanks, J. W. (2001). Group work with adolescent sexual offenders. *Journal of Individual Psychology*, *57*(1), 37–50.

Nicholl, D., Akhras, K. S., Diels, J., & Schadrack, J. (2010). Burden of schizophrenia in recently diagnosed patients: Healthcare utilization and cost perspective. Current Medical Research and Opinion, 26(4), 943–955. doi:10.1185/03007991003658956 PubMed doi:10.1185/03007991003658956 PMID:20163295

Nisbett, R. E., & Wilson, T. D. (1977). Telling more than we can know: Verbal reports on mental processes. *Psychological Review*, *84*(3), 231–259. doi:10.1037/0033-295X.84.3.231

Nizamie, A., Nizamie, S. H., & Shukla, T. R. (1992). Performance on Luria - Nebraska Neuropsychological Battery in Schhizophrenic Patients. *Indian Journal of Psychiatry*, *34*, 321–330. PMID:21776138

Njord, L., Merrill, R. M., Njord, R., Lindsay, R., & Pachano, J. D. R. (2010). Drug use among street children and non-street children in the Philippines. *Asia-Pacific Journal of Public Health*, *22*(2), 203–211. doi:10.1177/1010539510361515 PMID:20457649

Norcross, J. C. (2005). A primer on psychotherapy integration. In J. C. Norcross & M. R. Goldfried (Eds.), Handbook of psychotherapy integration (2nd ed.). New York: Oxford. doi:10.1093/med:psych/9780195165791.003.0001

Norcross, J. C., & Grencavage, L. M. (1989). Eclecticism and integration in psychotherapy: Major themes and obstacles. *British Journal of Guidance & Counselling*, *19*, 227–247.

Norman, R. M., Malla, A. K., Morrison, S. S. L., Helmes, E., Williamson, P. C., Thomas, J., & Cortese, L. (1997). Neuropsychological correlates of syndromes in schizophrenia. *The British Journal of Psychiatry*, *170*(2), 134–139. doi:10.1192/bjp.170.2.134 PMID:9093501

North, C. S., & Smith, E. M. (1993). A systematic study of mental health services utilization by homeless men and women. *Social Psychiatry and Psychiatric Epidemiology*, *28*(2), 77–83. doi:10.1007/BF00802096 PMID:8511667

Northern Ireland Association for Mental Health and The Sainsbury Centre for Mental Health Counting the Cost. (2007). *The Economic and Social Costs of Mental Health Problems in Northern Ireland*. Northern Ireland Association for Mental Health & Sainsbury Centre for Mental Health.

Novaco, R. W. (1979). *Therapist manual for stress inoculation training. Therapeutic interventions for anger problems*. Irvine, CA: University of California.

Nucho, A. O. (1987). The Psychocybernetic model of art therapy. Springfield, IL: Charlie C. Thomas.

Nuttall, J. (2002). Modes of therapeutic relationship in brief dynamic psychotherapy: A case study. *Psychodynamic Practice*, *8*(4), 505–523. doi:10.1080/1353333021000038854

Ochoa, S., Vilaplana, M., Haro, J., Villalta-Gil, V., Martínez, F., Cruz, M., & Autonell, J. et al. (2008). Do needs, symptoms, or disability of outpatients with Schizophrenia influence family burden? *Social Psychiatry and Psychiatric Epidemiology*, *43*(8), 612–618. doi:10.1007/s00127-008-0337-x PMID:18340397

Ogai, M., Iyo, M., Mori, N., & Takei, N. (2005). A right orbitofrontal region and OCD symptoms: A case report. *Acta Psychiatric Scandiavica,* (111), 74-7610.

Ogilvie, A. D., Morant, N., & Goodwin, G. M. (2005). The burden on informal caregivers of people with bipolar disorder. *Bipolar Disorders*, *7*(s1), 25–32. doi:10.1111/j.1399-5618.2005.00191.x PMID:15762866

Ohaeri, J. U. (2001). Caregiver burden and psychotic patients' perception of social support in a Nigerian setting. *Social Psychiatry and Psychiatric Epidemiology*, *36*(2), 86–93. doi:10.1007/s001270050294 PMID:11355450

Ohaeri, J. U. (2003). The burden of caregiving in families with a mental illness: A review of 2002. *Current Opinion in Psychiatry*, *16*(4), 457–465. doi:10.1097/01.yco.0000079212.36371.c0

Olfson, M., Mechanic, D., Hansell, S., Boyer, C. A., Walkup, J., & Weiden, P. J. (2000). Predicting medication non-compliance after hospital discharge among patients with schizophrenia. *Psychiatric Services (Washington, D.C.)*, *51*(2), 216–222. doi:10.1176/appi.ps.51.2.216 PMID:10655006

Olley, B. O. (2006). Social and health behaviors in youth of the streets of Ibadan, Nigeria. *Child Abuse & Neglect*, *30*(3), 271–282. doi:10.1016/j.chiabu.2005.10.011 PMID:16519940

Oquendo, M. A., Lizardi, D., Greenwald, S., Weissman, M. M., & Mann, J. J. (2004). Rates of lifetime suicide attempt and rates of lifetime major depression in different ethnic groups in the United States. Acta Psychiatrica Scandinavica, 110(6), 446–451. doi:10.1111/j.1600-0447.2004.00404.x PubMed doi:10.1111/j.1600-0447.2004.00404.x PMID:15521829

Orley, J., Saxena, S., & Herrman, H. (1998). Quality of life and mental illness: Reference from perspective of the WHO-QOL. *The British Journal of Psychiatry*, *172*(4), 291–293. doi:10.1192/bjp.172.4.291 PMID:9715330

Ormel, J., Von Korff, M., Burger, H., Scott, K., Demyttenaere, K., Huang, Y. Q., & Kessler, R. (2007). Mental disorders among persons with heart disease - results from World Mental Health surveys. General Hospital Psychiatry, 29(4), 325–334. doi:10.1016/j.genhosppsych.2007.03.009 PubMed doi:10.1016/j.genhosppsych.2007.03.009 PMID:17591509

Osher, F. C., & Kofoed, L. L. (1989). Treatment of patients with psychiatric and psychoactive substance abuse disorders. *Hospital & Community Psychiatry*, *40*(10), 1025–1030. PMID:2807202

Overall, J. E., & Gorham, D. R. (1962). The brief psychiatric rating scale. *Psychological Reports*, *10*(3), 799–812. doi:10.2466/pr0.1962.10.3.799

Oxford University Press. (2010). "Schizophrenia" Concise Medical Dictionary. Oxford Reference Online.

Padgett, D., Struening, E. L., & Andrews, H. (1990). Factors affecting the use of medical, mental health, alcohol, and drug treatment services by homeless adults. *Medical Care*, *28*(9), 805–821. doi:10.1097/00005650-199009000-00010 PMID:2402175

Palmer, B. W., Heaton, R. K., Paulsen, J. S., Kuck, J., Braff, D., Harris, M. J., & Jeste, D. V. et al. (1997). Is it possible to be schizophrenic yet neuropsychologically normal? *Neuropsychology*, *11*(3), 437–446. doi:10.1037/0894-4105.11.3.437 PMID:9223148

Pandey, G. N. (2013). Biological basis of suicide and suicidal behavior. *Bipolar Disorders*, *15*(5), 524–541. doi:10.1111/bdi.12089 PMID:23773657

Parkar, S. R. (2015). Elderly mental health: Needs. *Mens Sana Monographs*, *13*(1), 91–99. doi:10.4103/0973-1229.153311 PMID:25838727

Parker, G., Fairley, M., Greenwood, J., Jurd, S., & Silove, D. (1982). Parental representations of Schizophrenias and their association with onset and course of schizophrenia. *The British Journal of Psychiatry*, *141*(6), 573–581. doi:10.1192/bjp.141.6.573 PMID:7159804

Patel, V. (2009). The future of psychiatry in low- and middleincome countries. Psychological Medicine, 39(11), 1759–1762. doi:10.1017/S0033291709005224 PubMed doi:10.1017/S0033291709005224 PMID:20162837

Patterson, G. T. (2007). Examining missing person police reports to identify the service needs of runaway youth and their families. *Journal of Human Behavior in the Social Environment*, *16*(3), 73–88. doi:10.1300/10911350802107751

Patterson, P., Birchwood, M., & Cochrane, R. (2005). Expressed emotion as an adaptation to loss: Prospective study in Ist- episode psychosis. *The British Journal of Psychiatry*, *187*(48), s59–s64. doi:10.1192/bjp.187.48.s59 PMID:16055810

Patton, G. C., Coffey, C., Carlin, J. B., Degenhardt, L., Lynskey, M., & Hall, W. (2002). Cannabis use and mental health in young people: Cohort study. *British Medical Journal (Clinical Research Ed.)*, *325*(7374), 1195–1198. doi:10.1136/bmj.325.7374.1195 PMID:12446533

Patton, M. Q. (1970). *Qualitative Research and Evaluation Methods* (3rd ed.). Thousand Oaks, CA: Sage.

Paulsen, J. S., Heaton, R. K., Sadek, J. R., Perry, W., Delis, D. C., Braff, D., & Jeste, D. V. et al. (1995). The nature of learning and memory impairments in schizophrenia. *Journal of the International Neuropsychological Society*, *1*(01), 88–99. doi:10.1017/S135561770000014X PMID:9375213

Pavuluri, M. N., Henry, D. B., Devineni, B., Carbray, J. A., & Birmaher, B. (2006). Child mania rating scale: Development, reliability, and validity. *Journal of the American Academy of Child and Adolescent Psychiatry*, *45*(5), 550–560. doi:10.1097/01.chi.0000205700.40700.50 PMID:16601399

Pearlin, L. I., Mullan, J. T., Semple, S. J., & Skaff, M. M. (1990). Caregiving and the stress process: An overview of concepts and their measures. *The Gerontologist*, *30*(5), 583–594. doi:10.1093/geront/30.5.583 PMID:2276631

Peele, P. B., Xu, Y., & Kupfer, D. J. (2003). Insurance expenditures on bipolar disorder: Clinical and parity concerns. The American Journal of Psychiatry, 160(7), 1286–1290. doi:10.1176/appi.ajp.160.7.1286 PubMed doi:10.1176/appi.ajp.160.7.1286 PMID:12832243

Pekkala, E. T., & Merinder, L. B. (2002). *Psychoeducation for schizophrenia (Cochrane Review)*. Oxford, UK: Update Software.

Perlick, D. A., Rosenbeck, R. A., Clarkin, J. F., Maciejewski, P. K., Sirey, J., Struening, E., & Link, B. G. (2004). Impact of family burden and affective response on clinical outcome among patients with bipolar disorder. *Psychiatric Services (Washington, D.C.)*, *55*(9), 1029–1035. doi:10.1176/appi.ps.55.9.1029 PMID:15345763

Perlick, D. A., Rosenheck, R. A., Milkowitz, D. J., Kaczynski, R., Link, B., & Ketter, S. G. (2008). Caregiver burden and health in bipolar disorder: A Cluster analytic approach. *The Journal of Nervous and Mental Disease*, *196*(6), 484–491. doi:10.1097/NMD.0b013e3181773927 PMID:18552626

Perlick, D., Clarkin, J. F., Sirey, J., Raue, P., Greenfield, S., Struening, E., & Rosenheck, R. (1999). Burden experienced by care-givers of persons with bipolar affective disorder. *The British Journal of Psychiatry*, *175*(1), 56–62. doi:10.1192/bjp.175.1.56 PMID:10621769

Perlick, D., Rosenheck, R. A., Clarkin, J. F., Raue, P., & Sirey, J. (2001). Impact of family burden and patient symptom status on clinical outcome in bipolar affective disorder. *The Journal of Nervous and Mental Disease*, *189*(1), 31–37. doi:10.1097/00005053-200101000-00006 PMID:11206662

Perrin, T., & May, H. (2001). *Wellbeing in dementia: An occupational approach for therapists and carers*. Edinburgh, UK: Churchill Livingstone.

Perry, A., Tarrier, N., Morriss, R., McCarthy, E., & Limb, K. (1999). Randomized controlled trial of efficacy of teaching patients with bipolar disorder to identify early symptoms of relapse and obtain treatment. *British Medical Journal*, *318*(7177), 149–153. doi:10.1136/bmj.318.7177.149 PMID:9888904

Perry, B. D., Pollard, R. A., Blakley, T. L., Baker, W. L., & Vigilante, D. (1995). Childhood trauma, the neurobiology of adaptation and use-dependent development of the brain: How states become traits. *Infant Mental Health Journal*, *16*(4), 271–291. doi:10.1002/1097-0355(199524)16:4<271::AID-IMHJ2280160404>3.0.CO;2-B

Pescosolido, B. A., Martin, J. K., Long, J. S., Medina, T. R., Phelan, J. C., & Link, B. G. (2010). A disease like any other? A decade of change in public reactions to schizophrenia, depression, and alcohol dependence. *The American Journal of Psychiatry*, *16*(11), 1321–1330. doi:10.1176/appi.ajp.2010.09121743 PMID:20843872

Pesic, L. (2007). Social and health problems of the elderly. *ActaMedica Medianae*, *46*, 45–48.

Peterson, P. L., Baer, J. S., Wells, E. A., Ginzler, J. A., & Garrett, S. B. (2006). Short-term effects of a brief motivational intervention to reduce alcohol and drug risk among homeless adolescents. *Psychology of Addictive Behaviors*, *20*(3), 254–264. doi:10.1037/0893-164X.20.3.254 PMID:16938063

Petrakis, I. L., O'Malley, S., Rounsaville, B., Poling, J., McHugh-Strong, C., & Krystal, J. H. (2004). Naltrexone augmentation of neuroleptic treatment in alcohol abusing patients with schizophrenia. *Psychopharmacology*, *172*(3), 291–297. doi:10.1007/s00213-003-1658-9 PMID:14634716

Pharoah, F., Mari, J., Rathbone, J., & Wong, W. (2010). Family intervention for schizophrenia.[*Cochrane Database of Systematic Reviews*, (12): CD000088. PMID:21154340

Philip, R. (1976). When, what, and why? psychopharmacotherapy and other treatments in schizophrenia. *Comprehensive Psychiatry*, *17*(6), 683–693. doi:10.1016/0010-440X(76)90016-X PMID:186230

Phillips, M.R., Yang, G., Zhang, Y., Wang, L., Ji, H., & Zhou, M. (2002). Risk factors for suicide in China: a national case-control psychological autopsy study. *Lancet, 360*(9347), 1728-36.

Pigott, T. A., L' Heureux, F., Dubbert, B., Bernstein, S., & Murphy, D. L. (1994). Obsessive-compulsive disorder: Comorbid conditions. *The Journal of Clinical Psychiatry*, (55): 15–27. PMID:7961529

Pinzón-Rondón, A. M., Hofferth, S., & Briceño, L. (2008). Children working in the streets of Colombian cities: Different pathways to the street lead to different populations. *Children and Youth Services Review*, *30*(12), 1417–1424. doi:10.1016/j.childyouth.2008.04.009

Piselli, M., Elisei, S., Murgia, N., Quartesan, R., & Abram, K. M. (2009). Co-occurring psychiatric and substance use disorders among male detainees in Italy. *International Journal of Law and Psychiatry*, *29*, 370–385. PMID:19237198

Planansky, K., & Johnston, R. (1978). Depressive syndrome in schizophrenia. *Acta Psychiatrica Scandinavica*, *57*(3), 207–218. doi:10.1111/j.1600-0447.1978.tb06887.x PMID:645411

Pleasence, P & Balmer, N. (2007). *Mental health and the experience of problems involving rights*. Academic Press.

Pleasence, P., & Balmer, N. (2007). Mental health and the experience of housing problems involving rights. *People, Place and Policy Online*, *2*(1), 4–16. Retrieved from http://extra.shu.ac.uk/ppponline/issue_1_300108/documents/mental_health_housing_problems_rights.pdf

Pleasence, P., Balmer, N., & Buck, A. (2006). Causes of action: civil law and social justice (2nd ed.). London: Stationery Offifice. Retrieved from http:// www.lsrc.org.uk/publications/cofa2006.pdf

Pleasence, P., Buck, A., Balmer, N., O'Grady, A., Genn, H., & Smith, M. (2004b). Causes of action: civil law and social justice. Stationery Office, Norwich.

Pleasence, P., Balmer, N., & Buck, A. (2008). The health cost of civil-law problems: Further evidence of links between civil-law problems and morbidity, and the consequential use of health services'. *Journal of Empirical Legal Studies*, *5*(2), 351–373. doi:10.1111/j.1740-1461.2008.00127.x

Pleasence, P., Balmer, N., Buck, A., O'Grady, A., & Genn, H. (2004a). Civil law problems and morbidity'. *Journal of Epidemiology and Community Health*, *58*(7), 552–557. doi:10.1136/jech.2003.014076 PMID:15194714

Plummer, M. L., & Mustafa, K. (2007). Beginning street life: Factors contributing to children working and living on the streets of Khartoum, Sudan. *Children and Youth Services Review*, *29*(12), 1520–1536. doi:10.1016/j.childyouth.2007.06.008

Policies & Schemes. (2016). Retrieved January 18, 2016, from, Phttp://www.archive.india.gov.in/citizen/senior_citizen/senior_citizen.php?id=12

Posner, K., Brown, G. K., Stanley, B., Brent, D. A., Yershova, K. V., Oquendo, M. A., & Mann, J. J. et al. (2011). The Columbia–Suicide Severity Rating Scale: Initial Validity and Internal Consistency Findings From Three Multisite Studies With Adolescents and Adults. *The American Journal of Psychiatry*, *168*(12), 1266–1277. doi:10.1176/appi.ajp.2011.10111704 PMID:22193671

Posner, K., Oquendo, M. A., Gould, M., Stanley, B., & Davies, M. (2007). Columbia Classification Algorithm of Suicide Assessment (C-CASA): Classification of Suicidal Events in the FDA's Pediatric Suicidal Risk Analysis of Antidepressants. *The American Journal of Psychiatry*, *164*(7), 1035–1043. doi:10.1176/ajp.2007.164.7.1035 PMID:17606655

Poyurovsky, M., Faragian, S., Shabeta, A., & Kosov, A. (2008). Comparision of clinical characteristics, co-morbidity and pharmacotherapy in adolescents with and without obsessive-compulsive disorder. *Psychiatry Residence*, *159*, 133–139. doi:10.1016/j.psychres.2007.06.010

Praharaj, S. K., Verma, P., & Arora, M. (2008). Inhalant abuse (typewriter correction fluid) in street children. *Journal of Addiction Medicine*, *2*(4), 175–177. doi:10.1097/ADM.0b013e31817be5bc PMID:21768989

Prasad, J., Abraham, V. J., & Minz, S. (2006). Rates and factors associated with suicide in Kaniyambadi Block, Tamil Nadu, South India, 2000–2002. The International Journal of Social Psychiatry, 52(1), 65–71. doi:10.1177/0020764006061253 PubMed doi:10.1177/0020764006061253 PMID:16463596

Press note on poverty estimates of 2011-12. (2013). Planning Commission, Government of India.

Priebe, S., Roeder-Wanner, U.-U., & Kaiser, W. (2006). Quality of life in Ist admitted Schizophrenia patients: A follow up study. *Psychological Medicine*, *30*(1), 225–230. doi:10.1017/S0033291798008253 PMID:10722193

Prince, M., Patel, V., Saxena, S., Maj, M., Maselko, J., & Phillips, M.R. (2007). No health without mental health. *Lancet*, *370*(9590), 859-77.

Priscilla, E. (2005). *Gerontological nursing and healthy aging*. Elsevier Health Sciences.

Prison Statistics India. (2012). *Prison Statistics India is the eighteenth in the series of annual publication.* The National Crime Records Bureau, Ministry of Home Affairs.

Proctor, E. K., Landsverk, J., Aarons, G., Chambers, D., Glisson, C., & Mittman, B. (2009). Implementation research in mental health services: An emerging science with conceptual, methodological, and training challenges. Administration and Policy in Mental Health, 36(1), 24–34. doi:10.1007/s10488-008-0197-4 PubMed doi:10.1007/s10488-008-0197-4 PMID:19104929

PRS Legislative Research. (2014). *Legislative brief. The Rights of Persons with Disabilities Bill.* Retrieved March 12, 2015, from http://www.prsindia.org/uploads/media/Person%20with%20Disabilities/Legislative%20Brief%20%20-%20Disabilities%202014.pdf

Puig, O., Penades, R., Gasto, C., Catalan, R., Torres, A., & Salamero, M. (2008). Verbal memory, negative symptomatology and prediction of psychosocial functioning in schizophrenia. *Psychiatry Research, 158*(1), 11–17. doi:10.1016/j.psychres.2007.04.017 PMID:18001844

Qualls, S. H., & Kenny, M. (2008). *Caregiver Reaction Scale*. Unpublished assessment.

Radhakrishnan, R., & Andrade, C. (2012). Suicide: An Indian perspective. *Indian Journal of Psychiatry, 54*(4), 304–319. doi:10.4103/0019-5545.104793 PMID:23372232

Rai, A. (2008). Delhi City Report. In H. Mander (Ed.), *Living Rough Surviving City Streets- A study of Homeless Population in Delhi, Chennai, Patna and Madurai (2).* New Delhi, India: Planning Commission.

Rajkumar, A. P., Thangadurai, P., Senthilkumar, P., Gayathri, K., Prince, M., & Jacob, K. S. (2009). Nature, Prevalance and Factors Associated with Depression among the Elderly in Rural South Indian Community. *International Psychogeriatrics, 21*(2), 372–378. doi:10.1017/S1041610209008527 PMID:19243657

Rajkumar, R. P., Reddy, Y. C. J., & Kandavel, T. (2008). Clinical profile of "schizo-obsessive" disorder; a comparative study. *Comprehensive Psychiatry, 49*(3), 262–268. doi:10.1016/j.comppsych.2007.09.006 PMID:18396185

Rakshit, R. (2004). *An intervention study on the coping skills of the street children with substance abuse.* Bangalore: National Institute of Mental Health and Neuro Sciences.

Ramesh, K.G., & Sridhara, m.v. (2013). *Health Status of Elderly Living in the Old Age Homes: An Overview JMSD.* Academic Press.

Rangaswamy, S. M. (2001). Geneva, Switzerland: The World Health Organization; World Health Report on Mental Health: New understanding New Hope. *Indian Journal of Psychiatry, 43*(1), 1–4. PMID:21407829

Rani, M., Palani, G., & Sathiyasekaran, B. W. C. (2012). Morbidity profile of elders in OAH in Chennai. *National Journal of Community Medicine, 3*(3), 458–464.

Ran, M. S., Chan, C. L. W., Chen, E. Y. H., Xiang, M. Z., Caine, E. D., & Conwell, Y. (2006). Homelessness among patients with schizophrenia in rural China: A 10-year cohort study. *Acta Psychiatrica Scandinavica, 114*(2), 118–123. doi:10.1111/j.1600-0447.2006.00746.x PMID:16836599

Rao, P.G. (2010). An overview of Indian research in bipolar mood disorder. *Indian Journal of Psychiatry, 52*(1), 173-177.

Rao, V. A. (1965). Attempted suicide. *Indian Journal of Psychiatry, 7*, 253–264.

Rao, V. A. (1999). Toward suicide prevention. *Indian Journal of Psychiatry, 41*, 280–288. PMID:21430799

Rasanen, P., Tiilhonen, J., & Isohanni, M. (1998). Schizophrenia, Alcohol abuse and violent behaviour: A 26 year follow-up study of an unselected birth cohort. *Schizophrenia Bulletin*, *24*(3), 437–441. doi:10.1093/oxfordjournals.schbul.a033338 PMID:9718635

Rathod, S., Kingdom, D., Smith, P., & Turkington, D. (2005). Insight into schizophrenia: the effects of cognitive behavioural therapy on the components of insight and association with sociodemographics-data on a previously published randomized controlled trial. *Schizophrenia Research, 74*(2-3), 211-219.

Raune, D., Kuipers, E., & Bebbington, P. E. (2004). Expressed emotion at first episode-psychosis: Investigating a career appraisal model. *The British Journal of Psychiatry*, *184*(4), 321–326. doi:10.1192/bjp.184.4.321 PMID:15056576

Raveeshm, B. N., Anil, M. N., & Narendra, K. M. S. (2013). Law & Psychiatry in India: An Overview. *J Forensic Sci Criminol*, *1*, 203.

Ray, R. (1989). Alcohol diagnosis and phenomenology. *Proceedings of the Indo-US symposium on alcohol and drug use*. NIMHANS publication No 20 Bangalore.

Regier, D. A., Farmer, M. E., Rae, D. S., Locke, B. Z., Keith, S. J., Judd, L. L., & Goodwin, F. K. (1990). Comorbidity of mental disorders with alcohol and other drug abuse. Results from the Epidemiologic Catchment Area (ECA) Study. *Journal of the American Medical Association*, *264*(19), 2511–2518. doi:10.1001/jama.1990.03450190043026 PMID:2232018

Reichenberg, A. (2010). The assessment of neuropsychological functioning in schizophrenia. *Dialogues in Clinical Neuroscience*, *12*(3), 383–392. PMID:20954432

Reine, G., Lancon, C., Simeoni, M. C., Duplan, S., & Auquier, P. (2003). Caregiver burden in relatives of persons with schizophrenia: An overview of measure instruments. *L'Encéphale*, *29*(2), 137–147. PMID:14567165

Report, W. H. (2001). *Mental Health: New Understanding, New Hope*. Geneva: World Health Organization.

Rhodes, J., & Jason, L. (1988). *Preventing Substance Abuse Among young children and adolescents*. New York: Pergamon Press.

Rhyne, J. (1973/1995). *The Gestalt art experience*. Chicago: Magnolia Street.

Richardson, J. T. E. (1992). Imagery, mnemonics, and memory remediation. *Neurology*, *42*(2), 283–286. doi:10.1212/WNL.42.2.283 PMID:1736154

Rickels, K., Athanasiou, M., Robinson, D. S., Gibertini, M., Whalen, H., & Reed, C. R. (2009). Evidence for efficacy and tolerability of vilazodone in the treatment of major depressive disorder: A randomized, double-blind, placebo-controlled trial. *The Journal of Clinical Psychiatry*, *70*(3), 326–333. doi:10.4088/JCP.08m04637 PMID:19284933

Ridgely, M. S., Osher, F. C., & Goldman, H. H. (1987). Chronic Mentally Ill Young Adults With Substance Abuse Problems: A Review of Research, Treatment, and Training Issues. In *Report of the Task Force on Chronic Mentally Ill Young Adults With Substance Problems*. Baltimore, MD: University of Maryland, Department of Psychiatry.

Ries, R. K., Sloan, K. L., & Miller, N. S. (1997). Concept, diagnosis and treatment of dual diagnosis.[Philadelphia: W.B. Saunders.]. *Current Psychiatric Therapies*, *II*, 173–180.

Rihmer, Z., & Angst, J. (2005). Mood disorders: Epidemiology. In Kaplan & Sadock (Eds.), Comprehensive Textbook of Psychiatry (8th ed.; pp. 1646-1651). William & Wilkins.

Riley, S. (1999). *Contemporary art therapy with adolescents*. London: Jessica Kingsley.

Riley, S. (2001). *Group process made visible*. New York: Brunner-Routledge.

Riley, S., & Malchiodi, C. A. (1994). *Integrative approach to family art therapy*. Chicago: Magnolia Street.

Ristner, M., Modai, I., & Endicott, J. (2000). Differences in quality of life domains and psychopathologic and psychosocial factors in psychiatric patients. *The Journal of Clinical Psychiatry*, *61*(11), 880–889. doi:10.4088/JCP.v61n1113 PMID:11105747

Ristner, M., Modai, I., & Ponizovsky, A. (2002). Assessing psychological distress in psychiatric patients: Validation of the Talbieh Brief Distress Inventory. *Comprehensive Psychiatry*, *43*(3), 229–234. doi:10.1053/comp.2002.30800 PMID:11994843

Ritsner, M., Kurs, R., Gibel, A., Hirschmann, S., Shinkarenko, E., & Ratner, Y. (2003). Predictors of quality of life in major payshosis: A naturalistic follow- up study. *The Journal of Clinical Psychiatry*, *64*, 308–315. doi:10.4088/JCP.v64n0313 PMID:12716273

Robbins, T. W. (1990). The case for frontostriatal dysfunction in schizophrenia. *Schizophrenia Bulletin*, *16*(3), 391–402. doi:10.1093/schbul/16.3.391 PMID:2287930

Robertson, L., Connaughton, J., & Nicol, M. (1998). Life skills programmes for chronic mental illnesses. *Cochrane Database of Systematic Reviews*. doi:1.1002/14651858.CD000381

Robins, L., & Prince, R. K. (1991). Adult disorders predicted by childhood conduct problems: Results from the NIMH epidemiologic catchment area project. *Psychiatry*, *54*, 116–132. PMID:1852846

Robinson, D., Woerner, M. G., Alvir, J. M., Bilder, R., Goldman, R., Geisler, S., & Lieberman, J. A. et al. (1999). Predictors of relapse following response from a first episode of schizophrenia or schizoaffective disorder. *Archives of General Psychiatry*, *56*(3), 241–247. doi:10.1001/archpsyc.56.3.241 PMID:10078501

Rogers, N. (1993). *The Creative Connection*. Expressive Arts as Healing.

Rose, M. R. (1991). *Evolutionary Biology of Aging*. New York: Oxford University Press.

Rosenheck, R. A., Lam, J., Morrissey, J. P., Calloway, M. O., Stolar, M., & Randolph, F. (2002). Service systems integration and outcomes for mentally ill homeless persons in the ACCESS program: Access to Community Care and Effective Services and Supports. *Psychiatric Services (Washington, D.C.)*, *53*(8), 958–966. doi:10.1176/appi.ps.53.8.958 PMID:12161669

Rosenheck, R., Frisman, L., & Gallup, P. (1995). Effectiveness and cost of specific treatment elements in a program for homeless mentally ill veterans. *Psychiatric Services (Washington, D.C.)*, *46*(11), 1131–1139. doi:10.1176/ps.46.11.1131 PMID:8564501

Rubin, J. A. (1987/2001). *Approaches for art therapy* (J. A. Rubin, Ed.). Philadelphia: Brunner- Routledge.

Rubin, J. A. (2001). *Approaches to Art Therapy: Theory and techniques*. New York: Brunner Routledge.

Sadava, D., Hillis, D., Heller, C., & Berenbaum, M. (2011). *Life: The science of biology* (9th ed.). Sunderland, MA: Sinauer Associates Inc.

Sadock, B. J., & Sadock, V. (2003). *Kaplan and Sadock's Synopsis of Psychiatry* (9th ed.). Philadelphia: Lippincott Williams and Wilkins.

Safran, J. D., & Messer, S. B. (1997). Psychotherapy integration:Apostmodern critique. *Clinical Psychology: Science and Practice*, *4*(2), 140–192. doi:10.1111/j.1468-2850.1997.tb00106.x

Sahlem, G. L., Kalivas, B., Fox, J. B., Lamb, K., Roper, A., Williams, E. N., & Short, E. B. et al. (2014). Adjunctive triple chronotherapy (combined total sleep deprivation, sleep phase advance, and bright light therapy) rapidly improves mood and suicidality in suicidal depressed inpatients: An open label pilot study. *Journal of Psychiatric Research*, *59*, 101–107. doi:10.1016/j.jpsychires.2014.08.015 PMID:25231629

Salkovskis, P. M., & Kirk, J. (1988). Obsessional disorders: cognitive behaviour therapy for psychiatric problems A practical guide. Oxford University Press.

Salloum, I. M., Cornelius, J. R., Daley, D. C., Kirisci, L., Himmelhoch, J. M., & Thase, M. E. (2005). Efficacy of valproate maintenance in patients with bipolar disorder and alcoholism: A double-blind placebo-controlled study. *Archives of General Psychiatry*, *62*(1), 37–45. doi:10.1001/archpsyc.62.1.37 PMID:15630071

Salokangas, R. K., Vilkman, H., Ilonen, T., Taiminen, T., Bergman, J., Haaparanta, M., & Hietala, J. (2000). High levels of dopamine activity in the basal ganglia of cigarette smokers. *The American Journal of Psychiatry*, *157*(4), 632–634. doi:10.1176/appi.ajp.157.4.632 PMID:10739427

Salthouse, T. A. (1991). The processing-speed theory of adult age differences in cognition. *Psychological Review*, *103*(3), 403–428. doi:10.1037/0033-295X.103.3.403 PMID:8759042

Salvatore, S., Amelia, R., Marco, L., & Carmela, M. (2014). Caregiver's Burden and Quality of Life: Caring for Physical and Mental Illness. *International Journal Psychological Research*, *7*, 30–39.

Sanford, M., Boyle, M., Mccleary, Z., Miller, J., Steele, M., Duku, E., & Offord, D. (2006). A Pilot Study. *Mental Hygiene*, 27. PMID:16601642

Sansone, R. A., Watts, D. A., & Wiederman, M. W. (2014). Borderline personality symptomatology and legal charges related to drugs. *International Journal of Psychiatry in Clinical Practice*, *18*(2), 150–152. doi:10.3109/13651501.2013.847107 PMID:24059849

Saraceno, B., & Saxena, S. (2002). A mental health resources in the world: Results from Project Atlas of the WHO. *World Psychiatry; Official Journal of the World Psychiatric Association (WPA)*, *1*, 40–44. PMID:16946821

Saran, P. (2010). an overview of Indian Research in Personality Disorders. *Indian Journal of Psychiatry*, *52*(1), 250–254. doi:10.4103/0019-5545.69241 PMID:21180410

Sareen, J., Isaak, C., Katz, L.Y., Bolton, J., Enns, M.W, & Steinet M. B. (2014). Promising Strategies for Advancement in Knowledge of Suicide Risk Factors and Prevention. *American Journal of Preventive Medicine*, *47*(3S2), S257–S263.

Sareen, J., Chartier, M., Kjernisted, K. D., & Stein, M. B. (2001). Comorbidity of phobic disorders with alcoholism in a Canadian community sample. *Canadian Journal of Psychiatry*, *46*(8), 733–740. PMID:11692976

Sartorius, N. (2005). Stigma and discrimination because of schizophrenia: A summary of the WPA Global Programme Against Stigma and Discrimination because of Schizophrenia. *World Psychiatry; Official Journal of the World Psychiatric Association (WPA)*, *4*(1), 11–15.

Saunders, J. C. (2003). Families living with severe mental illness: A literature review. *Issues in Mental Health Nursing*, *24*(2), 175–198. doi:10.1080/01612840305301 PMID:12554427

Saykin, A. J., Gur, R. C., Gur, R. E., Mozley, P. D., Mozley, L. H., Resnick, S. M., & Stafiniak, P. et al. (1991). Neuropsychological function in schizophrenia. Selective impairment in memory and learning. *Archives of General Psychiatry*, *48*(7), 618–624. doi:10.1001/archpsyc.1991.01810310036007 PMID:2069492

Saykin, A. J., Shtasel, D. L., Gur, R. E., Kester, D. B., Mozley, L. H., Stafiniak, P., & Gur, R. C. (1994). Neuropsychological deficits in neuroleptic naïve patients with first- episode schizophrenia. *Archives of General Psychiatry, 51*(2), 124–131. doi:10.1001/archpsyc.1994.03950020048005 PMID:7905258

Scazufca, M., & Kuipers, E. (1996). Links between expressed emotion and burden of care in relatives of patients with schizophrenia. *The British Journal of Psychiatry, 168*(5), 580–587. doi:10.1192/bjp.168.5.580 PMID:8733796

Schacter, D. L., & Glisky, E. L. (1986). Memory remediation: Restoration, alleviation, and the acquisition of domain-specific knowledge. In B. Uzzell & Y. Gross (Eds.), Clinical neuropsychology of intervention (pp. 257-282). Boston: Martinus Nijhoff.

Schäfer, I., & Fisher, H. L. (2011). Childhood trauma and psychosis - what is the evidence? *Dialogues in Clinical Neuroscience, 13*(3), 360–365. PMID:22033827

Schaverian, J. (1992). *The Revealing Image: Analytical Art Psychotherapy in Theory and Practice.* Jessica Kingsley Publishers.

Schechter, M. D. (1960). *Fantasies and behaviour of the adopted child.* Beverly Hills, CA; Academic Press.

Schimmel, N. (2008). A humanistic approach to caring for street children: The importance of emotionally intimate and supportive relationships for the successful rehabilitation of street children. *Vulnerable Children and Youth Studies, 3*(3), 214–220. doi:10.1080/17450120802032883

Schonfeld, I., & Dupree, I. W. (1995). Treatment approaches for older problem drinkers. *The International Journal of the Addictions, 30*(13-14), 1819–1842. doi:10.3109/10826089509071057 PMID:8751320

Schore, A. (1994). *Affect regulation and the origin of the self.* Hillsdale, NJ: Erlbaum.

Schurink, E., & Tiba, M. (1993). Street children as a world phenomenon. In Schurink (Ed.), Street children. Pretoria: Human Sciences Research Council.

Schutt, R. K., Hough, R. L., Goldfinger, S. M., Lehman, A. F., Shern, D. L., Valencia, E., & Wood, P. A. (2009). Lessening homelessness among persons with mental illness: A comparison of five randomized treatment trials. *Asian Journal of Psychiatry, 2*(3), 100–105. doi:10.1016/j.ajp.2009.07.003 PMID:20161434

Scottish Association for Mental Health & Sainsbury Centre for Mental Health. (2007). Glasgow, UK: Scottish Association for Mental Health.

Seignourel, P. J., Kunik, M. E., & Snow, L. (2008). Anxiety in dementia: A critical review. *Clinical Psychology Review,* 7. PMID:18555569

Seitz, D. P., Brisbin, S., Herrmann, N., Rapoport, M. J., Wilson, K., Gill, S. S., & Conn, D. et al. (2012). Efficacy and feasibility of nonpharmacological interventions for neuropsychiatric symptoms of dementia in long term care: A systematic review. *Journal of American Medical Directorate Association, 13*(6), 503–506. doi:10.1016/j.jamda.2011.12.059 PMID:22342481

Sengupta, S. N., Das, P., Kamble, M. V., & Saxena, S. (1992). Dysmorphophobia with bipolar affective disorder: A case report. *Indian Journal of Psychiatry,* (34): 57–68. PMID:21776101

Sen, K. (1994). *Aging: Debates on Demographic Transition and Social Policy.* London: Zed Books Ltd.

Sethi, B. B. (1984). Need for Growth of Forensic Psychiatry. *Indian Journal of Psychiatry, 26,* 1–2. PMID:21965949

Seth, R., Kotwal, A., & Ganguly, K. K. (2005). Street and working children of Delhi, India, misusing toluene: An ethnographic exploration. *Substance Use & Misuse, 40*(11), 1659–1679. doi:10.1080/10826080500222792 PMID:16253933

Shadish, W. R., Jr., Lurigio, A. J., & Lewis, D. A. (1989). After deinstitutionalization: The present and future of mental health long-term care policy. The Journal of Social Issues, 45(3), 1–15. doi:10.1111/j.1540-4560.1989.tb01551.x doi:10.1111/j.1540-4560.1989.tb01551.x

Shakow, D. (1962). Segmental set: A theory of the formal psychological deficit in schizophrenia. *Archives of General Psychiatry*, *6*(1), 1–17. doi:10.1001/archpsyc.1962.01710190003001 PMID:13911157

Shamsi, S., Lau, A., Lencz, T., Burdick, K. E., DeRosse, P., Brenner, R., & Malhotra, A. K. et al. (2011). Cognitive and symptomatic predictors of functional disability in schizophrenia. *Schizophrenia Research*, *126*(1-3), 257–264. doi:10.1016/j.schres.2010.08.007 PMID:20828991

Shanmugiah, A., Varghese, M., & Khanna, S. (2002). Expressed emotions in obsessive compulsive disorder. *Indian Journal of Psychiatry*, *44*(1), 14–18. PMID:21206875

Sharma, G. (2013). *Mentally ill suffer a horrible fate in India*. Extracted from http://www.dw.com/en/mentally-ill-suffer-a-horrible-fate-in-india/a-17007499

Sharry, J., & Owens, C. (2000). The rules of engagement': A case study of a group with 'angry' adolescents. *Clinical Child Psychology and Psychiatry*, *5*(1), 53–62. doi:10.1177/1359104500005001006

Sheppard, B. A., Chavira, D., Azzam, A., Grados, M. A., Umana, P., Garrido, H., & Mathews, C. A. (2010). ADHD prevalence and association with hoarding behaviour in childhood-onset OCD. *Depression and Anxiety*, *27*(7), 667–674. doi:10.1002/da.20691 PMID:20583294

Shields, C. G., Franks, P., Harp, J. J., Campbell, T. L., & McDaniel, S. H. (1992). Development of the Family Emotional Involvement and Criticism, Scale (FEICS): A self-report scale to measure EE. *Journal of Marital and Family Therapy*, *18*, 395–407. doi:10.1111/j.1752-0606.1992.tb00953.x

Shields, C. G., Franks, P., Harp, J. J., McDaniel, S. H., & Campbell, T. L. (1992). Development of the Family Emotional Involvement and Criticism Scale (FEICS)- A self report scale to measure Expressed Emotions. *Journal of Marital and Family Therapy*, 18.

Shorter, E. (1997). A History of Psychiatry from the era of the Asylum to the age of Prozac. New York: Wiley.

Sideli, L., Mule, A., La Barbera, D., & Murray, R. M. (2012). Do child abuse and maltreatment increase risk of schizophrenia? *Psychiatry Investigation*, *9*(2), 87–99. doi:10.4306/pi.2012.9.2.87 PMID:22707958

Siegel, D. J. (1999). *The developing mind: Towards a neurobiology of interpersonal experience*. New York: Guilford Press.

Sierra, P., Livianos, L., & Rojo, L. (2005). Quality of life for patients with bipolar disorder: Relationship with clinical and demographic variables. *Bipolar Disorders*, *7*(2), 159–165. doi:10.1111/j.1399-5618.2005.00186.x PMID:15762857

Sikich, L., Hamer, R. M., Bashford, R. A., Sheitman, B. B., & Lieberman, J. A. (2004). A pilot study of risperidone, olanzapine, and haloperidol in psychotic youth: A double-blind, randomized, 8-week trial. *Neuropsychopharmacology*, *29*(1), 133–145. doi:10.1038/sj.npp.1300327 PMID:14583740

Silver, R. A. (2000). *Studies in art therapy (1962-2000)*. Sarasota, FL: Ablin Press.

Silverstein, S. M., & Wilkniss, S. M. (2004). At issue: The future of cognitive rehabilitation of schizophrenia. *Schizophrenia Bulletin*, *30*(4), 679–692. doi:10.1093/oxfordjournals.schbul.a007122 PMID:15954183

Silverstone, L. (1997). *Art Therapy - The Person-Centred Way: Art and the Development of the Person*. Jessica Kingsley Pub.

Sim, K., Mahendram, R., Siris, S. G., Heckers, S., & Chong, S. A. (2004). Subjective quality of life in first episode schizophrenia spectrum disorders with comorbid depression. *Psychiatry Research*, *15*(2), 141–147. doi:10.1016/j.psychres.2004.07.007 PMID:15590041

Singh, A., & Nizamie, S. H. (2004). Disability: the concept and related Indian legislations. *Mental Health Reviews*. Retrieved February 23, 2016 from http://www.psyplexus.com/mhr/disability_india.html

Singh, A. R., Verma, A. N., Verma, P. K., & Chaudhary, S. (2009). Subjective burden on spouses of schizophrenia patients. *Industrial Psychiatry Journal*, *18*(2), 97–100. doi:10.4103/0972-6748.62268 PMID:21180485

Singh, A., & Misra, N. (2009). A study on Loneliness, Depression and Sociability. *Industrial Psychiatry Journal*, *18*(1), 51–52. doi:10.4103/0972-6748.57861 PMID:21234164

Singh, G., & Verma, H. C. (1976). Murder in Punjab: A psychosocial study. *Indian Journal of Psychiatry*, *18*, 243–251.

Singleton, N., Bumpstead, R., O'Brien, M., Lee, A., & Meltzer, H. (2001). Psychiatric Morbidity among people living in private households in 2000. London: The Stationary Office.

Singleton, N., Meltzer, H., & Gatward, R. (1998). *Psychiatric Morbidity among Prisoners in England and Wales*. London: Stationery Office.

Sisask, M., & Varnik, A. (2012). Media roles in suicide prevention: A systematic review. *International Journal of Environmental Research and Public Health*, *9*(1), 123–138. doi:10.3390/ijerph9010123 PMID:22470283

Smith, S. L., & Howard, J. A. (1991). A comparative study of successful and disrupted adoptions. *The Social Service Review*, *65*(2), 248–261. doi:10.1086/603836

Smith, T., Weston, C., & Lieberman, J. (2010). Schizophrenia (maintenance treatment). *American Family Physician*, *75*(12), 1821–1829. PMID:20704164

Snyder, L. D., & Eisner, M. D. (2004). Obstructive Lung Disease among the Urban Homeless. *Chest*, *125*(5), 1719–1725. doi:10.1378/chest.125.5.1719 PMID:15136382

Sobol, B. (1982). Art therapy and strategic family therapy. *American Journal of Art Therapy*, 2.

Sohlberg, M. M., & Mateer, C. A. (1987). Effectiveness of an attention-training program. *Journal of Clinical and Experimental Neuropsychology*, *9*(2), 117–130. doi:10.1080/01688638708405352 PMID:3558744

Sokhlet, S., & Sharma, S. G. (1998). A study of psychiatric morbidity among heroin addicts. *Indian Journal of Psychiatry*, *40*, 18–19.

Solanki, R. K., Singh, P., Midha, A., & Chugh, K. (2008). Schizophrenia: Impact on quality of life. *Indian Journal of Psychiatry*, *50*(3), 181–186. doi:10.4103/0019-5545.43632 PMID:19742235

Somsundram, O. (1974). Crimes of persons with schizophrenia. *Indian Journal of Psychiatry*, *16*(2), 121–130.

Somsundram, O. (1997). Crimes of persons with affective disorders. *Indian Journal of Psychiatry*, *39*, 13–17. PMID:21584037

Soomro, G. M. (2012). Obsessive Compulsive disorder. *British Medical Journals. Clinical Evidence*, *1*(18), 1–25.

Sørensen, H. J., Jepsen, P. W., Haastrup, S., & Juel, K. (2005). Drug-use pattern, comorbid psychosis and mortality in people with a history of opioid addiction. *Acta Psychiatrica Scandinavica*, *111*(3), 244–249. doi:10.1111/j.1600-0447.2004.00445.x PMID:15701109

Spaulding, W. D., Fleming, S. K., Reed, D., Sullivan, M., Storzbach, D., & Lam, M. (1999). Cognitive functioning in schizophrenia: Implications for psychiatric rehabilitation. *Schizophrenia Bulletin*, *25*(2), 275–289. doi:10.1093/oxfordjournals.schbul.a033378 PMID:10416731

Spaulding, W. D., Reed, D., Sullivan, M., Richardson, C., & Weiler, M. (1999). Effects of cognitive treatment in psychiatric rehabilitation. *Schizophrenia Bulletin*, *25*(4), 657–676. doi:10.1093/oxfordjournals.schbul.a033409 PMID:10667738

Srinivasan, L., Thara, R., & Tirupati, S. N. (2005). Cognitive dysfunction and associated factors in patients with chronic schizophrenia. *Indian Journal of Psychiatry*, *47*(3), 139–143. doi:10.4103/0019-5545.55936 PMID:20814455

Srinivasan, L., & Tirupati, S. (2005). Relationship between cognition and work functioning among patients with schizophrenia in an urban area of India. *Psychiatric Services (Washington, D.C.)*, *56*(11), 1423–1428. doi:10.1176/appi.ps.56.11.1423 PMID:16282262

Sriram, G. T. (1990). Psychotherapy in developing countries: A public Health perspective. *Indian Journal of Psychiatry*, (2), 138–144. PMID:21927442

Stafford, M. R., Jackson, H., Mayo-Wilson, E., Morrison, A. P., & Kendall, T. (2013). Early interventions to prevent psychosis: Systematicreviewandmeta-analysis. *British Medical Journal*, *346*(jan18 1), f185. doi:10.1136/bmj.f185 PMID:23335473

Starkstein, S. E., Jorge, R., Petracca, G., & Robinson, R. G. (2007). The construct of generalized anxiety disorder in Alzheimer disease. *The American Journal of Geriatric Psychiatry*, *15*(1), 42–49. doi:10.1097/01.JGP.0000229664.11306.b9 PMID:17194814

Statistical Standard for Occupied Dwelling Type. (2009b). *Statistics New Zealand*. Wellington: Statistics New Zealand.

Steadman, H. J., Fabisiak, S., Dvoskin, J., & Holohean, E. J. (1987). Jr A survey of mental disability among state prison inmates. *Hospital & Community Psychiatry*, *38*(10), 1086–1090. PMID:3666699

Stektee, G., & Lam, J. (1993). Obsessive Compulsive Disorder. In Handbook of effective psychotherapy, (pp. 253-278). Springer US.

Stewart, S. E., Illmann, C., Geller, D. A., Leckman, J. F., King, R., & Pauls, D. L. (2009). A controlled family study of attention-deficit/hyperactivity disorder and Tourette's disorder. *Journal of the American Academy of Child and Adolescent Psychiatry*, *45*(11), 1354–1362. doi:10.1097/01.chi.0000251211.36868.fe PMID:17075358

Stohler, R., & Rossler, W. (2005). Dual Diagnosis. The evolving conceptual framework. Bibl Psychiatr., 172, 1-10. doi:10.1159/isbn.978-3-318-01002-2

Strachan, A. M., Leff, J. P., Goldstein, M., Doane, J. A., & Burtt, C. (1986). Emotional attributes and direct communication in the families of Schizophrenias: A cross national replication. *The British Journal of Psychiatry*, *149*(3), 279–287. doi:10.1192/bjp.149.3.279 PMID:3779290

Strachey, J. (1914). Mourning and melancholia, the standard edition of the complete psychological works of Sigmund Freud. London: Hogarth Press.

Strakowski, S. M., DelBello, M. P., Fleck, D. E., Adler, C. M., Anthenelli, R. M., Keck, P. E., & Amicone, J. (2005). Effects of co-occurring alcohol abuse on the course of bipolar disorder following a first hospitalization for mania. *Archives of General Psychiatry*, *62*(8), 851–858. doi:10.1001/archpsyc.62.8.851 PMID:16061762

Strakowski, S. M., DelBello, M. P., Fleck, D. E., Adler, C. M., Anthenelli, R. M., Keck, P. E., & Amicone, J. (2007). Effects of co-occurring cannabis use disorders on the course of bipolar disorder after a first hospitalization for mania. *Archives of General Psychiatry*, *64*(1), 57–64. doi:10.1001/archpsyc.64.1.57 PMID:17199055

Strategy in Mental Health of the National Health System. (2007). *Ministry of health and consumer affairs. Ministry of health and consumer affairs.* Publications center paseo del prado.

Struening, E. L., Perlick, D. A., Link, B. G., Hellman, F., Herman, D., & Sirey, J. A. (2001). Stigma as a barrier to recovery. The extent to which caregivers believe most people devalue consumers and their families. *Psychiatric Services (Washington, D.C.)*, *52*(12), 1633–1638. doi:10.1176/appi.ps.52.12.1633 PMID:11726755

Stuart, H. (2005). Why stigma matters and why it should be beaten. *World Psychiatry; Official Journal of the World Psychiatric Association (WPA)*, *4*(1), 4–5.

Substance Abuse and Mental Health Services Administration (SAMHSA). (n.d.). Retrieved from http://www.integration.samhsa.gov/clinical-practice/suicide-prevention

Sudhir, P. M. (2015). A practical Approach to cognitive behaviour therapy for adolescent. Springer.

Sullivan, G., Burnam, A., Koegel, P., & Hollenberg, J. (2000). Quality of life of homeless persons with mental illness: Results from the course of homelessness study. *Psychiatric Services (Washington, D.C.)*, *51*(9), 1135–1141. doi:10.1176/appi.ps.51.9.1135 PMID:10970916

Suresh, B. M., Pratima, M., Rajani, P., Naveen, K. C., & Madhusudhan, S. (2011). *Minds Imprisoned: Mental Health Care in Prisons. Publication, National Institute of Mental Health Neuro Sciences.* Bangalore: Common Mental Disorders in Prisons.

Swapna, B., Sudarshan, S. Y., & Shamshad, B. (2012). Burden on caregivers in Bipolar disorder and Alcohol. *International Journal of Biosocial and Medical Research*, *3*, 1992–1997.

Swartz, M. S., Perkins, D. O., Stroup, T. S., Davis, S. M., Capuano, G., Rosenheck, R. A., & Lieberman, J. A. et al. (2007). Effects of antipsychotic medications on psychosocial functioning in patients with chronic schizophrenia: Findings from the NIMH CATIE Study. *The American Journal of Psychiatry*, *164*(3), 428–436. doi:10.1176/ajp.2007.164.3.428 PMID:17329467

Switaj, P., Anczewska, M., Chrostek, A., Sabariego, C., Cieza, A., Bickenbach, J., & Chatterji, S. (2012). Disability and schizophrenia: A systematic review of experienced psychosocial difficulties. *BMC Psychiatry*, *12*(1), 193. doi:10.1186/1471-244X-12-193 PMID:23137171

Tabares-Seisdedos, R., Balanza-Martínez, V., Sanchez-Moreno, J., Martinez-Aran, A., Salazar-Fraile, J., Selva-Vera, G., & Vieta, E. et al. (2008). Neurocognitive and clinical predictors of functional outcome in patients with schizophrenia and bipolar I disorder at one-year follow-up. *Journal of Affective Disorders*, *109*(3), 286–299. doi:10.1016/j.jad.2007.12.234 PMID:18289698

Taiminen, T. J., Salokangas, R. K., Saarijarvi, S., Niemi, H., Lehto, H., Ahola, V., & Syvalahti, E. (1998). Smoking and cognitive deficits in schizophrenia: A pilot study. *Addictive Behaviors*, *23*(2), 263–266. doi:10.1016/S0306-4603(97)00028-2 PMID:9573430

Tamil Nadu Prevention of Begging Act. (1945). Complete Act- Bare Act.India.

Tamlyn, D., McKenna, P. J., Mortimer, A. M., Lund, C. E., Hammond, S., & Baddeley, A. D. (1992). Memory impairment in schizophrenia: Its extent, affiliations, and neuropsychological character. *Psychological Medicine*, *22*(01), 101–115. doi:10.1017/S0033291700032773 PMID:1349439

Tanay, E. (2007). Virginia Tech mass murder: A forensic psychiatrist's perspective. *The Journal of the American Academy of Psychiatry and the Law*, *35*, 152–153. PMID:17592159

Task Force on Civil Equal Justice Funding. (2003). *The Washington State civil legal needs study*. Washington State Supreme Court. Retrieved from <http://www.lri.lsc.gov/pdf/03/030185_lglndstudy093003.pdf>

Taylor, A., Goldberg, D., Hutchinson, S., Cameron, S., Gore, S. M., McMenamin, J., & Fox, R. et al. (2000). Prevalence of hepatitis C virus infection among injecting drug users in Glasgow 1990–1996: Are current harm reduction strategies working? *The Journal of Infection*, *40*(2), 176–183. doi:10.1053/jinf.2000.0647 PMID:10841096

Thane, P. (1978). The muddled history of retiring at 60 and 65. *New Society*, *45*(826), 234–236.

Thara, R. (2005). Measurement of psychiatric disability. The Indian Journal of Medical Research, 121, 723–724. PubMed PMID:16037616

Thara, R. (2004). Twenty-year course of schizophrenia: The Madras Longitudinal Study. *Canadian Journal of Psychiatry*, *49*, 564–569. PMID:15453106

Thara, R. (2005). Measurement of psychiatric disability. *The Indian Journal of Medical Research*, *121*, 723–724. PMID:16037616

Thara, R. (2012). Twenty-five years of schizophrenia: The Madras Longitudinal Study. *Indian Journal of Psychiatry*, *54*(2), 134–137. doi:10.4103/0019-5545.99531 PMID:22988319

Thara, R., Kamath, S., & Kumar, S. (1998). Women with schizophrenia and broken marriages-doubly disadvantaged? Part II: Family perspective. *The International Journal of Social Psychiatry*, *49*(3), 233–240. doi:10.1177/00207640030493009 PMID:14626366

Thara, R., Padmavati, R., Kumar, S., & Srinivasan, L. (1998). Instrument to assess burden on caregivers of chronic mentally ill. *Indian Journal of Psychiatry*, *40*, 21–29. PMID:21494438

Thara, R., & Patel, V. (2010). Role of non-governmental organizations in mental health in India. *Indian Journal of Psychiatry*, *52*(7), S389–S395. doi:10.4103/0019-5545.69276 PMID:21836712

Thara, R., & Rjkumar, S. (1993). Nature and course of disability in schizophrenia. *Indian Journal of Psychiatry*, *35*(1), 33–35. PMID:21776165

The Indian Succession Act. (1956). Bare Act; Eastern Book Company, Lucknow.

The Mental Health Act 1987 with Central and State Rules (1990). Delhi Law House, Delhi.

The national report on homelessness for Supreme Court of India. (2001). Supreme Court commissioners WR196/2001

The persons with disability (equal opportunities, protection of rights and full participation Act (1995). Bare Act; Eastern Book Company, Lucknow.

The Rehabilitation Committee of the Indian Psychiatric Society. (2002). IDEAS (Indian Disability Evaluation and Assessment Scale) - A scale for measuring and quantifying disability in mental disorders. Indian Psychiatric Society.

Thelma Beatriz, G.-C., Isela, J.-R., Alma, G., María Lilia, L.-N., & Carlos Alfonso, T.-Z. (2014). Association between HTR2C gene variants and suicidal behaviour: A protocol for the systematic review and meta-analysis of genetic studies. *BMJ Open*, *4*(9), e005423. doi:10.1136/bmjopen-2014-005423 PMID:25190618

Thirunavukarasu, M. (2011). Closing the treatment gap. *Indian Journal of Psychiatry*, *53*(3), 199–201. doi:10.4103/0019-5545.86803 PMID:22135436

Tidemalm, D., Langstrom, N., Lichtenstein, P., & Runeson, B. (2008). Risk of suicide after suicide attempt according to coexisting psychiatric disorder: Swedish cohort study with long term follow-up. *British Medical Journal*, *337*(nov18 3), a2205. doi:10.1136/bmj.a2205 PMID:19018040

Tiet, Q. Q., & Mausbach, B. (2007). Treatments for patients with dual diagnosis: A review. *Alcoholism, Clinical and Experimental Research*, *31*(4), 513–536. PMID:17374031

Till, B., Strauss, M., Sonneck, G., & Niederkrotenthaler, T. (2015). Determining the effects of films with suicidal content: A laboratory experiment. *The British Journal of Psychiatry*, *207*(1), 72–78. doi:10.1192/bjp.bp.114.152827 PMID:25906792

Timms, P., & Balazs, J. (1997). ABC of mental health. Mental health on the margins. *British Medical Journal*, *315*(7107), 536–539. doi:10.1136/bmj.315.7107.536 PMID:9329311

Tiwari, S. C. (2012). Geriatric Psychiatric Morbidity in Rural Northern India: Implications for the Future. *International Psychogeriatrics*, *12*(1), 35–48. doi:10.1017/S1041610200006189 PMID:10798452

Todd, J., Green, G., Harrison, M., Ikuesan, B. A., Self, C., Baldacchino, A., & Sherwood, S. (2004). Defining dual diagnosis of mental illness and substance misuse: Some methodological issues. *Journal of Psychiatric and Mental Health Nursing*, *11*(1), 48–54. doi:10.1111/j.1365-2850.2004.00683.x PMID:14723639

Torrens, M., Fonseca, F., Mateu, G., & Farre, M. (2005). Efficacy of antidepressants in substance use disorders with and without comorbid depression. A systematic review and meta-analysis. *Drug and Alcohol Dependence*, *78*(1), 1–22. doi:10.1016/j.drugalcdep.2004.09.004 PMID:15769553

Torres, A. R., Hoff, N. T., Padovani, C. R., & Ramos-Cerqueira, A. T. (2012). Dimensional analysis of burden in family caregivers of patients with obsessive–compulsive disorder. *Psychiatry and Clinical Neurosciences*, *66*(5), 432–441. doi:10.1111/j.1440-1819.2012.02365.x PMID:22834662

Torrey, E. F. (1994). Violent behavior by individuals with serious mental illness. *Hospital & Community Psychiatry*, *45*(7), 653–662. PMID:7927289

Torrey, E., Kennard, A., Eslinger, D., Lamb, R., & Pavle, J. (2010). *More Mentally Ill Persons are in Jails and Prisons than Hospitals: A Survey of the States*. Treatment Advocacy Center.

Toussieng, W. P. (1962). Disabilities in adopted children and adoptive parents, The National Committee for Mental Hygiene. *Mental Hygiene*, 27.

Tripathi, A., Nischal, A., Dalal, P. K., Agarwal, V., Agarwal, M., Trivedi, J. K., & Arya, A. et al. (2013). Sociodemographic and clinical profile of homeless mentally ill inpatients in a north Indian medical university. *Asian Journal of Psychiatry*, *6*(5), 404–409. doi:10.1016/j.ajp.2013.05.002 PMID:24011688

Tripathi, M. A., & Sridevi, G. (2014). CBT and remedial training in adolescent with writing difficulty and emotional problem: A case study, *Proceedings of International Conference on Developmental Disability*.

Trivedi, J. K., Goel, D., Sharma, S., Singh, A. P., Sinha, P. K., & Tandon, R. (2007). Cognitive functions in stable schizophrenia & euthymic state of bipolar disorder. *The Indian Journal of Medical Research*, *126*, 433–439. PMID:18160747

Trivedi, J. K., & Jilani, A. Q. (2011). Pathway of psychiatric care. *Indian Journal of Psychiatry*, *53*(2), 97–98. doi:10.4103/0019-5545.82530 PMID:21772640

Trowbridge, M. M. (1995). Graphic indicators of sexual abuse in children's drawings: A review of the literature. *The Arts in Psychotherapy*, *22*(5), 485–494. doi:10.1016/0197-4556(95)00052-6

Tynes, L. L., Salins, C., Skiba, W., & Winstead, D. K. (1992). A psychoeducational and support group for obsessive-compulsive disorder patients and their significant others. *Comprehensive Psychiatry, 33*(3), 197–201. doi:10.1016/0010-440X(92)90030-T PMID:1591912

U.S. Census Bureau. (2009). *Webinar on 2008 Income, Poverty, and Health Insurance Estimates from the Current Population Survey*. Retrieved February 13, 2012 (http://www.census.gov/newsroom/releases/archives/news_conferences/2009-09-10_remarks_johnson.html)

U.S. Department of Health and Human Services. (1999). *Mental health: A report of the Surgeon General*. Rockville, MD: U.S. Department of Health and Human Services, Substance Abuse and Mental Health Services Administration, Center for Mental Health Services, National Institutes of Health, National Institute of Mental Health.

U.S. Department of Health and Human Services. (2001). *Mental health: Culture, race, and ethnicity—A supplement to mental health: A report of the Surgeon General*. Rockville, MD: Author.

Ulak, B. J., & Cummings, A. L. (1997). Using clients' artistic expressions as metaphor in counselling: A pilot study. *Canadian Journal of Counselling, 31*(4), 305–316.

Ungvari, G. S., Caroff, S. N., & Gerevich, J. (2010). The catatonia conundrum: Evidence of psychomotor phenomena as a symptom dimension in psychotic disorders. *Schizophrenia Bulletin, 36*(2), 231–238. doi:10.1093/schbul/sbp105 PMID:19776208

UNICEF. (1993). *The state of the world's children* (1st ed.). New York: Oxford University.

UNICEF. (1998). *A background paper on street children*. Paper presented at the National Workshop on Street Children.

United Nations Population Division (UN). (2011). *World Population Prospects: The 2010 Revision*. Accessed at http://esa.un.org/unpd/wpp/index.htm

Ustun, T. B., Ayuso–Mateos, J. L., Chatterji, S., Mathers, C., & Murray, C. J. (2004). Global burden of depressive disorders in the year 2000. The British Journal of Psychiatry, 759–763. PubMed PMID:15123501

van Laar, M., van Dorsselaer, S., Monshouwer, K., & de Graaf, R. (2007). Does cannabis use predict the first incidence of mood and anxiety disorders in the adult population? *Addiction (Abingdon, England), 102*(8), 1251–1260. doi:10.1111/j.1360-0443.2007.01875.x PMID:17624975

Van Meter, A. R., Moreira, A. L., & Youngstrom, E. A. (2011). Meta-analysis of epidemiologic studies of pediatric bipolar disorder. *The Journal of Clinical Psychiatry, 72*(9), 1250–1256. doi:10.4088/JCP.10m06290 PMID:21672501

Van Noppen, B., Steketee, G., McCorkle, B. H., & Pato, M. (1997). Group and multifamily behavioral treatment for obsessive compulsive disorder: A pilot study. *Journal of Anxiety Disorders, 11*(4), 431–446. doi:10.1016/S0887-6185(97)00021-2 PMID:9276786

van Os, J., Bak, M., Hanssen, M., Bijl, R. V., de Graaf, R., & Verdoux, H. (2002). Cannabis use and psychosis: A longitudinal population-based study. *American Journal of Epidemiology, 156*(4), 319–327. doi:10.1093/aje/kwf043 PMID:12181101

Van, O. J., & Kapur, S. (2009). Schizophrenia. *Lancet, 374*(9690), 635–645. doi:10.1016/S0140-6736(09)60995-8 PMID:19700006

Vaughn, C., & Leff, P. (1976). The influence of family and social factors on the course of psychiatric illness. A comparison of schizophrenia and depressed neurotic patients. *The British Journal of Psychiatry, 129*(2), 125–137. doi:10.1192/bjp.129.2.125 PMID:963348

Veale, A., & Donà, G. (2003). Street children and political violence: A socio-demographic analysis of street children in Rwanda. *Child Abuse & Neglect*, *27*(3), 253–269. doi:10.1016/S0145-2134(03)00005-X PMID:12654324

Velligan, D. I., & Alphs, L. D. (2008). Negative Symptoms in Schizophrenia: The Importance of Identification and Treatment. *Psychiatric Times*, *25*(3), 1–6. PMID:19590742

Velligan, D. I., Bow-Thomas, C. C., Mahurin, R. K., Miller, A. L., & Halgunseth, L. C. (2000). Do specific neurocognitive deficits predict specific domains of community function in schizophrenia? *The Journal of Nervous and Mental Disease*, *188*(8), 518–524. doi:10.1097/00005053-200008000-00007 PMID:10972571

Vern, L. B., & Norella, P. (2009). *Handbook of theories of aging*. Springer Publishing Company.

Vijayakumar, L., & Rajkumar, S. (1999). Are risk factors for suicide universal? A case-control study in India. Acta Psychiatrica Scandinavica, 99(6), 407–411. doi:10.1111/j.1600-0447.1999.tb00985.x PubMed doi:10.1111/j.1600-0447.1999.tb00985.x PMID:10408261

Vijayakumar, L. (2007). Suicide and its prevention: The urgent need in India. *Indian Journal of Psychiatry*, *49*(2), 81–84. doi:10.4103/0019-5545.33252 PMID:20711387

Vijayakumar, L. (2010). Indian research on suicide. *Indian Journal of Psychiatry*, *52*(711), S291–S296. doi:10.4103/0019-5545.69255 PMID:21836697

Voice, O. (2009). *Shaping our aging society*. Help the Aged and Age Concern.

Vojta, C., Kinosian, B., Glick, H., Altshuler, L., & Bauer, M. S. (2001). Self-reported quality of life across mood states in bipolar disorder. *Comprehensive Psychiatry*, *42*(3), 190–195. doi:10.1053/comp.2001.23143 PMID:11349236

Voruganti, L. N., Heslegrave, R. J., & Awad, A. G. (1997). Neuroleptic dysphoria may be the missing link between schizophrenia and substance abuse. *The Journal of Nervous and Mental Disease*, *185*(7), 463–465. doi:10.1097/00005053-199707000-00008 PMID:9240366

Wahl, O. F. (2003). News media portrayal of mental illness. *The American Behavioral Scientist*, *46*(12), 1594–1600. doi:10.1177/0002764203254615

Waldman, A. (2004). Police struggle with approach to the mentally ill: recent killings have led to calls for better tracking and treatment of the mentally ill and more training for officers. *The Christian Science Monitor.* Accessible at www.csmonitor. com/2004/0317/p11s02-usju.htm

Walmsley, R. (2005). *The World Female Imprisonment*. The International Centre for Prison Studies (ICPS).

Walmsley, R. (2009). *World Prison Population List* (8th ed.). King's College London International Centre for Prison Studies.

Wang, P. S., Lane, M., Olfson, M., Pincus, H. A., Wells, K. B., & Kessler, R. C. (2005). Twelve-month use of mental health services in the United States: Results from the National Comorbidity Survey Replication. *Archives of General Psychiatry*, *62*(6), 629–640. doi:10.1001/archpsyc.62.6.629 PMID:15939840

Warner, R., & Atkinson, M. (1988). The relationship between Schizophrenia patients' perceptions of their parents and the course of their illness. *The British Journal of Psychiatry*, *153*(3), 344–353. doi:10.1192/bjp.153.3.344 PMID:3250671

Washington State Legislature Definitions. (2016). *Definitions*. Retrieved on 04 January, 2016 from http://apps.leg.wa.gov/rcw/default.aspx?cite=24.06.005

Watanabe, N., Hunot, V., Omori, I. M., Churchill, R., & Furukawa, T. A. (2007). Psychotherapy for depression among children and adolescents: A systematic review. *Acta Psychiatrica Scandinavica*, *116*(2), 84–95. doi:10.1111/j.1600-0447.2007.01018.x PMID:17650269

Weir, F. (1987). The role of symbolic expression in its relation to art therapy: A Kleinian approach. In Images of art therapys. London: Routledge.

Weiss, M. G., Ramakrishna, J., & Somma, D. (2006). Health-related stigma: Rethinking concepts and interventions. *Psychology Health and Medicine*, *11*(3), 277–287. doi:10.1080/13548500600595053 PMID:17130065

Weisz, J. R., McCarty, C. A., & Valeri, S. M. (2006). Effects of psychotherapy for depression in children and adolescents a meta-analysis. *Psychological Bulletin*, *132*(1), 132–149. doi:10.1037/0033-2909.132.1.132 PMID:16435960

Weisz, J. R., Weiss, B., Han, S. S., Granger, D. A., & Morton, T. (1995). Effects of psychotherapy with children and adolescents revisited: A meta-analysis of treatment outcome studies. *Psychological Bulletin*, *117*(3), 450–468. doi:10.1037/0033-2909.117.3.450 PMID:7777649

Wen, C. K., Hudak, P. L., & Hwang, S. W. (2007). Homeless people's perceptions of welcomeness and unwelcomeness in health-care encounters. *Journal of General Internal Medicine*, *22*(7), 1011–1017. doi:10.1007/s11606-007-0183-7 PMID:17415619

Wenger, T., Moldrich, G., & Furst, S. (2003). Neuromorphological background of cannabis addiction. *Brain Research Bulletin*, *61*(2), 125–128. doi:10.1016/S0361-9230(03)00081-9 PMID:12831997

WHO. (2000). *Working with street children: A training package on substance use, sexual and reproductive health including HIV/AIDS and STDs*. Geneva: WHO- Department of Mental Health and Substance Dependence.

WHO. (2005). *Resource Book on Mental Health, Human Rights and Legislation*. World Health Organization.

WHO. (2006). *Constitution of the World Health Organization*. WHO.

WHO. (2007). *Mental health in prisons*. Retrieved from http://www.who.int/mental_health/policy/services/en/index.html

WHO. (2010). *mhGAP-IG*. Retrieved from http://whqlibdoc.who.int/publications/ 2010/9789241548069_eng.pdf

WHO. (2012). *Dementia: a public health priority*. World Health Organization, Alzheimer's disease International. Retrieved from http://apps.who.int/ iris/bitstream/10665/75263/1/9789241564458_eng.pdf

WHO. (2012). *Risks to mental health: An overview of vulnerabilities and risk factors*. Retrieved from www.who.int/about/copyright

Wig, N. N., & Murthy, S. (1994). From Mental Illness to Mental Health. *Health for the Millions*, 2–4.

Wikler, A. (1973). Dynamics of drug dependence: Implications of a conditioning theory for research and treatment. *Archives of General Psychiatry*, *28*(5), 611–616. doi:10.1001/archpsyc.1973.01750350005001 PMID:4700675

Wilcox, H. C., Conner, K. R., & Caine, E. D. (2004). Association of alcohol and drug use disorders and completed suicide: An empirical review of cohort studies. *Drug and Alcohol Dependence*, *76*(Suppl), S11–S19. doi:10.1016/j.drugalcdep.2004.08.003 PMID:15555812

Wild, T. C., el-Guebaly, N., Fischer, B., Brissette, S., Brochu, S., Bruneau, J., & Mun, P. (2005). Comorbid depression among untreated illicit opiate users: Results from a multisite Canadian study. *Canadian Journal of Psychiatry*, *50*(9), 512–518. PMID:16262105

Wiley, B. (2003). Schizophrenia. Author.

Wilson, C. S., Bennett, M. E., & Bellack, A. S. (2013). Impact of Family History in Persons With Dual Diagnosis. *Journal of Dual Diagnosis*, *9*(1), 30–38. doi:10.1080/15504263.2012.744937 PMID:23538687

Wilson, D. R. (2010). Health consequences of childhood sexual abuse. *Perspectives in Psychiatric Care*, *46*(1), 56–64. doi:10.1111/j.1744-6163.2009.00238.x PMID:20051079

Wintersteen, R. T. (1986). Rehabilitating the chronically mentally ill: Social work's claim to leadership. Social Work, 31, 332–337.

Wittchen, H. U., & Jacobi, F. (2005). Size and burden of mental disorders in Europe: A critical appraisal of 27 studies. European Neuropsychopharmacology, 21, 655–679. doi:10.1016/j.euroneuro.2011.07.018 PubMed doi:10.1016/j.euroneuro.2011.07.018 PMID:15961293

Wittchen, H. U., Kessler, R. C., & Beesdo, K. (2002). Generalized anxiety and depression in primary care: Prevalence, recognition, and management. *The Journal of Clinical Psychiatry*, *63*(8), 24–34. PMID:12044105

Wolberg, L. R. (1995). *The techniques of psychotherapy* (4th ed.). Jason Aronson Inc.

Wolthaus, J., Dingemans, P., Schene, A., Linszen, D., Wiersma, D., Bosch, R., & Hijman, R. (2002). Caregiver burden in recent - onset schizophrenia and spectrum disorders: The influence of symptoms and personality traits. *The Journal of Nervous and Mental Disease*, *190*(4), 241–247. doi:10.1097/00005053-200204000-00005 PMID:11960085

Wong, S. E. (2014). A Critique of the Diagnostic Construct Schizophrenia. *Research on Social Work Practice*, *24*(1), 132–141. doi:10.1177/1049731513505152

World Bank. (1993). *World Development Report. Investing in Health.* New York: Oxford University Press.

World Drug Report. (2006). Retrieved 9 February, 2016, from https://www.unodc.org/unodc/en/data-and-analysis/WDR-2006.html

World Federation of Mental Health (WFMH). (2010). *Caring for the caregiver: Why your mental health matters when you are caring for others.* Woodbridge, VA: WFMH.

World Health Organization, World Health Report. (2001). *Mental Health: New Understanding, New Hope.* WHO.

World Health Organization. (1979). Schizophrenia: An International Follow-up Study. WHO.

World Health Organization. (1992). *The ICD-10 classification of mental and behavioural disorders: clinical descriptions and diagnostic guidelines.* Geneva: World Health Organization.

World Health Organization. (1992–94). *International Statistical Classification of Diseases and Related Health Problems.* WHO.

World Health Organization. (1993). *WHO programme on substance abuse, 'one way street': A report on phase I of street children project.* Geneva: WHO.

World Health Organization. (1999). *The 'Newly Defined' Burden of Mental Problems. Fact Sheet No. 217.* Geneva: World Health Organization.

World Health Organization. (2001). *International Classification of Functioning.* Geneva: Disability and Health.

World Health Organization. (2001). *Project Atlas: Mapping mental health resources around the world.* Retrieved March 12, 2015, from http://www.who.int/ whr/2001/media_centre/en/ whr01_fact_sheet3_ en.pdf

World Health Organization. (2003). The burden of mental disorders is expected to rise significantly over the next 20 years: Are we doing enough to address the growing mental health challenges. WHO.

World Health Organization. (2008). The Global Burden of Disease: 2004 Update. Geneva, Switzerland: WHO Press.

World Health Organization. (2015). *Preventing suicide: a global imperative*. World Health Organization. Retrieved from http://www.who.int/mental_health/suicide-prevention/world_report_2014/en/

Wright, N. M. J., Campbell, T. L., & Tompkins, C. N. E. (2002). Comparison of conventional and accelerated hepatitis B immunization schedules for homeless drug users. *Communicable Disease and Public Health*, *5*, 324–326. PMID:12564251

Wright, N. M. J., & Tompkins, C. N. E. (2006). How can health services effectively meet the health needs of homeless people? *The British Journal of General Practice*, *56*, 286–293. PMID:16611519

Wyatt, R. J. (1997). Research in schizophrenia and the discontinuation of antipsychotic medications. *Schizophrenia Bulletin*, *23*(1), 3–9. doi:10.1093/schbul/23.1.3 PMID:9050108

Wykes, T., Reeder, C., Corner, J., Williams, C., & Everitt, B. (1999). The effects of neurocognitive remediation on executive processing in patients with schizophrenia. *Schizophrenia Bulletin*, *25*(2), 291–307. doi:10.1093/oxfordjournals.schbul.a033379 PMID:10416732

Wykes, T., Reeder, C., Landau, S., Everitt, B., Knapp, M., Patel, A., & Romeo, R. (2007). Cognitive remediation therapy in schizophrenia Randomised controlled trial. *The British Journal of Psychiatry*, *190*(5), 421–427. doi:10.1192/bjp.bp.106.026575 PMID:17470957

Xue, Z. (2009). Urban street children in China: A social exclusion perspective. *International Social Work*, *52*(3), 401–408. doi:10.1177/0020872808102072

Yamamoto, H., Tsuchida, H., Nakamae, T., Seiji, N., Sakai, Y., Fujimori, A., & Narumoto, J. (2012). Relationship between severity of obsessive-compulsive symptoms and schizotypy in obsessive-compulsive symptoms and schizotypy in obsessive-compulsive disorder. *Neuropsychiatric Disease and Treatment*, *8*, 579–583. doi:10.2147/NDT.S38450 PMID:23248572

Yesavage, J. A., Rose, T. L., & Spiegel, D. (1982). Relaxation training and memory improvement in elderly normals: Correlations of anxiety rating and recall improvement. *Experimental Aging Research*, *8*(4), 1982. doi:10.1080/03610738208260365 PMID:6762966

Yip, P. S., Caine, E., Yousuf, S., Chang, S. S., Wu, K. C., & Chen, Y. Y. (2012). Means restriction for suicide prevention. *Lancet*, *379*(9834), 2393–2399. doi:10.1016/S0140-6736(12)60521-2 PMID:22726520

Young, K. W. (2004). Quality of life of people with long- term psychiatric illness living in residential home. *International Journal of Psychosocial Rehabilitation*, *9*, 133–145.

Zachariah, e. t. k. c., Mathew, s., & Irudaya, r. (2000). *Socio-Economic and Demographic Consequenes of Migration in Kerala*. Academic Press.

Zammit, S., Allebeck, P., Andreasson, S., Lundberg, I., & Lewis, G. (2002). Self reported cannabis use as a risk factor for schizophrenia in Swedish conscripts of 1969: Historical cohort study. *BMJ (Clinical Research Ed.)*, *325*(7374), 1199. doi:10.1136/bmj.325.7374.1199 PMID:12446534

Zarit, S. H., Reever, K. E., & Bach-Peterson, J. (1980). Relatives of the impaired elderly: Correlates of feelings of burden. *The Gerontologist*, *20*(6), 649–655. doi:10.1093/geront/20.6.649 PMID:7203086

Zergaw, A., Hailemariam, D., Alem, A., & Kebede, D. (2008). A longitudinal comparative analysis of economic and family caregiver burden due to bipolar disorder. *Bipolar Disorders*, *11*, 191–198. PMID:19588042

Ziedonis, D. M., & Trudeau, K. (1997). Motivation to quit using substances among individuals with schizophrenia: Implications for a motivation-based treatment model. *Schizophrenia Bulletin*, *23*(2), 229–238. doi:10.1093/schbul/23.2.229 PMID:9165633

Zimberg, S. (1999). A dual diagnosis typology to improve diagnosis and treatment of dual disorder patients. *Journal of Psychoactive Drugs*, *31*(1), 47–51. doi:10.1080/02791072.1999.10471725 PMID:10332638

Zohar, J., Fostick, L., & Juyen-Wetzler, E. (2009). Obsessive compulsive disorder. In New Oxford Textbook of Psychiatry (2nd ed.; pp. 765-773). New York: Oxford University Press.

About the Contributors

Barre Vijay Prasad He completed Master's Degree in Psychology from Andhra University, he later went to acquire his first M Phil in Rehabilitation Psychology from National Institute for the Mentally Handicapped (NIMH) in Secunderabad. Thereafter, he went on to acquire his second M Phil in Clinical Psychology from one of the most reputed institutes in India - Institute of Human Behaviour and Allied Sciences- [IHBAS] Shahdra, Delhi). He is the first psychologist to have accreditation as a dually trained professional psychologist with qualifications as a Clinical Psychologist and a Rehabilitation Psychologist from Rehabilitation Council of India (RCI) – Delhi. He is a Professional Life Member of Indian Association of Clinical Psychology (IACP). He has awarded Doctoral Degree in Psychology from Centre for Health Psychology, University of Hyderabad. He has been awarded: Centenary Merit award during beginning of his professional psychology career. Currently he is working as Associate Professor and HoD in the Department of Clinical Psychology at Dharwad Institute of Mental Health and Neurosciences (DIMHANS-India). He is now working to produce ways of working manuals for reducing psychological distress amongst mentally ill and patients with cancer in the field of Psycho-oncology. He is trained at conducting various assessments such as Psycho-diagnostics, neuropsychological profiling, personality assessments amongst other skills. Not only does he work on assessments he is proficient in providing interventions using multi-modal approaches. He is trained in providing support for various initiatives disability rehabilitation, promotion of mental health and wellbeing. He specializes in cognitive behavioral therapies and behavioral interventions for various clinical disorders. He has published many articles in national and international journals, book chapters as well, and presented several conference papers on mental health, disability rehabilitation and psycho-oncology. He is also working on writing a book on "21st Century Eminent Psychologists- Biography".

* * *

Ashfak Ahamed Currently he is working as a Clinical Psychologist in NIMHANS Bengaluru, after his fellowship programme in psychiatric rehabilitation. He completed MPhil cognitive sciences from University of Hyderabad and MPhil Clinical psychology from Central Institute of Psychiatry Ranchi. He had two publications in his credit.

Shamsi Akbar completed her post-graduation in clinical psychology from Rohilkhand University Bareilly. She worked as a Clinical Psychologist Chandra Psychiatric center Bareilly. Thereafter in 2011 she moved to Lucknow and joined the Dept. of Geriatric Mental Health, King Georges Medical University Lucknow to perusing PhD. In 2013 she got best Poster presentation award in 9th Annual National

Conference of Indian Association for Geriatric Mental Health (IAGMH). In 2014 she developed a 1st scale in India for older adults "Scale for Satisfaction and Expectation of Older Adults in Old Age Homes." In 2015 she received the "Best Research Paper" among medical science section K G's Medical University Lucknow. In 2015 "Best Researcher Award" in the Department of Geriatric Mental Health K.G s Medical University Lucknow. In 2015 she got IAGMH / INTAS award in National Conference of Indian Association for Geriatric Mental Health (IAGMH). She has number of publications in National and International Journals, Chapters in Books and has enlisted many presentation/participations at national and international conferences.

Deepali Bedi she is a qualified Clinical Psychologist with RCI recognized degree in M. Phil. Clinical Psychology, and having a decade of experience in her field. She worked with reputed Hospitals like Max Mental Health Department, Lady Harding Medical College, Air Force CME and Delhi Psychiatric Centre. She also worked with many multinationals, consumer based companies, software industry, engineering based companies, also banks. Apart from these, she has worked with various reputed schools. Presently working with Sukoon Psychotherapy Center wherein her involvement in psychometric testing, Individual, Family and Group Psychotherapy for stress, work life balance, relationship issues, marital issues, woman cell issues, other gender issues and various psychiatric and non-psychiatric problems. Currently she is an associate member with the Indian psychoanalytical society. She have been involved in various research projects including: Case study on "The effectiveness of Music Therapy with the diagnoses of Autism" likewise many her credentials.

Poornima C. She is a Clinical Psychologist currently working as a Senior Research Fellow in Department of Clinical Psychology NIMHANS. She completed her M.Phil in Clinical Psychology from NIMHANS. She had worked as a Junior Research Fellow in the Department of Child and Adolescent Psychiatry at NIMHANS.

Sushma C. She completed her Msc in Psychology, Bangalore University, Bangalore. Currently working as Clinical psychologist in Department of psychology, Dharwad Institute of Mental Health and Neurosciences (DIMHANS) Dharwad. State of Karnataka, India. Research interests and specialties: 1. Child and Adolescent psychiatry 2. Women mental health 3. Personality disorders 4. Marital therapy 5. Parapsychology. She had two national and four international journals to her credentials.

Lakshmana G. has been working as an Assistant Professor at Central University of Karnataka, Kalaburagi. He has published many research articles in international and national journals. He has few projects to his credit as well. His areas of research interest are health and mental health and working with vulnerable population.

Amit Garg he completed a post-graduation degree in Psychiatry from Maulana Azad Medical College, latter he joined as Senior Resident in Institute of Human Behavior and Allied Sciences (IHBAS), Delhi. After finishing his tenure, he has been selected as Assistant Professor, in department of psychiatry at IHBAS. He holds special interest in the field if De-addiction and Dual Diagnosis disorders including Psycho-pharmacology.

Bhavuk Garg completed MBBS, MD, DNB, he is currently working as a Senior Resident in Department of Psychiatry at Institute of Human Behaviour and Allied Sciences (IHBAS), NABH accredited Hospital based Autonomous Institute under Govt. of Delhi. He completed his MBBS from the prestigious Maulana Azad Medical College, New Delhi in 2009. He did his post graduation (MD Psychiatry) from IHBAS, New Delhi in 2013. He also obtained DNB in Psychiatry from National Board of Examinations. He is actively involved in post graduate teaching and research in the fields of child psychiatry, biological psychiatry and addiction psychiatry.

Shobit Garg received his DPM and MD from CIP, Ranchi. He is an assistant professor in the department of Psychiatry, Shri Guru Ram Rai Institute of Medical and Health Sciences (SGRRIM) since 2013. He was senior residence in CIP, Ranchi. He has various national and international publications and has presented papers in national conference.

Susmita Halder is Clinical Psychologist with over 8 years of clinical and teaching experiences. Currently she is faculty at Amity University, Rajasthan. Her major area of interest is cognitive assessment and training in dofferent conditions. She is having more than 20 publications in national and international journals and member of various psychological and psychiatric associations.

Shailesh Jha has completed his M.B.B.S (2009) from Pt. J.N.M. Medical College, Raipur (C.G) and received his M.D Psychiatry (2013) from India's premier institute i.e. All India Institute of Medical Sciences (AIIMS), New Delhi. He is currently working as a senior resident, Department of Psychiatry, Institute of Human Behavior and Allied Sciences (IHBAS), Delhi since 2013. He is a member of The Indian Association for Social Psychiatry (IASP). He has various national and international publications and has presented multiple papers at national conferences.

Pratima Kaushik has been awarded Ph.D. degree from Delhi University. She is currently teaching at Amity University, Noida, U.P., India for more than 3 years. Prior to this she worked as freelancing clinical psychologist at several renowned psychiatric hospitals in New Delhi. Her areas of specialization are Clinical Psychology, Research Methodology, Statistics, Neuropsychology and Psychotherapy. She has many national and international publications in her credit.

Amit Khanna currently working as Assistant Professor in the Department of Psychiatry at the Institute of Human Behaviour and Allied Sciences (IHBAS) in Delhi. Has received his M.D Degree in Psychiatry from IHBAS and has over 7 years of experience in the field of Psychiatry. His areas of specialization are psychopathology, women mental health, child and adolescent Psychiatry and dual diagnosis.

Prerna Khanna she is working as a Consultant Clinical Psychologist at Max Superspeciality hospital, Vaishali since 2009. Has worked as Assistant Professor at Gargi College and Keshav Mahavidyalay, Delhi University. Over 8 years of rich experience in providing counselling and psychotherapy for various mental health issues and behaviour problems. Education and Training, PhD (Psychology) awarded from Delhi University, M.Phil (Clinical Psychology) from IHBAS, affiliated to Delhi University. M. A., B.A., from Indraprastha College for Women, Delhi University and Certificate in Guidance, IGNOU. She cleared her UGC- NET and qualified trained in HIV/AIDS counselling, certified by NACO. Her specialties of interest are Child and Adolescent Mental Health Issues, management of Psychological

Disorders, Couple and Marital therapy. Her Professional memberships are Registered Clinical Psychologist in Rehabilitation Council of India and Member of Indian Psychiatric Society. She had many national and international publications are additional credentials.

Hitesh Khurana currently Professor in Department of Psychiatry, at Pt. B.D. Sharma PGIMS, Rohtak, Haryana.

Srinivas Kosgi graduated from Kasturba Medical College Mangalore in 1998 and worked as Medical Officer of Health, Primary Health Center, Matmari, and Raichur - Karnataka. He worked as junior resident in Department of Oncology IRCH, All India Institute of Medical Sciences New Delhi, during 1999-2000. He had postgraduate degree in Psychological Medicine from National Institute of Mental health and Neurosciences Bangalore and Diplomat in National Board (DNB) in Psychiatry from National Board of Examinations, New Delhi. During his tenure he was instrumental in setting up of Center for Psychiatric Research and has credit of conducting 34 Multicenter International Clinical trials in the capacity of Sub-Investigator and Principal Investigator. Since March 2012 he is working as Associate Professor in Department of Psychiatry, Dharwad Institute of Mental Health and Neurosciences (DIMHANS) - Dharwad. He has six publications in National and International Journals. He is also peer reviewer for Journal of Neurosciences in Rural Practice (JNRP). His area of interest is Wilson's disease, Speech and language deficits in schizophrenia, child and adolescent problems and De-addiction.

Prerna Kukreti she completed her MBBS, MD (psychiatry), IDMHLHR (International Diploma in Mental Health Law and Human Rights), currently she is working as a Assistant professor in Department of Psychiatry at Hamdard Institute of Medical Sciences and Research (HIMSR), Jamia Hamdard, Delhi 110062, India. Her areas of interests are forensic psychiatry, community psychiatry and neuropsychiatry.

Akash Mahato is a registered Clinical Psychologist and faculty at Amity University Rajasthan. His area of interest is researching neurocognitive correlates of functioning in different clinical populations; and CBT.

B. P. Mishra has received his M.Phil (1991) and Ph.D (1995) in clinical psychology from CIP, Ranchi. He is a professor and In charge of Clinical Psychology in the Department of Psychiatry, Dayanand Medical College and Hospital, Ludhiana, Punjab. He is a fellow member of IACP and also registered in RCI. He was a member of expert committee of RCI from 2009-2012 and a member of editorial board of Indian Journal of Clinical Psychology from 2007-2010. He has various national and international publications and has presented papers in national conferences. He has delivered various lectures on the academic front and community level.

Preeti Mishra received her Ph.D (clinical psychology) from Central Institute of Psychiatry (CIP), Ranchi in 2013. She has worked as a Research officer at CIP in a project "HIFAZAT". She has various publications and has presented papers in national conference. She has delivered various lectures at the community level. She is now working as a Clinical Psychologist in the Department of Psychiatry at SMI Medical College and Hospital, Dehradun.

Raveesh B N presently he is the director of Dharwad Institute of Mental Health and Neurosciences (DIMHANS) Dharwad. State Karnataka, India. Prior to this, he is a recognized postgraduate teacher in Rajiv Gandhi University of Health Sciences, Bangalore and evaluator for various Universities. He served National Indian Psychiatry Society as Assistant Editor and Editor for Indian Psychiatry Society Karnataka Chapter. He had organized State, Regional and International conferences related to Law& Psychiatry. He has more than 250 presentations, 4 chapters in International Psychiatry books and 38 publications. He received Young Teacher award by Indian Psychiatry Society, Karnataka Chapter and many academic awards like International Associateship (Royal College of Psychiatry, UK), Special scholarship (Greece, 2005), Young Scientist (Biological Psychiatry, Vienna, 2005), ICMD grant (Turkey, 2006), Young Fellowship (WPA, Venezuela, 2006) and Young Psychiatrist (WPA, Germany, 2007). He also a member of legal cell of Indian Psychiatry Society Karnataka Chapter and Member of Community cell of Karnataka State Mental Health Task Force, Government of Karnataka. Currently, President – Elect of Indian Psychiatry Society Karnataka Chapter and first Asian member for European Violence in Psychiatry Research Group (EViPRG).

Jyoti Mishra Pandey received her M.Phil in medical and social psychology (M.M&SP) from Central Institute of Psychiatry (CIP), Ranchi in 2011. She has been awarded as a first rank holder in her M.Phil (M&SP). She has worked as Assistant Professor in the Department of Clinical Psychology at Central Institute of Psychiatry (CIP). She has also worked as a Clinical Psychologist in the Department of Psychiatry and Pediatric at Bharati Vidyapeeth Medical College and Hospital, Pune. She is a Professional member of Indian Association of Clinical Psychology (IACP) and also registered in RCI. She has various publications and has presented papers in national conference. She has delivered various lectures and conducted workshops on the academic and community level. She is pursuing Ph.D from Ranchi Institute of Neuro-psychiatry and Allied Sciences (RINPAS), Ranchi. Currently she is doing private practice.

Ashwini R. Patil, Clinical Psychologist, completed her masters in Psychology, University of Mysore and she went on to acquire her M. Phil in Psychology from Shri Venkateswara University from Tirupati. Currently she is working as a Clinical Psychologist at Dharwad Institute of Mental Health and Neurosciences (DIMHANS)-Dharwad-Karnataka – India. She specializes in cognitive behavioral therapies and behavioral interventions for various clinical disorders; OCD, anxiety and depression, adaptation of integrated psychological therapy (IPT) for wives of schizophrenia. She is also interested in the application of these interventions in lifestyle disorders, chronic medical conditions such as hypertensions, diabetes, TTH, migraine, infertility and pain relief issues. Her research interest is in the broad area of women's mental health, family psychotherapy, promotion of mental health in vulnerable populations. She also published chapters and articles in various national and international books and journals.

Tej Bahadur Singh is Founder (1996) Chairman and Professor of the Department of Clinical Psychology at IHBAS, Delhi. Training of Clinical Psychologists commenced in the year 2004. On an average 15 Clinical Psychologists are qualifying every year at this centre. Now the department (the only training centre of Government Sector in the northern region of the country) is a thoroughly known, well reciprocated by aspirant students of Psychology and comparable to any other leading training centre; of the country. He earned a postgraduate in Psychology (1975) from Ranchi University pursued his studies for his professional qualification at Central Institute of Psychiatry under the same University. He was awarded postgraduate Diploma in Psychiatric Social Work (Academic Sessions: 1977-1979), Diploma in Medical and Social Psychology (Academic Sessions: 1979-1981) and Doctoral degree (1990) by CIP Ranchi. He joined Institute of Human Behaviour and Allied Sciences as Assistant Professor Clinical Psychology, in the year 1996(October) and superannuated as Professor and Head: Department of Clinical Psychology in the year 2012(June). In the year 2008 he was appointed Dean; IHBAS. Department of Clinical Psychology of IHBAS, professionally and academically is comparable to any other existing Clinical Psychology department of the country. IHBAS; a training centre of excellence, is producing 18 (from the year 2006 onwards) Clinical Psychologists every year. As Dean (Institute of Behavioural Science) and Professor; Clinical Psychology he also served Institute of Behavioural science, Gujarat Forensic Sciences University, Gandhi Nagar, Gujarat (2013). He was appointed (Feb.2014) as Faculty and Consultant Clinical Psychologist in the Department of Psychiatry, Institute of Medical Sciences, by Banaras Hindu University and superannuated from the services of BHU in the year 2015(June). Currently he is serving Centre for Psychological Sciences under Central University of South Bihar; Patna, as Professor: Psychology (from Dec. 2015 onwards). Delhi Psychiatric Society (Life Member) and Indian Psychiatric Society (Life Associate Member). He was a member on the Editorial Board (1987 to 2012) of International Journal of Rehabilitation Research (U.K.). Currently he is a member on the Editorial Board of Disabilities & Impairments (India). There are 64 research publications and 21 research monographs and chapters in books to his credit published in various national and international journals. As senior faculty and chief/joint investigator he supervised research projects (15); research work of 20 students at doctoral and post graduate level in Clinical Psychology. He provided leadership to Indian Association of Clinical Psychologists for two years (2008-2009) as President of the Association.

Pallavi Sinha is currently working as Senior Resident in the Department of Psychiatry at Institute of Human Behavior and Allied Sciences (IHBAS), Delhi. After completing her post-graduation from IHBAS, she also cleared DNB examination in Psychiatry. Her interests in the field of Psychiatry include De-addiction and Dual Diagnosis disorders.

Shikha Soni she is a Clinical Psychologist currently working as a Senior Research Fellow in Department of Clinical Psychology NIMHANS. She had completed her M.Phil in Clinical Psychology from Central Institute of Psychiatry. Thereafter, she worked as an intern in Department of Neuropsychology in Medanta Gurgaon.

Godishala Sridevi has received her M.Phil (2009) in Rehabilitation Psychology from Sweekaar Academy of Rehabilitation Sciences, Hyderabad. She received her PhD (2013) in Rehabilitation Psychology from The Open International University of Medicina Alternativa, SriLanka. She worked as a lecturer in rehabilitation psychology in the Department of Clinical Psychology at Sweekaar Academy of Rehabilitation Sciences, Hyderabad. She worked as a Head of the Department in GEMS Health Care, Hyderabad. She is pursuing her full time PhD from Osmania University since 2013 with ICSSR Doctoral Fellowship. She is a life associate member of IACP since 2013 and also registered in RCI since 2009. She has various national and international book publications and journal publications (40 publications) with 23 journal citations and 18.4417 Impact Factor. She is a reviewer for Journal of Disability Studies, India. She has presented papers in national and international conferences and attended various national and international conferences and workshops. She assisted and guided trainees in various Research Projects under M.Phil in rehabilitation psychology and PG Diploma in Rehabilitation Psychology (PGDRP) examinations.

Deepika Srivastav is a registered clinical psychologist by rehabilitation council of India (RCI), residing in Delhi. She completed her M.Phil. From one of the most reputed institute in India, Institute of Human Behaviour and Allied Sciences (IHBAS), Delhi. She is doing her PhD in psychology on "Effect of cognitive behaviour therapy on Parkinson's Disease" at university of Delhi. She is a consultant clinical Psychologist at Nulife Hospital, Delhi and is also associated with various hospitals and private clinics in Delhi. She has her contribution in the development of Wechsler Abbreviated Scale of Intelligence-second Edition (WASI-IV) as an examiner with Pearson Clinical and talent Assessment (Bangalore), India. She is working as a psychologist at Jawaharlal Nehru University, Delhi. She is a visiting faculty at IGNOU, Department of Psychology. She has various publications in national and international journals that include various case studies related with Psychological treatment in Neurological and psychiatric disorder.

Meghamala S. Tavaragi she completed her MBBS, DPM (Diploma in Psychiatry), JJM Medical college Davanagere. Currently she is working as Senior Resident in Department of psychiatry, Dharwad Institute of Mental Health and Neurosciences (DIMHANS) Dharwad. State of Karnataka, India. Research interests and specialties: 1. Alcohol/ Drug abuses, De-Addiction and Psychosocial rehabilitation 2. Child and women sexual abuse related psychiatric illness 3. Forensic psychiatry 4. Women mental health 5. Personality disorders 6. Child and Adolescents Mental Health issues 7. Parapsychology 8. Complimentary medicine: Music and Relaxation, aroma therapy 9. Food and psychiatry 10. Psycho-social interventions: Patients with Affective disorders, schizophrenia and their care givers. She had three national and six international journals to her credentials.

M. A. Tripathi is a registered Cinical Psychologist, presently working as Assistant Professor in Department of Clinical Psychology, Sweekaar Academy of Rehabilitation Sciences, Secunderabad, India. He has over 10 years of teaching experience at undergraduate level to psychology students. He also worked as a counsellor with street children on HIV/AIDS project and also has experience as a sports psychologist. His area of interest is cognitive behaviour therapy.

Index

E

F

G

H

I

L

M

N

O

P

Q

R

S

T

U

W

www.ingramcontent.com/pod-product-compliance
Lightning Source LLC
LaVergne TN
LVHW060401300926
849162LV00006B/1318